# Adaptive Design Theory and Implementation Using SAS and R

## Second Edition

# Chapman & Hall/CRC Biostatistics Series

Published Titles

Chapman & Hall/CRC Biostatistics Series

# Adaptive Design Theory and Implementation Using SAS and R

## Second Edition

### Mark Chang

AMAG Pharmaceuticals, Inc.

Lexington, Massachusetts, USA

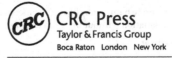

CRC Press
Taylor & Francis Group
Boca Raton   London   New York

CRC Press is an imprint of the
Taylor & Francis Group, an **informa** business

A CHAPMAN & HALL BOOK

CRC Press
Taylor & Francis Group
6000 Broken Sound Parkway NW, Suite 300
Boca Raton, FL 33487-2742

First issued in paperback 2016

© 2014 by Taylor & Francis Group, LLC
CRC Press is an imprint of Taylor & Francis Group, an Informa business

No claim to original U.S. Government works

Version Date: 20141022

ISBN 13: 978-1-138-03423-5 (pbk)
ISBN 13: 978-1-4822-5659-8 (hbk)

**Visit the Taylor & Francis Web site at**
**http://www.taylorandfrancis.com**

**and the CRC Press Web site at**
**http://www.crcpress.com**

To those who are striving toward a better way

# Series Introduction

The primary objectives of the Biostatistics Book Series are to provide useful reference books for researchers and scientists in academia, industry, and government, and also to offer textbooks for undergraduate and/or graduate courses in the area of biostatistics. This book series will provide comprehensive and unified presentations of statistical designs and analyses of important applications in biostatistics, such as those in biopharmaceuticals. A well-balanced summary will be given of current and recently developed statistical methods and interpretations for both statisticians and researchers/scientists with minimal statistical knowledge who are engaged in the field of applied biostatistics. The series is committed to providing easy-to-understand, state-of-the-art references and textbooks. In each volume, statistical concepts and methodologies will be illustrated through real world examples.

In the past several decades, it has been recognized that increasing spending of biomedical research does not reflect an increase of the success rate of pharmaceutical (clinical) development. As a result, the United States Food and Drug Administration (FDA) kicked off a Critical Path Initiative to assist the sponsors in identifying the scientific challenges underlying the medical product pipeline problems. In 2006, the FDA released a Critical Path Opportunities List that outlines 76 initial projects (six broad topic areas) to bridge the gap between the quick pace of new biomedical discoveries and the slower pace at which those discoveries are currently developed into therapies. Among the 76 initial projects, the FDA calls for advancing innovative trial designs, especially for the use of prior experience or accumulated information in trial design. Many researchers interpret it as the encouragement for the use of adaptive design methods in clinical trials.

In clinical trials, it is not uncommon to modify trial and/or statistical procedures during the conduct of the trials based on the review of interim data. The purpose is not only to efficiently identify clinical benefits of the test treatment under investigation, but also to increase the probability of success of clinical development. The use of adaptive design methods for modifying the trial and/or statistical procedures of on-going clinical trials based on accrued data has been practiced for years in clinical research. However, it is a concern whether the $p$-value or confidence interval regarding the treatment effect obtained after the modification is reliable or correct. In addition, it is also a concern that the use of adaptive design methods in a clinical trial may lead to a totally different trial that is unable to address scientific/medical questions that the trial is intended to answer. In their book, Chow and Chang (2006) provide a comprehensive summarization of statistical methods for the use of adaptive design methods in clinical trials. This volume provides useful approaches for implementation of adaptive design methods in clinical trials through the application of statistical software such as SAS and R. It covers statistical methods for various adaptive designs such as adaptive group sequential design, adaptive dose-escalation design, adaptive seamless phase-II/III trial design (drop-the-losers design), and biomarker-adaptive design. It would be beneficial to practitioners such as biostatisticians, clinical scientists, and reviewers in regulatory agencies who are engaged in the areas of pharmaceutical research and development.

**Shein-Chung Chow**
Editor-in-Chief

# Preface to the Second Edition

There have been remarkable advancements in methodological study and application of adaptive trials since the publication of the first edition in 2007. I have been thinking about the revision for years and finally I complete the revision today.

In this revision, I have added 12 new chapters, including Chapter 6, Adaptive Noninferiority Design with Paired Binary Data; Chapter 7, Adaptive Design with Incomplete Paired Data; Chapter 12, Blinded and Semi-Blinded Sample-Size Reestimation Design; Chapter 13, Adaptive Design with Coprimary Endpoint; Chapter 15, Pick-the-Winners Design; Chapter 16, The Add-Arm Design for Unimodal Response; Chapter 18, Biomarker-Informed Adaptive Design; Chapter 23, Bayesian Design for Efficacy-Toxicity Trade-Off and Drug Combination; Chapter 24, Bayesian Approach to Biosimilarity Trial; Chapter 25, Adaptive Multiregional Trial Design; Chapter 26, SAS and R Modules for Group Sequential Design; and Chapter 27, Data Analysis of Adaptive Trial.

I have also made major changes to the following chapters: For Chapter 8, $K$-Stage Adaptive Designs, analytical methods in addition to the simulation methods are now included. For Chapter 11, Unblinded Sample-Size Reestimation Design, the focus is on the comparisons between and discussions on different methods using simulations. I have completely rewritten Chapter 14, Multiple-Endpoint Adaptive Design and Chapter 19, Survival Modeling and Adaptive Treatment Switching, using analytical methods instead of simulation methods. Sequential parallel designs with rerandomization are added in Chapter 20, Response-Adaptive Allocation Design. For Chapter 22, Adaptive Dose-Escalation Trial, I have included the skeleton approach. In the Appendices, some utility SAS code and SAS macros for the add-arm designs are included, and the modified R function for CRM to include the skeleton approach is also provided. In this revision, we have added nearly 20 new SAS macros and R functions. We have enhanced the exercises or problems in end of each chapter. We want to remind readers that some of the exercises are different from those you would find in a typical textbook of elementary statistics, where all necessary information for solving the problem is exactly given, no more or no less. Some exercises in the book often mimic practical situations, you might be given only the basic information to solve the problem, you need to figure out which information is necessary, what kind of information is missing, and where to get it or how to make assumptions. Those exercises are helpful before you design a real life adaptive trial.

I hope with these revisions and enhancements, readers will find the book useful in designing adaptive trials.

I want to thank Dr. Sandeep Menon for using this book and providing me valuable feedback. I very much appreciate my students, Dr. Jing Wang, Dr. Joseph Wu, Mr. Mike Pickard, Mr. Zhaoyang Teng, and Dr. Yansong Cheng for their creative thinking and hard work. Their contributions are reflected in various chapters. I also thank students in my adaptive design class at Boston University for their engagement and feedback, and thanks to Dr. Sandeep Menon for co-teaching the class with me.

**Mark Chang**

# Preface to the First Edition

This book is about adaptive clinical trial design and computer implementation. Compared to a classical trial design with static features, an adaptive design allows for changing or modifying the characteristics of a trial based on cumulative information. These modifications are often called adaptations. The word *adaptation* is so familiar to us because we constantly make adaptations in our daily lives according to what we learn over time. Some of the adaptations are necessary for survival, while others are made to improve our quality of life. We should be equally smart in conducting clinical trials by making adaptations based on what we learn as the trial progresses. These adaptations are made because they can improve the efficiency of the trial design, provide earlier remedies, and reduce the time and cost of drug development. An adaptive design is also ethically important. It allows for stopping a trial earlier if the risk to subjects outweighs the benefit, or when there is early evidence of efficacy for a safe drug. An adaptive design may allow for randomizing more patients to the superior treatment arms and reducing exposure to inefficacious, but potentially toxic, doses. An adaptive design can also be used to identify better target populations through early biomarker responses.

The aims of this book are to provide a unified and concise presentation of adaptive design theories, furnish the reader with computer programs in SAS and R (also available at www.statisticians.org) for the design and simulation of adaptive trials, and offer (hopefully) a quick way to master the different adaptive designs through examples that are motivated by real issues in clinical trials. The book covers broad ranges of adaptive methods with an emphasis on the relationships among different methods. As Dr. Simon Day pointed out, there are good and bad adaptive designs; a design is not necessarily good just because it is adaptive. There are many rules and issues that must be considered when implementing adaptive designs.

This book has included most current regulatory views as well as discussions of challenges in planning, execution, analysis, and reporting for adaptive designs.

From a "big picture" view, drug development is a sequence of decision processes. To achieve ultimate success, we cannot consider each trial as an isolated piece; instead, a drug's development must be considered an integrated process, using Bayesian decision theory to optimize the design or program as explained in Chapter 21. It is important to point out that every action we take at each stage of drug development is not with the intent of minimizing the number of errors, but minimizing the impact of errors. For this reason, the power of a hypothesis test is not the ultimate criterion for evaluating a design. Instead, many other factors, such as time, safety, and the magnitude of treatment difference, have to be considered in a utility function. From an even bigger-picture view, we are working in a competitive corporate environment, and statistical game theory will provide the ultimate tool for drug development. In the last chapter of the book, I will pursue an extensive discussion of the controversial issues about statistical theories and the fruitful avenues for future research and application of adaptive designs.

Adaptive design creates a new landscape of drug development. The statistical methodology of adaptive design has been greatly advanced by literature in recent years, and there are an increasing number of trials with adaptive features. The PhRMA and BIO adaptive design working groups have made great contributions in promoting innovative approaches to trial design. In preparing the manuscript of this book, I have benefited from discussions with following colleagues: Shein-Chung Chow, Michael Krams, Donald Berry, Jerry Schindler, Michael Chernick, Bruce Turnbull, Barry Turnbull, Sue-Jane Wang (FDA), Vladimir Dragalin, Qing Liu, Simon Day (MHRA), Susan Kenley, Stan Letovsky, Yuan-Yuan Chiu, Jonca Bull, Gorden Lan, Song Yang, Gang Chen, Meiling Lee, Alex Whitmore, Cyrus Mehta, Carl-Fredrik Burman, Richard Simon, George Chi, James Hung (FDA), Aloka Chakravarty (FDA), Marc Walton (FDA), Robert O'Neill (FDA), Paul Gallo, Christopher Jennison, Jun Shao, Keaven Anderson, Martin Posch, Stuart Pocock, Wassmer Gernot, Andy Grieve, Christy Chung, Jeff Maca, Alun Bedding, Robert Hemmings (MHRA), Jose Pinheiro, Jeff Maca, Katherine Sawyer, Sara Radcliffe, Jessica Oldham, Christian Sonesson, Inna Perevozskaya, Anastasia Ivanova, Brenda Gaydos, Frank Bretz, Wenjin Wang, Suman Bhattacharya, and Judith Quinlan.

I would like to thank Hua Liu, PhD; Hugh Xiao, PhD; Andy Boral, MD; Tracy Zhang, MS; MingXiu Hu, PhD; Alun Bedding, PhD; and Jing Xu, PhD for their careful review and many constructive comments. Thanks to Steve Lewitzky, MS; Kate Rinard, MS; Frank Chen, MS; Hongliang Shi, MS; Tracy Zhang, MS; and Rachel Neuwirth, MS for support. I wish to express my gratitude to the following individuals for sharing their clinical, scientific, and regulatory insights about clinical trials: Andy Boral, MD; Iain Web, MD; Irvin Fox, MD; Jim Gilbert, MD; Ian Walters, MD; Bill Trepicchio, PhD; Mike Cooper, MD; Dixie-Lee Esseltine, MD; Jing Marantz, MD; Chris Webster, and Robert Pietrusko, Pharm D.

Thanks to Jane Porter, MS; Nancy Simonian, MD; and Lisa Aldler, BA for their support during the preparation of this book. Special thanks to Lori Engelhardt, MA, ELS, for careful reviews and many editorial comments.

From Taylor and Francis, I would like to thank David Grubbs, Sunil Nair, Jay Margolis, and Amber Donley for providing me the opportunity to work on this book.

**Mark Chang**
Millennium Pharmaceuticals, Inc.
Cambridge, Massachusetts, USA
www.statisticians.org

# Contents

*Contents*

| 19.2.3 | Parameter Estimation and Inference | 396 |
| 19.2.4 | Applications of First-Hitting-Time Model | 397 |
| 19.2.5 | Multivariate Model with Biomarkers | 398 |
| 19.3 | Multistage Model | 401 |
| 19.3.1 | General Framework of Multistage Model | 401 |
| 19.3.2 | Covariates and Treatment Switching | 403 |
| 19.4 | Summary and Discussion | 405 |
| **20** | **Response-Adaptive Allocation Design** | **409** |
| 20.1 | Opportunities | 409 |
| 20.2 | Traditional Randomization Methods | 410 |
| 20.3 | Basic Response-Adaptive Randomizations | 411 |
| 20.3.1 | Play-the-Winner Model | 411 |
| 20.3.2 | Randomized Play-the-Winner Model | 412 |
| 20.3.3 | Optimal Randomized Play-the-Winner | 413 |
| 20.4 | Adaptive Design with Randomized Play-the-Winner | 414 |
| 20.5 | General Response-Adaptive Randomization | 418 |
| 20.5.1 | SAS Macro for $K$-Arm RAR with Binary Endpoint | 418 |
| 20.5.2 | SAS Macro for $K$-Arm RAR with Normal Endpoint | 420 |
| 20.5.3 | RAR for General Adaptive Designs | 423 |
| 20.6 | Sequential Parallel Comparison Design | 423 |
| 20.7 | Summary and Discussion | 425 |
| **21** | **Introductory Bayesian Approach in Clinical Trial** | **427** |
| 21.1 | Introduction | 427 |
| 21.2 | Bayesian Learning Mechanism | 428 |
| 21.3 | Bayesian Basics | 429 |
| 21.3.1 | Bayes' Rule | 429 |
| 21.3.2 | Conjugate Family of Distributions | 431 |
| 21.4 | Trial Design | 432 |
| 21.4.1 | Bayesian for Classical Design | 432 |
| 21.4.2 | Bayesian Power | 434 |
| 21.4.3 | Frequentist Optimization | 435 |
| 21.4.4 | Bayesian Optimal Adaptive Designs | 437 |
| 21.5 | Trial Monitoring | 441 |
| 21.6 | Analysis of Data | 442 |
| 21.7 | Interpretation of Outcomes | 444 |

# List of Figures

# List of Tables

# List of Examples

# List of SAS Macros and R Functions

# Chapter 1

# Introduction

## 1.1 Motivation

Investment in pharmaceutical research and development has more than doubled in the past decade; however, the increase in spending for biomedical research does not reflect an increased success rate of pharmaceutical development. (Figure 1.1). Reasons for this include the following: (1) a diminished margin for improvement escalates the level of difficulty in proving drug benefits; (2) genomics and other new sciences have not yet reached their full potential; (3) mergers and other business arrangements have decreased candidates; (4) easy targets are the focus as chronic diseases are more difficult to study; (5) failure rates have not improved; and (6) rapidly escalating costs and complexity decrease willingness/ability to bring many candidates forward into the clinic (Woodcock, 2004).

There are several critical areas for improvement in drug development. One of the obvious areas for improvement is the design, conduct, and analysis of clinical trials. Improvement of the clinical trials process includes (1) the development and utilization of biomarkers or genomic markers, (2) the establishment of quantitative disease models, and (3) the use of more informative designs such as adaptive and/or Bayesian designs. In practice, the use of clinical trial simulation, the improvement of clinical trial monitoring, and the adoption of new technologies for prediction of clinical outcome will also help in increasing the probability of success in the clinical development of promising candidates. Most importantly, we should not use the evaluation tools and infrastructure of the last century to develop this century's advances. Instead, an innovative approach using adaptive design methods for clinical development must be implemented.

In the next section, we will provide the definition of adaptive design and brief descriptions of commonly used adaptive designs. In Section 1.2.8,

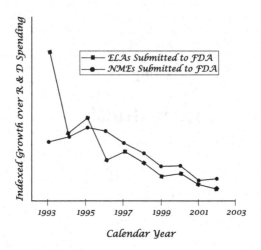

Figure 1.1:   Trends in NDAs Submitted to FDA (Data Source: PAREXEXL, 2003)

the importance of computer simulation is discussed. In Section 1.4, we will provide the roadmap for this book.

## 1.2   Adaptive Design Methods in Clinical Trials

An adaptive design is a clinical trial design that allows adaptations or modifications to aspects of the trial after its initiation without undermining the validity and integrity of the trial (Chang, 2005a; Chow, Chang, and Pong, 2005). The PhRMA Working Group defines an adaptive design as a clinical study design that uses accumulating data to decide how to modify aspects of the study as it continues, without undermining the validity and integrity of the trial (Dragalin, 2006; Gallo et al., 2006).

The adaptations may include, but are not limited to, (1) a group sequential design, (2) an sample-size adjustable design, (3) a drop-losers design, (4) an adaptive treatment allocation design, (5) an adaptive dose-escalation design, (6) a biomarker-adaptive design, (7) an adaptive treatment-switching design, (8) an adaptive dose-finding design, and (9) a combined adaptive design. An adaptive design usually consists of multiple stages. At each stage, data analyses are conducted, and adaptations are taken based on updated information to maximize the probability of success. An adaptive design is also known as a flexible design (EMEA, 2002).

An adaptive design has to preserve the validity and integrity of the trial. The validity includes internal and external validities. *Internal validity* is the degree to which we are successful in eliminating confounding variables and establishing a cause–effect relationship (treatment effect) within the study itself. A study that readily allows its findings to generalize to the population at large has high *external validity*. *Integrity* involves minimizing operational bias, creating a scientifically sound protocol design, adhering firmly to the study protocol and standard operating procedures (SOPs), executing the trial consistently over time and across sites or countries, providing comprehensive analyses of trial data and unbiased interpretations of the results, and maintaining the confidentiality of the data.

### 1.2.1  *Group Sequential Design*

A group sequential design (GSD) is an adaptive design that allows for premature termination of a trial due to efficacy or futility, based on the results of interim analyses. GSD was originally developed to obtain clinical benefits under economic constraints. For a trial with a positive result, early stopping ensures that a new drug product can be exploited sooner. If a negative result is indicated, early stopping avoids wasting resources. Sequential methods typically lead to savings in sample size, time, and cost when compared with the classical design with a fixed sample size. Interim analyses also enable management to make appropriate decisions regarding the allocation of limited resources for continued development of a promising treatment. GSD is probably one of the most commonly used adaptive designs in clinical trials.

Basically, there are three different types of GSDs: early efficacy stopping design, early futility stopping design, and early efficacy/futility stopping design. If we believe (based on prior knowledge) that the test treatment is very promising, then an early efficacy stopping design should be used. If we are very concerned that the test treatment may not work, an early futility stopping design should be employed. If we are not certain about the magnitude of the effect size, a GSD permitting early stopping for both efficacy and futility should be considered. In practice, if we have a good knowledge regarding the effect size, then a classical design with a fixed sample-size would be more efficient.

### 1.2.2  *Sample-Size Reestimation Design*

A sample-size reestimation (SSR) design refers to an adaptive design that allows for sample-size adjustment or reestimation based on the review of interim analysis results (Figure 1.2). The sample-size requirement for a trial is sensitive to the treatment effect and its variability. An inaccurate estimation of the effect size and its variability could lead to an underpowered or overpowered design, neither of which is desirable. If a trial is underpowered, it will not be able to detect a clinically meaningful difference, and consequently could prevent a potentially effective drug from being delivered to patients. On the other hand, if a trial is overpowered, it could lead to unnecessary exposure of many patients to a potentially harmful compound when the drug, in fact, is not effective. In practice, it is often difficult to estimate the effect size and variability because of many uncertainties during protocol development. Thus, it is desirable to have the flexibility to reestimate the sample size in the middle of the trial.

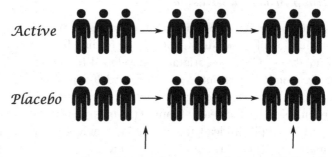

*Interim results may indicate additional*
*patients required to preserve the power*

Figure 1.2:   Sample-Size Reestimation Design

There are two types of sample-size reestimation procedures, namely, sample-size reestimation based on blinded data and sample-size reestimation based on unblinded data. In the first scenario, the sample adjustment is based on the (observed) pooled variance at the interim analysis to recalculate the required sample size, which does not require unblinding the data. In this scenario, the type-I error adjustment is practically negligible. In the second scenario, the effect size and its variability are reassessed, and sample size is adjusted based on the updated information. The statistical method for adjustment could be based on effect size or the conditional power.

Note that the flexibility in SSR is at the expense of a potential loss of power. Therefore, it is suggested that an SSR be used when there are no good estimates of the effect size and its variability. In the case where there is some knowledge of the effect size and its variability, a classical design would be more efficient.

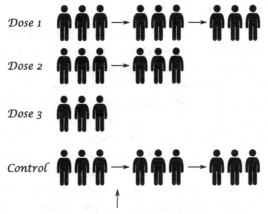

Dose 1

Dose 2

Dose 3

Control

*Interim results indicate: some doses are*
*inferior and can be dropped from the study*

Figure 1.3: Drop-Loser Design

### 1.2.3 *Drop-Loser Design*

A drop-loser design (DLD) is an adaptive design consisting of multiple stages. At each stage, interim analyses are performed and the losers (i.e., inferior treatment groups) are dropped based on prespecified criteria (Figure 1.3). Ultimately, the best arm(s) are retained. If there is a control group, it is usually retained for the purpose of comparison. This type of design can be used in phase-II/III combined trials. A phase-II clinical trial is often a dose-response study, where the goal is to assess whether there is treatment effect. If there is treatment effect, the goal becomes finding the appropriate dose level (or treatment groups) for the phase-III trials. This type of traditional design is not efficient with respect to time and resources because the phase-II efficacy data are not pooled with data from phase-III trials, which are the pivotal trials for confirming efficacy. Therefore, it is desirable to combine phases II and III so that the data can be used efficiently, and the time required for drug development can be reduced. Bauer and Kieser (1999) provide a two-stage method for this purpose, where investigators can terminate the trial entirely or drop a subset of treatment groups for lack of efficacy after the first stage. As pointed out by Sampson and Sill (2005), the procedure of dropping the losers is highly flexible, and the distributional assumptions are kept to a minimum. However, because of the generality of the method, it is difficult to construct confidence intervals. Sampson and Sill derived a uniformly most powerful, conditionally unbiased test for a normal endpoint.

### 1.2.4   *Adaptive Randomization Design*

An adaptive randomization/allocation design (ARD) is a design that allows modification of randomization schedules during the conduct of the trial. In clinical trials, randomization is commonly used to ensure a balance with respect to patient characteristics among treatment groups. However, there is another type of ARD, called response-adaptive randomization (RAR), in which the allocation probability is based on the response of the previous patients. RAR was initially proposed because of ethical considerations (i.e., to have a larger probability to allocate patients to a superior treatment group); however, response randomization can be considered a drop-loser design with a seamless allocation probability of shifting from an inferior arm to a superior arm. The well-known response-adaptive models include the randomized play-the-winner (RPW) model (see Figure 1.4), an optimal model that minimizes the number of failures. Other response-adaptive randomizations, such as utility-adaptive randomization, also have been proposed and are combinations of response-adaptive and treatment-adaptive randomization (Chang and Chow, 2005).

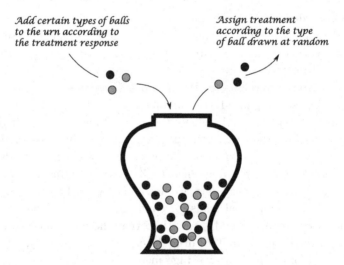

Figure 1.4:   Response Adaptive Randomization

### 1.2.5   *Adaptive Dose-Finding Design*

Dose escalation is often considered in early phases of clinical development for identifying maximum tolerated dose (MTD), which is often considered the optimal dose for later phases of clinical development. An adaptive dose-finding (or dose-escalation) design is a design in which the dose level used to treat the next-entered patient is dependent on the toxicity of the previous patients, based on some traditional escalation rules (Figure 1.5). Many early dose-escalation rules are adaptive, but the adaptation algorithm is somewhat ad hoc. Recently more advanced dose-escalation rules have been developed using modeling approaches (frequentist or Bayesian framework) such as the continual reassessment method (CRM) (O'Quigley, Pepe, and Fisher, 1990; Chang and Chow, 2005) and other accelerated escalation algorithms. These algorithms can reduce the sample-size and overall toxicity in a trial and improve the accuracy and precision of the estimation of the MTD. Note that CRM can be viewed as a special response-adaptive randomization.

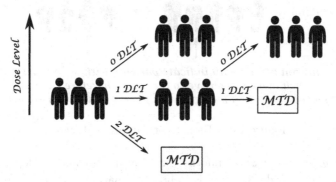

*A group of 3 patients initially treated at each dose level; toxicity measured by DLTs*

Figure 1.5:    Dose Escalation for Maximum Tolerated Dose

## 1.2.6    *Biomarker-Adaptive Design*

Biomarker-adaptive design (BAD) refers to a design that allows for adaptations using information obtained from biomarkers. A biomarker is a characteristic that is objectively measured and evaluated as an indicator of normal biologic or pathogenic processes or pharmacologic response to a therapeutic intervention (Chakravarty, 2005). A biomarker can be a classifier, prognostic, or predictive marker.

*A classifier biomarker* is a marker that usually does not change over the course of the study, such as DNA markers. Classifier biomarkers can be used to select the most appropriate target population, or even for personalized treatment. Classifier markers can also be used in other situations. For example, it is often the case that a pharmaceutical company has to make a decision whether to target a very selective population for whom the test drug likely works well or to target a broader population for whom the test drug is less likely to work well. However, the size of the selective population may be too small to justify the overall benefit to the patient population. In this case, a BAD may be used, where the biomarker response at interim analysis can be used to determine which target populations should be focused on (Figure 1.6).

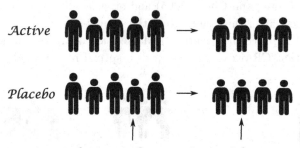

*Interim results may indicate patients with gene x are much more responsive to the drug; therefore, at the second stage only patients with gene x will be recruited.*

Figure 1.6:    Biomarker-Adaptive Design

*A prognostic biomarker* informs the clinical outcomes, independent of treatment. It provides information about the natural course of the disease in individuals who have or have not received the treatment under study. Prognostic markers can be used to separate good- and poor-prognosis patients at the time of diagnosis. If expression of the marker clearly separates patients with an excellent prognosis from those with a poor prognosis, then the marker can be used to aid the decision about how aggressive the therapy needs to be.

*A predictive biomarker* informs the treatment effect on the clinical endpoint. Compared to a gold-standard endpoint, such as survival, a biomarker can often be measured earlier, more easily, and more frequently. A biomarker is less subject to competing risks and less affected by other treatment modalities, which may reduce sample size due to a larger effect size. A biomarker could lead to faster decision making. However, validating predictive biomarkers is challenging. BAD simplifies this challenge. In a BAD, "softly" validated biomarkers are used at the interim analysis to assist in decision making, while the final decision can still be based on a gold-standard endpoint, such as survival, to preserve the type-I error (Chang, 2005b).

### 1.2.7 Adaptive Treatment-Switching Design

An adaptive treatment-switching design (ATSD) is a design that allows the investigator to switch a patient's treatment from the initial assignment if there is evidence of lack of efficacy or a safety concern (Figure 1.7).

To evaluate the efficacy and safety of a test treatment for progressive diseases, such as cancers and HIV, a parallel-group, active-control, randomized clinical trial is often conducted. In this type of trial, qualified patients are randomly assigned to receive either an active control (a standard therapy or a treatment currently available in the marketplace) or a test treatment under investigation. Due to ethical considerations, patients are allowed to switch from one treatment to another if there is evidence of lack of efficacy or disease progression. In practice, it is not uncommon that up to 80% of patients may switch from one treatment to another. Sommer and Zeger (1991) referred to the treatment effect among patients who complied with treatment as "biological efficacy." Branson and Whitehead (2002) widened the concept of biological efficacy to encompass the treatment effect as if all patients adhered to their original randomized treatments in clinical studies allowing treatment switching. Despite allowing a switch in treatment, many clinical studies are designed to compare the test treatment with the active control agent as if no patients had ever been switched. This certainly has an impact on the evaluation of the efficacy of the test treatment, because the response-informative switching causes the treatment effect to be confounded. The power for the methods without considering the switching is often lost dramatically because many patients from two groups have eventually taken the same drugs (Shao, Chang, and Chow, 2005). Currently, more approaches have been proposed, which include mixed exponential mode (Chang, 2006a; Chow and Chang, 2006) and a mixture of the Wiener processes (Lee, Chang, and Whitmore, 2008).

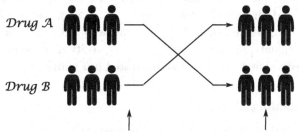

*Treatments are switched when the disease is progressed due to ethical considerations.*

Figure 1.7: Adaptive Treatment Switching

### 1.2.8 *Clinical Trial Simulation*

Clinical trial simulation (CTS) is a process that mimics clinical trials using computer programs. CTS is particularly important in adaptive designs for several reasons: (1) the statistical theory of adaptive design is complicated with limited analytical solutions available under certain assumptions; (2) the concept of CTS is very intuitive and easy to implement; (3) CTS can be used to model very complicated situations with minimum assumptions, and type-I error can be strongly controlled; (4) using CTS, not only can we calculate the power of an adaptive design, but we can also generate many other important operating characteristics such as expected sample-size, conditional power, and repeated confidence interval—ultimately this leads to the selection of an optimal trial design or clinical development plan; (5) CTS can be used to study the validity and robustness of an adaptive design in different hypothetical clinical settings, or with protocol deviations; (6) CTS can be used to monitor trials, project outcomes, anticipate problems, and suggest remedies before it is too late; (7) CTS can be used to visualize the dynamic trial process from patient recruitment, drug distribution, treatment administration, and pharmacokinetic processes to biomarkers and clinical responses; and finally, (8) CTS has minimal cost associated with it and can be done in a short time.

CTS was started in the early 1970s and became popular in the mid 1990s due to increased computing power. CTS components include (1) a trial Design Mode, which includes design type (parallel, crossover, traditional, adaptive), dosing regimens or algorithms, subject selection criteria, and time, financial, and other constraints; (2) an Execution Model, which models the human behaviors that affect trial execution (e.g., protocol compliance, cooperation culture, decision cycle, regulatory authority, inference of opinion leaders); (3) a Response Model, which includes disease models that imitate the drug behavior (PK and PD models) or intervention mechanism, and an infrastructure model (e.g., timing and validity of the assessment, diagnosis tool); and (4) an Evaluation Model, which includes criteria for evaluating design models, such as utility models and Bayesian decision theory. The CTS model is illustrated in Figure 1.8.

### 1.2.9 *Regulatory Aspects*

The FDA's Critical Path initiative is a serious attempt to bring attention and focus to the need for targeted scientific efforts to modernize the techniques and methods used to evaluate the safety, efficacy, and quality of

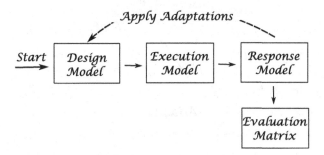

Figure 1.8: Clinical Trial Simulation Model

medical products as they move from product selection and design to mass manufacture. Critical Path is NOT about the drug discovery process. The FDA recognizes that improvement and new technology are needed. The National Institutes of Health (NIH) is getting more involved via the "roadmap" initiative. Critical Path is concerned with the work needed to move a candidate all the way to a marketed product. It is clear that the FDA supports and encourages innovative approaches in drug development. The regulatory agents feel that some adaptive designs are encouraging, but are cautious about others, specially for pivotal studies (EMEA, 2006; Hung, O'Neill, Wang, and Lawrence, 2006; Hung, Wang, and O'Neill, 2006; Temple, 2006).

"Adaptive designs should be encouraged for Phases I and II trials for better exploration of drug effects, whether beneficial or harmful, so that such information can be more optimally used in latter stages of drug development. Controlling false positive conclusions in exploratory phases is also important so that the confirmatory trials in latter stages achieve their goals. The guidance from such trials properly controlling false positives may be more informative to help better design confirmatory trials" (Hung et al., 2006). As pointed out by FDA statistician Dr. Stella Machado, "The two major causes of delayed approval and nonapproval of phase III studies is poor dose selection in early studies and phase III designs [that] don't utilize information from early phase studies" ("The Pink Sheet," Dec. 18, 2006, p. 24). The FDA is granting industry a great deal of leeway in adaptive design in the early learning phase, while at the same time suggesting that emphasis be placed on dose-response and exposure risk. Dr. O'Neill said that learning about the dose-response relationship lies at the heart of adaptive designs. Companies should begin a dialogue about adaptive designs with FDA medical officers and statisticians as early as a year before beginning a trial as suggested by Dr. Robert Powell from the FDA.

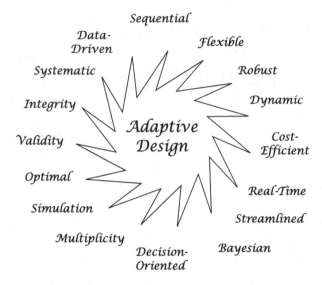

Figure 1.9:   Characteristics of Adaptive Designs

### 1.2.10   *Characteristics of Adaptive Designs*

Adaptive design is a sequential data-driven approach. It is a dynamic process that allows for real-time learning. It is flexible and allows for modifications to the trial, which make the design cost-efficient and robust against the failure. Adaptive design is a systematic way to design different phases of trials, thus streamlining and optimizing the drug development process. In contrast, the traditional approach is composed of weakly connected phase-wise processes. Adaptive design is a decision-oriented, sequential learning process that requires up-front planning and a great deal of collaboration among the different parties involved in the drug development process. To this end, Bayesian methodology and computer simulation play important roles. Finally, the flexibility of adaptive design does not compromise the validity and integrity of the trial or the development process (Figure 1.9).

Adaptive design methods represent a revolution in pharmaceutical research and development. Using adaptive designs, we can increase the chances for success of a trial with a reduced cost. Bayesian approaches provide an ideal tool for optimizing trial designs and development plans. Clinical trial simulations offer a powerful tool to design and monitor trials. Adaptive design, the Bayesian approach, and trial simulation combine to form an ultimate statistical instrument for the most successful drug development programs.

## 1.3 FAQs about Adaptive Designs

The following questions collected from several journalists from scientific and technological journals (Nature Biotechnology, BioIT World, Contract Pharms, etc.) during the interviews eight years ago are still valuable to discuss today.

1. *What is the classification of an adaptive clinical trial? Is there a consensus in the industry regarding what adaptive trials entail?*

After many conferences and discussions, there is more or less a consensus on the definition of adaptive design. A typical definition is as follows:

An adaptive design is a design that allows modifications to aspects of the trial after its initiation without undermining the validity and integrity of the trial. All adaptive designs involve interim analyses and adaptations or decision making based on the interim results.

There are many ways to classify adaptive designs. The following are common examples of adaptive trials:

• Sample size reestimation design to increase the probability of success

• Early stopping due to efficacy or futility design to reduce cost and time

• Response adaptive randomization design to give patients a better chance of being assigned to superior treatment

• Drop-loser design for adaptive dose finding to reduce sample size by dropping the inferior treatments earlier

• Add-arm design featuring adaptive selection of treatment groups (arms) to reduce the exposure and shorten the study

• Adaptive dose escalation design to minimize toxicity while at the same time acquiring information on maximum tolerated dose

• Adaptive seamless design combining two traditional trials in different phases into a single trial, reducing cost and time to market

• Biomarker enrichment design to have earlier efficacy or safety readout to select better target populations or subpopulation

2. *What challenges does the adaptive trial model present?*

Adaptive designs can reduce time and cost, minimize toxicity, help select the best dose for the patients, and better target populations. With adaptive design, we can develop better science for testing new drugs and, in turn, better science for prescribing them.

There are challenges associated with adaptive design. Statistical methods are available for most common adaptive designs, but for more complicated adaptive designs, the methodologies are still in development.

Operationally, an adaptive design often requires real-time or near real-time data collection and analysis. In this regard, data standardizations, such as CDISC and electronic data capture (EDC), are very helpful in data cleaning and reconciliation. Note that not all adaptive designs require perfectly clean data at interim analysis, but the cleaner the data are, the more efficient the design is. Adaptive designs require the ability to rapidly integrate knowledge and experiences from different disciplines into the decision-making process and, hence, require a shift to a more collaborative working environment among disciplines.

There is no regulatory guidance for adaptive designs at the moment. Adaptive trials are reviewed on a case-by-case basis. Naturally there are fears that a protocol using this innovative approach may be rejected, causing a delay.

The interim unblinding may potentially cause bias and put the integrity of the trial at risk. Therefore, the unblinding procedure should be well established before the trial starts, and frequent unblinding should be avoided. Also, unblinding the premature results to the public could jeopardize the trial.

3. *How would adaptive trials affect traditional phases of drug development? How are safety and efficacy measured in this type of trial?*

Adaptive designs change the way we conduct clinical trials. Trials in different phases can be combined to create a seamless study. The final safety and efficacy requirements are not reduced because of adaptive designs. In fact, with adaptive designs, the efficacy and safety signals are collected and reviewed earlier and more often than in traditional designs. Therefore, we may have a better chance of avoiding unsafe drug exposure to large patient populations. A phase-II and -III combined seamless design, when the trial is carried out to the final stage, has longer-term patient efficacy and safety data than traditional phase-II, phase-III trials; however, precautions should be taken at the interim decision making when data are not mature.

4. *If adaptive trials become widely adopted, how would it impact clinical trial materials and the companies that provide them?*

Depending on the type of adaptive design, there might be requirements for packaging and shipping to be faster and more flexible. Quick and accurate efficacy and safety readouts may also be required. The electronic drug packages with an advanced built-in recording system will be helpful.

If adaptive trials become widely adopted, the drug manufacturers who can provide the materials adaptively will have a better chance of success.

5. *What are some differences between adaptive trials and the traditional trial model with respect to the supply of clinical trial materials?*

For a traditional or classical design, the amount of material required is fixed and can be easily planned before the trial starts. However, for some adaptive trials, the exact amount of required materials is not clear until later stages of the trial. Also the next dosage for a site may not be fully determined until the time of randomization; therefore, vendors may need to develop a better drug distribution strategy.

6. *What areas of clinical development would experience cost/time savings with the adaptive trial model?*

Adaptive design can be used in any phase, even in the preclinical and discovery phases. Drug discovery and development is a sequence of decision processes. The traditional paradigm breaks this into weakly connected fragments or phases. An adaptive approach will eventually be utilized for the whole development process to get the right drug to the right patient at the right time.

Adaptive design may require fewer patients, less trial material, sometimes fewer lab tests, less work for data collection, and fewer data queries to be resolved. However, an adaptive trial requires much more time during up-front planning and simulation studies.

7. *What are some of the regulatory issues that need to be addressed for this type of trial?*

Regulatory documents related to the adaptive clinical trials were issued between 2007 to 2012. They are

(1) European Medicines Agency (EMEA)—Reflection Paper on Methodological Issues in Confirmatory Clinical Trials Planned with an Adaptive Design (October 2007)
(2) U.S. Food and Drug Administration (FDA)—Draft Guidance—Guidance for Industry Adaptive Design Clinical Trials for Drugs and Biologics (February 2010)
(3) U.S. Food and Drug Administration (FDA)—Guidance for the Use of Bayesian Statistics in Medical Device Clinical Trials (February 2010)
(4) U.S. Food and Drug Administration (FDA)—Draft Guidance—Guidance for Industry on Enrichment Strategies for Clinical Trials to Support Approval of Human Drugs and Biological Products (December 2012)

If the adaptive design is submitted with solid scientific support and strong ethical considerations and is operationally feasible, there should not be any fears of rejection of such a design. On the other hand, with a significant increase in adaptive trials in NDA submissions, regulatory bodies may face a temporary shortage of resources for reviewing such designs. Adaptive designs are relatively new to the industry and to regulatory bodies; therefore, there is a lot to learn by doing them. For this reason, it is a good idea to start with adaptive designs in earlier stages of drug development.

## 1.4   Roadmap

Chapter 2, Classical Design: The classical design and issues raised from the traditional approaches are reviewed. The statistical design methods discussed include one- and two-group designs, multiple-group dose-response designs, as well as equivalence and noninferiority designs.

Chapter 3, Theory of Hypothesis-Based Adaptive Design: Unified theory for adaptive designs, which covers four key statistical elements in adaptive designs: stopping boundary, adjusted $p$-value, point estimation, and confidence interval is introduced. Discuss how different approaches can be developed under this unified theory and what the common adaptations are.

Chapter 4, Method with Direct Combination of $p$-values: Using the unified formulation discussed in Chapter 3, the method with an individual stagewise $p$-value and the methods with the sum and product of the stagewise $p$-values are discussed in detail for two-stage adaptive designs. Trial examples and step-by-step instructions are provided.

Chapter 5, Method with Inverse-Normal $p$-values: The inverse-normal method generalizes the classical group sequential method. The method can also be viewed as weighted stagewise statistics and includes several other methods as special cases. Mathematical formulations are derived and examples are provided regarding how to use the method for designing a trial.

Chapter 6, Adaptive Noninferiority Design with Paired Binary Data: Classical and adaptive noninferiority designs with paired binary data are discussed. Examples of sensitivity and specificity studies are provided.

Chapter 7, Adaptive Design with Incomplete Paired Data: When partial paired data is missing, the trial data become a mixture of paired and unpaired data. We discuss how to design an adaptive trial to consider missing paired data.

Chapter 8, $K$-Stage Adaptive Designs: Chapters 4 and 5 are mainly focused on two-stage adaptive designs because these designs are simple and usually have a closed-form solution. In Chapter 8, we use analytical and simulation approaches to generalize the methods to $K$-stage designs using analytical methods, SAS macros, and R functions.

Chapter 9, Conditional Error Function Method and Conditional Power: The conditional error function method is a very general approach. We discuss in particular the Proschan-Hunsberger method and the Muller-Schafer method. We will compare the conditional error functions for various other methods and study the relationships between different adaptive design methods through the conditional error functions and conditional power.

Chapter 10, Recursive Adaptive Design: The recursive two-stage adaptive design not only offers a closed-form solution for $K$-stage designs, but also allows for very broad adaptations. We first introduce two powerful principles, the error-spending principle and the conditional error principle, from which we further derive the recursive approach. Examples are provided to illustrate the different applications of this method.

Chapter 11, Unblinded Sample-Size Reestimation Design: This chapter is devoted to the commonly used adaptation, unblinded sample-size reestimation. Various sample-size reestimation methods are evaluated and compared. The goal is to demonstrate a way to evaluate different methods under different conditions and to optimize the trial design that fits a particular situation. Practical issues and concerns are also addressed.

Chapter 12, Blinded and Semi-Blinded Sample-Size Reestimation Design: In contrast to unblinded analysis, in this chapter we will discuss the sample-size reestimation without unblinding the treatment code. We will first discuss different methods to estimate the treatment effect without unblinding the randomization code, then discuss the different sample-size reestimation methods. Finally we will see an effective sample size reestimation method with a mixture of blinded and unblinded methods.

Chapter 13, Adaptive Design with Coprimary Endpoint: We will discuss how to control type-I error in an adaptive trial with coprimary endpoints, the stopping boundary, the power, and the conditional power, from both analytically and simulation perspective. R-functions are provided.

Chapter 14, Multiple-Endpoint Adaptive Design: One of the most challenging issues is the multiple-endpoint analysis with adaptive design. We will briefly review the multiplicity issues and commonly used methods in classical trials. Then motivated by an actual adaptive design in an oncology trial, we will discuss the methods for the multiple-endpoint issues with coprimary endpoints in adaptive trials.

Chapter 15, Pick-the-Winners Design: We will first discuss the opportunities for phase-II and -III trials combinations. Two adaptive design methods will be discussed, the common pick-the-winner design and the adaptive Dunnett test.

Chapter 16, The Add-Arm Design for Unimodal Response: In a classical drop-loser (or drop-arm) design, patients are randomized into all arms (doses) and at the interim analysis, inferior arms are dropped. Therefore, compared to the traditional dose-finding design, this adaptive design can reduce the sample size by not carrying over all doses to the end of the trial or by dropping the losers earlier. However, given a unimodal response, we discuss a more efficient design, the add-arm design.

Chapter 17, Biomarker-Enrichment Design: In this chapter, adaptive design methods are developed for classifier, diagnosis, and predictive markers. SAS macros have been developed for biomarker-adaptive designs. The improvement in efficiency is assessed for difference methods in different scenarios.

Chapter 18, Biomarker-Informed Adaptive Design: The conventional approach uses the patient-level correlation model, together with historical knowledge, to describe the relationship between the biomarker and the primary endpoint. However, this approach ignores the important factor in the relationship between the mean of biomarker response and the primary endpoint; without this consideration, the models turn out to have little effect of biomarker on the primary endpoint. In this chapter, we will discuss a more advanced method that will incorporate the relationships at patient level and the aggregate level.

Chapter 19, Survival Modeling and Adaptive Treatment Switching: Response-adaptive treatment switching and crossover are statistically challenging. Treatment switching is not required for the statistical efficacy of a trial design; rather, it is motivated by an ethical consideration. Several methods are discussed, including the time-dependent exponential, the mixed exponential, and a mixture of Wiener models.

Chapter 20, Response-Adaptive Allocation Design: Response-adaptive randomizations/allocations have many different applications. They can be used to reduce the overall sample-size and the number of patients exposed to ineffective or even toxic regimens. We will discuss some commonly used adaptive randomizations, such as randomized play-the-winner. The sequential parallel design with rerandomization is also discussed.

Chapter 21, Introductory Bayesian Approach in Clinical Trial: The philosophical differences between the Bayesian and frequentist approaches are discussed. Through many examples, the two approaches are compared in terms of design, monitoring, analysis, and interpretation of results. More importantly, how to use Bayesian decision theory to further improve the efficiency of adaptive designs is discussed with examples.

Chapter 22, Adaptive Dose-Escalation Trial: The adaptive dose-finding designs, or dose-escalation designs, are discussed in this chapter. The goals are to reduce the overall sample size and the number of patients exposed to ineffective or even toxic regimens and to increase the precision and accuracy of MTD (maximum tolerated dose) assessment. We will discuss oncology dose-escalation trials with traditional and Bayesian continual reassessment methods

Chapter 23, Bayesian Design for Efficacy-Toxicity Trade-off and Drug Combination: In this chapter, we will study the more complex Bayesian dose-finding models in two dimensions. Either the outcome has two dimensions, efficacy and toxicity, or the treatment has two dimensions, drug combinations.

Chapter 24, Bayesian Approach to Biosimilarity Trial: Unlike small molecule drug products, for which we can make generic versions that contain the exact same active ingredient as the brand-name drug, biological drugs, such as protein, are large molecule products that are generally produced using a living system or organism, and may be manufactured through biotechnology, derived from natural sources, or produced synthetically. Following the FDA's stepwise totality evidence approach, we will discuss statistical methods and designs that combine different sources of information to provide the totality of the evidence for biosimilar drug approval.

Chapter 25, Adaptive Multiregional Trial Design: A global multiregional clinical trial (MRCT) is an international clinical trial conducted in multiple countries with a uniform study protocol. Its goal is to get the drug approval in multiple countries. We will discuss some regulatory requirements, optimal adaptive MRCT design, and the Bayesian approach.

Chapter 26, SAS and R Modules for Group Sequential Design: We introduce the SAS procedures for group sequential designs and discuss simple examples.

Chapter 27, Data Analysis of Adaptive Trial: Data analyses of an adaptive trial include point and confidence parameter estimates, and adjusted p-values. We discuss the controversial issues surrounding these topics and different types of biases and their adjustments.

Chapter 28, Planning, Execution, Analysis, and Reporting: In this chapter, we discuss the logistic issues with adaptive designs. The topics cover planning, monitoring, analysis, and reporting for adaptive trials. It also includes the most concurrent regulatory views and recommendations.

Chapter 29, Debates in Adaptive Designs: We will present very broad discussions of the challenges and controversies presented by adaptive designs from philosophical and statistical perspectives.

Appendix A: Random Number Generation

Appendix B: A Useful Utility

Appendix C: SAS Macros for Add-Arm Designs

Appendix D: Implementing Adaptive Designs in R

**Computer Programs**

Most adaptive design methods have been implemented and tested in SAS version 9, and major methods have also been implemented in R. These computer programs are compact (often fewer than 50 lines of SAS code) and ready to use. For convenience, electronic versions of the programs have been made available at **www.statisticians.org**.

The SAS code is enclosed in >>**SAS Macro x.x**>> and <<**SAS**<< or in >>**SAS**>> and <<**SAS**<<. R programs are presented in Appendix B.

**Problems**

**1.1** What are the main differences between classical clinical trial design and adaptive trial design?

**1.2** Describe the objectives of different adaptive designs and when different types of adaptive designs should be used.

**1.3** What challenges may we face when we adopt the adaptive design? Provide some examples for which a classical instead of an adaptive design should be used.

# Chapter 2

# Classical Design

## 2.1 Overview of Drug Development

Pharmaceutical medicine uses all the scientific, clinical, statistical, regulatory, and business knowledge available to provide a challenging and rewarding career. On average, it costs about $1.8 billion to take a new compound to market and only one in 10,000 compounds ever reaches the market. There are three major phases of drug development: (1) preclinical research and development, (2) clinical research and development, and (3) after the compound is on the market, a possible "post-marketing" phase.

The preclinical phase represents bench work (in vitro) followed by animal testing, including kinetics, toxicity, and carcinogenicity. An investigational new drug application (IND) is submitted to the FDA seeking permission to begin the heavily regulated process of clinical testing in human subjects. The clinical research and development phase, representing the time from the beginning of human trials to the new drug application (NDA) submission that seeks permission to market the drug, is by far the longest portion of the drug development cycle and can last from 2 to 10 years (Tonkens, 2005).

Clinical trials are usually divided into three phases. The primary objectives of phase I are (1) to determine the metabolism and pharmacological activities of the drug, the side effects associated with increasing dose, and early evidence of effectiveness, and (2) to obtain sufficient information regarding the drug's pharmacokinetics and pharmacological effects to permit the design of well-controlled and scientifically valid phase-II clinical studies (21 CFR 312.21). Unless it is an oncology study, where the maximum tolerated dose (MTD) is primarily determined by a phase-I dose-escalation study, the dose-response or dose-finding study is usually conducted in phase II, and efficacy is usually the main focus. The choice of study design and study population in a dose-response trial will depend on the phase of development, therapeutic indication under investigation, and severity of the disease in the patient population of interest (ICH Guideline E4, 1994). Phase-III trials are considered confirmative trials.

The FDA does not actually approve the drug itself for sale. It approves the labeling, the package insert. United States law requires truth in labeling, and the FDA ensures that claims that a drug is safe and effective for treatment of a specified disease or condition have, in fact, been proven. All prescription drugs must have labels, and without proof of the truth of its label, a drug may not be sold in the United States.

In addition to mandated conditional regulatory approval and post-marketing surveillance trials, other reasons sponsors may conduct post-marketing trials include comparing their drug with that of competitors, widening the patient population, changing the formulation or dose regimen, or applying a label extension. A simplified view of the NDA is shown in Figure 2.1 (Tonkens, 2005).

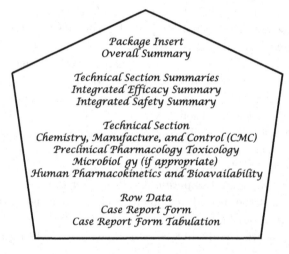

Figure 2.1:    A Simplified View of the NDA

In classical trial designs, power and sample-size calculations are a major task. The sample-size calculations for two-group designs have been studied by many scholars, among them Julious (2004), Chow, Shao, and Wang (2003), Machin, et al. (1997), Campbell, Julious, and Altman (1995), and Lachin and Foukes (1986).

In what follows, we will review a unified formulation for sample-size calculation in classical two-arm designs including superiority, noninferiority, and equivalence trials. We will also discuss some important concepts and issues with the designs that are often misunderstood. We will first discuss two-group superiority and noninferiority designs in Section 2.2. Equivalence studies will be discussed in Section 2.3. Three different types of equivalence studies (average, population, and individual equivalences) are reviewed. We will discuss dose-response studies in Section 2.4. The sample-size calculations for various endpoints are provided based on the contrast test.

## 2.2 Two-Group Superiority and Noninferiority Designs

### 2.2.1 *General Approach to Power Calculation*

When testing a null hypothesis $H_0 : \varepsilon \leq 0$ against an alternative hypothesis $H_a : \varepsilon > 0$, where $\varepsilon$ is the treatment effect (difference in response), the type-I error rate function is defined as

$$\alpha(\varepsilon) = \Pr\left\{\text{reject } H_0 \text{ when } H_0 \text{ is true}\right\}.$$

Note: alternatively, the type-I error rate can be defined as $\sup_{\varepsilon \in H_0} \{\alpha(\varepsilon)\}$. Similarly, the type-II error rate function $\beta$ is defined as

$$\beta(\varepsilon) = \Pr\left\{\text{fail to reject } H_0 \text{ when } H_a \text{ is true}\right\}.$$

For hypothesis testing, knowledge of the distribution of the test statistic under $H_0$ is required. For sample-size calculation, knowledge of the distribution of the test statistic under a particular $H_a$ is also required. To control the overall type-I error rate at level a constant level $\alpha^*$ under any point of the $H_0$ domain, the condition $\alpha(\varepsilon) \leq \alpha^*$ for all $\varepsilon \leq 0$ must be satisfied, where $\alpha^*$ is a threshold that is usually larger than 0.025 unless it is a phase-III trial. If $\alpha(\varepsilon)$ is a monotonic function of $\varepsilon$, then the maximum type-I error rate occurs when $\varepsilon = 0$, and the rejection region should be derived under this condition (for this reason we will simply use constant $\alpha$ instead of $\alpha^*$). For example, for the null hypothesis $H_0 : \mu_2 - \mu_1 \leq 0$, where $\mu_1$ and $\mu_2$ are the means of the two treatment groups, the maximum type-I error rate occurs on the boundary of $H_0$ when $\mu_2 - \mu_1 = 0$. Let $T = \frac{\hat{\mu}_2 - \hat{\mu}_1}{\hat{\sigma}}$, where $\hat{\mu}_i$ and $\hat{\sigma}$ are the sample mean and pooled sample standard deviation, respectively. Further, let $\Phi_o(T)$ denote the cumulative distribution function (cdf) of the test statistic on the boundary of the null hypothesis domain, and let $\Phi_a(T)$ denote the cdf under $H_a$. Given this information, under the large sample assumption, $\Phi_o(T)$ is the cdf of the standard normal distribution, $N(0,1)$, and $\Phi_a(T)$ is the cdf of $N(\frac{\sqrt{n}\varepsilon}{2\sigma}, 1)$, where $n$ is the total sample-size and $\sigma$ is the common standard deviation (Figure 2.2).

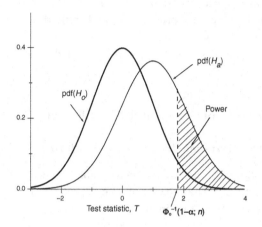

Figure 2.2:   Power as a Function of $\alpha$ and $n$

The power of the test statistic $T$ under a particular $H_a$ can be expressed as follows:

$$\text{Power}(\varepsilon) = \Pr(T \geq \Phi_o^{-1}(1-\alpha;n)|H_a) = 1 - \Phi_a(\Phi_o^{-1}(1-\alpha;n);n),$$

which is equivalent to

$$\text{Power}(\varepsilon) = \Phi\left(\frac{\sqrt{n}\varepsilon}{2\sigma} - z_{1-\alpha}\right), \tag{2.1}$$

where $\Phi$ is the cdf of the standard normal distribution, $\varepsilon$ is treatment difference, and $z_{1-\alpha}$ are the percentiles of the standard normal distribution. Figure 2.2 is an illustration of the power function of $\alpha$ and the sample size $n$. The total sample-size is given by

$$n = \frac{4(z_{1-a} + z_{1-\beta})^2\sigma^2}{\varepsilon^2}. \tag{2.2}$$

More generally, for an imbalanced design with sample-size ratio $r = n_1/n_2$ and a margin $\delta$ ($\delta > 0$ for superiority test and $\delta < 0$ for noninferiority test), the sample size is given by

$$n_2 = \frac{(z_{1-\alpha} + z_{1-\beta})^2\sigma^2(1+1/r)}{(\varepsilon - \delta)^2}. \tag{2.3}$$

Table 2.1: Sample Sizes for Different Types of Endpoints

| Endpoint | Sample-Size | Variance |
|---|---|---|
| One mean | $n = \frac{(z_{1-a}+z_{1-\beta})^2 \sigma^2}{\varepsilon^2}$ | |
| Two means | $n_1 = \frac{(z_{1-a}+z_{1-\beta})^2 \sigma^2}{(1+1/r)^{-1}\varepsilon^2}$ | |
| One proportion | $n = \frac{(z_{1-a}+z_{1-\beta})^2 \sigma^2}{\varepsilon^2}$ | $\sigma^2 = p(1-p)$ |
| Two proportions | $n_1 = \frac{(z_{1-a}+z_{1-\beta})^2 \sigma^2}{(1+1/r)^{-1}\varepsilon^2}$ | $\sigma^2 = \bar{p}(1-\bar{p});$ $\bar{p} = \frac{n_1 p_1 + n_2 p_2}{n_1 + n_2}.$ |
| One survival curve | $n = \frac{(z_{1-a}+z_{1-\beta})^2 \sigma^2}{\varepsilon^2}$ | $\sigma^2 = \lambda_0^2 \left(1 - \frac{e^{\lambda_0 T_0}-1}{T_0 \lambda_0 e^{\lambda_0 T_s}}\right)^{-1}$ |
| Two survival curves | $n_1 = \frac{(z_{1-a}+z_{1-\beta})^2 \sigma^2}{(1+1/r)^{-1}\varepsilon^2}$ | $\sigma^2 = \frac{r\sigma_1^2 + \sigma_2^2}{1+r},$ $\sigma_i^2 = \lambda_i^2 \left(1 - \frac{e^{\lambda_i T_0}-1}{T_0 \lambda_i e^{\lambda_i T_s}}\right)^{-1}$ |

Note: $r = \frac{n_2}{n_1}$. $\lambda_0 =$ expected hazard rate, $T_0 =$ uniform patient accrual time, and $T_s =$ trial duration. Logrank-test is used for comparison of the two survival curves.

Equation (2.3) is a general sample-size formulation for the two-group designs with a normal, binary, or survival endpoint. When using the formulation, the corresponding "standard deviation" $\sigma$ should be used, examples of which have been listed in Table 2.1 for commonly used endpoints (Chang and Chow, 2006b).

We now derive the standard deviation for the time-to-event endpoint. Under an exponential survival model, the relationship among hazard ($\lambda$), median ($T_{median}$), and mean ($T_{mean}$) survival time is very simple:

$$T_{Median} = \frac{\ln 2}{\lambda} = (\ln 2)T_{mean}.$$

Let $\lambda_i$ be the population hazard rate for group $i$. The corresponding variance $\sigma_i^2$ can be derived in several different ways. Here we use Lachin and Foulkes' maximum likelihood approach (Lachin and Foulkes, 1986; Chow, et al., 2003).

Let $T_0$ and $T_s$ be the accrual time period and the total trial duration, respectively. We can then prove that the variance for uniform patient entry is given by

$$\sigma^2(\lambda_i) = \lambda_i^2 \left[1 + \frac{e^{-\lambda_i T_s}(1 - e^{\lambda_i T_0})}{T_0 \lambda_i}\right]^{-1}.$$

Let $a_{ij}$ denote the uniform entry time of the $j$th patient of the $i$th group, i.e., $a_{ij} \sim \frac{1}{T_0}$, $0 \leq a_{ij} \leq T_0$. Let $t_{ij}$ be the time-to-event starting from the time of the patient's entry for the $j$th patient in the $i$th group, $i = 1, ..., k$, $j = 1, ..., n_i$. It is assumed that $t_{ij}$ follows an exponential distribution with a hazard rate of $\lambda_i$. The information observed is $(x_{ij}, \delta_{ij})$ $= (\min(t_{ij},\ T_s - a_{ij}),\ I\{t_{ij} \leq T_s - a_{ij}\})$. For a fixed $i$, the joint likelihood for $x_{ij}$, $j = 1, ..., n_i$ can be written as

$$L(\lambda_i) = \frac{1}{T_0^{n_i}} \lambda_i^{\sum_{j=1}^{n_i} \delta_{ij}} e^{-\lambda_i \sum_{j=1}^{n_i} x_{ij}}.$$

Taking the derivative with respect to $\lambda_i$ and letting it equal zero, we can obtain the maximum likelihood estimate (MLE) for $\lambda_i$, which is given by $\hat{\lambda}_i = \frac{\sum_{j=1}^{n_i} \delta_{ij}}{\sum_{j=1}^{n_i} x_{ij}}$. According to the Central Limit Theorem, we have

$$\sqrt{n_i}(\hat{\lambda}_i - \lambda_i) = \sqrt{n_i} \frac{\sum_{j=1}^{n_i}(\delta_{ij} - \lambda_i x_{ij})}{\sum_{j=1}^{n_i} x_{ij}}$$

$$= \frac{1}{\sqrt{n_i} E(x_{ij})} \sum_{j=1}^{n_i} (\delta_{ij} - \lambda_i x_{ij}) + o_p(1)$$

$$\xrightarrow{d} N(0, \sigma^2(\lambda_i)),$$

where

$$\sigma^2(\lambda_i) = \frac{var(\delta_{ij} - \lambda_i x_{ij})}{E^2(x_{ij})}$$

and $\xrightarrow{d}$ denotes convergence in distribution. Note that

$$E(\delta_{ij}) = E(\delta_{ij}^2) = 1 - \int_0^{T_0} \frac{1}{T_0} e^{-\lambda_i(T_s - a)} da = 1 + \frac{e^{-\lambda_i T_s}(1 - e^{\lambda_i T_0})}{T_0 \lambda_i}$$

$$E(x_{ij}) = \frac{1}{\lambda_i} E(\delta_{ij}), \text{ and } E(x_{ij}^2) = \frac{2E(\delta_{ij} x_{ij})}{\lambda_i}.$$

Hence,

$$\sigma^2(\lambda_i) = \frac{var(\delta_{ij} - \lambda_i x_{ij})}{E^2(x_{ij})} = \frac{1}{E^2(x_{ij})} \left( E(\delta_{ij}^2) - 2\lambda_i E(\delta_{ij} x_{ij}) + \lambda_i^2 E(x_{ij}^2) \right)$$

$$= \frac{E(\delta_{ij}^2)}{E^2(x_{ij})} = \frac{\lambda_i^2}{E(\delta_{ij})} = \lambda_i^2 \left[ 1 + \frac{e^{-\lambda_i T_s}(1 - e^{\lambda_i T_0})}{T_0 \lambda_i} \right]^{-1}.$$

**Example 2.1    Arteriosclerotic Vascular Disease Trial**

Cholesterol is the main lipid associated with arteriosclerotic vascular disease. The purpose of cholesterol testing is to identify patients at risk for arteriosclerotic heart disease. The liver metabolizes cholesterol to its free form and transports it to the bloodstream via lipoproteins. Nearly 75% of the cholesterol is bound to low-density lipoproteins (LDLs)—"bad cholesterol"—and 25% is bound to high-density lipoproteins (HDLs)—"good cholesterol." Therefore, cholesterol is the main component of LDLs and only a minimal component of HDLs. LDL is the substance most directly associated with increased risk of coronary heart disease (CHD).

Suppose we are interested in a trial for evaluating the effect of a test drug on cholesterol in patients with CHD. A two-group parallel design is chosen for the trial with LDL as the primary endpoint. The treatment difference in LDL is estimated to be 5% with a standard deviation of 0.3. For power = 90% and one-sided $\alpha = 0.025$, the total sample can be calculated using (2.2):

$$n = \frac{4(1.96 + 1.28)^2 \left(0.3^2\right)}{0.05^2} = 1512.$$

For a noninferiority test, with a margin $\delta = -0.01$ (the determination of $\delta$ is a complicated issue and will not be discussed here.), the total sample-size is given by

$$n = \frac{4(1.96 + 1.28)^2 \left(0.3^2\right)}{(0.05 + 0.01)^2} = 1050.$$

We can see that the required sample size is smaller for the noninferiority test than for a superiority test.

### 2.2.2    *Powering Trials Appropriately*

During the design, $\varepsilon$ ($\delta_{true}$) and $\sigma$ are unknowns, but they can be estimated. Therefore, the power is just an estimation of the probability of achieving statistical significance, and its precision is dependent on the precision of the initial estimate of $\varepsilon$ and $\sigma$. When lacking information, a minimum clinically or commercially meaningful treatment difference $\delta_{min}$ is often used. However, this strategy is not as good as it appears to be for the following reasons: (1) Power is not probability of success. The common phrase "90% power to detect a difference of $\delta$" does not mean that there is a 90% probability of proving statistically that the treatment effect is larger than $\delta_{min}$. What it really means is that if the true treatment difference is $\delta_{min}$, then there is a 90% probability of proving a treatment difference $> 0$ (*zero*) at $\alpha$ level (Figure 2.3). (2) If the trial is designed based on $\delta_{\min}$, then as long as the observed treatment difference $\hat{\delta} > 0.61\,\delta_{\min}$, there is a statistical significance. The trial is overpowered if the statistical significance is achieved even when there is no clinically or commercially meaningful magnitude of treatment effect. (3) If the true treatment difference is equal to $\delta_{\min}$, then there is 50% chance that the observed treatment difference $\hat{\delta} > \delta_{\min}$ regardless of the sample-size (Figure 2.4). (4) $\delta_{\min}$ is difficult to know. Using the following formulation for the real superior design is too conservative:

$$n_2 = \frac{(z_{1-\alpha} + z_{1-\beta})^2\, \sigma^2\, (1 + 1/r)}{(\varepsilon - \delta_{\min})^2}. \tag{2.4}$$

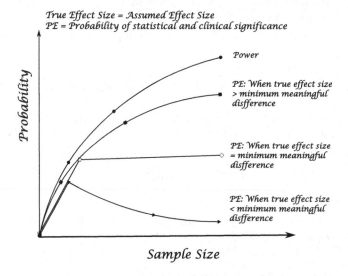

Figure 2.3:   Power and Probability of Efficacy (PE)

The selections of the type-I error rate $\alpha$ and the type-II error rate $\beta$ should be based on study objectives that may vary from phase to phase in clinical trials. It depends on efficacy, safety, and other aspects of the trial. From a safety perspective, the number of patients should be gradually increased from early phases to later phases due to the potential toxicity of the test drug. From an efficacy point-of-view, for early phases, there is more concern about missing good drug candidates and less concern about the false positive rate. In this case, a larger $\alpha$ is recommended. For later phases, a smaller $\alpha$ should be considered to meet regulatory requirements.

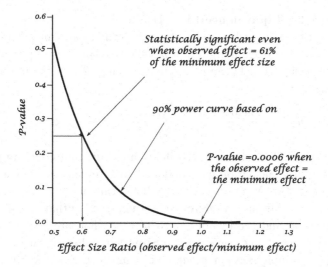

Figure 2.4: *p*-value versus Observed Effect Size

In practice, it is suggested that the benefit–risk ratio should be taken into consideration when performing sample-size calculations. In such a case, Bayesian decision theory is a useful tool.

## 2.3 Two-Group Equivalence Trial

### 2.3.1 *Equivalence Test*

The equivalence test for the two parallel groups can be stated as

$$H_0 : |\mu_1 - \mu_2| \geq \delta \quad \text{versus} \quad H_a : |\mu_1 - \mu_2| < \delta, \tag{2.5}$$

where the subscripts 1 and 2 refer to the test and reference groups, respectively. If the null hypothesis is rejected, then we conclude that the test drug and the reference drug are equivalent.

For a large sample size, the null hypothesis is rejected if

$$T_1 = \frac{\bar{x}_1 - \bar{x}_2 - \delta}{\sigma\sqrt{\frac{1}{n_1} + \frac{1}{n_2}}} < -z_{1-\alpha} \text{ and } T_2 = \frac{\bar{x}_1 - \bar{x}_2 + \delta}{\sigma\sqrt{\frac{1}{n_1} + \frac{1}{n_2}}} > z_{1-\alpha}. \tag{2.6}$$

The approximate sample size is given by (Chow et al., 2003)

$$n_2 = \frac{\left(z_{1-\alpha} + z_{1-\beta/2}\right)^2 \sigma^2 \left(1 + 1/r\right)}{\left(|\varepsilon| - \delta\right)^2}, \tag{2.7}$$

where $r = n_1/n_2$.

## Example 2.2    Equivalence LDL Trial

For the LDL trial in Example 2.1, assume the treatment difference $\varepsilon = 0.01$ and an equivalence margin of $\delta = 0.05$, the sample size per group for a balanced design ($r = 1$) can be calculated using (2.7) with 90% power at $\alpha = 0.05$ level:

$$n_2 = \frac{(1.6446 + 1.6446)^2 \, (0.3^2) \, (1 + 1/1)}{(0.01 - 0.05)^2} = 1217.$$

Note that (2.7) is just an approximation even with a large sample size, but an accurate calculation can be done using simulation. For a normal endpoint, the SAS Macro 2.1 which follows can be used for power and sample-size calculations for equivalence studies. Note that the confidence interval method and the two one-sided tests method are equivalent. The SAS variables are defined as follows: **nSims** = number of simulation runs; **nPerGrp** = sample size per group; **ux** = mean in group x; **uy** = mean in group y; **delta** = the equivalence margin; **sigmax** and **sigmay** = standard deviation for groups x and y, respectively; **alpha** = type-I error rate control; **xMean** and **yMean** = the simulated means in group x and y, respectively; **powerCI** = power based on the confidence interval method; and **powerTest** = power based on the two one-sided tests method.

>>**SAS Macro 2.1:    Equivalence Trial with Normal Endpoint**>>
```
%Macro EquivCI(nSims=1000, nPerGrp=200, ux=0, uy=1, delta=1.2,
sigmax=1, sigmay=1.2, alpha=0.05);
Data TwoGVars;
Keep xMean yMean powerCI powerTest;
powerCI=0; powerTest=0;
Do iSim=1 To &nSims;
 xMean=0; yMean=0; s2x=0; s2y=0;
 Do iObs=1 To &nPerGrp;
xNOR=Rannor(7362); xMean=xMean+xNor; s2x=s2x+xNor**2;
yNOR=Rannor(2637); yMean=yMean+yNor; s2y=s2y+yNor**2;
End;
xMean=xMean*&sigmax/&nPerGrp+&ux;
yMean=yMean*&sigmay/&nPerGrp+&uy;
sp=((s2x*&sigmax**2+s2y*&sigmay**2)/(2*&nPerGrp-2))**0.5;
se=sp/(&nPerGrp/2)**0.5;
 * CI method;
ICW=Probit(1-&alpha)*se;
If Abs(yMean-xMean)+ICW < &delta Then
```

```
powerCI=powerCI+1/&nSims;
 *Two one-sided test method;
T1=(xMean-yMean-&delta)/se;
T2=(xMean-yMean+&delta)/se;
If T1=Probit(1-&alpha) & T2>Probit(1-&alpha) Then
powerTest=powerTest+1/&nSims;
End;
Output;
Run;
Proc Print Data=TwoGVars(obs=1); Run;
%Mend EquivCI;
<<SAS<<
```

The following SAS statements are examples of simulations under the null and alternative hypotheses.

```
>>SAS>>
Title "Equivalence test with normal response: Alpha under Ho";
%EquivCI(nSims=10000, nPerGrp=1000, ux=0.2, uy=0, delta=0.2, sigmax=1,
sigmay=1, alpha=0.05);
Title "Equivalence test with normal response: Power under Ha";
%EquivCI(nSims=10000, nPerGrp=198, ux=0, uy=1, delta=1.2, sigmax=0.8,
sigmay=0.8, alpha=0.05);
<<SAS<<
```

For a binary endpoint, the power and sample-size for an equivalence test can be simulated using the SAS Macro 2.2 below. Note that the confidence interval method and the two one-sided tests method are equivalent. The SAS variables are defined as follows: **nSims** = number of simulation runs; **nPerGrp** = sample-size per group; **px** = response rate in group x; **py** = response rate in group y; **delta** = the equivalence margin; **sigmax** and **sigmay** = standard deviation for groups x and y, respectively; **alpha** = type-I error rate control; **xMean** and **yMean** = the simulated means in group x and y, respectively; **powerCI** = power based on the confidence interval method; and **powerTest** = power based on the two one-sided tests method.

### >>SAS Macro 2.2: Equivalence Trial with Binary Endpoint>>

```
%Macro   TwoSamZTest(nSims=100000,   nPerGrp=100,   px=0.3,   py=0.4,
delta=0.3, alpha=0.05);
Data TwoGVars;
KEEP powerCI powerTest;
```

```
powerCI=0; powerTest=0;
Do iSim=1 To &nSims;
PxObs=Ranbin(733,&nPerGrp,&px)/&nPerGrp;
PyObs=Ranbin(236,&nPerGrp,&py)/&nPerGrp;
se=((PxObs*(1-PxObs)+PyObs*(1-PyObs))/&nPerGrp)**0.5;
*CI method;
ICW=Probit(1-&alpha)*se;
IF Abs(PxObs-PyObs)+ICW < &delta Then
powerCI=powerCI+1/&nSims;
 *Two one-sided tests method;
T1=(PyObs-PxObs-&delta)/se;
T2=(PyObs-PxObs+&delta)/se;
IF T1=Probit(1-&alpha) & T2>Probit(1-&alpha) Then
powerTest=powerTest+1/&nSims;
End;
Output;
Run;
Proc Print; Run;
%Mend TwoSamZTest;
```
<<**SAS**<<

>>**SAS**>>
```
Title "Equivalence test with binary response: Alpha under Ho";
%TwoSamZTest(nPerGrp=100, px=0.1, py=0.2, delta=0.1, alpha=0.05);
Title "Equivalence test with binary response: Power under Ha";
%TwoSamZTest(nPerGrp=100, px=0.3, py=0.3, delta=0.2, alpha=0.05);
```
<<**SAS**<<

### 2.3.2 Average Bioequivalence

Pharmacokinetics (PK) is the study of the body's absorption, distribution, metabolism, and elimination of a drug. An important outcome of a PK study is the bioavailability of the drug. The bioavailability of a drug is defined as the rate and extent to which the active drug ingredient or therapeutic moiety is absorbed and becomes available at the site of drug action. As bioavailability cannot be easily measured directly, the concentration of the drug that reaches the circulating bloodstream is taken as a surrogate. Therefore, bioavailability can be viewed as the concentration of the drug that is in the blood. Two drugs are bioequivalent if they have the same bioavailability. There are a number of instances in which trials are conducted to show that two drugs are bioequivalent (Jones and Kenward, 2003): (1) when different formulations of the same drug are to be marketed, for instance, in solid-tablet or liquid-capsule form; (2) when a generic version of an innovator drug is to be marketed; and (3) when production of a drug is scaled up; and the new production process needs to be shown to produce drugs of equivalent strength and effectiveness as the original process.

At the present time, average bioequivalence (ABE) serves as the current international standard for bioequivalence (BE) testing using a $2 \times 2$ crossover design (Chow and Liu, 2008). The PK parameters used for assessing ABE are area under the curve (AUC) and peak concentration (Cmax). The recommended statistical method is the two one-sided tests procedure to determine if the average values for the PK measures determined after administration of the T (test) and R (reference) products were comparable. This approach is termed ABE. It is equivalent to the so-called confidence interval method, which involves the calculation of a 90% confidence interval for the ratio of the averages (population geometric means) of the measures for the T and R products. To establish BE, the calculated confidence interval should fall within a BE limit, usually 80%–125% for the ratio of the product averages. The 1992 FDA guidance has also provided specific recommendations for logarithmic transformation of PK data, methods to evaluate sequence effects, and methods to evaluate outlier data.

In practice, people also use parallel designs and the 90% confidence interval for nontransformed data. To establish BE, the calculated confidence interval should fall within a BE limit, usually 80%–120% for the difference of the product averages.

The hypothesis for ABE in a $2 \times 2$ crossover design with log-transformed data can be written as

$$H_{01} : \mu_T - \mu_R \leq -\ln 1.25,$$
$$H_{02} : \mu_T - \mu_R \geq \ln 1.25.$$

The asymptotic power is given by (Chow et al., 2003)

$$n = \frac{\left(z_{1-\alpha} + z_{1-\beta/2}\right)^2 \sigma_{1,1}^2}{2 \left(\ln 1.25 - |\varepsilon|\right)^2},$$

where the variance for the intrasubject comparison is estimated using

$$\hat{\sigma}_{1,1}^2 = \frac{1}{n_1 + n_2 - 2} \sum_{j=1}^{2} \sum_{i=1}^{n_j} \left(y_{i1j} - y_{i2j} - \bar{y}_{1j} + \bar{y}_{2j}\right)^2,$$

$y_{ikj}$ is the log-transformed PK measure from the $i$th subject in the $j$th sequence at the $k$th dosing period, and $\bar{y}_{kj}$ is the sample mean of the observations in the $j$th sequence at the $k$th period.

## Example 2.3    Average Bioequivalence Trial

Suppose we are interested in establishing ABE between an inhaled formulation and a subcutaneously injected formulation of a test drug. The PK parameter chosen for this bioequivalence test is a log-transformation of the 24-hour AUC (i.e., the raw data is log-normal). Assume that the difference between the two formulations in $\log(\text{AUC})$ is $\varepsilon = 0.04$ and the standard deviation for the intrasubject comparison is $\sigma_{1,1}^2 = 0.55$ with $\alpha = 0.05$ and $\beta = 0.2$, the sample size per sequence is given by

$$n = \frac{(1.96 + 0.84)^2 (0.55)^2}{2 (0.223 - 0.04)^2} = 36.$$

For a small sample, the bioequivalence test can be obtained using the following SAS Macro Power2By2ABE. The purpose of this macro is to calculate sample size for an average BE trial featuring a $2 \times 2$ crossover design with a normal endpoint. The power formulation was derived by Jones and Kenward (2003, p. 336). The SAS variables are defined as follows: **sWithin** = Within-subject standard deviation on log-scale; **uRatio** = ratio of two treatment means; **n** = total sample-size; and **power** = power of the test.

**>>SAS Macro 2.3:    Crossover Bioequivalence Trial>>**

```
%Macro Power2By2ABE(totalN=24, sWithin=0.355, uRatio=1);
Data ABE; Keep sWithin uRatio n power;
n=&totalN; sWithin=&sWithin; uRatio=&uRatio;
* Err df for AB/BA crossover design;
n2=n-2;
t1=tinv(1-0.05,n-2); t2=-t1;
nc1=Sqrt(n)*log(uRatio/0.8)/Sqrt(2)/sWithin;
nc2=Sqrt(n)*log(uRatio/1.25)/Sqrt(2)/sWithin;
df=Sqrt(n-2)*(nc1-nc2)/(2*t1);
Power=Probt(t2,df,nc2)-Probt(t1,df,nc1);
Run;
Proc Print; Run;
%Mend Power2By2ABE;
```
**<<SAS<<**

An example of how to use the macro is presend in the following:

>>**SAS**>>
%Power2By2ABE(totalN=58, sWithin=0.355, uRatio=1)
<<**SAS**<<

### 2.3.3 *Population and Individual Bioequivalence*

An FDA 2001 guidance describes two new approaches, termed population bioequivalence (PBE) and individual bioequivalence (IBE). PBE is concerned with assessing if a patient who has not yet been treated with R or T can be prescribed either formulation. IBE is a criterion for deciding if a patient who is currently being treated with R can be switched to T. The ABE method does not assess a subject-by-formulation interaction variance, that is, the variation in the average T and R difference among individuals. In contrast, PBE and IBE approaches include comparisons of both averages and variances of the measure. The PBE approach assesses total variability of the measure in the population. The IBE approach assesses within-subject variability for the T and R products, as well as the subject-by-formulation interaction. For PBEs and IBEs, the 95% confidence intervals are recommended with the same BE limits as those for ABE.

Statistical analyses of PBE and IBE data typically require a higher-order crossover design such as [RTR,TRT] or [RTRT,TRTR]. The statistical model is often a hierarchical model. PBE and IBE approaches, but not the ABE approach, allow two types of scaling: reference scaling and constant scaling. Reference scaling means that the criterion used is scaled to the variability of the R product, which effectively widens the BE limit for more variable reference products. Although generally sufficient, use of reference scaling alone could unnecessarily narrow the BE limit for drugs and/or drug products that have low variability but a wide therapeutic range. This guidance, therefore, recommends mixed scaling for the PBE and IBE approaches. With mixed scaling, the reference-scaled form of the criterion should be used if the reference product is highly variable; otherwise, the constant-scaled form should be used.

The hypothesis test for IBE is given by

$$H_0 : \begin{cases} (\mu_T - \mu_R)^2 + \sigma_D^2 + \sigma_{WT}^2 - 3.49\sigma_{WR}^2 \geq 0 & \text{if } \sigma_{WR}^2 > 0.04, \\ (\mu_T - \mu_R)^2 + \sigma_D^2 + \sigma_{WT}^2 - \sigma_{WR}^2 - 0.996 \geq 0 & \text{if } \sigma_{WR}^2 \leq 0.04, \end{cases}$$

where $\sigma_{WT}^2$ and $\sigma_{WR}^2$ are the within-subject variances for T and R, respectively; $\sigma_{BT}^2$ and $\sigma_{BR}^2$ are the between-subject variances for T and R; and $\sigma_D^2 = \sigma_{BT}^2 + \sigma_{BR}^2 - 2\rho\sigma_{BT}^2\sigma_{BR}^2$ is the subject-by-formulation interaction, where $\rho$ is the between-subject correlation of T and R. The mean of T and R are denoted by $\mu_T$ and $\mu_R$, respectively.

The hypothesis test for PBE is given by

$$H_0 : \begin{cases} (\mu_T - \mu_R)^2 + \sigma_T^2 - 3.49\sigma_R^2 \geq 0 & \text{if } \sigma_R^2 > 0.04, \\ (\mu_T - \mu_R)^2 + \sigma_T^2 - \sigma_R^2 - 0.996 \geq 0 & \text{if } \sigma_R^2 \leq 0.04, \end{cases}$$

where $\sigma_T^2 = \sigma_{WT}^2 + \sigma_{BT}^2$ and $\sigma_R^2 = \sigma_{WR}^2 + \sigma_{BR}^2$.

Further details can be found in Jones and Kenward (2003) and Chow and Liu (2003). SAS programs for IBE and PBE are available from Jones and Kenward.

## 2.4   Dose-Response Trials

Dose-response trials are also called dose-finding trials. Four questions are often of interest in a dose-response trial (Ruberg, 1995): (1) Is there any evidence of drug effect? (2) What doses exhibit a response different from the control response? (3) What is the nature of the dose-response? and (4) What is the optimal dose? A phase-II dose-response trial is typically a multiple-arm parallel design with a control group. There are a variety of approaches to statistical analysis for a dose-response study; for examples, see Chuang and Agresti (1997) and Stewart and Ruberg (2000). A commonly used and conservative approach is to compare each active dose to the control using Dunnett's test or a stepwise test. As pointed out by Stewart and Ruberg, the contrast will detect certain expected dose-response features without forcing those expected features into the analysis model. Commonly used contrast procedures include Dunnett's test (Dunnett, 1955), the regression test of Tukey et al. (Tukey and Ciminera, 1885), Ruberg's basin contrast (Ruberg, 1989), Williams's test (Williams, 1971, 1972), and the Cochran–Armitage test (Cochran, 1954; Amitage, 1955). For multiple contrast tests, there are usually multiplicity adjustment requirements (Hsu and Berger, 1999). The sample size formulation is available for multi-arm dose-response trials for binary endpoints based on contrast tests (Nam, 1987). For ordered categorical data, Whitehead (1993) derived a formulation for sample size calculation based on a proportional-odds model.

The objective of this section is to provide a unified formulation and a user-friendly SAS macro for calculating the power and sample size for multiple-arm superiority and noninferiority trials with continuous, binary, or survival endpoints (Chang, 2006b; Chang and Chow, 2006b).

### 2.4.1 *Unified Formulation for Sample-Size*

In multiple-arm trials, a general one-sided hypothesis testing problem can be stated as a contrast test:

$$H_0 : L(\mathbf{u}) \leq 0; \text{ vs. } H_a : L(\mathbf{u}) = \varepsilon > 0, \tag{2.8}$$

where the operator or function $L(\cdot)$ is often linear; $\mathbf{u} = \{u_i\}$; $u_i$ can be the mean, proportion, or hazard rate for the $i$th group depending on the study endpoint; and $\varepsilon$ is a constant.

A test statistic can be defined as

$$T = \frac{L(\hat{\mathbf{u}})}{\sqrt{var_{\varepsilon=0}(L(\hat{\mathbf{u}}))}}, \tag{2.9}$$

where $\hat{\mathbf{u}}$ is an unbiased estimator of $\mathbf{u}$.

A linear operator of $L(\cdot)$ is particularly interesting and will be used in the rest of the chapter:

$$L(\mathbf{u}) = \sum_{i=1}^{k} c_i u_i - \delta, \tag{2.10}$$

where the contrast coefficient $c_i$ satisfies the equation $\sum_{i=1}^{k} c_i = 0$ ($c_1 = 1$ for a single-arm trial). Without losing generality, assume that $c_i u_i > 0$ indicates efficacy; then, for a superiority design, $\delta \geq 0$, and for a noninferiority design, $\delta < 0$. Note that if $\delta = 0$ and $H_0$ defined by (2.8) is rejected for some $\{c_i\}$ satisfying $\sum_{i=1}^{k} c_i = 0$, then there is a difference among $u_i$ ($i = 1, ..., k$).

Let $\hat{\mathbf{u}}$ be the mean for a continuous endpoint, proportion for a binary endpoint, and maximum likelihood estimator (MLE) of the hazard rate for a survival endpoint; then, the asymptotic distributions of the test statistic can be obtained from the central limit theorem:

Under the null hypothesis, the test statistic is given by

$$T = \frac{L_{\varepsilon=0}(\hat{\mathbf{u}})}{v_o} \sim N(0, 1) \tag{2.11}$$

and under the specific alternative hypothesis associated with $\varepsilon$, the test statistic is given by

$$T = \frac{L(\hat{\mathbf{u}})}{v_o} \sim N(\frac{\varepsilon}{v_o}, \frac{v_a^2}{v_o^2}), \tag{2.12}$$

where

$$\varepsilon = E(L(\hat{u}), \tag{2.13}$$

$$\begin{cases} v_o^2 = var_{\varepsilon=0}(L(\hat{u})) \\ v_a^2 = var(L(\hat{u})) \end{cases} . \tag{2.14}$$

Because of (2.10), (2.14) can be written as

$$\begin{cases} v_o^2 = \sum_{i=1}^{k} c_i^2 var_{\varepsilon=0}(\hat{u}_i) = \sigma_o^2 \sum_{i=1}^{k} \frac{c_i^2}{n_i} = \frac{\theta_o^2}{n} \\ v_a^2 = \sum_{i=1}^{k} c_i^2 var(\hat{u}_i) = \sum_{i=1}^{k} \frac{c_i^2 \sigma_i^2}{n_i} = \frac{\theta_a^2}{n} \end{cases} , \tag{2.15}$$

where

$$\begin{cases} \theta_o^2 = \sigma_o^2 \sum_{i=1}^{k} \frac{c_i^2}{f_i} \\ \theta_a^2 = \sum_{i=1}^{k} \frac{c_i^2 \sigma_i^2}{f_i} \end{cases} , \tag{2.16}$$

where $n_i$ is the sample size for the $i$th arm, $f_i = \frac{n_i}{n}$ is the size fraction, $n = \sum_{i=0}^{k} n_i$, $\sigma_o^2$ is the variance of the response under $H_0$, and $\sigma_i^2$ is the variance under $H_a$ for the $i$th arm.

From (2.12) and (2.15), it is immediately obtained that under the specific alternative hypothesis, the test statistic $T$ is normally distributed with a mean of $\frac{\sqrt{n}\varepsilon}{\theta_o}$ and a variance of $\frac{\theta_a^2}{\theta_o^2}$. Therefore, similar to (2.1), the power considering heterogeneity of variances can be obtained as

$$\text{power} = \Phi\left(\frac{\varepsilon\sqrt{n} - \theta_o z_{1-\alpha}}{\theta_a}\right). \tag{2.17}$$

Similar to (2.2), the sample-size with the heterogeneous variances is given by

$$n = \frac{(z_{1-\alpha}\theta_o + z_{1-\beta}\theta_a)^2}{\varepsilon^2}. \tag{2.18}$$

Note that $\varepsilon$ defined by (2.13) is the treatment difference $\Delta$—the non-inferior/superiority margin $\delta$. When $\delta = 0$, $\varepsilon$ is simply the treatment difference.

Equations (2.16) through (2.18) are applicable to any $k$-arm design ($k \geq 1$). The asymptotic variance $\sigma_i^2$ can be estimated by

$$\hat{\sigma}_i^2 = \hat{p}_i(1 - \hat{p}_i) \tag{2.19}$$

for a binary endpoint with an estimated response rate of $\hat{p}_i$, and

$$\hat{\sigma}_i^2 = \hat{\lambda}_i^2 \left[1 + \frac{e^{-\hat{\lambda}_i T_s}(1 - e^{\hat{\lambda}_i T_0})}{T_0 \hat{\lambda}_i}\right]^{-1} \tag{2.20}$$

for an exponentially distributed survival endpoint with an estimated hazard rate of $\hat{\lambda}_i$. These two variances can be used to calculate $\theta_o^2$ and $\theta_a^2$ in (2.16) when the sample size is large. It can be seen that (2.17) and (2.18) have included the common one-arm and two-arm superiority and noninferiority designs as special cases: for a one-arm design, $c_1 = 1$, and for a two-arm design, $c_1 = -1$ and $c_2 = 1$.

### 2.4.2 Application Examples

Three examples (all modified from the actual trials) will be used to demonstrate the utility of the proposed method for clinical trial designs. The first example is a multiple-arm trial with a continuous endpoint. In the second example, both superiority and noninferiority designs are considered for a multiple-arm trial with a binary endpoint. The third example is an application of the proposed method for designing a multiple-arm trial with a survival endpoint, where different sets of contrasts and balanced, as well as unbalanced, designs are compared. For convenience, the SAS macro for sample-size calculation is provided.

### Example 2.4 Dose-Response Trial with Continuous Endpoint

In a phase-II asthma study, a design with 4 dose groups (0 mg, 20 mg, 40 mg, and 60 mg) of the test drug is proposed. The primary efficacy endpoint is the percent change from baseline in forced expiratory volume in the first second (FEV1). From previous studies, it has been estimated that there will be 5%, 12%, 13%, and 14% improvements over baseline for the control, 20 mg, 40 mg, and 60 mg groups, respectively, and a homogeneous standard deviation of $\sigma = 22\%$ for the FEV1 change from baseline. To be consistent with the response shape, let the contrast $c_i = 100(\mu_i - \frac{1}{4}\sum_{i=1}^{4}\mu_i)$, i.e., $c_1 = -6$, $c_2 = 1$, $c_3 = 2$, $c_4 = 3$, where $\mu_i$ is the estimated FEV1 improvement in the $i$th group. It can be seen that any set of contrasts with multiples of the above $\{c_i\}$ will lead to the same sample size. Thus, it can be obtained that $\varepsilon = \sum_{i=1}^{4} c_i\mu_i = 50\%$. Using a balanced design ($f_i = 1/4$) with a one-sided $\alpha = 0.05$, the sample size required to detect a true difference of $\varepsilon = 0.5$ with 80% power is given by

$$n = \left[\frac{(z_{1-\alpha} + z_{1-\beta})\sigma}{\varepsilon}\right]^2 \sum_{i=1}^{4} \frac{c_i^2}{f_i}$$

$$= \left[\frac{(1.645 + 0.842)(0.22)}{0.50}\right]^2 4((-6)^2 + 1^2 + 2^2 + 3^2)$$

$$= 240.$$

Thus, a total sample size of 240 is required for the trial.

## Example 2.5    Dose-Response Trial with Binary Endpoint

A trial is to be designed for patients with acute ischemic stroke of recent onset. The composite endpoint (death and miocardial infarction [MI]) is the primary endpoint. There are four dose levels planned with event rates of 14%, 13%, 12%, and 11%, respectively. The first group is the active control group (14% event rate). We are interested in both superiority and noninferiority tests comparing the test drug to the active control. Notice that there is no need for multiplicity adjustment for the two tests because of the closed-set test procedure. The comparisons are made between the active control and the test groups; therefore, the contrast for the active control should have a different sign than the contrasts for the test groups. Let $c_1 = -6$, $c_2 = 1$, $c_3 = 2$, and $c_4 = 3$. It is assumed that the noninferiority margin for the event rate is $\delta = 0.5\%$, and the event rate is $p_o = 0.14$ under the null hypothesis. Because it is a noninferiority design and the noninferiority margin is usually defined based on a two-arm design, to make this noninferiority margin usable in the multiple-arm design, the contrasts need to be rescaled to match the two-arm design, i.e., set the contrast for the control group $c_1 = -1$. The final contrasts used in the trial are given by $\left\{ c_1 = -1,\ c_2 = \frac{1}{6},\ c_3 = \frac{1}{3},\ c_4 = \frac{1}{2} \right\}$. Based on this information, it can be obtained that $\varepsilon = \sum_{i=1}^{k} c_i p_i - \delta = -0.02333 - 0.005 = -0.02833$, where $p_i$ is the estimated event rate in the $i$th group. Using a balanced design ($f_i = 1/4$), the two key parameters, $\theta_o^2$ and $\theta_a^2$, can be calculated as follows:

$$\begin{cases} \theta_o^2 = p_o(1 - p_o) \sum_{i=1}^{k} \frac{c_i^2}{f_i} = 0.6689 \\ \theta_a^2 = \sum_{i=1}^{k} \frac{c_i^2\, p_i(1-p_i)}{f_i} = 0.639 \end{cases}.$$

Using a one-sided $\alpha = 0.025$ and a power of 90%, the sample-size required for the noninferiority test is given by

$$n = \left[ \frac{(z_{1-\alpha}\theta_o + z_{1-\beta}\theta_a)}{\varepsilon} \right]^2$$

$$= \left[ \frac{(1.96\sqrt{0.6689} + 1.2815\sqrt{0.639})}{-0.02833} \right]^2$$

$$= 8600.$$

Thus a total sample-size of 8600 patients is required for the noninferiority test. With 8600 patients, the power for the superiority test ($\delta = 0, \varepsilon =$

0.0233) is 76.5%, which is calculated as follows:

$$\text{power} = \Phi_o \left( \frac{\varepsilon\sqrt{n} - \theta_o z_{1-\alpha}}{\theta_a} \right)$$

$$= \Phi_o \left( \frac{0.0233\sqrt{8600} - 1.96\sqrt{0.6689}}{\sqrt{0.639}} \right)$$

$$= \Phi_o (0.6977) = 76\%.$$

Note that different contrasts can be explored to minimize the sample size.

An interesting note is that the Cochran–Armitage linear trend test is a special case of the contrast test in which the contrast $c_i = d_i - \bar{d}$, where $d_i$ is the $i$th dose and $\bar{d}$ is the average dose.

### Example 2.6 Dose-Response Trial with Survival Endpoint

Let $\lambda_i$ be the population hazard rate for group $i$. The contrast test for multiple survival curves can be written as $H_0 : \sum_{i=0}^{k} c_i \lambda_i \leq 0$. This null hypothesis is assumed in the following example.

In a four-arm (active control, lower dose of test drug, higher dose of test drug, and combined therapy), phase-II oncology trial, the objective is to determine if there is treatment effect with time-to-progression as the primary endpoint. Patient enrollment duration is estimated to be $T_0 = 9$ months and the total trial duration is $T_s = 16$ months. The estimated median times for the four groups are 14, 20, 22, and 24 months with the corresponding hazard rates of 0.0459, 0.0347, 0.0315, and 0.0289/month, respectively (under the exponential survival distribution, $\lambda T_{Median} = ln2$). The hazard rate under the null hypothesis is assumed to be 0.03525. A power of 80% and a one-sided $\alpha$ of 0.025 are proposed for the trial. The small $\alpha$ is used due to the consideration of potential accelerated approval using this trial. In order to achieve the most efficient design (i.e., minimum sample size), sample sizes from different contrasts and various designs (balanced and unbalanced) are compared. The results are presented in Table 2.2, where the optimal design is the minimum variance design in which the number of patients assigned to each group is proportional to the variance of the group. It can be seen that the optimal design with sample-size fractions (0.343, 0.244, 0.217, and 0.197) is generally the most powerful and requires fewer patients regardless of the shape of the contrasts. The contrasts with a linear trend also work well for the optimal design. Although the optimal design with linear contrasts seems attractive with a total sample size of 646 subjects, in practice, more patients being assigned to the control group

Table 2.2:   Sample Sizes for Different Contrasts (Balanced Design)

| Scenario | Contrast | | | | Total n | |
|---|---|---|---|---|---|---|
| | | | | | Balance | Optimal |
| Average dose effect | −3 | 1 | 1 | 1 | 838 | 690 |
| Linear response trend | −6 | 1 | 2 | 3 | 759 | 646 |
| Median time trend | −6 | 0 | 2 | 4 | 742 | 664 |
| Hazard-rate trend | 10.65 | −0.55 | −3.75 | −6.35 | 742 | 651 |

Note: Sample-size fractions for the optimal design = 0.343, 0.244, 0.217, and 0.197.

presents an ethical concern, and it is desirable to obtain more information on the test groups. Therefore, a balanced design with contrasts (10.65, −0.55, −3.75, and −6.35) is recommended with a total sample size of 742 subjects.

### 2.4.3   *Determination of Contrast Coefficients*

There are two criteria that need to be considered when selecting contrasts: (1) The selected contrasts must lead to a clinically meaningful hypothesis test, and (2) the selected contrasts should provide the most powerful test statistic after criterion 1.

To use a contrast test, the selection of contrasts should be practically meaningful. If one is interested in a treatment difference among any groups, then any contrasts can be applied. If one is only interested in the comparison between dose-level 1 and other dose levels, then one should make the contrast for dose-level 1 have a different sign from that of the contrasts for other dose groups. Otherwise, efficacy may not be concluded even when the null hypothesis $H_0$ is rejected, because the rejection of $H_0$ could be due simply to the opposite effects (some positive and some negative) of different dose levels of the test drug.

To study how the different combinations of response shapes and contrasts may affect the sample-size and power, the following five different shapes (Table 2.3) are considered.

Table 2.3:   Response and Contrast Shapes

| Shape | $u_1$ | $u_2$ | $u_3$ | $u_4$ | $c_1$ | $c_2$ | $c_3$ | $c_4$ |
|---|---|---|---|---|---|---|---|---|
| Linear | 0.1 | 0.3 | 0.5 | 0.7 | −3.00 | −1.00 | 1.00 | 3.00 |
| Step | 0.1 | 0.4 | 0.4 | 0.7 | −3.00 | 0.00 | 0.00 | 3.00 |
| Umbrella | 0.1 | 0.4 | 0.7 | 0.5 | −3.25 | −0.25 | 2.75 | 0.75 |
| Convex | 0.1 | 0.1 | 0.1 | 0.6 | −1.25 | −1.25 | −1.25 | 3.75 |
| Concave | 0.1 | 0.6 | 0.6 | 0.6 | −3.75 | 1.25 | 1.25 | 1.25 |

Note: $c_i = b\left(u_i - \frac{1}{4}\Sigma_{i=1}^4 u_i\right)$, b = any constant.

Sample sizes required under a balanced design for different combinations of responses and contrasts are presented in Table 2.4. It can be seen that under a balanced design, when response and contrasts have the same shape, a minimal sample size is required. If an inappropriate contrast set is used, the sample size could be 30 times larger than the optimal design.

Table 2.4: Sample Size per Group for Various Contrasts

| Response | Linear | Step | Contrast Umbrella | Convex | Concave |
|---|---|---|---|---|---|
| Linear | 31 | 35 | 52 | 52 | 52 |
| Step | 39 | 35 | 81 | 52 | 52 |
| Umbrella | 55 | 74 | 33 | 825 | 44 |
| Convex | 55 | 50 | 825 | 33 | 297 |
| Concave | 55 | 50 | 44 | 297 | 33 |

Note: $\sigma = 1$, one-sided $\alpha = 0.05$

In fact, under a balanced design, homogenous variance under $H_0$ and $H_a$ and $\delta = 0$, the minimum sample size or maximum power is achieved when the following equation is satisfied (assume $\bar{u} = \sum_{i=1}^{k} u_i = 0$):

$$\frac{\partial n}{\partial c_i} = 0. \tag{2.21}$$

Under the given conditions, (2.21) is equivalent to

$$\frac{\partial}{\partial c_i} \left( \frac{\sum_{i=1}^{M} c_i^2}{\left[\sum_{i=1}^{M} c_i u_i\right]^2} \right) = 0. \tag{2.22}$$

It is obvious that the solution to (2.22) is $c_i = u_i$ $(i = 1, ..., k)$. If $\bar{u} \neq 0$, we can make a linear transformation $u_i^* = u_i - \bar{u}$; hence, $c_i = u_i^*$ or $c_i = u_i - \bar{u}$ for minimum sample size.

### 2.4.4   *SAS Macro for Power and Sample-Size*

For convenience, the sample-size calculation formulation (2.18) has been implemented in SAS macro AsympN. This SAS macro can be used to calculate the sample size for multiple-arm superiority and noninferiority trial designs with continuous, binary, or survival endpoints. The parameters are defined as follows:   **endpoint** = "normal", "binary", or "survival"; **alpha** = one-sided significance level; **nArms** = number of groups; **delta** ($> 0$) = superiority margin, and **delta** ($< 0$) = noninferiority margin; **tAcr** = patient enrollment duration; **tStd** = study duration; **u{i}** are treatment mean, proportions of response, or hazard rates for the $i$th group; **s{i}** =

standard deviations for a continuous endpoint; $c\{i\}$ = the contrasts; and $f\{i\}$ = sample-size fractions among treatment groups. Note that **tAcr** and **tStd** are for a survival endpoint only, and $\Sigma c\{i\}$=0. The standard deviation under the null hypothesis is assumed to be the average standard deviation over all groups.

## >>SAS Macro 2.4:    Sample Size for Dose-Response Trial>>

```
%Macro AsympN(endpoint="normal", alpha=0.025, power=0.8, nArms=5,
delta=0, tStd=12, tAcr=4);
Data contrastN; Set dInput;
Keep Endpoint nArms alpha power TotalSampleSize;
Array u{&nArms}; Array s{&nArms}; Array f{&nArms};
Array c{&nArms}; endpoint=&endpoint; delta=&delta;
alpha=&alpha; power=&power; nArms=&nArms;
epi = 0; s0 = 0;
Do i =1 To nArms; epi = epi + c{i}*u{i}- &delta/nArms; End;
If &endpoint = "normal" Then Do;
Do i =1 To nArms; s0 = s0 + s{i}/nArms; End;
End;
If &endpoint = "binary" Then Do;
Do i = 1 To nArms;
s{i} = (u{i}*(1-u{i}))**0.5;
s0=s0 + s{i}/nArms;
End;
End;
If &endpoint = "survival" Then Do;
Do i = 1 To nArms;
s{i} = u{i}*(1+exp(-u{i}*&tStd)*(1-exp(u{i}*&tAcr))/(&tAcr*u{i}))**(-0.5);
s0 = s0 + s{i}/nArms;
End;
End;
sumscf0 = 0; sumscf = 0;
Do i = 1 To nArms; sumscf0 = sumscf0 + s0**2*c{i}*c{i}/f{i}; End;
Do i = 1 To nArms; sumscf = sumscf + s{i}**2*c{i}*c{i}/f{i}; End;
n  =  ((PROBit(1-&alpha)*sumscf0**0.5  +  Probit(&power)*sumscf**0.5)/
epi)**2;
TotalSampleSize = round(n);
Run;
Proc print;
Run;
```

%Mend AsympN;
<<**SAS**<<

The following example shows how to call this SAS macro for sample-size calculations with normal, binary, and survival endpoints.

>>**SAS**>>
Title " = s of How to Use the SAS Macros";
Data dInput;
Array u{4}(.46, .35, .32, .3);      ** Responses;
Array s{4}(2, 2, 2, 2);    ** Standard deviation for normal endpoint;
Array c{4}(-4, 1, 1, 2);              ** Contrasts;
Array f{4} (.25, .25 ,.25, .25);    ** Sample size fractions;
%AsympN(endpoint="normal", alpha=0.025, power=0.8, nArms=4);
%AsympN(endpoint="binary", alpha=0.025, power=0.8, nArms=4);
%AsympN(endpoint="survival", alpha=0.025, power=0.8, nArms=4, delta=0, tStd=2, tAcr=.5);
Run;
<<**SAS**<<


## 2.5   Summary and Discussion

In this chapter, we reviewed commonly used classical trial design methods. The methods derived from a contrast test can be used for power and sample-size calculations for $k$-arm trials ($k \geq 1$). They can be used for superiority or noninferiority designs with continuous, binary, or survival endpoints. The selection of contrasts is critical. The selected contrasts must lead to a clinically meaningful hypothesis test and should lead to a powerful test statistic. The examples above provided details about the use of these methods. Contrast testing can be used to detect treatment difference. The most (or least) responsive arm can be considered superior or noninferior to the control and can be selected for studies in the next phase. As far as the response shape is concerned, model approaches or multiple-contrast tests can be used to establish the confidence intervals or predictive intervals of the response for each dose level under study. The optimal dose is more complicated because the safety aspect has to be considered.

It is important to remember that the power very much relies on the assumption of the estimated effect size at the time of study design. It is even more critical to fully understand these three different concepts about effect size: true size, estimated size, and minimum meaningful effect size, and their impacts on trial design. Last but not least, trial design involves many different aspects of medical/scientific, statistical, commercial, regulatory, operational, and data management functions. A statistician cannot view the achievement of a design with the greatest power or smallest sample size as the ultimate goal. Further, a trial design cannot be viewed as an isolated task. Instead, drug development should be viewed as an integrated process in which a sequence of decisions are made. We will discuss more on this throughout the book.

## Problems

**2.1** A clinical design team is discussing the trial design for a phase-III asthma study. Based on the results of a phase-II trial, the percent increase from baseline in FEV is 6%, 11%, and 15% for placebo, 400 mg, and 800 mg dose groups, respectively. The common standard deviation is 18%. No safety concerns have been raised based on the phase-II data. The medical research and commercial groups in the company believe that the clinically and commercially meaningful minimum treatment difference is 7% between active group and placebo because a commercial product with 7% mean FVE1 improvement over placebo is available on the market with a good safety profile.

Design this phase-III trial (type of design, number of groups and dose levels, sample size). Justify your design, determine the $p$-value if the observed is 6.9%, 7%, and 7.1%, and discuss the implications of these $p$-values to your design.

**2.2** An Oncology Trial Design. Design the following trial and recommend a sample size.

Consider a two-arm oncology trial comparing a test treatment to an active control with respect to the primary efficacy endpoint, time to disease progression (TTP). Based on data from previous studies, the median TTP is estimated to be 10 months (hazard rate = 0.0693) for the control group, and 13 months (hazard rate = 0.0533) for the test treatment group. Assume that there is a uniform enrollment with an accrual period of 10 months and that the total study duration is expected to be 24 months.

**2.3** Some Commonly Used Formulas

(1) For PK/PD and Bioequivalence studies, log-transformation is often used.

(a) Prove the following:

$$\sigma_{\ln X} = \sqrt{\ln (1 + CV_X)} \quad \text{if } \ln X \text{ is normal.}$$

(b) Prove the following relationship under a general condition with a small $CV$:

$$\ln X \simeq \ln \mu + \frac{X - \mu}{\mu} \sim N \left( \ln \mu, \ CV^2 \right).$$

(2) For a survival analysis, the power is often based on the number of events instead of the number of patients. Therefore, we can use the exponential model to predict the time when a certain number of events is reached. This is very useful for operational planning. Prove the following

relationships under the assumption of exponential distribution:

$$D = \begin{cases} R\left(T - \frac{1}{\lambda} + \frac{1}{\lambda}e^{-\lambda T}\right) & \text{if } T \leq T_0, \\ R\left[T_0 - \frac{1}{\lambda}\left(e^{\lambda T_0} - 1\right)e^{-\lambda T}\right] & \text{if } T > T_0, \end{cases}$$

and

$$T = \begin{cases} -\frac{1}{\lambda}\ln\left(\frac{\lambda D}{R} - \lambda T + 1\right) & \text{if } T \leq T_0, \\ -\frac{1}{\lambda}\ln\left[\lambda\left(T_0 - \frac{D}{R}\right)\left(e^{\lambda T_0} - 1\right)^{-1}\right] & \text{if } T > T_0, \end{cases}$$

where $T_0$ = enrollment duration, $T$ = the time of interesting from randomization, $D$ = number of deaths, $R$ = uniform enrollment rate, $\lambda$ = hazard rate.

Also prove the following under exponential distribution:

$$T_{median} = \frac{\ln 2}{\lambda} = T_{mean}\ln 2$$

and the two-sided $(1 - \alpha)\%$ confidence interval for the hazard $\lambda$:

$$\left[\frac{\hat{\lambda}}{2D}\chi^2_{2D,\ 1-\alpha/2}, \ \frac{\hat{\lambda}}{2D}\chi^2_{2D,\ \alpha/2}\right],$$

where $T_{median}$ = median time, $T_{mean}$ = mean time, $\hat{\lambda}$ = MLE of $\lambda$.

**2.4** Power and Sample Size Formulation for a Model-Based Approach to Dose-Response Trials

Test-based approaches are fine for detecting evidence against the null hypothesis in the direction of a positive trend. However, they do not provide much insight into the form of the relationship. A model-based perspective is better for this purpose. A good-fitting model describes the nature of the association, provides parameters for describing the strength of the relationship, provides predicted probabilities for the response categories at any dose, and helps us to determine the optimal dose. It also yields the hypothesis of no treatment effect if a frequentist approach is used for the modeling. However, the results from model-based approaches are heavily dependent on the accuracy of the model to the natural phenomenon.

Whitehead (1993; Chuang and Agresti, 1997) developed the sample-size formulation for an ordinal response based on the proportional odds model (logistic model) for two groups. The total sample size for a one-sided test is given by

$$N = \frac{2(r+1)^2(z_{1-\alpha} + z_{1-\beta})^2}{r(\ln R)^2(1 - \sum \bar{p}_i^3)},$$

where $r$ is sample-size ratio, $R$ is odd ratio which can be obtained from logistic regression with or without covariates, and $\bar{p}_i$ is the anticipated marginal proportion in the response category $i$.

The power is given by

$$power = \Phi \left( \sqrt{\frac{N\,r\,(\ln R)^2(1 - \sum \bar{p}_i^3)}{2(r+1)^2}} - z_{1-\alpha} \right).$$

Generalize the formulations for sample size and power for dose-response models other than logistic model.

**2.5** Reproduction

Consider a trial with two parallel arms comparing the mean difference. Assume that the known variance $\sigma^2 = 1$ and the true treatment difference is $\delta$. The estimated treatment difference is $\delta_0$. The trial was design at level $\alpha$ with $(1 - \beta)$ power and sample-size $n$. In other words, $P_{\delta=0}\,(p \leq \alpha) = \alpha$, $P_{\delta=\delta_0}\,(p \leq \alpha) = 1 - \beta$. If the observed treatment difference $\hat{\delta}$ at the end of the trial is less than, equal to, or larger than the true difference $\delta$, what is in each case the probability (reproductivity) that the next trial will show statistical significance with sample size $n$. Can we use the reproductivity of 50% when $\delta = \hat{\delta}$ to argue that $\alpha = 0.025\%$ is too unconservative? Why?

**2.6** Correlation between response difference and common variance

Equation (2.23) is valid when $\hat{\delta}$ is not related to $\hat{\sigma}$, Draw a function (or graphically via simulation) to reveal the relationship between $\hat{\delta}$ and $\hat{\sigma}$ for Normal, binary, and survival endpoint with finite sample size.

# Chapter 3

# Theory of Hypothesis-Based Adaptive Design

## 3.1 Introduction

As indicated early in Chapter 1, an adaptive design is a design that allows adaptations or modifications to some aspects of a trial after its initiation without undermining the validity and integrity of the trial. The adaptations may include, but are not limited to, sample-size reestimation, early stopping for efficacy or futility, response-adaptive randomization, and dropping inferior treatment groups. Adaptive designs usually require unblinding data and invoke a dependent sampling procedure. Therefore, theory behind adaptive design is much more complicated than that behind classical design. Validity and integrity have been strongly debated from statistical, operational, and regulatory perspectives during the past several years. However, despite different views, most scholars and practitioners believe that adaptive design could prove to be an efficient tool for drug development if used properly. The issues of validity and integrity will be discussed in depth in Chapter 28.

Many interesting methods for adaptive design have been developed. Virtually all methods can be viewed as some combination of stagewise $p$-values. The stagewise $p$-values are obtained based on the subsample from each stage; therefore, they are mutually independent and uniformly distributed over [0,1] under the null hypothesis. The first method uses the same stopping boundaries as a classical group sequential design (O'Brien and Fleming, 1979; Pocock, 1977) and allows stopping for early efficacy or futility. Lan and DeMets (1983) proposed the error spending method (ESM), in which the timing and number of analyses can be changed based on a prespecified error-spending function. ESM is derived from Brownian motion. The method has been extended to allow for sample-size reestimation (SSR) (Cui, Hung, and Wang, 1999). It can be viewed as a fixed-weight method (i.e., using fixed weights for z-scores from the first and second stages regardless of sample-size change). Lehmacher and Wassmer (1999) further degeneralized this weight method by using the inverse-normal method, in which the z-score is not necessarily taken from a normal endpoint, but from the inverse-normal function of stagewise $p$-values. Hence, the method can be used for any type of endpoint.

The second method is based on a direct combination of stagewise $p$-values. Bauer and Kohne (1994) use the Fisher combination (product) of stagewise $p$-values to derive the stopping boundaries. Chang (2006a) used the sum of the stagewise $p$-values to construct a test statistic and derived a closed form for determination of stopping boundaries and $p$-value calculations as well as conditional power for trial monitoring.

The third method is based on the conditional error function. Proschan and Hunsberger (1995) developed an adaptive design method based on the conditional error function for two-stage designs with normal test statistics. Müller and Schäfer (2001) developed the conditional error method where the conditional error function is avoided and replaced with a conditional error that is calculated on fly. Instead of a two-stage design, Müller and Schäfer's method can be applied to a K-stage design and allows for many adaptations.

The fourth method is based on recursive algorithms such as Brannath-Posch-Bauer's recursive combination tests (Brannath, Posch and Bauer, 2002), Müller-Schäfer's decision-function method (Müller and Schäfer, 2004), and Chang's (2006e) recursive two-stage adaptive design (RTAD). All four recursive methods are developed for K-stage designs allowing for general adaptations. RTAD is the simplest and most powerful method and the calculations of stopping boundary, conditional power, sample-size modification, $p$-values, and other operating characteristics can be performed manually without any difficulties.

In the next several chapters we will cover these methods in detail, but now let's introduce the general framework for an adaptive design. Under this general framework, we can easily study the different methods, perform comparisons, and look into the relationships that exist among the different methods. This chapter will focus on three major issues: type-I error control, analysis including point and confidence interval estimations, and design evaluations.

This chapter might seem a bit too theoretical or abstract to readers who are new to adaptive designs, but I hope you can read it adaptively, that is, just pay attention to the logic, ignoring the mathematical details. You should revisit this chapter from time to time after you read more in later chapters.

## 3.2  General Theory

There are four major components of adaptive designs in the frequentis paradigm: (1) type-I error rate or $\alpha$-control: determination of stopping boundaries, (2) type-II error rate $\beta$: calculation of power or sample-size, (3) trial monitoring: calculation of conditional power or futility index, and (4) analysis after the completion of a trial: calculations of adjusted $p$-values, unbiased point estimates, and confidence intervals.

### 3.2.1  *Stopping Boundary*

Consider a clinical trial with $K$ stages and at each stage a hypothesis test is performed followed by some actions that are dependent on the analysis results. Such actions can be early futility or efficacy stopping, sample-size reestimation, modification of randomization, or other adaptations. The objective of the trial (e.g., testing the efficacy of the experimental drug) can be formulated using a global hypothesis test, which is the intersection of the individual hypothesis from the interim analyses.

$$H_0 : H_{01} \cap ... \cap H_{0K}, \tag{3.1}$$

where $H_{0k}$ $(k = 1, ..., K)$ is the null hypothesis at the $k$th interim analysis. Let's denote the sample-size per group for the subsample at the $k$th stage as $n_k$. In practice, all $H_{0k}$ use usually the same as $H_0$ and our discussion will be limited to this situation for now. In the rest of the chapter, $H_{0k}$ testing will be based on subsamples from previous stages with the corresponding test statistic denoted as $T_k$ which will be a combination of $p_i (i = 1, ..., k)$, where $p_i$ is the $p$-value from the subsample obtained at the $i$th stage. A one-sided test is always used in this book unless otherwise specified.

The stopping rules are given by

$$\begin{cases} \text{Stop for efficacy} & \text{if } T_k \leq \alpha_k \,, \\ \text{Stop for futility} & \text{if } T_k > \beta_k, \\ \text{Continue with adaptations if } \alpha_k < T_k \leq \beta_k, \end{cases} \tag{3.2}$$

where $\alpha_k < \beta_k$ $(k = 1, ..., K - 1)$, and $\alpha_K = \beta_K$. For convenience, $\alpha_k$ and $\beta_k$ are called the efficacy and futility boundaries, respectively.

To reach the $k$th stage, a trial has to pass the 1th to $(k-1)$th stages. Therefore, the probability of rejecting the null hypothesis $H_0$ or simply, the rejection probability at the $k$th stage is given by $\psi_k(\alpha_k)$, where

$$\psi_k(t) = \Pr(\alpha_1 < T_1 < \beta_1, ..., \alpha_{k-1} < T_{k-1} < \beta_{k-1}, T_k < t)$$
$$= \int_{\alpha_1}^{\beta_1} \cdots \int_{\alpha_{k-1}}^{\beta_{k-1}} \int_{-\infty}^{t} f_{T_1...T_k}\, dt_k\, dt_{k-1}...dt_1, \qquad (3.3)$$

where $f_{T_1...T_k}$ is the joint pdf of $T_1, ...,$ and $T_k$.

Note that because the sequential adaptive designs control the overall alpha under a global null hypotheses (3.1), it is very important to properly form the hypotheses at each stage such that they are consistent and rejecting any of them will lead to the same clinical implication. This is particularly important when making hypothesis adaptations.

### 3.2.2    *Formula for Power and Adjusted p-value*

**Definition 3.1:** The $p$-value associated with a test is the smallest significance level $\alpha$ for which the null hypothesis is rejected (Robert, 1997, p. 196).

Let

$$p_c(t; k) = \psi_k(t|H_0). \qquad (3.4)$$

The error rate ($\alpha$ spent) at the $k$th stage is given by

$$\pi_k = \psi_k(\alpha_k|H_0). \qquad (3.5)$$

The power of rejecting $H_0$ at the $k$th stage is given by

$$\varpi_k = \psi_k(\alpha_k|H_a). \qquad (3.6)$$

When efficacy is claimed at a certain stage, the trial is stopped. Therefore, the type-I errors at different stages are mutually exclusive. Hence, the experiment-wise type-I error rate can be written as

$$\alpha = \sum_{k=1}^{K} \pi_k. \qquad (3.7)$$

Similarly, the power is given by

$$power = \sum_{k=1}^{K} \varpi_k. \qquad (3.8)$$

Equation (3.5) is the key to determining the stopping boundaries' adaptive designs as illustrated in the next several chapters. When $\Sigma_{i=1}^{k}\pi_i$ is reviewed as a function of information time or stage $k$, it is the so-called error-spending function.

It is interesting to define an adjusted $p$-value by

$$p_a(t; k) = \min\left\{1, \sum_{i=1}^{k-1}\pi_i + p_c(t; k)\right\}. \tag{3.9}$$

An important characteristic of this adjusted $p$-value is that when the test statistic $t$ is on stopping boundary $a_k$, $p_k$ must be equal to alpha spent so far.

Note that the adjusted $p$-value is a measure of overall statistical strength against $H_0$. The later the $H_0$ is rejected, the larger the adjusted $p$-value is, and the weaker the statistical evidence (against $H_0$) is. A late rejection leading to a larger $p$-value is reasonable because the alpha at earlier stages has been spent.

### 3.2.3 *Selection of Test Statistics*

Without losing generality, assume $H_{0k}$ is a null hypothesis for the efficacy of the experimental drug, which can be written as

$$H_{0k} : \eta_{k1} \geq \eta_{k2} \quad \text{vs.} \quad H_{ak} : \eta_{k1} < \eta_{k2}, \tag{3.10}$$

where $\eta_{k1}$ and $\eta_{k2}$ are the treatment responses (mean, proportion, or survival) in the two comparison groups at the $k$th stage.

It is desirable to chose $T_k$ such that $f_{T_1...T_k}$ has a simple form. Notice that when $\eta_{k1} = \eta_{k2}$, the $p$-value $p_k$ from the subsample at the $k$th stage is uniformly distributed on [0,1] under $H_0$. This desirable property can be used to construct test statistics for adaptive designs.

There are many possible combinations of the $p$-values such as (1) linear combination (Chang, 2006a):

$$T_k = \Sigma_{i=1}^{k} w_{ki} p_i, \quad k = 1, ..., K, \tag{3.11}$$

(2) product of stagewise $p$-values (Fisher combination, Bauer and Kohne, 1994):

$$T_k = \prod_{i=1}^{k} p_i, \quad k = 1, ..., K, \tag{3.12}$$

and (3) linear combination of inverse-normal stagewise $p$-values (Cui et al., 1999, Lan and DeMets, 1983, Lehmacher and Wassmer, 1999):

$$T_k = \Sigma_{i=1}^{k} w_{ki} \Phi^{-1} \left(1 - p_i\right), \ k = 1, ..., K, \tag{3.13}$$

where weight $w_{ki} > 0$ can be constant or a function (ESM) of data from previous stages, and $K$ is the number of analyses planned in the trial.

### 3.2.4  *Polymorphism*

After selecting the type of test statistic, we can determine the stopping boundaries $\alpha_k$ and $\beta_k$ by using (3.3), (3.5), and (3.7) under the global null hypothesis (3.1). Once the stopping boundaries are determined, the power and sample size under a particular $H_a$ can be numerically calculated using (3.3), (3.6), and (3.8).

The polymorphism refers to the fact that the stopping boundaries (and other operating characteristics) can be constructed in many different ways, all with type-I error control.

After selecting the test statistic, we can choose one of the following approaches to fully determine the stopping boundaries:

(1) Choose certain types of functions for $\alpha_k$ and $\beta_k$. The advantage of using a stopping boundary function is that there are only limited parameters in the function to be determined. After the parameters are determined, the stopping boundaries are then fully determined using (3.3), (3.5), and (3.7), regardless of the number of stages. The commonly used boundaries are OB-F (O'Brien and Fleming, 1979), Pocock's (1977), and Wang–Tsiatis' boundaries (Wang and Tsiatis, 1987).

(2) Choose certain forms of functions for $\pi_k$ such that $\Sigma_{k=1}^{K} \pi_k = \alpha$. Traditionally, the cumulative quantity $\pi_k^* = \Sigma_{i=1}^{k} \pi_i$ is called the error-spending function, which can be either a function of stage $k$ or the so-called information time based on sample-size fraction. After determining the function $\pi_k$ or equivalently $\pi_k^*$, the stopping boundaries $\alpha_k$ and $\beta_k$ ($k = 1, ..., K$) can be determined using (3.3), (3.5), and (3.7).

The so-called error-spending approach, which uses a predetermined error-spending function, allows for changing the number and timing of interim analyses. It is interesting to know that there is usually an equivalent stopping boundary function (at least implicitly) for any error-spending function (Lan and DeMets, 1983).

(3) Choose nonparametric stopping boundaries, i.e., no function is assumed, instead, use computer simulations to determine the stopping boundaries via a trial-and-error method. The nonparametric method does not

allow for the changes to the number and timing of the interim analyses.

(4) Using the conditional error function method, one can rewrite the stagewise error rate for a two-stage design (see Chapter 8 for general multiple-stage designs) as

$$\pi_2 = \psi_2(\alpha_2|H_0) = \int_{\alpha_1}^{\beta_1} A(p_1)\,dp_1, \qquad (3.14)$$

where $A(p_1)$ is called the conditional error function. For a given $\alpha_1$ and $\beta_1$, by carefully selecting $A(p_1)$, the overall $\alpha$ control can be met (Proschan and Hunsberger, 1995). However, finding a good $A(p_1)$ isn't always easy. Therefore, the following method was developed.

(5) The conditional error method is similar to the conditional error function method, but in this method, for a given $\alpha_1$ and $\beta_1$, $A(p_1)$ is calculated on the fly or in real-time, and only for the observed $\hat{p}_1$ under $H_0$. Adaptations can be made under the condition that keep $A(p_1|H_0)$ unchanged.

Note that $\alpha_k$ and $\beta_k$ are usually functions of only stage $k$ or information time, but they can be functions of response data from previous stages, i.e., $\alpha_k = \alpha_k(t_1, ..., t_{k-1})$ and $\beta_k = \beta_k(t_1, ..., t_{k-1})$. In fact using variable transformations of the test statistic to another test statistic, the stopping boundaries often change from response-independent to response-dependent. Bauer and Kohne (1994) actually use a response-dependent boundary for the second stage $\alpha_2/p_1$.

(6) Recursive two-stage design (Chang, 2006) is a simple and powerful approach to a general $N$-stage design. It is considered an $N$-stage adaptive design and is a composite of many overlapped two-stage designs that use the conditional error principal to derive the closed forms for the $N$-stage design (see Chapter 8 for details).

If you feel you have had enough math, you can skip to the next chapter and come back to this chapter after completing Chapter 7.

### 3.2.5  *Adjusted Point Estimates*

Estimation problems deserve a bit of philosophical discussion before we proceed to how to calculate them. We have focused our discussion within the frequentist paradigm, which is constructed fundamentally on the concept of repeated experiments. There are at least three types of unbiased point estimates, corresponding to four different sample spaces: (1) Unconditional point estimate (UE) in which the corresponding sample space consists of all possible results from a repeated experiments with a given design. Usually only the sponsor can see these results. (2) Conditional estimate (CE) is based on the positive or statistically significant results; the corresponding sample space consists of all results with statistical significance. Regulatory authorities and patients usually see only this set of results. (3) Stagewise estimate (SE) is based on trial stopping at each stage; the corresponding sample space is all possible results from repeated experiments when they stop at a given stage K.

Theoretically, the sponsor (pharmaceutical company) can see all POSSIBLE results from a trial (equivalent to all results from repeated experiments with a given design); sponsors usually submit only positive trial results to regulatory agencies, and the agencies weigh the benefit–risk ratio and select a subset of the positive results for approval for marketing. For a classical, single-stage design, what sponsors see is the unconditional estimate. What the regulatory agencies and patients see are roughly the conditional estimates.

**Conditional Estimate**

Let's take a hypothesis testing two group means as an example. Here we will discuss CE ($\delta_c$) and UE ($\delta$) for both classical and adaptive designs. For a normal response, the CE is the mean under the condition that the null hypothesis of no treatment effect is rejected. It can be derived that the relative bias of the conditional mean for a classical design with two independent groups is given by

$$\frac{\delta - \delta_c}{\delta} = \frac{1}{1 - \beta} \frac{\sigma}{\delta\sqrt{\pi n}} \exp\left(-\frac{1}{2}z_{1-\beta}^2\right), \tag{3.15}$$

where $\beta$ is the type-II error rate, $\sigma$ is the standard deviation, and $n$ is the sample size per group. It is true that what we submit to the regulatory reviewers is a conditional mean that is biased. For $\beta = 0.2$, there is about a 12% bias for a classical design (see Table 3.1). Whether a conditional or unconditional mean is submitted to regulatory authorities, the approval will be based on the conditional mean. Therefore, what patients see is the most biased mean. Statisticians are often faced with the question of whether to report the conditional or unconditional mean. Should the conditional mean be adjusted because it is reported to patients and is biased for both classical and adaptive designs?

Which mean should be used under which condition? If the conditional mean is the most important because it is what sponsors show the FDA and patients, then it should be adjusted regardless of classical or adaptive design because it is biased in both designs. Because the conditional mean (CM) is biased for both classical and adaptive designs, there is no reason to adjust it for an adaptive design but not for a classical design.

Table 3.1: Conditional and Unconditional Means

| Design | True mean difference | Unconditional mean difference | Conditional mean difference |
|---|---|---|---|
| Classical | 1 | 1 | 1.12 |
| Adaptive | 1 | 1.05 | 1.25 |

Note: Standard deviation $= 2.5$; $N_{max} = N_{fix} = 100/$group

## Unconditional Estimate

If the unconditional mean is the most important, then it should be adjusted for an adaptive design, but not for a classical design. A general method for obtaining an unbiased point estimate is described as follows:

Let $\delta_B$ be a biased estimate for an adaptive design and $\delta$ be the true value for the parameter of interest. The bias can be expressed as a function of $\delta$:

$$\xi(\delta) = \delta - \bar{\delta}_B, \qquad (3.16)$$

where $\bar{\delta}_B$ is the expectation of $\delta_B$:

$$\bar{\delta}_B = \delta - \xi(\delta). \qquad (3.17)$$

From (3.17) we obtain

$$\delta = \eta^{-1}(\bar{\delta}_B), \qquad (3.18)$$

where $\eta^{-1}(\delta)$ is the inverse function of $\eta(\delta) = \delta - \xi(\delta) = (I - \xi)(\delta)$, $I =$ identity mapping. An unbiased estimate can be given by

$$\delta_u = \delta_B + \xi(\delta) = \delta_B + \xi\left((I - \xi)^{-1}(\bar{\delta}_B)\right). \qquad (3.19)$$

The challenge is that we don't know $\delta$ and $\xi(\cdot)$. However, we can use linear approximation to $\xi(\delta)$ to solve the problem.

Assume

$$\xi(\delta) = c_0 + c_1\delta, \qquad (3.20)$$

where $c_i$ $(i = 0, 1)$ are constants. Substituting (3.20) into (3.17) and solving for $\delta$, we can obtain

$$\delta = \frac{c_0 + \bar{\delta}_B}{1 - c_1}. \qquad (3.21)$$

Because $c_i(i = 0, 1)$ is a constant, we can immediately obtain an unbiased estimator from (3.21):

$$\delta_u = \frac{c_0 + \delta_B}{1 - c_1}. \qquad (3.22)$$

The monotonic relationship $\xi(\delta) = c_0 + c_1\delta$ usually holds at least in a small range of $\delta \in (\delta - \varepsilon, \delta + \varepsilon)$.

By trying several (at least 2) $\delta = \delta_m$ around $\delta_B$ and using simulation to calculate the bias $\xi(\delta_m) = \delta_m - \bar{\bar{\delta}}_{B_m}$ for each $\delta_m$, we get

$$\xi(\delta_m) = c_0 + c_1\delta_m. \tag{3.23}$$

We can solve for $m = 2$ or estimate $c_0$ and $c_1$ from (3.23).

The reasons to choose the values of $\delta_m$ near the best guessed value of $\delta_B$ are obvious. If $\delta_B$ is near $\delta$, then (3.23) works well; if $\delta_B$ is far away from the true $\delta$, adjusting is not important anyway. If we name (3.23) the first-order bias adjustment, then the zero-order bias adjustment is a degeneralized case when letting $c_1 = 0$ in (3.23).

**Stagewise Estimates**

The research papers on adjusted stagewise estimates are Lawrence and Hung (2003), Wassmer (2005), Posch et al. (2006), Brannath, Koenig, and Bauer (2006), among others. The sample space for the stagewise estimate at the $k$th stage consists of all possible outcomes when the trial is stopped at the $k$th stage.

Consider the following estimate:

$$\delta_{sw} = \sum_{i=1}^{k} w_{ki}\delta_i, \text{ if trial stops at the } k\text{th stage}, \tag{3.24}$$

where $\delta_i$ is the stagewise unbiased estimate of treatment difference $\delta$ based on the subsample from the $i$th stage; $k$ is the stage where the trial stops; and $w_{ki}$ is a constant weight that usually, but not necessarily, satisfies $\Sigma_{i=1}^{k} w_{ki} = 1$.

If the trial design does not allow for early stopping, e.g., an interim analysis (IA) for sample-size adjustment only, then (3.24) is an unbiased estimator of $\delta$. This is because

$$E(\delta_{sw}) = \sum_{i=1}^{k} w_{ki}E(\delta_i) = \sum_{i=1}^{k} w_{ki}\delta = \delta \sum_{i=1}^{k} w_{ki} = \delta. \tag{3.25}$$

However, most adaptive clinical trials do allow for early stopping and $\delta_{sw}$ from (3.24) is biased in general. A simple solution to get unconditionally unbiased estimates is to add a few subjects (at least two) even if the trial has been stopped early. These few subjects will not be used for $p$-value calculation, but only to get an unbiased estimation.

### 3.2.6 *Derivation of Confidence Intervals*

Consider the null hypothesis:

$$H : \delta = \delta_0. \tag{3.26}$$

For $\delta_0 = 0$, we use the test statistic $T$. In general, we use the test statistic

$$\tilde{T} = T - T_0(\delta_0), \tag{3.27}$$

where the function $T_0(\delta_0)$ is the expectation of $T$ under $H$ and $T_0(0) = 0$.

A $100(1-\alpha)\%$ confidence interval consists of all the $\delta_0$ such that the null hypothesis (3.26) would not be rejected, given the observed value $\hat{T}$ of the test statistic $\tilde{T}$. Therefore, the upper and lower bounds of this confidence interval are found by equating $\tilde{T} = \alpha_k$ at the $k$th stage (Assume that $\tilde{T}$ under $\delta = \delta_0$ and $T$ under $\delta = 0$ have the same distribution; therefore, the same stopping boundary $\alpha_k$ can be used.). This leads to

$$T - T_0(\delta_0) = \pm\alpha_k. \tag{3.28}$$

Equation (3.28) can be solved for $\delta_0$ to obtain the confidence limits:

$$\delta_0 = T_0^{-1}\left(\hat{T} \mp \alpha_k\right). \tag{3.29}$$

If the adjusted $p$-value is used, then (3.29) is also numerically equal to the $(1 - \Sigma_{i=1}^k \pi_i)\%$ confidence limits if the trial is stopped at the $k$th stage.

For an adaptive design, if the test statistic at the $k$th stage is given by

$$T = \sum_{i=1}^k w_{ki}\frac{\delta_i}{\sigma}\sqrt{\frac{n_i}{2}}, \tag{3.30}$$

where $\Sigma_{i=1}^K w_{ki}^2 = 1$, then we have

$$T_o(\delta_0) = \sum_{i=1}^k w_{ki}\frac{\delta_0}{\sigma}\sqrt{\frac{n_i}{2}}. \tag{3.31}$$

For symmetrical stopping boundaries (i.e., two-sided $\alpha$, one efficacy boundary and one futility boundary that are symmetrical), the lower and upper limits of a $(1 - \Sigma_{i=1}^k \pi_i)\%$ confidence interval at the $k$th stage are given by

$$\delta_0 = \frac{\sum_{i=1}^k w_{ki}\frac{\delta_i}{\sigma}\sqrt{\frac{n_i}{2}} \mp \alpha_k}{\sum_{i=1}^k w_{ki}\frac{1}{\sigma}\sqrt{\frac{n_i}{2}}}. \tag{3.32}$$

Also, because of symmetry, the point estimate is given by

$$\delta_0 = \frac{\sum_{i=1}^{k} w_{ki} \delta_i \sqrt{\frac{n_i}{2}}}{\sum_{i=1}^{k} w_{ki} \sqrt{\frac{n_i}{2}}}. \tag{3.33}$$

For a one-sided confidence limit, one of the limits is set at infinity, and (3.32) and (3.33) hold approximately. Note that in calculation, we can replace $\sigma$ by $\hat{\sigma}$. (3.32) can be viewed as the $(1 - \alpha)\%$ repeated confidence interval (RCI).

## 3.3    Design Evaluation—Operating Characteristics

### 3.3.1    *Stopping Probabilities*

The stopping probability at each stage is an important property of an adaptive design, because it provides the time-to-market and the associated probability of success. It also provides information on the cost (sample size) of the trial and the associated probability. In fact, the stopping probabilities are used to calculate the expected samples that present the average cost or efficiency of the trial design and the duration of the trial.

There are two types of stopping probabilities: unconditional probability of stopping to claim efficacy (reject $H_0$) and unconditional probability of futility (accept $H_0$). The former refers to the efficacy stopping probability (ESP), and the latter refers to the futility stopping probability (FSP). From (3.3), it is obvious that the ESP at the $k$th stage is given by

$$ESP_k = \psi_k(\alpha_k) \tag{3.34}$$

and the FSP at the $k$th stage is given by

$$FSP_k = \psi_{k-1}(\beta_{k-1}) - \psi_{k-1}(\alpha_{k-1}) - \psi_k(\beta_k). \tag{3.35}$$

### 3.3.2    *Expected Duration of an Adaptive Trial*

The stopping probabilities can be used to calculate the expected trial duration, which is definitely an important feature of an adaptive design. The conditionally (on the efficacy claim) expected trial duration is given by

$$\bar{t}_e = \sum_{k=1}^{K} ESP_k \, t_k, \tag{3.36}$$

where $t_k$ is the time from the first-patient-in to the $k$th interim analysis.

The conditionally (on the futility claim) expected trial duration is given by

$$\bar{t}_f = \sum_{k=1}^{K} FSP_k \, t_k. \tag{3.37}$$

The unconditionally expected trial duration is given by

$$\bar{t} = \sum_{k=1}^{K} \left( ESP_k + FSP_k \right) t_k. \tag{3.38}$$

### 3.3.3 *Expected Sample Sizes*

The expected sample size is a commonly used measure of the efficiency (cost and timing of the trial) of the design. The expected sample size is a function of the treatment difference and its variability, which are unknowns. Therefore, expected sample size is really based on hypothetical values of the parameters. For this reason, it is beneficial and important to calculate the expected sample size under various critical or possible values of the parameters. The total expected sample size per group can be expressed as

$$N_{\text{exp}} = \sum_{k=1}^{K} N_k \left( ESP_k + FSP_k \right). \tag{3.39}$$

It can also be written as

$$N_{\text{exp}} = \sum_{k=1}^{K} N_k \left( \psi_k(\alpha_k) + \psi_{k-1}(\beta_{k-1}) - \psi_k(\beta_k) - \psi_{k-1}(\alpha_{k-1}) \right), \tag{3.40}$$

where $N_k = \sum_{i=1}^{k} n_i$ is the cumulative sample size per group.

### 3.3.4 *Conditional Power and Futility Index*

The conditional power is the conditional probability of rejecting the null hypothesis during the rest of the trial based on the observed interim data. The conditional power is commonly used for monitoring an ongoing trial. Similar to the ESP and FSP, conditional power is dependent on the population parameters or treatment effect and its variability. The conditional power at the $k$th stage is the sum of the probability of rejecting the null hypothesis at stage $k + 1$ to $K$ ($K$ does not have to be predetermined), given the observed data from stages 1 through $k$.

$$cP_k = \sum_{j=k+1}^{K} \Pr\left(\cap_{i=k+1}^{j-1}(a_i < T_i < \beta_i) \cap T_j \leq \alpha_j \mid \cap_{i=1}^{k} T_i = t_i\right), \quad (3.41)$$

where $t_i$ is the observed test statistic $T_i$ at the $i$th stage. For a two-stage design, the conditional power can be expressed as

$$cP_1 = \Pr\left(T_2 \leq \alpha_2 | t_1\right). \quad (3.42)$$

The futility index is defined as the conditional probability of accepting the null hypothesis:

$$FI_k = 1 - cP_k. \quad (3.43)$$

### 3.3.5 *Utility and Decision Theory*

It is important to realize that the choice of a design should not be based on power only. In fact power may not be a good criterion for evaluating a design, especially when it comes to adaptive designs. In many situations, time is more important than power. Also, a design with high power to detect a small and clinically irrelevant difference is not desirable.

Decision theory is a body of knowledge that assists a decision maker in choosing among a set of alternatives in light of their possible consequences. Decision theory is based on the concept of utility or, equivalently, the loss function. The decision maker's preferences for the mutually exclusive consequences of an alternative are described by a utility function that permits calculation of the expected utility for each alternative using Bayesian theory. The alternative with the highest expected utility is considered the most preferable. The Bayesian decision theory is illustrated in Figure 3.1.

For an adaptive trial with sample-size reestimation, the Bayesian decision theory can be briefly stated as follows:

Define the utility $U(\hat{\delta}, n)$ and the prior distribution $\pi(\delta)$. Denote the posterior by $\pi(\delta|\hat{\delta}_1)$ and the interim observed treatment difference by $\hat{\delta}_1$.

The expected utility at the design stage is given by

$$EU(n) = \int \int U\left(\hat{\delta}, n\right) \pi\left(\delta\right) \Pr\left(\hat{\delta}|\delta\right) d\delta \, d\hat{\delta}$$

The expected utility at the interim analysis is given by

$$EU(n) = \int \int U\left(\hat{\delta}, n\right) \pi\left(\delta|\hat{\delta}_1\right) \Pr\left(\hat{\delta}|\delta\right) d\delta \, d\hat{\delta}$$

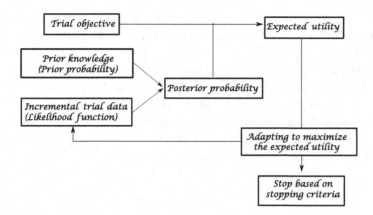

Figure 3.1: Bayesian Decision Approach

The Bayesian decision approach is to determine an action (i.e., sample size $n$) that maximizes the expected utility under certain constraints:

$$\frac{\partial EU\left(n\right)}{\partial n} = 0.$$

Decision theory can be viewed as one-person game theory, involving a game with a single player against nature. This refers to a situation where the result of a decision depends on the action of another player (nature). For example, if the decision to make is to carry an umbrella or not, the result (get wet or not) depends on what action nature takes. An important feature of this model is that the returns affect only the decision maker, not nature. However, in game theory, both players have an interest in the outcome. Note that we can treat our problems using utility theory because a decision maker's action does not materially affect nature. In the modern drug development age, pharmaceutical companies face many competitors. Therefore, strictly speaking, game theory is more applicable than utility theory in this competing–cooperative environment. Fortunately, utility theory can take the competition into consideration by constructing a utility that includes the result of the competitor's action (if it is relatively static), although this approach is not as good as game theory. We will discuss later in detail how to generate optimal designs using Bayesian decision theory in Chapter 21.

## 3.4 Summary

In this chapter, we have provided a uniform formulation for adaptive designs and the polymorphism, i.e., how the uniform formulation can be used to develop various adaptive design methods. In the next several chapters, we will illustrate this in detail, derive different methods, and apply them to different trials. We have also discussed the estimation issues and the general methods. In Chapter 8, we will discuss estimation again in great detail with trial examples. Evaluation of trial designs is obviously important. We have reviewed many operating characteristics of adaptive designs. Keep in mind that we should not misunderstand power to be the sole criterion when judging a trial design. Instead, think of drug development as an integrated process—decision or game theory is the ultimate tool for trial evaluation.

## Problems

**3.1** Based on Equation (3.2), explicitly write out the stopping rules at each stage for a two-stage adaptive trial and a three-stage adaptive trial.

**3.2** Suppose we define: $T_1 = p_1$ and $T_2 = p_1 p_2$.

Assume the stagewise $p$-value $p_i$ uniformly distributed in $[0,1]$ and no futility stopping boundary used.

Derive formulations for

(1)    the efficacy stopping probabilities ($ESP_k$) under $H_0$,

(2)    the expected sample size under $H_0$.

**3.3** Prove that the bias of conditional estimate (conditional on $p$-value$\leq \alpha$) can be expressed by Equation (3.15) for a classical two-group design.

# Chapter 4

# Method with Direct Combination of $p$-values

In this chapter, we will use the theory developed in the previous chapter with several different test statistics based on direct combination of stagewise $p$-values, which include (1) method based on individual $p$-values (MIP), (2) method based on the sum of $p$-values (MSP), and (3) method based on the product of $p$-values (MPP). We will focus on two-stage designs and derive the closed forms for determination of stopping boundaries and adjusted $p$-values. Many different examples are presented, in which power and sample-size calculations are based on computer simulations. The methods are very general, meaning that they can be applied to broad adaptations. However, the examples provided will focus on classical group sequential designs and sample-size reestimation (SSR).

## 4.1 Method Based on Individual $p$-values

This method refers to MIP, in which the test statistic is defined as

$$T_k = p_k, \tag{4.1}$$

where $p_k$ is the stagewise $p$-value from the $k$th stage subsample.

Using Equations (3.3), (3.5), and (3.7), a level-$\alpha$ test requires

$$\alpha = \sum_{k=1}^{K} \alpha_k \prod_{i=1}^{k-1} (\beta_i - \alpha_i). \tag{4.2}$$

When the upper bound exceeds the lower bound in (4.2), define $\prod_{i=1}^{0}(\cdot) = 1$.

Using (4.2), the stopping boundary $(\alpha_i, \beta_i)$ can be determined. For a two-stage design, (4.2) becomes

$$\alpha = \alpha_1 + \alpha_2(\beta_1 - \alpha_1). \tag{4.3}$$

For convenience, examples of stopping boundaries from (4.2) are tabulated for a one-sided $\alpha = 0.025$ (Table 4.1).

Table 4.1:    Stopping Boundaries $\alpha_2$ with MIP

| | $\alpha_1$ | 0.000 | 0.0025 | 0.005 | 0.010 | 0.015 | 0.020 |
|---|---|---|---|---|---|---|---|
| $\beta_1$ | | | | | | | |
| 0.15 | | 0.1667 | 0.1525 | 0.1379 | 0.1071 | 0.0741 | 0.0385 |
| 0.20 | | 0.1250 | 0.1139 | 0.1026 | 0.0789 | 0.0541 | 0.0278 |
| 0.25 | | 0.1000 | 0.0909 | 0.0816 | 0.0625 | 0.0426 | 0.0217 |
| 0.30 | $\alpha_2$ | 0.0833 | 0.0756 | 0.0678 | 0.0517 | 0.0351 | 0.0179 |
| 0.35 | | 0.0714 | 0.0647 | 0.0580 | 0.0441 | 0.0299 | 0.0152 |
| 0.50 | | 0.0500 | 0.0452 | 0.0404 | 0.0306 | 0.0206 | 0.0104 |
| 1.00 | | 0.0250 | 0.0226 | 0.0201 | 0.0152 | 0.0102 | 0.0051 |

Note: One-sided $\alpha = 0.025$.

The $p$-value defined by Equation (3.9) is given by

$$p(t; k) = \begin{cases} t, & k = 1, \\ \alpha_1 + t(\beta_1 - \alpha_1) & k = 2 \end{cases}. \tag{4.4}$$

MIP is useful in the sense that it is very simple and can serve as the "baseline" for comparing different methods. MIP does not use combined data from different stages, while most other adaptive designs do.

SAS Macro 4.1 below has been implemented for simulating two-arm adaptive trials with a binary endpoint and allowing for sample-size reestimation. The test statistic can be based on individual stagewise $p$-values, or the sum or product of the stagewise $p$-values (details provided later in this chapter). The SAS variables are defined as follows: **Px** and **Py** are true proportions of response in the groups x and y, respectively; **DuHa** = the estimate for the true treatment difference under the alternative $H_a$; **N** = sample-size per group; **alpha1** = early efficacy stopping boundary (one-sided); **beta1** = early futility stopping boundary (one-sided); and **alpha2** = final efficacy stopping boundary (one-sided). The null hypothesis test is $H_0$: $\delta+$**NId** $< 0$, where $\delta =$ **Py** $-$ **Px** is the treatment difference and **NId** = noninferiority margin (NId $\leq 0$ for superiority and NId $> 0$ for noninferiority test). **nSims** = the number of simulation runs, **alpha** = one-sided overall type-I error rate, and **beta** = type-II error rate. **nAdj** = "N" for the case without sample-size reestimation and **nAdj** = "Y" for the case with sample size adjustment, **Nmax** = maximum sample size allowed, **N0** = the initial sample size at the final analysis, **nInterim** = sample size for the interim analysis, **a** = the parameter in (4.17) for the sample size adjustment, **FSP** = futility stopping probability, **ESP** = efficacy stopping probability, **AveN** = average sample size, **Power** = power of the hypothesis testing, **nClassic** = sample size for the corresponding classical design, and **Model** = "ind," "sum," or "prd" for the methods, MIP, MSP, and MPP, respectively.

\>\>**SAS Macro 4.1: Two-Stage Adaptive Design with Binary Endpoint**\>\>

```
%Macro DCSPbinary(nSims=1000000, Model="ind," alpha=0.025, beta=0.2,
NId=0, Px=0.2, Py=0.4, DuHa=0.2, nAdj="N," Nmax=100, N0=100,
nInterim=50, a=2, alpha1=0.01, beta1=0.15, alpha2=0.1071);
Data DCSPbinary; Keep Model FSP ESP AveN Power nClassic;
seedx=2534; seedy=6762; Model=&model; NId=&NId;
Nmax=&Nmax; N1=&nInterim; Px=&Px; Py=&Py;
eSize=abs((&DuHa+NId)/((Px*(1-Px)+Py*(1-Py))/2)**0.5);
nClassic=Round(2*((probit(1-&alpha)+probit(1-&beta))/eSize)**2);
FSP=0; ESP=0; AveN=0; Power=0;
Do isim=1 To &nSims;
nFinal=N1;
Px1=Ranbin(seedx,N1,px)/N1;
Py1=Ranbin(seedy,N1,py)/N1;
sigma=((Px1*(1-Px1)+Py1*(1-Py1))/2)**0.5;
T1 = (Py1-Px1+NId)*Sqrt(N1/2)/sigma;
p1=1-ProbNorm(T1);
If p1>&beta1 Then FSP=FSP+1/&nSims;
If p1<=&alpha1 Then Do;
Power=Power+1/&nSims; ESP=ESP+1/&nSims;
End;
If p1>&alpha1 and p1<=&beta1 Then Do;
eRatio=abs(&DuHa/(abs(Py1-Px1)+0.0000001));
nFinal=Min(&Nmax,Max(&N0,eRatio**&a*&N0));
If &nAdj="N" then nFinal=&Nmax;
If nFinal>N1 Then Do;
N2=nFinal-N1;
Px2=Ranbin(seedx,N2,px)/N2;
Py2=Ranbin(seedy,N2,py)/N2;
sigma=((Px2*(1-Px2)+Py2*(1-Py2))/2)**0.5;
```

```
T2 = (Py2-Px2+NId)*Sqrt(N2/2)/sigma;
p2=1-ProbNorm(T2);
If Model="ind" Then TS2=p2;
If Model="sum" Then TS2=p1+p2;
If Model="prd" Then TS2=p1*p2;
If .<TS2<=&alpha2 then Power=Power+1/&nSims;
End;
End;
AveN=AveN+nFinal/&nSims;
End;
Output;
Run;
Proc Print Data=DCSPbinary; Run;
%Mend DCSPbinary;
```
<<**SAS**<<

## Example 4.1    Adaptive Design for Acute Ischemic Stroke Trial

A phase-III trial is to be designed for patients with acute ischemic stroke of recent onset. The composite endpoint (death and MI) is the primary endpoint, and the event rate is 14% for the control group and 12% for the test group. Based on a large sample assumption, the sample size for a classical design is 5937 per group, which has 90% power to detect the difference at the one-sided alpha = 0.025. Using MIP, an interim analysis is planed based on a response assessment of 50% of the patients. We use SAS macro 4.1 to design the trial as follows:

(1) Choose stopping boundaries at the first stage: $\alpha_1 = 0.01$, $\beta_1 = 0.25$; then from Table 4.1, obtain $\alpha_2 = 0.0625$.

(2) Check the stopping boundary to make sure that the familywise error is controlled. We run simulations under the null hypothesis (14% event rate for both groups) using the following SAS code:

>>**SAS**>>
```
%DCSPbinary(Model="ind", alpha=0.025, beta=0.1, Px=0.14, Py=0.14,
DuHa=0.02, nAdj="N", Nmax=7000, nInterim=3500, alpha1=0.01, beta1=0.25,
alpha2=0.0625);
```
<<**SAS**<<

The simulated familywise error rate is $\alpha = 0.0252$; therefore, the stopping boundaries are confirmed.

(3) Calculate power or sample size under the alternative hypothesis (14% and 12% event rates for the control and the test groups, respectively) using the following SAS code:

```
>>SAS>>
%DCSPbinary(Model="ind", alpha=0.025, beta=0.1, Px=0.12, Py=0.14,
DuHa=0.02, nAdj="N", Nmax=7000, nInterim=3500, alpha1=0.01, beta1=0.25,
alpha2=0.0625);
<<SAS<<
```

(4) Perform sensitivity analyses (under condition $H_s$). Because the treatment difference is unknown, it is desirable to perform simulations under different assumptions about treatment difference, e.g., treatment difference = 0.015 (14% versus 12.5%). For the sensitivity analysis, we simply use the following SAS macro call:

```
>>SAS>>
%DCSPbinary(Model="ind", alpha=0.025, beta=0.1, Px=0.125, Py=0.14,
DuHa=0.015, nAdj="N", Nmax=7000, nInterim=3500, alpha1=0.01,
beta1=0.25, alpha2=0.0625);
<<SAS<<
```

We now can summarize the simulation outputs of the three scenarios in Table 4.2.

Table 4.2: Operating Characteristics of a GSD with MIP

| Simulation condition | FSP | ESP | N | $N_{max}$ | Power (alpha) |
|---|---|---|---|---|---|
| $H_o$ | 0.750 | 0.010 | 4341 | 7000 | (0.025) |
| $H_a$ | 0.035 | 0.564 | 4905 | 7000 | 0.897 |
| $H_s$ | 0.121 | 0.317 | 5468 | 7000 | 0.668 |

From Table 4.2, we can see that the design has a smaller expected sample size ($\bar{N}$) under $H_0$ and $H_a$ (4341, 4905) than the classical design (5937). However, the group sequential design has a larger maximum sample-size (7000) than the classical design (5937). The early futility stopping probability (FSP) and early efficacy stopping probability (ESP) are also shown in Table 4.2. The sensitivity analysis shows a large power loss when treatment difference is lower than expected, i.e., the group sequential design does not protect the power when the initial effect size is overestimated. To protect power, we can use the sample-size reestimation method, which will be discussed later in this chapter.

Note that the MIP design is different from the sequence of two sepa-

rate trials because MIP can use the early futility boundary in constructing a later stopping boundary. We will discuss this issue in great detail
later.

Now let's calculate adjusted $p$-values. Assume that the trial is finished,
with the stagewise $p$-value $p_1 = 0.012$ (which is larger than $\alpha_1 = 0.01$ and
not significant; therefore the trial continues to the second stage) and $p_2$
$= 0.055 < \alpha_2 = 0.0625$. Therefore, the null hypothesis is rejected, and the
test drug is significantly better than the control.

The $p$-value can be calculated from (4.4) using $t = p_2$ :

$$p = \alpha_1 + p_2(\beta_1 - \alpha_1) = 0.01 + 0.055(0.25 - 0.01) = 0.0232.$$

## 4.2  Method Based on the Sum of $p$-values

Chang (2006a) proposed an adaptive design method, in which the test
statistic is defined as the sum of the stagewise $p$-values. This method is
referred to as MSP. At the $k$th stage, the test statistic is defined as

$$T_k = \Sigma_{i=1}^k p_i, \ k = 1, ..., K. \tag{4.5}$$

The key to derive the stopping boundary is to calculate the probability
function $\psi_k(t)$ defined in (3.3) under the null hypothesis and the decision
rules defined in (3.2)

For a two stage design, the stopping rules are

$$\text{At Stage 1,} \begin{cases} \text{Reject } H_0 & \text{if } T_1 \leq \alpha_1, \\ \text{Accept } H_0 & \text{if } T_1 > \beta_1, \\ \text{Continue with adaptations if } \alpha_1 < T_1 \leq \beta_1, \end{cases} \tag{4.6}$$

where $0 < \alpha_1 < \beta_1 \leq 1$.

$$\text{At Stage 2,} \begin{cases} \text{Reject } H_0 \text{ if } T_2 \leq \alpha_2 \\ \text{Accept } H_0 \text{ if } T_2 > \alpha_2 \end{cases}. \tag{4.7}$$

Noticing that $p_i$ is often uniformly distributed in $[0,1]$ under the null hy-
potheis, for the first stage we have

$$\psi_1(t|H_0) = \int_0^t dt_1 = t. \tag{4.8}$$

For the second stage, we have

$$\psi_2(t|H_0) = \int_{\alpha_1}^{\beta_1} \int_0^t f_{T_1 T_2} \, dt_2 dt_1. \tag{4.9}$$

Noticing that $p_1$ and $p_2$ are indepedent, we have $f_{T_1 T_2} = f(T_2|T_1) f(T_1) = f(p_1 + p_2|p_1) f(p_1) = 1$. We will prove that

$$\psi_2(t|H_0) = \begin{cases} \frac{1}{2}(t - \alpha_1)^2, & \text{when } \alpha_1 < t \le \beta_1 \\ (\beta_1 - \alpha_1)t - \frac{1}{2}(\beta_1^2 - \alpha_1^2), & \text{when } \beta_1 < t \le \alpha_1 + 1 \\ t - \alpha_1 + t\beta_1 - \frac{1}{2}t^2 - \frac{1}{2}\beta_1^2 - \frac{1}{2}, & \text{when } \alpha_1 + 1 < t \le 2 \\ 0, & \text{otherwise} \end{cases} \tag{4.10}$$

**Proof.**

$$\psi_2(t|H_0) = \int_{\alpha_1}^{\min(\beta_1,t)} \int_{t_1}^{\min(t_1+1,t)} dt_2 dt_1.$$

(1) When $\alpha_1 < t \le \beta_1$, we have

$$\psi_2(t|H_0) = \int_{\alpha_1}^{t} \int_{t_1}^{t} dt_2 dt_1 = \frac{1}{2}(t - \alpha_1)^2;$$

(2) when $\beta_1 < t \le \alpha_1 + 1$, we have

$$\psi_2(t|H_0) = \int_{\alpha_1}^{\beta_1} \int_{t_1}^{t} dt_2 dt_1 = (\beta_1 - \alpha_1)t - \frac{1}{2}(\beta_1^2 - \alpha_1^2).$$

(3) When $\alpha_1 + 1 < t \le 2$, we have

$$\psi_2(t|H_0) = \int_{\alpha_1}^{\beta_1} (\min(t_1 + 1, t) - t_1) dt_1 = \int_{\alpha_1}^{t-1} dt_1 + \int_{t-1}^{\beta_1} (t - t_1) dt_1$$

$$= \int_{\alpha_1}^{t-1} dt_1 + \int_{t-1}^{\beta_1} (t - t_1) dt_1 = t - \alpha_1 + t\beta_1 - \frac{1}{2}t^2 - \frac{1}{2}\beta_1^2 - \frac{1}{2}.$$

$\square$

To calculate the stopping boundaries in (4.6) and (4.7), we let $\pi_1$ and $\pi_2$ be the $\alpha$ spent at stage 1 and stage 2 $(\pi_1 + \pi_2 = \alpha)$, that is,

$$\pi_1 = \psi_1(\alpha_1|H_0) \tag{4.11}$$

and

$$\pi_2 = \psi_2(\alpha_2|H_0), \tag{4.12}$$

respectively.

For simplicity, we let $\beta_1 = \alpha_2$ for the moment. Given that, from (4.10)–(4.12) we obtain

$$\begin{cases} \alpha_1 = \pi_1 \\ \pi_2 = \frac{1}{2}(\alpha_2 - \alpha_1)^2. \end{cases}$$

Solving for $\alpha_2$, we obtain

$$\alpha_2 = \sqrt{2\pi_2} + \alpha_1.$$

Since $\pi_2 = \alpha - \pi_1$, the previous equation can be written as

$$\alpha_2 = \sqrt{2(\alpha - \pi_1)} + \pi_1. \tag{4.13}$$

We give some numerical examples in Table 4.3.

Table 4.3:  Stopping Boundaries with MSP

| $\alpha_1$ | 0.0000 | 0.00250 | 0.0050 | 0.0100 | 0.0150 | 0.0200 |
|---|---|---|---|---|---|---|
| $\alpha_2$ | 0.22361 | 0.21463 | 0.20500 | 0.18321 | 0.15642 | 0.12000 |

Note: One-sided $\alpha = 0.025$ and $\beta_1 = \alpha_2$.

In general, after choosing $\alpha_1$ (or $\pi_1$) and $\beta_1$ for the first stage, the stopping boundary $\alpha_2$ can be easily determined by the following formulation:

$$\alpha = \alpha_1 + \psi_2(\alpha_2|H_0), \tag{4.14}$$

where

$$\psi_2(\alpha_2|H_0) = \begin{cases} \frac{1}{2}(\alpha_2 - \alpha_1)^2, & \text{when } \alpha_2 \leq \beta_1 \\ (\beta_1 - \alpha_1)\alpha_2 - \frac{1}{2}(\beta_1^2 - \alpha_1^2), & \text{when } \alpha_2 > \beta_1 \end{cases}$$

See Table 4.4 for examples of the stopping boundaries based on (4.14).

It is interesting to know that when $p_1 > \alpha_2$, there is no point in continuing the trial because $p_1 + p_2 > p_1 > \alpha_2$, and futility should be claimed. Therefore, statistically it is always good idea to choose $\beta_1 < \alpha_2$. However, because the non-binding futility rule is adopted currently by the regulatory bodies, it is better to use the stopping boundaries with $\beta_1 = \alpha_2$.

Table 4.4:  Stopping Boundaries $\alpha_2$ with MSP

| | $\alpha_1$ | 0.000 | 0.0025 | 0.005 | 0.010 | 0.015 | 0.020 |
|---|---|---|---|---|---|---|---|
| $\beta_1$ | | | | | | | |
| 0.05 | | 0.5250 | 0.4999 | 0.4719 | 0.4050 | 0.3182 | 0.2017 |
| 0.10 | | 0.3000 | 0.2820 | 0.2630 | 0.2217 | 0.1751 | 0.1225 |
| 0.15 | $\alpha_2$ | 0.2417 | 0.2288 | 0.2154 | 0.1871 | 0.1566 | 0.1200 |
| 0.20 | | 0.2250 | 0.2152 | 0.2051 | 0.1832 | 0.1564 | 0.1200 |
| >0.25 | | 0.2236 | 0.2146 | 0.2050 | 0.1832 | 0.1564 | 0.1200 |

Note: One-sided $\alpha = 0.025$.

Giving the stopping boundary $\alpha_1$ and $\beta_1$, $p_a(k)$ the adjusted $p$-value as indicated by (3.9) in Chapter 3. For two-stage design, $\psi_k(t|H_0)$ is explicitely given by (4.10).

SAS Macro 4.2 below is implemented for simulating two-arm adaptive designs with a normal endpoint. The adaptive method can be based on individual stagewise $p$-values, or the sum or product of the stagewise $p$-values (see details later in this chapter). The SAS variables are defined as follows: **ux** and **uy** are true treatment means in the x and y groups, respectively. **DuHa** = the estimate for the true treatment difference under the alternative $H_a$. **alpha1** = early efficacy stopping boundary (one-sided), **beta1** = early futility stopping boundary (one-sided), and **alpha2** = final efficacy stopping boundary (one-sided). The null hypothesis test is $H_0$: $\delta + \mathbf{NId} < 0$, where $\delta = \mathbf{uy} - \mathbf{ux}$ is the treatment difference, and **NId** = noninferiority margin. **nSims** = the number of simulation runs, **alpha** = one-sided overall type-I error rate, and **beta** = type-II error rate. **nAdj** = "N" for the case without sample-size reestimation and **nAdj** = "Y" for the case with sample-size adjustment, **Nmax** = maximum sample size allowed, **N0** = the initial sample size at the final analysis, **nInterim** = sample size for the interim analysis, **a** = the parameter in (4.22) for the sample-size adjustment, **FSP** = futility stopping probability, **ESP** = efficacy stopping probability, **AveN** = average sample-size, **Power** = power of the hypothesis testing, **nClassic** = sample-size for the corresponding classical design, and **Model** = "ind," "sum," or "prd" for the methods MIP, MSP, and MPP, respectively.

## >>SAS Macro 4.2: Two-Stage Adaptive Design with Normal Endpoint>>

```
%Macro DCSPnormal(nSims=1000000, Model="sum", alpha=0.025, beta=0.2,
sigma=2, NId=0, ux=0, uy=1,
nInterim=50, Nmax=100, N0=100, DuHa=1, nAdj="Y", a=2, alpha1=0.01,
beta1=0.15, alpha2=0.1871);
Data DCSPnormal; Keep Model FSP ESP AveN Power nClassic;
seedx=1736; seedy=6214; alpha=&alpha; NId=&NId; Nmax=&Nmax;
ux=&ux; uy=&uy; sigma=&sigma; model=&Model; N1=&nInterim;
eSize=abs(&DuHa+NId)/sigma;
nClassic=round(2*((probit(1-alpha)+probit(1-&beta))/eSize)**2);
FSP=0; ESP=0; AveN=0; Power=0;
Do isim=1 To &nSims;
nFinal=N1;
ux1 = Rannor(seedx)*sigma/Sqrt(N1)+ux;
uy1 = Rannor(seedy)*sigma/Sqrt(N1)+uy;
T1 = (uy1-ux1+NId)*Sqrt(N1)/2**0.5/sigma;
p1=1-ProbNorm(T1);
```

If p1>&beta1 then FSP=FSP+1/&nSims;
If p1<=&alpha1 then do;
Power=Power+1/&nSims; ESP=ESP+1/&nSims;
End;
If p1>&alpha1 and p1<=&beta1 Then Do;
eRatio = abs(&DuHa/(abs(uy1-ux1)+0.0000001));
nFinal = min(&Nmax,max(&N0,eRatio**&a*&N0));
If &DuHa*(uy1-ux1+NId) < 0 Then nFinal = N1;
If &nAdj = "N" then nFinal = &Nmax;
If nFinal > N1 Then Do;
ux2 = Rannor(seedx)*sigma/Sqrt(nFinal-N1)+ux ;
uy2 = Rannor(seedy)*sigma/Sqrt(nFinal-N1)+uy;
T2 = (uy2-ux2+NId)*Sqrt(nFinal-N1)/2**0.5/sigma;
p2=1-ProbNorm(T2);
If Model="ind" Then TS2=p2;
If Model="sum" Then TS2=p1+p2;
If Model="prd" Then TS2=p1*p2;
If .<TS2<=&alpha2 Then Power=Power+1/&nSims;
End;
End;
AveN=AveN+nFinal/&nSims;
End;
Output;
Run;
Proc Print Data=DCSPnormal; run;
%Mend DCSPnormal;
<<**SAS**<<

## Example 4.2    Adaptive Design for Asthma Study

In a phase-III asthma study with 2 dose groups (control and active), the primary efficacy endpoint is the percent change from baseline in FEV1. The estimated FEV1 improvement from baseline is 5% and 12% for the control and active groups, respectively, with a common standard deviation of $\sigma = 22\%$. Based on a large sample assumption, the sample size for a fixed design is 208 per group, which has 90% power to detect the difference at a one-sided alpha = 0.025. Using MSP, an interim analysis is planned based on the response assessments of 50% of the patients. To design an adaptive trial (GSD), we can use the SAS macro DCSPnormal, described as follows:

(1) Choose stopping boundaries at the first stage: $\alpha_1 = 0.01$, $\beta_1 = 0.15$; then from Table 4.4, we can obtain $\alpha_2 = 0.1871$.

(2) Check the stopping boundary to make sure that the familywise error is controlled by submitting the following SAS statement:

>>**SAS**>>
%DCSPnormal(Model="sum", alpha=0.025, beta=0.1, sigma=0.22, ux=0.05, uy=0.05, nInterim=155, Nmax=310, DuHa=0.07, nAdj="N", alpha1=0.01, beta1=0.15, alpha2=0.1871);
<<**SAS**<<

The simulated familywise error rate $\alpha = 0.0253$. Therefore the stopping boundaries are confirmed.

(3) Calculate power or sample size required using the following SAS statement:

>>**SAS**>>
%DCSPnormal(Model="sum", alpha=0.025, beta=0.1, sigma=0.22, ux=0.05, uy=0.12, nInterim=155, Nmax=310, DuHa=0.07, nAdj="N", alpha1=0.01, beta1=0.15, alpha2=0.1871);
<<**SAS**<<

(4) Perform the sensitivity analysis (under condition $H_s$) with treatment means of 0.05 and 0.1 for the control and test groups, respectively, by submiting the following SAS statement:

>>**SAS**>>
%DCSPnormal(Model="sum", alpha=0.025, beta=0.1, sigma=0.22, ux=0.05, uy=0.10, nInterim=155, Nmax=310, DuHa=0.07, nAdj="N", alpha1=0.01, beta1=0.15, alpha2=0.1871);
<<**SAS**<<

The simulation results are summarized in Table 4.5.

Table 4.5: Operating Characteristics of a GSD with MSP

| Simulation condition | FSP | ESP | N | $N_{max}$ | Power (alpha) |
|---|---|---|---|---|---|
| $H_o$ | 0.849 | 0.010 | 177 | 310 | (0.025) |
| $H_a$ | 0.039 | 0.682 | 198 | 310 | 0.949 |
| $H_s$ | 0.167 | 0.373 | 226 | 310 | 0.743 |

From Table 4.5, we can see that the design has a smaller expected sample size $(\bar{N})$ under $H_0$ and $H_a$ (177, 198) than the classical design (208). If the trial stops early, only 155 patients per group are required. However,

the group sequential design has a larger maximum sample size (310) than
the classical design (208). The early FSP and early ESP are also shown in
Table 4.5. The sensitivity analysis shows a large power loss when treatment
difference is slightly lower than expected. To protect power, we can use the
sample-size reestimation method.

Now let's calculate the conditional $p$-values. Assume the trial is finished
with the stagewise $p$-value (unadjusted, based on subsample from the stage)
for the first stage of $p_1 = 0.012$ (which is larger than $\alpha_1 = 0.01$, therefore
the trial continues to the second stage) and the stagewise $p$-value for the
second stage of $p_2 = 0.18$. The test statistic at stage 2 is $t = p_1 + p_2$
$= 0.012 + 0.18 = 0.192 > \alpha_2 = 0.1871$. Therefore, we failed to reject the
null hypothesis and cannot claim superior efficacy of the test drug.

From (3.4) and (4.10), we have

$$p_c(2) = (\beta_1 - \alpha_1)t - \frac{1}{2}\left(\beta_1^2 - \alpha_1^2\right)$$

$$= (0.15 - 0.01)\,0.192 - \frac{1}{2}\left(0.15^2 - 0.01^2\right)$$

$$= 0.015\,68.$$

The adjusted $p$-value is

$$p_a(2) = \pi_1 + p_c(2) = 0.01 + 0.015\,68 = 0.02568 > \alpha = 0.025,$$

which leads to the same conclusion of failing to reject $H_0$.

Being equivalent to MSP, we can define the test statistic as the mean
(instead of the sum) of stagewise $p$-values. At the $k$th stage, the test statistic is defined as

$$T_k = \frac{1}{k}\Sigma_{i=1}^{k}p_i, \quad k = 1, ..., K. \tag{4.15}$$

Since the $p$-value can be viewed as the evidence against the null hypothesis, the notion of this method is to equally weight the evidence against the
null hypothesis. Let's call this method the method based on mean of $p$-
values or MMP.

In general, we can define the test statistic as a linear combination of
stagewise $p$-values:

$$T_k = \sum_{i=1}^{k} w_{ki}p_i, \tag{4.16}$$

where constant $w_{ki} > 0$ and $\sum_{i=1}^{k} w_{ki} = 1$, $k = 1, ..., K$.

## 4.3 Method with Product of *p*-values

This method is referred to as MPP. The test statistic in this method is based on the product of the stagewise *p*-values from the subsamples. For two-stage designs, the test statistic is defined as

$$T_k = \Pi_{i=1}^k p_i, \ k = 1, 2. \tag{4.17}$$

The $\alpha$ spent in the two stages is given by

$$\pi_1 = \int_0^{\alpha_1} dt_1 = \alpha_1 \tag{4.18}$$

and

$$\pi_2 = \int_{\alpha_1}^{\beta_1} \int_0^{\alpha_2} \frac{1}{t_1} dt_2 dt_1. \tag{4.19}$$

Carrying out the integrations in (4.19) and substituting the results into (3.7), we can obtain the following formulation for determining stopping boundaries:

$$\alpha = \alpha_1 + \alpha_2 \ln \frac{\beta_1}{\alpha_1}, \ \alpha_1 < \beta_1 \le 1. \tag{4.20}$$

Note that the stopping boundaries based on Fisher's criterion are special cases of (4.20), where $\alpha_2 = \exp\left[-\frac{1}{2}\chi_4^2(1-\alpha)\right]$, i.e., $\alpha_2 = 0.00380$ for $\alpha = 0.025$. To calculate the stopping boundaries, one can predetermine $\alpha$, $\alpha_1$, and $\beta_1$, then solve (4.20) for $\alpha_2$. See Table 4.6 for examples.

Table 4.6: Stopping Boundaries $\alpha_2$ with MPP

| $\beta_1$ | $\alpha_1$ | 0.001 | 0.0025 | 0.005 | 0.010 | 0.015 | 0.020 |
|---|---|---|---|---|---|---|---|
| 0.15 | | 0.0048 | 0.0055 | 0.0059 | 0.0055 | 0.0043 | 0.0025 |
| 0.20 | | 0.0045 | 0.0051 | 0.0054 | 0.0050 | 0.0039 | 0.0022 |
| 0.25 | | 0.0043 | 0.0049 | 0.0051 | 0.0047 | 0.0036 | 0.0020 |
| 0.30 | $\alpha_2$ | 0.0042 | 0.0047 | 0.0049 | 0.0044 | 0.0033 | 0.0018 |
| 0.35 | | 0.0041 | 0.0046 | 0.0047 | 0.0042 | 0.0032 | 0.0017 |
| 0.40 | | 0.0040 | 0.0044 | 0.0046 | 0.0041 | 0.0030 | 0.0017 |
| 0.50 | | 0.0039 | 0.0042 | 0.0043 | 0.0038 | 0.0029 | 0.0016 |
| 1.00 | | 0.0035 | 0.0038 | 0.0038 | 0.0033 | 0.0024 | 0.0013 |

Note: One-sided $\alpha = 0.025$.

The *p*-value can be obtained using

$$p(t; k) = \begin{cases} t, & k = 1, \\ \alpha_1 + t \ln \frac{\beta_1}{\alpha_1}, & k = 2, \end{cases} \tag{4.21}$$

where $t = p_1$ if the trial stops at stage 1 ($k = 1$) and $t = p_1 p_2$ if the trial stops at stage 2 ($k = 2$).

It is interesting to know that when $p_1 < \alpha_2$, there is no point in continuing the trial because $p_1 p_2 < p_1 < \alpha_2$ and efficacy should be claimed. Therefore, it is suggested that we should choose $\beta_1 > \alpha_1 > \alpha_2$.

SAS Macro 4.3 below has been implemented for simulating two-arm adaptive designs with survival endpoint. The adaptive method can be based on individual stagewise $p$-values, or the sum or product of the stagewise $p$-values. The SAS variables are defined as follows: **ux** and **uy** are true hazard rates in the x and y groups, respectively. **DuHa** = the estimate for the true treatment difference under the alternative $H_a$, and **N** = sample-size per group. **alpha1** = early efficacy stopping boundary (one-sided), **beta1** = early futility stopping boundary (one-sided), and **alpha2** = final efficacy stopping boundary (one-sided). The null hypothesis test is $H_0$: $\delta +$ **NId** < 0, where $\delta =$ **uy** $-$ **ux** is the treatment difference and **NId** = noninferiority margin. **nSims** = the number of simulation runs, **alpha** = one-sided overall type-I error rate, and **beta** = type-II error rate. **nAdj** = "N" for the case without sample-size reestimation and **nAdj** = "Y" for the case with sample-size adjustment, **Nmax** = maximum sample size allowed, **N0** = the initial sample-size at the final analysis, **nInterim** = sample-size for the interim analysis, **a** = the parameter in (4.17) for the sample-size adjustment, **FSP** = futility stopping probability, **ESP** = efficacy stopping probability, **AveN** = average sample size, **Power** = power of the hypothesis test, **nClassic** = sample-size for the corresponding classical design, **Model** = "ind," "sum," or "prd" for the methods, MIP, MSP, and MPP, respectively.

### >>SAS Macro 4.3: Two-Stage Adaptive Design with Survival Endpoint>>

```
%Macro DCSPSurv(nSims=1000000, Model="sum", alpha=0.025, beta=0.2,
NId=0, tStd=12, tAcr=4, ux=0, uy=1, DuHa=1, nAdj="Y", Nmax=100,
N0=100, nInterim=50, a=2, alpha1=0.01, beta1=0.15, alpha2=0.1871);
Data DCSPSurv; Keep Model FSP ESP AveN Power nClassic;
seedx=2534; seedy=6762; alpha=&alpha; NId=&NId;
Nmax=&Nmax; ux=&ux; uy=&uy; N1=&nInterim; model=&model;
Expuxd=exp(-ux*&tStd);  Expuyd=exp(-uy*&tStd);
sigmax=ux*(1+Expuxd*(1-exp(ux*&tAcr))/(&tAcr*ux))**(-0.5);
sigmay=uy*(1+Expuyd*(1-exp(uy*&tAcr))/(&tAcr*uy))**(-0.5);
sigma=((sigmax**2+sigmay**2)/2)**0.5;
eSize=abs(&DuHa+NId)/sigma;
nClassic=Round(2*((probit(1-alpha)+Probit(1-&beta))/eSize)**2);
```

```
FSP=0; ESP=0; AveN=0; Power=0;
Do isim=1 To &nSims;
nFinal=N1;
ux1 = Rannor(seedx)*sigma/Sqrt(N1)+ux;
uy1 = Rannor(seedy)*sigma/Sqrt(N1)+uy;
T1 = (uy1-ux1+NId)*Sqrt(N1)/2**0.5/sigma;
p1=1-ProbNorm(T1);
If p1>&beta1 Then FSP=FSP+1/&nSims;
If p1<=&alpha1 Then do;
Power=Power+1/&nSims; ESP=ESP+1/&nSims;
End;
If p1>&alpha1 and p1<=&beta1 Then Do;
eRatio=Abs(&DuHa/(Abs(uy1-ux1)+0.0000001));
nFinal=min(Nmax,max(&N0,eRatio**&a*&N0));
If &DuHa*(uy1-ux1+NId)<0 then nFinal=N1;
If &nAdj="N" then nFinal=Nmax;
If nFinal>N1 Then Do;
ux2 = Rannor(seedx)*sigma/Sqrt(nFinal-N1)+ux ;
uy2 = Rannor(seedy)*sigma/Sqrt(nFinal-N1)+uy;
T2 = (uy2-ux2+NId)*Sqrt(nFinal-N1)/2**0.5/sigma;
p2=1-ProbNorm(T2);
If Model="ind" Then TS2=p2;
If Model="sum" Then TS2=p1+p2;
If Model="prd" Then TS2=p1*p2;
If .<TS2<=&alpha2 Then Power=Power+1/&nSims;
End;
End;
AveN=AveN+nFinal/&nSims;
End;
Output;
Run;
Proc Print Data=DCSPSurv; Run;
%Mend DCSPSurv;
```
<<**SAS**<<

## Example 4.3   Adaptive Design for Oncology Trial

In a two-arm comparative oncology trial, the primary efficacy endpoint is time-to-progression (TTP). The median TTP is estimated to be 8 months (hazard rate = 0.08664) for the control group, and 10.5 months (hazard rate = 0.06601) for the test group. Assume a uniform enrollment with an accrual period of 9 months and a total study duration of 24 months. The log-rank test will be used for the analysis. An exponential survival distribution is assumed for the purpose of sample-size calculation. The classical design requires a sample size of 323 subjects per group.

We design the trial with one interim analysis when 40% of patients have been enrolled. The interim analysis for efficacy is planned based on TTP, but it does not allow for futility stopping. Using MPP, we choose the following boundaries: $\alpha_1 = 0.005$, $\beta_1 = 1$ ($\beta_1 = 1$ implies no futility stopping), and $\alpha_2 = 0.0038$ from Table 4.6. Again, we follow the same steps as for the two previous examples using the SAS macro **DCSPSurv**: Note that in SAS Macro 4.3, we again assume that the stagewise $p$-values are mutually independent. The steps for the simulations are

(1) Choose stopping boundaries at the first stage: $\alpha_1 = 0.005$, $\beta_1 = 1$; then from Table 4.6, we can obtain $\alpha_2 = 0.0038$.

(2) Check the stopping boundary to make sure that the familywise error is controlled by submitting the following SAS statement:

\>\>**SAS**\>\>
%DCSPSurv(Model="prd", alpha=0.025, beta=0.15, tStd=24, tAcr=9, ux=0.08664, uy=0.08664, DuHa=0.02063, nAdj="N", Nmax=344, N0=344, nInterim=138, alpha1=0.005, beta1=1, alpha2=0.0038);
\<\<**SAS**\<\<

The simulated familywise error rate $\alpha = 0.0252$. Therefore, the stopping boundaries are confirmed.

(3) Calculate power or sample size required using the following SAS macro call:

\>\>**SAS**\>\>
%DCSPSurv(Model="prd", alpha=0.025, beta=0.15, tStd=24, tAcr=9, ux=0.06601, uy=0.08664, DuHa=0.02063, nAdj="N", Nmax=344, N0=344, nInterim=138, alpha1=0.005, beta1=1, alpha2=0.0038);
\<\<**SAS**\<\<

We modified the sample size until it reached the desired power. It turns out that the maximum sample size is 344 and the sample size for the interim analysis is 138 per group.

(4) Perform a sensitivity analysis under the condition $H_s$. Because a 2.5-month difference in median TTP is a conservative estimate, the obvious question is: What is the early stopping probability if the true treatment difference in median TTP is, for example, 3 months (8 months versus 11 months or hazard rate = 0.06301)? To answer this question, we issue the

following SAS statement with hazard rates of 0.08664 and 0.06301 for the control and test groups, respectively.

>>**SAS**>>
%DCSPSurv(Model="prd", alpha=0.025, beta=0.15, tStd=24, tAcr=9, ux=0.06301, uy=0.08664, DuHa=0.02363, nAdj="N", Nmax=344, N0=344, nInterim=138, alpha1=0.005, beta1=1, alpha2=0.0038);
<<**SAS**<<

We now summarize the simulation outputs for the three scenarios in Table 4.7.

Table 4.7: Operating Characteristics of a GSD with MPP

| Simulation condition | FSP | ESP | N | $N_{max}$ | Power (alpha) |
|---|---|---|---|---|---|
| $H_o$ | 0 | 0.005 | 343 | 344 | 0.025 |
| $H_a$ | 0 | 0.268 | 289 | 344 | 0.851 |
| $H_s$ | 0 | 0.381 | 265 | 344 | 0.937 |

From Table 4.7, we can see that the design has a smaller expected sample size ($\bar{N}$) under $H_a$ (289/group) than the classical design (323/group). If the trial stops early, only 138 patients per group are required. However, the group sequential design has a larger maximum sample-size (344) than the classical design (323). The early FSP and early ESP are also shown in Table 4.7. The sensitivity analysis shows that the early stopping probability increases from 26.8% to 38.1% if the difference in median TTP is 3 months instead of 2.5 months. This indicates a time savings, too. Also, the power will be 93.7% if the difference in median TTP is 3 months instead of 2.5 months. We can see that the group sequential design is very advantageous when the effect size is larger than our initial estimate. We will discuss this in a later chapter on choosing adaptive designs.

Now let's calculate adjusted $p$-values. If the trial is stopped at the first stage with $p_1 = 0.002$, then the conditional and overall $p$-values are the same and equal to 0.002. If the first stagewise $p$-value $p_1 = 0.05$ (which is larger than $\alpha_1 = 0.005$ and not significant; therefore the trial continued to the second stage) and $p_2 = 0.07$, the test statistic at stage 2 is $t = p_1 p_2 = (0.05)(0.07) = 0.0035 < \alpha_2 = 0.0038$. Therefore, we reject the null hypothesis and claim the efficacy of the test drug. The probability defined by (3.4) is

$$p_c(2) = t \ln \frac{\beta_1}{\alpha_1} = 0.0185,$$

and the adjusted $p$-value is

$$p_a = \alpha_1 + p_c(2) = 0.005 + 0.0185 = 0.0235 < \alpha = 0.025.$$

Therefore, the $H_0$ should be rejected.

## Example 4.4  Early Futility Stopping Design with Binary Endpoint

We use an early example. A phase-III trial is to be designed for patients with acute ischemic stroke of recent onset. The composite endpoint (death and MI) is the primary endpoint, and event rate is 14% for the control group and 12% for the test group. Based on a large sample assumption, the sample size for a fixed design is 5937 per group, which provides 90% power to detect the difference at one-sided alpha = 0.025. An interim analysis for futility stopping is planed based on 50% patients' response assessments. The interim look is for futility stopping. We can use both MIP and MSP, but we don't recommend MPP in this case because MPP doesn't allow for futility early stopping only. Because the regulatory agency may be concerned that in the current practice, the futility boundary may not be followed, i.e., the trial did continue when in fact the futility boundary had been crossed. To protect type-I error, it was suggested that the futility boundary should not be used for determining the stopping boundaries at later stages. We know that MIP and MSP have used the futility boundary in determination of the subsequent boundaries. However, we will propose a better procedure in which the stopping boundaries are different depending on whether the futility boundary is followed or not. Let's illustrate this with MSP for this trial.

(1) Choose futility stopping boundaries from Table 4.4: $\alpha_1 = 0$ (implying no early efficacy stopping), $\beta_1 = 0.15$, $\alpha_2 = 0.2417$. If the futility boundary has not been followed, the first stage subsample will not be used in the final analysis and $\alpha_2 = 0.025$ will be used. Alternatively, we can conservatively use $\alpha_1 = 0$, $\beta_1 = 0.15$, $\alpha_2 = 0.2236$ (This $\alpha_2$ is corresponding to $\alpha_1 = 0$ and $\beta_1 = 1$).

(2) Run simulations to obtain the sample size required and the operating characteristics under $H_a$ with $\alpha = 0.025$ and $\beta = 0.1$ (power = 0.9). By trying different maximum sample size ($N_{\max}$) in the following SAS statement, we found that 7360 gives the desired power (the classical design requires $n$ = 5937 per group):

>>**SAS**>>
%DCSPbinary(Model="sum", alpha=0.025, beta=0.1, Px=0.12, Py=0.14,
DuHa=0.02, Nmax=7360, nInterim=3680, alpha1=0, beta1=0.15,
alpha2=0.2417);
<<**SAS**<<

(3) To obtain the operating characteristics under $H_0$, submit the following
SAS statement:

>>**SAS**>>
%DCSPbinary(Model="sum", alpha=0.025, beta=0.1, Px=0.14, Py=0.14,
DuHa=0.02, Nmax=7360, nInterim=3680, alpha1=0, beta1=0.15,
alpha2=0.2417);
<<**SAS**<<

The simulation results are presented in Table 4.8.

Table 4.8:  Operating Characteristics of a GSD with MSP

| Simulation condition | FSP | ESP | N | $N_{max}$ | Power (alpha) |
|---|---|---|---|---|---|
| $H_o$ | 0.851 | 0 | 4232 | 7360 | 0.025 |
| $H_a$ | 0.065 | 0 | 7124 | 7360 | 0.899 |

Note that the futility design is used because there is a great concern
that the drug may not have efficacy. In such a case, the expected sample size is 4229/group which is much smaller than the classical design
(5937/group).

If the conservative stopping boundaries ($\alpha_1 = 0$, $\beta_1 = 0.15$, and $\alpha_2 =$
0.2236) are used, the simulated power is 89.4% with the same sample-size
(Nmax = 7360) by submitting the following SAS statement:

>>**SAS**>>
%DCSPbinary(Model="sum", alpha=0.025, beta=0.1, Px=0.12, Py=0.14,
DuHa=0.02, Nmax=7360, nInterim=3680, alpha1=0, beta1=0.15,
alpha2=0.2236);
<<**SAS**<<

Using the conservative boundaries, the $\alpha$ is actually controlled at a
0.0224 level. In this example, there is minimal difference in power between
the two methods.

**Example 4.5   Noninferiority Design with Binary Endpoint**
Let's consider a noninferiority/superiority design for the trial in Example 4.4. If superiority is not achieved, we will perform a noninferiority test.

Because of the closed testing procedure, no alpha adjustment is required for the two hypothesis tests. The noninferiority boundary is decided to be 0.5%. For the purpose of comparison, we use the same sample-size and stopping boundaries as in Example 4.4.

(1) Choose futility stopping boundaries from Table 4.4: $\alpha_1 = 0$, $\beta_1 = 0.15$, and $\alpha_2 = 0.2417$.

(2) Perform simulations by using the following SAS statement to obtain the sample-size required and the operating characteristics under $H_a$ with $\alpha = 0.025$ and Nmax $= 7360$ per group:

>>**SAS**>>
%DCSPbinary(Model="sum", alpha=0.025, beta=0.1,  NId=0.005, Px=0.12, Py=0.14, DuHa=0.02, Nmax=7360, nInterim=3680, alpha1=0, beta1=0.15, alpha2=0.2417);
<<**SAS**<<

(3) Obtain the operating characteristics under $H_0$ by running simulations under $H_0$:

>>**SAS**>>
%DCSPbinary(Model="sum", alpha=0.025, beta=0.1,  NId=0.005, Px=0.145, Py=0.14,  DuHa=0.02,  Nmax=7360,     nInterim=3680,   a=2,   alpha1=0, beta1=0.15, alpha2=0.2417);
<<**SAS**<<

Note that the futility design is used because there is great concern that the drug may not have efficacy. In such a case, the expected sample size is 4923/group.

(4) Perform the sensitivity analysis under the condition that the event rate is 12.5%. The power for the noninferiority test under this condition is 89.5%, which is obtained by submitting the following SAS statement:

>>**SAS**>>
%DCSPbinary(Model="sum", alpha=0.025, beta=0.1, NId=0.005, Px=0.125, Py=0.14, DuHa=0.02, Nmax=7360, nInterim=3680, alpha1=0, beta1=0.15, alpha2=0.2417);
<<**SAS**<<

The simulation results are presented in Table 4.9.

**Example 4.6   Sample-Size Reestimation with Normal Endpoint**
    In a phase-III asthma study with 2 dose groups (control and active), the primary efficacy endpoint is the percent change from baseline in FEV1.

Table 4.9: Operating Characteristics of a GSD with MSP

| Simulation condition | FSP | ESP | N | $N_{max}$ | Power (alpha) |
|---|---|---|---|---|---|
| $H_o$ | 0.850 | 0 | 4232 | 7360 | 0.025 |
| $H_a$ | 0.010 | 0 | 7302 | 7360 | 0.977 |
| $H_s$ | 0.068 | 0 | 7110 | 7360 | 0.895 |

The estimated FEV1 improvements from baseline are 5% and 12% for the control and active groups, respectively, with a common standard deviation of $\sigma = 22\%$. Based on a large sample assumption, the sample size for a fixed design is 208 per group with 95% power and a one-sided alpha = 0.025. Using MSP, an interim analysis is planned based on the response assessments of 50% of the patients. The interim analysis is used for sample-size reestimation and also for futility stopping. We follow the steps below to design the adaptive trial.

(1) Choose stopping boundaries at the first stage: $\alpha_1 = 0$, $\beta_1 = 0.25$, then from Table 4.4, we obtain $\alpha_2 = 0.2236$.

(2) Determine the rule for sample-size reestimation:

$$N = \left(\frac{E_0}{E}\right)^a N_0, \qquad (4.22)$$

where $N$ is the newly estimated sample size, $N_0$ = initial sample size, $a$ is a constant and often chosen to be 2, and $E_0$ and $E$ are predetermined and observed effect sizes or treatment differences, respectively. Choose $N_0 = 242$, which is suggested to be close to but larger than the sample size for the classical design. The choice of $N_0$ should be dependent on the operating characteristics of the design; therefore, several iterations may be required before a satisfactory $N_0$ is chosen.

(3) Perform simulations without SSR using the following SAS statement:

```
>>SAS>>
%DCSPnormal(Model="sum", alpha=0.025, beta=0.1, sigma=0.22, ux=0.05,
uy=0.12, nInterim=121, Nmax=242, N0=242, DuHa=0.07, alpha1=0,
beta1=0.25, alpha2=0.2236);
<<SAS<<
```

(4) Perform simulations with SSR using the following SAS statement:

```
>>SAS>>
%DCSPnormal(Model="sum", alpha=0.025, beta=0.1, sigma=0.22, ux=0.05,
uy=0.12, nInterim=121, Nmax=350, N0=242, DuHa=0.07, nAdj="Y",
alpha1=0, beta1=0.25, alpha2=0.2236);
<<SAS<<
```

(5) Perform simulations for sensitivity analysis without SSR using the following SAS statement:

>>**SAS**>>
%DCSPnormal(Model="sum", alpha=0.025, beta=0.1, sigma=0.22, ux=0.05, uy=0.105, nInterim=121, Nmax=242, N0=242, DuHa=0.07, alpha1=0, beta1=0.25, alpha2=0.2236);
<<**SAS**<<

(6) Perform simulations for sensitivity analysis with SSR (note that DuHa = 0.07 for sensitivity analysis):

>>**SAS**>>
%DCSPnormal(Model="sum", alpha=0.025, beta=0.1, sigma=0.22, ux=0.05, uy=0.105, nInterim=121, Nmax=350, N0=242, DuHa=0.07, nAdj="Y", alpha1=0, beta1=0.25, alpha2=0.2236);
<<**SAS**<<

The simulation results are presented in Table 4.10. Note that we set the futility boundary at $\beta_1 = 0.25$ due to the consideration that if the treatment effect is very small (such that $p_1 > 0.25$), the required sample size to be adjusted is very large and not feasible.

Table 4.10: Operating Characteristics of a GSD with MSP

| Simulation condition | Method | FSP | N | $N_{max}$ | Power |
|---|---|---|---|---|---|
| | classical | 0 | 208 | 208 | 0.025 |
| $H_0$ | without SSR | 0.750 | 151 | 242 | 0.025 |
| | with SSR | 0.750 | 177 | 350 | 0.025 |
| | classical | 0 | 208 | 208 | 0.900 |
| $H_a$ | without SSR | 0.036 | 238 | 242 | 0.900 |
| | with SSR | 0.036 | 278 | 350 | 0.928 |
| | classical | 0 | 208 | 208 | 0.722 |
| $H_s$ | without SSR | 0.102 | 230 | 242 | 0.733 |
| | with SSR | 0.102 | 285 | 350 | 0.804 |

From Table 4.10, we can see that the adaptive design has a smaller expected sample size $(\bar{N})$ under $H_0$ than the classical design (208). When using the sample-size reestimation mechanism, the power is protected to a certain degree (72.2% for the classical vs. 73.3% for adaptive design without SSR and 80.4% with SSR). Of course, this power protection is at the cost of sample size. Note the average n = 285/group with sample-size adjustment when the effect is 5% versus 10.5%. If this sample size is used in a classical design, the power would be 84.7%. The sample-size reestimation has lost its efficiency in this sense, though there is a saving in sample size under $H_0$.

**Example 4.7    Sample-Size Reestimation with Survival Endpoint**

In this example we will compare MIP, MSP, and MPP and illustrate how to calculate the adjusted $p$-values with these 3 different methods.

Suppose in a two-arm comparative oncology trial, the primary efficacy endpoint is TTP. The median TTP is estimated to be 8 months (hazard rate = 0.08664) for the control group, and 10.5 months (hazard rate = 0.06601) for the test group. Assume uniform enrollment with an accrual period of 9 months and a total study duration of 24 months. The log-rank test will be used for the analysis. An exponential survival distribution is assumed for the purpose of sample-size calculation.

To generate the operating characteristics using MIP, MSP, and MPP, we use the following SAS macro calls, respectively:

**>>SAS>>**

%DCSPsurv(model="ind", alpha=0.025, beta=0.15, tStd=24, tAcr=9, ux=0.06601, uy=0.08664, DuHa=0.02063, nAdj="Y", Nmax=400, N0=350, nInterim=200, alpha1=0.01, beta1=0.25, alpha2=0.0625);

%DCSPsurv(model="sum", alpha=0.025, beta=0.15, NId=0, tStd=24, tAcr=9, ux=0.06601, uy=0.08664, DuHa=0.02063, nAdj="Y", Nmax=400, N0=350, nInterim=200, alpha1=0.01, beta1=0.25, alpha2=0.1832);

%DCSPsurv(model="prd", alpha=0.025, beta=0.15, tStd=24, tAcr=9, ux=0.06601, uy=0.08664, DuHa=0.02063, nAdj="Y", Nmax=400, N0=350, nInterim=200, a=2, alpha1=0.01, beta1=0.25, alpha2=0.00466);

**<<SAS<<**

When there is a 10.5-month median time for the test group, the classical design requires a sample-size of 323 per group with 85% power at a level of significance (one-sided) $\alpha = 0.025$. To increase efficiency, an adaptive design with an interim sample-size of 200 patients per group is used. The interim analysis allows for early efficacy or futility stopping with stopping boundaries (from Tables 4.1, 4.3, and 4.5) $\alpha_1 = 0.01$, $\beta_1 = 0.25$, and $\alpha_2 = 0.0625$ for MIP, 0.1832 for MSP, and 0.00466 for MPP. The sample-size adjustment is based on (4.17). The maximum sample size allowed for adjustment is $N_{max} = 400$. The parameter for sample-size adjustment $N_o$ is 350 ($N_o$ is usually chosen to be close to the sample size from the classical design so that the adaptive design will have similar power to the classical design.). The simulation results are presented in Table 4.11.

Note that power is the probability of rejecting the null hypothesis. Therefore, when the null hypothesis is true, the power is the type-I error rate $\alpha$. From Table 4.10, it can be seen that the one-sided $\alpha$ is controlled at a 0.025 level as expected for all three methods. The expected sample sizes

Table 4.11:   Operating Characteristics of Adaptive Methods

| Median time | | | | Expected | Power (%) |
|---|---|---|---|---|---|
| Test | Control | ESP | FSP | N | MIP/MSP/MPP |
| 8 | 8 | 0.010 | 0.750 | 248 | 2.5/2.5/2.5 |
| 10.5 | 8 | 0.512 | 0.046 | 288 | 86.3/87.3/88.8 |

Note: 1,000,000 simulation runs.

under both $H_0$ and $H_a$ are smaller than the sample size for the classical design (290/group). The power is 86.3%, 87.3%, and 88.8% for MIP, MSP, and MPP, respectively. All three designs have the same expected sample size of 288/group which is smaller than the sample size (323/group) for the classical design with 85% power. In adaptive design, conditional power is more important than power.

## 4.4   Event-Based Adaptive Design

The methods discussed for survival analyses so far are based on the number of patients at each stage, instead of number of events. The reason for this is that the methods are based on the assumption of independent stagewise statistics. Therefore, the first $N_1$ patients enrolled will be used for the first interim analysis regardless of their having the event or not. Strictly speaking, the commonly used log-rank test statistics based on number of events,

$$T\left(\hat{D}_k\right) = \sqrt{\frac{\hat{D}_k}{2}} \ln \frac{\hat{\lambda}_1}{\hat{\lambda}_2} \sim N\left(\sqrt{\frac{D_k}{2}} \ln \frac{\lambda_1}{\lambda_2}, 1\right), \qquad (4.23)$$

are not independent, where $D_k$ is the number of events at the $k$th stage. However, Breslow and Haug (1977) and Canner (1997) showed that the independent normal approximation works well for small $D_k$. The relationship between the number of deaths and number of patients is given in Problem 2.3 in Chapter 2. Using (4.23), we can implement adaptive design for survival based on the number of events as follows.

SAS Macro 4.4 below has been implemented for simulating two-arm group sequential designs with survival endpoint. The adaptive method can be based on individual stagewise $p$-values, or the sum or product of the stagewise $p$-values. The SAS variables are defined as follows: **ux** and **uy** are true hazard rates in the x and y groups, respectively. **N** = sample-size per group. **alpha1** = early efficacy stopping boundary (one-sided), **beta1** = early futility stopping boundary (one-sided), and **alpha2** = final efficacy stopping boundary (one-sided). **nSims** = the number of simulation runs, **alpha** = one-sided overall type-I error rate, and **beta** = type-II error rate. **InfoTime** = sample-size ratio for the interim analysis, **FSP** = futility stopping probability, **ESP** = efficacy stopping probability, **AveDs** = average total number of events, **Power** = power of the hypothesis test, **Model** = "ind," "sum," or "prd" for the methods, MIP, MSP, and MPP, respectively, **tStd** = study duration, and **tAcr** = accrual time.

## >>SAS Macro 4.4:   Event-Based Adaptive Design>>

```
%Macro DCSPSurv2(nSims=1000000, Model="sum", alpha=0.025, beta=0.2,
tStd=12, tAcr=4, ux=0.08, uy=0.1, N=100, InfoTime=0.5, alpha1=0.01,
beta1=0.15, alpha2=0.1871);
Data DCSPSurv; Keep Model FSP ESP Power AveDs N;
seed1=2534; seed2=2534; alpha=&alpha; N=&N; ux=&ux;
uy=&uy; model=&model; infoTime=&infoTime; tAcr=&tAcr;
FSP=0; ESP=0; AveDs=0; Power=0; u=(ux+uy)/2;
Ds=2*N/&tAcr*(&tAcr-(exp(u*&tAcr)-1)/u*exp(-u*&tStd));
Ds1=Ds*infoTime;
Do isim=1 To &nSims;
nFinal=Ds1;
T1 = Rannor(seed1)+Sqrt(Ds1/2)*log(uy/ux);
p1=1-ProbNorm(T1);
If p1>&beta1 Then FSP=FSP+1/&nSims;
If p1<=&alpha1 Then do;
Power=Power+1/&nSims; ESP=ESP+1/&nSims;
End;
If p1>&alpha1 and p1<=&beta1 Then Do;
nFinal=Ds;
T2 = Rannor(seed2)+Sqrt((Ds-Ds1)/2)*log(uy/ux);
p2=1-ProbNorm(T2);
If Model="ind" Then TS2=p2;
If Model="sum" Then TS2=p1+p2;
If Model="prd" Then TS2=p1*p2;
If .<TS2<=&alpha2 Then Power=Power+1/&nSims;
End;
AveDs=AveDs+nFinal/&nSims;
End;
Output;
Run;
Proc Print Data=DCSPSurv; Run;
```

%Mend DCSPSurv2;

<<**SAS**<<

An example of using this SAS macro is presented as follows:

>>**SAS**>>

%DCSPSurv2(nSims=100000, model="sum", alpha=0.025, beta=0.2, tStd=24, tAcr=9,   ux=0.06601,  uy=0.08664,  N=180,  InfoTime=0.5,  alpha1=0.01, beta1=0.15, alpha2=0.1871);

<<**SAS**<<

Whether based on the number of events or patients, the results are very similar. SAS Macro 4.4 can be extended to general adaptive design with sample-size reestimation. Other methods for adaptive design with a survival endpoint can be found from work by Li, Shih, and Wang (2005). Practically, the accrual has to continue in most cases when collecting the data and performing the interim analysis; it is often the case that at the time when interim analysis is done, most or all patients are enrolled. What is the point of having the interim analysis? The answer is a positive interim analysis would allow the drug to be on the market earlier.

## 4.5    Adaptive Design for Equivalence Trial

In Chapter 2, we have studied the equivalence test for the two parallel groups:

$$H_0 : |\mu_T - \mu_R| \geq \delta \text{ versus } H_a : |\mu_T - \mu_R| < \delta. \tag{4.24}$$

If the null hypothesis is rejected, then we conclude that the test drug and the reference drug are equivalent.

For a large sample size, the null hypothesis is rejected if

$$T_1 = \frac{\bar{x}_R - \bar{x}_T - \delta}{\hat{\sigma}\sqrt{\frac{2}{n}}} < -z_{1-\alpha} \text{ and } T_2 = \frac{\bar{x}_R - \bar{x}_T + \delta}{\hat{\sigma}\sqrt{\frac{2}{n}}} > z_{1-\alpha}. \tag{4.25}$$

The approximate sample size per group is given by (see Chapter 2)

$$n = \frac{2\left(z_{1-\alpha} + z_{1-\beta/2}\right)^2 \sigma^2}{\left(|\varepsilon| - \delta\right)^2}. \tag{4.26}$$

Equation (4.25) is equivalent to the following condition:

$$p = \max\{p_{01}, p_{02}\} \leq \alpha \tag{4.27}$$

where $p_{01} = \Phi(T_1)$ and $p_{02} = \Phi(-T_2)$.

We now discuss the two-stage adaptive design that allows for sample-size adjustment based on information at the first stage. The key for the adaptive equivalence trial is to define an appropriate stagewise $p$-value. We can use a $p$-value similar to (4.27) but based on subsample from the $k$th stage, i.e.,

$$p_k = \max\left\{\Phi\left(T_{k1}\right), \Phi\left(-T_{k2}\right)\right\}, \tag{4.28}$$

where

$$T_{k1} = \frac{\bar{x}_{kR} - \bar{x}_{kT} - \delta}{\hat{\sigma}_k \sqrt{\frac{2}{n_k}}} \text{ and } T_{k2} = \frac{\bar{x}_{kR} - \bar{x}_{kT} + \delta}{\hat{\sigma}_k \sqrt{\frac{2}{n_k}}}. \tag{4.29}$$

Using the stagewise $p$-values defined in (4.28), we can use MIP, MSP, and MPP to design adaptive equivalence trial without any difficulty. For convenience, let's implement the method in SAS.

SAS Macro 4.5 below has been implemented for simulating two-arm equivalence trial with normal endpoint. The adaptive method can be based on individual stagewise $p$-values, or the sum or product of the stagewise $p$-values. The SAS variables are defined as follows: **ux** and **uy** are true proportions of response in the x and y groups, respectively. **DuHa** = the estimate for the true treatment difference under the alternative $H_a$, and **N** = sample-size per group. **alpha1** = early efficacy stopping boundary (one-sided), **beta1** = early futility stopping boundary (one-sided), and **alpha2** = final efficacy stopping boundary (one-sided). The null hypothesis test is given by (4.24). **NId** = equivalence margin, **nSims** = the number of simulation runs, **alpha** = one-sided overall type-I error rate, and **beta** = type-II error rate. **nAdj** = "N" for the case without sample-size reestimation and **nAdj** = "Y" for the case with sample-size adjustment, **Nmax** = maximum sample-size allowed, **N0** = the initial sample-size at the final analysis, **nInterim** = sample size for the interim analysis, **a** = the parameter in (4.22) for the sample-size adjustment, **FSP** = futility stopping probability, **ESP** = efficacy stopping probability, **AveN** = average sample size, **Power** = power of the hypothesis testing, and **Model** = "ind," "sum," or "prd" for the methods MIP, MSP, and MPP, respectively.

### >>SAS Macro 4.5:    Adaptive Equivalence Trial Design>>

```
%Macro DCSPEqNormal(nSims=1000000,Model= "sum", alpha=0.05, beta=0.2,
sigma=0.3, NId=0.2, ux=0, uy=0.1, nInterim=50, Nmax=100, N0=100,
DuHa=1, nAdj= "Y", a= -2, alpha1=0, beta1=0.2, alpha2=0.3);
Data DCSPEqNormal; Keep Model FSP ESP AveN Power;
```

```
seedx=1736; seedy=6214; alpha=&alpha; NId=&NId; Nmax=&Nmax;
ux=&ux; uy=&uy; sigma=&sigma; model=&Model; N1=&nInterim;
eSize=abs(&DuHa+NId)/sigma;
FSP=0; ESP=0; AveN=0; Power=0;
Do isim=1 To &nSims;
nFinal=N1;
ux1 = Rannor(seedx)*sigma/Sqrt(N1)+ux;
uy1 = Rannor(seedy)*sigma/Sqrt(N1)+uy;
T11 = (uy1-ux1-NId)*sqrt(N1/2)/sigma;
T12 = (uy1-ux1+NId)*sqrt(N1/2)/sigma;
p11=Probnorm(T11);
p12=Probnorm(-T12);
p1=max(p11,p12);
If p1>&beta1 then FSP=FSP+1/&nSims;
If p1<=&alpha1 then do;
Power=Power+1/&nSims; ESP=ESP+1/&nSims;
End;
If p1>&alpha1 and p1<=&beta1 Then Do;
eRatio = abs(&DuHa/(abs(uy1-ux1)+0.0000001));
nFinal = min(&Nmax,max(&N0,eRatio**&a*&N0));
If &DuHa*(uy1-ux1+NId) < 0 Then nFinal = N1;
If &nAdj = "N" then nFinal = &Nmax;
If nFinal > N1 Then Do;
ux2 = Rannor(seedx)*sigma/sqrt(nFinal-N1)+ux ;
uy2 = Rannor(seedy)*sigma/sqrt(nFinal-N1)+uy;
T21 = (uy2-ux2-NId)*sqrt(nFinal-N1)/2**0.5/sigma;
T22 = (uy2-ux2+NId)*sqrt(nFinal-N1)/2**0.5/sigma;
p21=Probnorm(T21);
p22=Probnorm(-T22);
p2=max(p21,p22);
If Model="ind" Then TS2=p2;
If Model="sum" Then TS2=p1+p2;
If Model="prd" Then TS2=p1*p2;
If .<TS2<=&alpha2 Then Power=Power+1/&nSims;
End;
End;
AveN=AveN+nFinal/&nSims;
End;
Output;
```

Run;
Proc Print Data=DCSPEqNormal; run;
%Mend DCSPEqNormal;
<<**SAS**<<

This SAS Macro can also be used for binary and survival endpoints as long as one provides the corresponding "standard deviation" as shown in Table 2.1.

### Example 4.8    Adaptive Equivalence LDL Trial

We use the LDL trial in Example 2.2; the equivalence margin is assumed to be $\delta = 5\%$; the treatment difference in LDL is $1\%$ ($70\%$ versus $71\%$) with a standard deviation of $30\%$. Suppose we decide to use $\alpha = 0.05$ and initial sample size $N_0 = 1200$ per group, the maximum sample size $N_{max} = 2000$ per group, and the interim analysis sample size $N_1 = 600$ per group. The SSR algorithm is given by (4.22) with the parameter $a = -2$. Using MSP, we choose $\alpha_1 = 0$ and $\beta_1 = 0.2$, then $\alpha_2 = 0.35$ from (4.14).

To study the operating characteristics, we use the following SAS macro calls for the design:

>>**SAS**>>
Title " Check alpha under Ho with alpha = 0.05";
%DCSPEqNormal(Model="sum", alpha=0.05, beta=0.2, sigma=.3, NId=0.05, ux=0.70,   uy=0.75,   nInterim=600,   Nmax=2000,   N0=1200,   DuHa=0.01, nAdj="Y", a=-2, alpha1=0.0, beta1=.2, alpha2=0.35);
Title " Simulate the Power under Ha";
%DCSPEqNormal(Model="sum", alpha=0.05, beta=0.2, sigma=.3, NId=0.05, ux=0.70,   uy=0.71,   nInterim=600,   Nmax=2000,   N0=1200,   DuHa=0.01, nAdj="Y", a=-2, alpha1=0.0, beta1=.2, alpha2=0.35);
Title " Sensitivity Analysis (without SSR)";
%DCSPEqNormal(Model="sum", alpha=0.05, beta=0.2, sigma=.3, NId=0.05, ux=0.70,   uy=0.72,   nInterim=600,   Nmax=1200,   N0=1200,   DuHa=0.01, nAdj="N", a=-2, alpha1=0.0, beta1=.2, alpha2=0.35);
Title " Sensitivity Analysis (with SSR)";
%DCSPEqNormal(Model="sum", alpha=0.05, beta=0.2, sigma=.3, NId=0.05, ux=0.70,   uy=0.72,   nInterim=600,   Nmax=2000,   N0=1200,   DuHa=0.01, nAdj="Y", a=-2, alpha1=0.0, beta1=.2, alpha2=0.35);
<<**SAS**<<

The simulation results are summarized as follows: under the null condition ($u_x = 0.70$, $u_y = 0.75$), the average sample-size is $\bar{N} = 868$/group and $\alpha = 0.050$; under the alternative condition ($u_x = 0.70$, $u_y = 0.71$),

$\bar{N} = 1552$ and power $= 0.91$; if the treatment difference is bigger, e.g., 2% ($u_x = 0.70$, $u_y = 0.72$), the average sample-size $\bar{N} = 1088$ and power $= 0.72$ for the design without SSR, and $\bar{N} = 1515$ and power $= 0.78$ for the design with SSR. There is about 6% power increase by using SSR.

## 4.6   Summary

We have derived the closed forms for stopping boundaries using stagewise $p$-values based on subsamples from each stage, in which we have assumed the $p$-values are independent and uniformly distributed without proof or precisely the $p$-values are p-clud (see Chapter 10). The test statistics corresponding to the three methods (MIP, MSP, and MPP) are individual stagewise $p$-values without combining the data from different stages, the sum of the stagewise $p$-values, and the product of the stagewise $p$-values. Note that MIP is different from classical design because the early futility boundaries are used to construct the stopping boundaries for later stages. By comparing the results from MSP, MPP, or other methods with MIP, we can study how much efficacy is gained by combining data from different stages. It is strongly suggested that sufficient simulations be performed using SAS macros provided in this chapter or R programs in Appendix D before determining which method should be used (the electronic versions of the simulation programs can be obtained at www.statisticians.org). There are practical issues that need to be considered too, and these will be addressed in later chapters. Finally, although the examples of adaptive design in this chapter involve mainly sample-size reestimation, MIP, MSP, and MPP are general adaptive design methods and can be used for a variety of adaptive designs (see later chapters of this book).

## Problems

**4.1** Suppose the median times for the two treatment groups in Example 4.7 are 9 months and 12 months. Design an adaptive trial and justify the adaptive design method (MIP, MSP, or MPP) and the design you have chosen.

**4.2** Derive stopping boundaries and $p$-value for two-stage adaptive design based on the following test statistics:

$$T_k = \frac{1}{k} \sum_{i=1}^{k} p_i \text{ for k=1 and 2,}$$

where $p_i$ is the stagewise $p$-value based on subsample from the $i$th stage.

**4.3** Investigate the independence of the stagewise test statistics (4.16) under exponential survival distribution using analytical or simulation approach.

# Chapter 5

# Method with Inverse-Normal $p$-values

In this chapter we will study the method based on inverse-normal $p$-values (MINP), in which the test statistic at the $k$th stage $T_k$ is a linear combination of the weighted inverse-normal of the stagewise $p$-values. The weight can be fixed or a function of information time. MINP can be viewed as a general method including the group sequential method, the Lan–DeMets error-spending method, the Lehmacher–Wassmer method, the Fisher–Shen self-design method, and the Cui–Hung–Wang SSR method as special cases.

## 5.1 Method with Linear Combination of z-Scores

Let $z_k$ be the stagewise normal test statistic at the $k$th stage. In a group sequential design, the test statistic can be expressed as

$$T_k^* = \sum_{i=1}^{k} w_{ki} z_i, \qquad (5.1)$$

where the weights satisfy the equality $\sum_{i=1}^{k} w_{ki}^2 = 1$ and the stagewise Normal statistic $z_i$ is based on the subsample for the $i$th stage. The weights $w_{ki}$ can be functions of information time or sample-size fraction. Note that for fixed weights, $T_k^*$ in (5.1) has a normal distribution. For weights that are a function of information time, $T_k^*$ in (5.1) forms a Brownian motion. Utilization of (5.1) with constant weights allows for changes in the timing (information time) of the interim analyses and the total sample size, while the incorporation of functional weights allows for changes in timing and in the number of analyses. Their combination will allow broader adaptations.

Note that when $w_{ki}$ is fixed, the standard multivariate normal distribution of $\{T_1^*, ..., T_k^*\}$ will not change regardless of adaptations as long as $z_i$ $(i = 1, ..., k)$ has the standard normal distribution. To be consistent with the unified formations in Chapter 3, in which the test statistic is on $p$-scale, we use the transformation $T_k = 1 - \Phi(T_k^*)$ such that

$$T_k = 1 - \Phi\left(\sum_{i=1}^{k} w_{ki} z_i\right), \tag{5.2}$$

where $\Phi$ = cdf of the standard normal distribution.

Unlike MIP, MSP, and MPP, the stopping boundary and power in MINP can be calculated using only numerical integration or computer simulation. Numerical integration is complicated (Jennison and Turnbull, 2000b; CTriSoft, 2002), but the determination of stopping boundaries through simulation is straightforward and precise. The stopping boundaries based on the test statistic defined by (5.2) can be generated using SAS Macro 5.1.

SAS Macro 5.1 below is implemented for computing stopping boundaries with MINP. The SAS variables are defined as follows: **nSims** = number of simulations, **Model** = "fixedW" for constant weights; otherwise, the weights are dependent on information time. For the constant weights, values are specified by **w1** and **w2**. **alpha** = familywise $\alpha$, **nInterim** = sample size per group for the interim analysis, and **Nmax** = maximum sample size allowed for the trial. **alpha1**, **beta1**, and **alpha2** are the stopping boundaries. **Power** is the probability of rejecting the null hypothesis. Therefore, the boundaries should be adjusted during the simulation until the power is equal to **alpha**.

### >>SAS Macro 5.1: Stopping Boundaries with Adaptive Designs>>

```
%Macro SB2StgMINP(nSims=100000, Model= "fixedW", w1=0.5, w2=0.5, alpha
=.025, nInterim=50, Nmax=100, alpha1=0.01, beta1=0.15, alpha2=0.1871);
Data SB2StgMINP; Keep Model Power;
alpha=&alpha; Nmax=&Nmax; Model=&model;
w1=&w1; w2=&w2; n1=&nInterim; Power=0; seedx=231;
Do isim=1 To &nSims;
nFinal=N1;
T1 = Rannor(seedx);
p1=1-ProbNorm(T1);
If p1<=&alpha1 then do;
Power=Power+1/&nSims;
End;
if p1>&alpha1 and p1<=&beta1 then do;
T2 = Rannor(seedx);
If Model^= "fixedW" Then do
```

```
w1=Sqrt(n1/nFinal);
w2=Sqrt((1-n1/nFinal));
End;
Z2=(w1*T1+w2*T2)/Sqrt(w1*w1+w2*w2);
p2=1-ProbNorm(Z2);
If .<p2<=&alpha2 then Power=Power+1/&nSims;
End;
End;
Output;
Run;
Proc Print data=SB2StgMINP; Run;
%Mend SB2StgMINP;
```
<<**SAS**<<

To determine the stopping boundaries, the predetermined **alpha1** and **beta1**, and try different **alpha2** until **Power** from the SAS output is close enough to alpha. An example of calling SAS Macro 5.1 is presented in the following:

>>**SAS**>>
```
Title "Stopping Boundaries by Simulations";
%SB2StgMINP(Model="fixedW", w1=0.5, w2=0.5, alpha=0.025, nInterim=50,
Nmax=100, alpha1=0, beta1=0.15, alpha2=0.0327);
```
<<**SAS**<<

Examples of stopping boundaries for a two-stage design with equal weights are presented in Table 5.1.

Table 5.1: Stopping Boundaries $\alpha_2$ with Equal Weights

| $\beta_1$ | $\alpha_1$ | 0.000 | 0.0025 | 0.005 | 0.010 | 0.015 | 0.020 |
|---|---|---|---|---|---|---|---|
| 0.15 | | 0.0327 | 0.0315 | 0.0295 | 0.0244 | 0.0182 | 0.0105 |
| 0.20 | | 0.0295 | 0.0284 | 0.0267 | 0.0221 | 0.0165 | 0.0097 |
| 0.25 | | 0.0279 | 0.0267 | 0.0250 | 0.0209 | 0.0156 | 0.0092 |
| 0.30 | | 0.0268 | 0.0257 | 0.0241 | 0.0202 | 0.0152 | 0.0090 |
| 0.35 | $\alpha_2$ | 0.0262 | 0.0251 | 0.0236 | 0.0197 | 0.0148 | 0.0089 |
| 0.50 | | 0.0253 | 0.0243 | 0.0228 | 0.0191 | 0.0144 | 0.0087 |
| 0.70 | | 0.0250 | 0.0240 | 0.0226 | 0.0189 | 0.0143 | 0.0086 |
| 1.00 | | 0.0250 | 0.0240 | 0.0225 | 0.0188 | 0.0143 | 0.0086 |

Note: One-sided $\alpha = 0.025$ and 10,000,000 simulation runs

## 5.2    Lehmacher and Wassmer Method

To extend the method with linear combination of $z$-scores, Lehmacher and Wassmer (1999) proposed the test statistic at the $k$th stage that results from the inverse-normal method of combining independent stagewise $p$-values (Hedges and Olkin, 1985):

$$T_k^* = \sum_{i=1}^{k} w_{ki} \Phi^{-1} (1 - p_i),  \qquad (5.3)$$

where the weights satisfy the equality $\sum_{i=1}^{k} w_{ki}^2 = 1$ and $\Phi^{-1}$ is the inverse function of $\Phi$, the standard normal cdf Under the null hypothesis, the stagewise $p_i$ is usually uniformly distributed over [0,1]. The random variables $z_i = \Phi^{-1} (1 - p_i)$ and $T_k^*$ have the standard normal distribution. Lehmacher and Wassmer (1999) suggested using equal weights, i.e., $w_{ik} \equiv \frac{1}{\sqrt{k}}$.

Again, to be consistent with the unified formulations proposed in Chapter 3, transform the test statistic to the $p$-scale, i.e.,

$$T_k = 1 - \Phi \left( \sum_{i=1}^{k} w_{ki} \Phi^{-1} (1 - p_i) \right).  \qquad (5.4)$$

With (5.4), the stopping boundary is on the $p$-scale and easy to compare with other methods regarding operating characteristics. In this book, (5.4) is implemented in SAS and R, instead of (5.3).

When the test statistic defined by (5.4) is used, the classical group sequential boundaries are valid regardless of the timing and sample-size adjustment that may be based on the observed data at the previous stages. Note that under the null hypothesis, $p_i$ is usually uniformly distributed over [0,1], and hence, $z_i = \Phi^{-1} (1 - p_i)$ has the standard normal distribution. The Lehmacher–Wassmer (L-W) method provides a broad method for different endpoints as long as the $p$-value under the null hypothesis is uniformly distributed over [0,1].

The Lehmacher–Wassmer Inverse-Normal method has been implemented in SAS and R (see SAS Macro 5.2). The SAS variables are defined as follows: **nSims** = number of simulations. **Model** = "fixedW" for constant weights, and **Model** = "InfoFun" for functional weights. **alpha** = overall alpha level, **sigma** = the equivalent standard deviation, **NId** = the noninferiority margin, and **ux** and **uy** = the responses in groups x and y, respectively. **nInterim** = sample size for the interim analysis, **Nmax** = maximum sample size, **N0** = initial sample size at the final analysis, and

**DuHa** = the treatment difference under alternative hypothesis. **nAdj** = "Y" for sample-size adjustment; for no SSR, **nAdj** = "N." **a** = the parameter in the sample-size adjustment algorithm in Chapter 11, and **alpha1**, **beta1**, and **alpha2** = stopping boundaries as defined earlier. **FSP** = futility stopping probability, **ESP** = efficacy stopping probability, **AveN** = average sample size, **Power** = power from simulations, and **nClassic** = sample size for the corresponding classical design.

## >>SAS Macro 5.2: Two-Stage Design with Inverse-Normal Method>>

```
%Macro MINP(nSims=1000000, Model="fixedW", w1=0.5, w2=0.5, alpha=0.025, beta=0.2, sigma=2, NId=0, ux=0, uy=1, nInterim=50, Nmax=100, N0=100, DuHa=1, nAdj="N", a=2, alpha1=0.01, beta1=0.15, alpha2=0.1871);
Data MINP; Keep Model FSP ESP AveN Power nClassic PAdj;
seedx=1736; seedy=6214; alpha=&alpha; NId=&NId;
Nmax=&Nmax; Model=&model; w1=&w1; w2=&w2; ux=&ux;
uy=&uy; sigma=&sigma; N1=&nInterim;
eSize=abs(&DuHa+NId)/sigma;
nClassic=Round(2*((Probit(1-alpha)+Probit(1-&beta))/eSize)**2);
FSP=0; ESP=0; AveN=0; Power=0;
Do isim=1 To &nSims;
nFinal=N1;
ux1 = Rannor(seedx)*sigma/Sqrt(N1)+ux;
uy1 = Rannor(seedy)*sigma/Sqrt(N1)+uy;
T1 = (uy1-ux1+NId)*Sqrt(N1)/2**0.5/sigma;
p1=1-ProbNorm(T1);
If p1>&beta1 Then FSP=FSP+1/&nSims;
If p1<=&alpha1 Then Do;
Power=Power+1/&nSims; ESP=ESP+1/&nSims;
End;
If p1>&alpha1 and p1<=&beta1 Then Do;
eRatio=Abs(&DuHa/(Abs(uy1-ux1)+0.0000001));
nFinal=min(&Nmax,max(&N0,eRatio**&a*&N0));
If &DuHa*(uy1-ux1+NId)<0 Then nFinal=N1;
If &nAdj="N" Then nFinal=&Nmax;
If nFinal>N1 Then Do;
ux2 = Rannor(seedx)*sigma/Sqrt(nFinal-N1)+ux ;
uy2 = Rannor(seedy)*sigma/Sqrt(nFinal-N1)+uy;
T2 = (uy2-ux2+NId)*Sqrt(nFinal-N1)/2**0.5/sigma;
If Model^="fixedW" Then Do
```

```
w1=Sqrt(N1/nFinal);
w2=Sqrt((1-N1/nFinal));
End;
Z2=(w1*T1+w2*T2)/Sqrt(w1*w1+w2*w2);
p2=1-ProbNorm(Z2);
If .<p2<=&alpha2 Then Power=Power+1/&nSims;
End;
End;
AveN=AveN+nFinal/&nSims;
End;
PAdj=&alpha1+power-ESP;  ** Stagewise ordering p-value;
Output;
Run;
Proc Print Data=MINP; Run;
%Mend MINP;
```
<<**SAS**<<

### Example 5.1   Inverse-Normal Method with Normal Endpoint

Let's use an earlier example of an asthma study. Suppose a phase-III asthma study with 2 dose groups (control and active) with the percent change from baseline in FEV1 as the primary efficacy endpoint. The estimated FEV1 improvement from baseline is 5% and 12% for the control and active groups, respectively, with a common standard deviation of $\sigma = 22\%$. Based on a large sample assumption, the sample size for a fixed design is 208 per group with 90% power and a one-sided alpha = 0.025. Using MIP, an interim analysis is planned based on the response assessment for 50% of the patients. We now use SAS Macro 5.2 to assist in the adaptive design, described as follows:

(1) Choose stopping boundaries at the first stage: $\alpha_1 = 0.01$, $\beta_1 = 1$; then from Table 5.1, we obtain the corresponding $\alpha_2 = 0.019$.

(2) Check the stopping boundary to make sure that the familywise error is controlled by using the following SAS statement:

>>**SAS**>>
```
%MINP(Model="fixedW", w1=0.5, w2=0.5, alpha=0.025, beta=0.1,
sigma=0.22, ux=0.05, uy=0.05, nInterim=100, Nmax=200,
DuHa=0.07, nAdj="N", alpha1=0.01, beta1=1, alpha2=0.019);
```
<<**SAS**<<

The simulated familywise error rate $\alpha = 0.0253$. Therefore, the stopping boundaries are confirmed.

(3) Calculate power or sample size required using the following SAS statement:

>>**SAS**>>
%MINP(Model= "fixedW", w1=0.5, w2=0.5, alpha=0.025, beta=0.1,
sigma=0.22, ux=0.05, uy=0.12, nInterim=100, Nmax=200,
DuHa=0.07, nAdj= "N", alpha1=0.01, beta1=1, alpha2=0.019);
<<**SAS**<<

(4) Perform the sensitivity analysis under the condition $H_s$: 0.05 versus 0.1 by submitting the following SAS code:

>>**SAS**>>
%MINP(Model= "fixedW", w1=0.5, w2=0.5, alpha=0.025, beta=0.1,
sigma=0.22, ux=0.05, uy=0.10, nInterim=100, Nmax=200,
DuHa=0.07, nAdj= "N", alpha1=0.01, beta1=1, alpha2=0.019);
<<**SAS**<<

We now summarize the simulation outputs of the three scenarios in Table 5.2.

Table 5.2: Operating Characteristics of GSD with MINP

| Simulation condition | FSP | ESP | N | $N_{max}$ | Power (alpha) |
|---|---|---|---|---|---|
| $H_o$ | 0 | 0.010 | 199 | 200 | (0.025) |
| $H_a$ | 0 | 0.470 | 153 | 200 | 0.873 |
| $H_s$ | 0 | 0.237 | 176 | 200 | 0.597 |

Note that OBF boundary is for early efficacy stopping only and the corresponding error spending for a one-sided test is $\alpha_1 = 0.0025$, $\beta_1 = 1$, and $\alpha_2 = 0.0240$.

We now calculate the adjusted $p$-values (See Chapter 3). If the trial stopped at the first stage, then the $p$-value does not need any adjustment. Suppose the trial is finished, with a stagewise $p$-value for the first stage of $p_1 = 0.012$ (which is larger than $\alpha_1 = 0.01$ and not significant; therefore, the trial continued to the second stage) and the stagewise $p$-value for the second stage of $p_2 = 0.015 < \alpha_2 = 0.019$. Therefore the null hypothesis is rejected. However, $p_2 = 0.015$ is the naive or unadjusted $p$-value. The adjusted $p$-value at stage 2 can be obtained through simulation, which is illustrated as follows:

The conditional (on trial stopping at stage 2) $p$-value is the probability of the stagewise $p$-value at stage 2 being smaller than the observed stagewise $p$-value. Therefore, we can use the same SAS Macro 5.2 for the power calculation to calculate the conditional $p$-value. To do this, we use the observed stagewise $p$-value $p_2$ to replace $\alpha_2$ in SAS Macro 5.2; then $p$-value is $p_{adj} = \alpha_1 + p_c$ from the SAS output. The following is the SAS call to generate (under $H_0$) the adjusted $p$-value:

>>**SAS**>>
%MINP(Model= "fixedW", w1=0.5, w2=0.5, alpha=0.025, beta=0.1,
sigma=0.22, ux=0.05, uy=0.05, nInterim=155, Nmax=310,
DuHa=0.07, nAdj= "N", alpha1=0.01, beta1=1, alpha2=0.015);
<<**SAS**<<

From the SAS outputs, the $p$-value is $p_{adj} = 0.0215 < \alpha$.

**Example 5.2    Inverse-Normal Method with SSR**

Now suppose we want to do sample-size reestimation (SSR) and the interim analysis is planed for 100 patients/group. The SSR rule is given by (4.17) with the parameter of a $= 2$. We present two designs with equal weights: (1) The trial does not allow for early stopping and the interim analysis is for sample-size reestimation only. The stopping boundaries are $\alpha_1 = 0$, $\beta_1 = 1$, and $\alpha_2 = 0.025$; and (2) The interim analysis is for early futility stopping and sample-size reestimation. The stopping boundaries are $\alpha_1 = 0$, $\beta_1 = 0.5$, and $\alpha_2 = 0.0253$. For SSR, the maximum sample-size is $N_{max} = 400$/group, and the initial sample size is $N_0 = 200$/group. We are going to assess the $n$-reestimation mechanism when the treatment difference is small (5% versus 10%) using SAS Macro 5.2.

For design 1, the simulations can be performed using the following SAS macro call:

>>**SAS**>>
%MINP(Model= "fixedW", w1=1, w2=1, alpha=0.025, beta=0.1, sigma=0.22,
ux=0.05, uy=0.1, nInterim=100, Nmax=400, N0=200, nAdj= "Y", DuHa=0.07,
alpha1=0, beta1=1, alpha2=0.025);
<<**SAS**<<

For design 2, the simulations can be performed using the following SAS macro call:

>>**SAS**>>
%MINP(Model= "fixedW", w1=1, w2=1, alpha=0.025, beta=0.1, sigma=0.22,
ux=0.05, uy=0.1, nInterim=100, Nmax=400, N0=200, nAdj= "Y", DuHa=0.07,
alpha1=0, beta1=0.5, alpha2=0.0253);
<<**SAS**<<

We now summarize the simulation results in Table 5.3.

Table 5.3:   Operating Characteristics of an SSR with MSP

| Design | FSP | ESP | N | $N_{max}$ | Power |
|---|---|---|---|---|---|
| Without SSR | 0.167 | 0.237 | 176 | 200 | 0.597 |
| SSR only | 0 | 0 | 304 | 400 | 0.823 |
| SSR & futility stopping | 0.054 | 0 | 304 | 400 | 0.825 |

Note that the results for the design without SSR (i.e., classical group sequential design) are from the sensitivity analysis in Table 5.2. From Table 5.3, we can see that there are similar operating characteristics between the two designs with SSR. Both designs increase the power from 59.7 for the classical group sequential design to over 82%.

## 5.3   Classical Group Sequential Method

In classical group sequential design (GSD), the stopping boundaries are usually specified by a function of stage $k$. The commonly used such functions are Pocock and O'Brien-Fleming boundary functions. Wang and Tsiatis (1987) proposed a family of two-sided tests with a shape parameter $\Delta$, which includes Pocock's and O'Brien-Fleming's boundary functions as special cases. Because W-T boundary is based on $z$-scale, for consistent, we can convert them to $p$-scale. The W-T boundary on $p$-scale is given by

$$a_k > 1 - \Phi\left(\alpha_K \tau_k^{\Delta-1/2}\right), \tag{5.5}$$

where $\tau_k = \frac{k}{K}$ or $\tau_k = \frac{n_k}{n_K}$ (information time), $\alpha_K$ is the stopping boundary at the final stage and a function of the number of stages $K, \alpha,$ and $\Delta$.

Note that the normal statistic $T_k$ from the cumulative sample at the $k$th stage in GSD can be written in the combination of stagewise normal $z$-statistics $(z_i, i = 1, ..., k)$:

$$T_k = \frac{1}{\sqrt{N_k}} \sum_{j=1}^{N_k} (y_j - x_j) = \frac{1}{\sqrt{N_k}} \sum_{i=1}^{k} \sum_{j=1}^{n_i} (y_{i_j} - x_{i_j})$$

$$= \sum_{i=1}^{k} \frac{1}{\sqrt{n_i}} \sum_{j=1}^{n_i} (y_{i_j} - x_{i_j}) \sqrt{\frac{n_i}{N_k}} = \sum_{i=1}^{k} z_i \sqrt{\eta_{ki}},$$

where $x_i$ and $y_i$ are the $i$th observations in group x and y, respectively, $n_i$ = stagewise sample size at stage $i$, $N_k = \Sigma_{j=1}^{k} n_j$ is the cumulative sample size at stage $k$, and the information fraction (not information time!) $\eta_{ki} = \frac{n_i}{N_k} = w_{ki}^2$, and $z_i = \frac{1}{\sqrt{n_i}} \sum_{j=1}^{n_i} (y_{i_j} - x_{i_j})$. For simplicity, we have assumed $\sigma = 1$ in the derivation.

Therefore, in classical GSD method, we can write the test statistic at the $k$th stage as

$$T_k = \sum_{i=1}^{k} w_{ki} z_i, \tag{5.6}$$

where the weights

$$w_{ki} = \sqrt{\eta_{ki}}. \tag{5.7}$$

The method can be extended to other endpoints using the inverse-normal transform, i.e.,

$$T_k = \sum_{i=1}^{k} \sqrt{\eta_{ki}} \Phi^{-1} (1 - p_i). \tag{5.8}$$

For a two-stage design with two independent groups, (5.6) becomes

$$\begin{cases} T_1 = z_1 \\ T_2 = z_1 \sqrt{\frac{n_1}{n_1+n_2}} + z_2 \sqrt{\frac{n_2}{n_1+n_2}} \end{cases}. \tag{5.9}$$

For a group sequential design without SSR the weights $w_{ki} = \sqrt{\eta_{ki}}$ are a prefixed constant, which is basically the same as the L-W method from the previous section. However, it allows for SSR; $\sqrt{\eta_{ki}}(i > 1)$ is a function of $z_j (j = 1, ..., i - 1)$. Therefore, $T_k$ is not a linear combination of $z_i$; hence, it is usually not normal. Consequently, the stopping boundaries for the classical group sequential designs cannot be used in the case with sample-size reestimation. In other words, when the test statistic is defined by (5.6), a new set of stopping boundaries has to be determined using computer simulation when the trial allows for SSR.

The following are the numerical examples of this method used with and without SSR.

## Example 5.3  Group Sequential Design

We will use the asthma trial example again: a phase-III asthma study with 2 dose groups (control and active) with the percent change from baseline in FEV1 as the primary efficacy endpoint. The estimated FEV1 improvement from baseline is 5% and 12% for the control and active groups, respectively, with a common standard deviation of $\sigma = 22\%$. The interim analysis is performed based on the first 100 patients in each group. A futility design is used with $\alpha_1 = 0, \beta_1 = 0.5$, and $\alpha_2 = 0.0253$.

In simulations with the SAS Macro 5.2, the model is specified as "GSD." Again, we study the sensitivity by assuming 5% versus 10% FEV1 change in the control and test groups, respectively. (Note that DuHa = 0.07 not 0.05 should be used for the sensitivity analysis)

(1) Design without sample-size adjustment

Because this is not equal weights design and the interim analysis was not performed for 50% of the patients, we cannot use the stopping boundaries in Table 5.1. The stopping boundaries can be determined using simulations. By fixing $\alpha_1 = 0$, $\beta_1 = 0.5$, and trying different values for $\alpha_2$, we find that $\alpha_1 = 0$, $\beta_1 = 0.5$, and $\alpha_2 = 0.0266$ satisfy the requirement of overall alpha = 0.025. Here is the final SAS macro call to obtain the stopping boundaries:

```
>>SAS>>
%MINP(Model="GSD", alpha=0.025, beta=0.1, sigma=0.22, ux=0.05,
uy=0.05, nInterim=100, Nmax=310, DuHa=0.07, nAdj="N", alpha1=0,
beta1=0.5, alpha2=0.0266);
<<SAS<<
```

The power of the design can be obtained by using the following SAS statement:

```
>>SAS>>
%MINP(Model="GSD", alpha=0.025, beta=0.1, sigma=0.22, ux=0.05,
uy=0.10, nInterim=100, Nmax=310, DuHa=0.07, nAdj="N", alpha1=0,
beta1=0.5, alpha2=0.0266);
<<SAS<<
```

(2) Design with sample-size adjustment

For the design with sample-size adjustment, we have to first determine the stopping boundaries using simulations. By fixing $\alpha_1 = 0$, $\beta_1 = 0.5$, and trying different $\alpha_2$, we find that $\alpha_1 = 0$, $\beta_1 = 0.5$, and $\alpha_2 = 0.0265$ satisfy the overall alpha = 0.025 requirement. We use the following SAS code to determine the stopping boundaries and obtain the power:

```
>>SAS>>
%MINP(Model="GSD", alpha=0.025, beta=0.1, sigma=0.22,
ux=0.05, uy=0.05, nInterim=100, Nmax=400, N0=310, DuHa=0.07, alpha1=0,
nAdj="Y", beta1=0.5, alpha2=0.0265);
%MINP(Model="GSD", alpha=0.025, beta=0.1, sigma=0.22, ux=0.05,
uy=0.10, nInterim=100, Nmax=400, N0=310, DuHa=0.07, nAdj="Y",
alpha1=0, beta1=0.5, alpha2=0.0265);
<<SAS<<
```

The simulation results are presented in Table 5.4.

Table 5.4: Operating Characteristics of a GSD with MSP

| Design | FSP | ESP | N | $N_{max}$ | Power |
|---|---|---|---|---|---|
| Group sequential | 0.054 | 0 | 299 | 310 | 0.795 |
| Adaptive SSR | 0.054 | 0 | 356 | 400 | 0.861 |

## 5.4 Cui–Hung–Wang Method

Cui, Hung, and Wang (1999) developed a method for an adaptive design allowing for sample-size reestimation based on the unblinded results of the interim analysis. Consider a group sequential trial with two groups and one interim analysis.

$$T_2^* = w_1 z_1 + w_2 z_2, \tag{5.10}$$

where the weights $w_i = \sqrt{\frac{n_i}{n_1+n_2}}$, in which the sample size $n_1$ and $n_2$ are the original sample sizes. Because the original $n_2$ can be arbitrarily chosen, the weight $w_i > 0$ can actually be any prefixed positive value satisfying $w_1^2 + w_2^2 = 1$. It is important to remember that the weights are dependent on the originally planned sample size not the modified sample size. When there is actually no modification of sample size, the test statistic is the same as for the classical group sequential design.

There are many possible sample-size adjustment algorithms. Cui et al. (1999) suggest using the following formulation for new sample size at the second stage:

$$n_2^* = \left(\frac{\delta}{\hat{\delta}_1}\right)^2 (n_1 + n_2) - n_1, \tag{5.11}$$

where $\delta$ and $\hat{\delta}$ are the initial estimated treatment difference and the observed difference at stage 1, respectively. The stopping boundaries for Ciu-Hung-Wang's method are the same as for a classical GSD.

## 5.5 Lan–DeMets Method

The Lan–DeMets method (Lan and DeMets, 1983) is an early and very interesting adaptive design method, the error-spending approach, in which they elegantly use the properties of Brownian (Wiener) motion.

### 5.5.1 *Brownian Motion*

Brownian motion (Figure 5.1) has been widely studied and the results are ready to use for sequential designs in clinical trials.

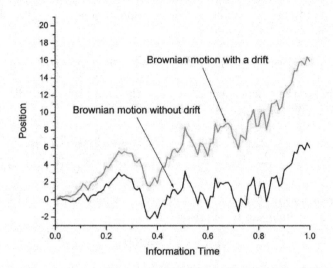

Figure 5.1: Examples of Brownian motion

**Definition 5.1:** A stochastic process $\{X(t), t \geq 0\}$ is said to be a Brownian motion with a drift $\mu$ if

(1) $X(0) = 0$;

(2) $\{X(t), t \geq 0\}$ has a stationary and independent increment;

(3) for every $t > 0, X(t)$ is normally distributed with mean $\mu t$ and variance $\sigma^2 t$, i.e.,

$$X(t) \sim \frac{1}{\sqrt{2\pi\sigma^2 t}} \exp\left(-\frac{(x - \mu t)^2}{2\sigma^2 t}\right). \tag{5.12}$$

The covariance of the Brownian motion is $\text{cov}[X(t), X(s)] = \sigma^2 \min\{s, t\}$.

The standard Brownian motion $B(t)$ is the Brownian motion with $\mu = 0$ and $\sigma^2 = 1$. The conditional probability density function of $B(t)$ is given by

$$p\left(x_2, t | x_1\right) = \frac{1}{\sqrt{2\pi t}} \exp\left(-\frac{1}{2t}\left(x_2 - x_1\right)^2\right), \tag{5.13}$$

where $x_1 = x_1\left(t_1\right)$, $x_2 = x_2\left(t_2\right)$, and $t_2 > t_1$.

The conditional probability of the position at time $t + s$ given the position at time $s$ can be written as

$$\Pr\left\{B\left(t + s\right) \le y | B\left(s\right) = x\right\} = \Phi\left(\frac{y - x}{\sqrt{t}}\right). \tag{5.14}$$

Because of the independent increment, the joint probability distribution of $X\left(t_1\right), ..., X\left(t_n\right)$ is given by

$$f\left(x_1, ..., x_n\right) = \sum_{i=1}^{n} f_{t_i - t_{i-1}}\left(x_i - x_{i-1}\right) = \frac{\exp\left(-\frac{1}{2}\sum_{i=1}^{n}\frac{(x_i - x_{i-1})^2}{t_i - t_{i-1}}\right)}{(2\pi)^{n/2}\sqrt{\Pi_{i=1}^{n}\left(t_i - t_{i-1}\right)}}. \tag{5.15}$$

The relationship between the standard Brownian motion and Brownian motion with drift $\mu$ can be expressed as

$$X\left(t\right) = \mu t + \sigma B\left(t\right). \tag{5.16}$$

The cumulative probability is given by

$$\Pr\left\{X\left(t\right) \le y | X\left(0\right) = x\right\} = \Phi\left(\frac{y - x - \mu t}{\sigma\sqrt{t}}\right). \tag{5.17}$$

**The First Hitting of Standard Brownian Motion:**

Let $C$ be a horizontal boundary (Figure 5.1) and $M(t)$ be the maximum of the standard Brownian motion with time $t$, i.e., $M(t) = \max_{0 \le u \le t} B(u)$. It can be proved, using the reflection principle (Taylor and Karlin, 1998, p. 491–493), that the probability of the first passing (the boundary) before time $t > 0$ can be expressed as

$$\Pr\left\{M\left(t\right) \ge C\right\} = 2\left[1 - \Phi\left(\frac{C}{\sqrt{t}}\right)\right]. \tag{5.18}$$

Equation (5.18) can be used directly to control type-I error (see next subsection).

**Remarks:** There are many examples of Brownian motion. Einstein showed that the solution $\nu$ for the diffusion or permeability equation $\frac{\partial \nu}{\partial t} = \frac{1}{2}\sigma^2\frac{\partial^2 \nu}{\partial x^2}$ is the Brownian motion (5.12) with a unit diffusion coefficient. Random-walk with a varied step length forms a Brownian motion.

Brownian motion is also known as a memoryless process. The independence of the increment process also implies that we can predict the future as long as we know the current status. However, in many cases, to predict the future, we have to know not only the present, but also the past.

### 5.5.2 Lan–DeMets Error-Spending Method

Brownian motion was first introduced by Lan and DeMets (1983) to the adaptive design with a prefixed error spending function, which allows for changing the timing and the number of analyses.

We know from (5.6) and (5.7) that the test statistic based on the cumulative sample size at the $k$th stage can be written as

$$Z_k = \Sigma_{i=1}^k z_i \sqrt{\eta_{ki}}. \tag{5.19}$$

When the maximum sample size $N$ is fixed, i.e., without SSR, the Brownian motion can be constructed as follows:

$$B_k = Z_k \sqrt{\tau_k}, \tag{5.20}$$

where the information time $\tau_k = \frac{N_k}{N}$, $N_k = \Sigma_{i=1}^k n_i$.

From (5.20), the following properties can be obtained using simple calculations:

(1) $E[B_N(\tau)] = \theta \sqrt{N}$

(2) $var(B_N(\tau)) = \tau$

(3) $cov(B_N(\tau_1), B_N(\tau_2)) = \min(\tau_1, \tau_2)$

Note that $B_k$ is a linear function of information time $\tau_k \in [0, 1]$. Because the Brownian motion is not observable between two interim analyses, we can assign an accumulated crossing probability to the information time point $\tau_k$.

Brownian motion is formed only if the trial continues without any early stopping. However, if we are interested in the first pass (efficacy or futility), then Brownian motion results can be used for the trial with early stopping.

We can see that the Brownian motion can be viewed as weighted stage-wise $z$-scores, where the weights are

$$w_{ki} = \sqrt{\tau_k \eta_{ki}}. \tag{5.21}$$

The Lan–DeMets method is similar to, but different from, the L–W method because the weights $w_{ki} = \sqrt{\tau_k \eta_{ki}}$ are not a prefixed constant. Instead, they are a prefixed function of information time. Note that the Lan–DeMets method uses the same stopping boundaries as a classical GSD, because for each fixed information time, the test statistic is the same as a classical GSD. For the two-stage design, the stopping boundaries and power can be obtained through simulation using SAS Macros 5.1 and 5.2.

We now use Brownian motion to illustrate the error-spending method because Lan and DeMets (1983) originally proposed the error-spending approach using Brownian motion.

If $H_0$ is rejected whenever the position of the Brownian motion first crosses the boundary $C$, then we can control overall $\alpha$ by letting the maximum crossing probability $\Pr\{M(1) \geq C\} = \alpha$ and solving (5.18) for $C$. In other words, from $2[1 - \Phi(C)] = \alpha$, we can immediately obtain $C = z_{1-\alpha/2} = \Phi^{-1}(1 - \alpha/2)$. We now designate the error-spending function to be the first passing probability (5.18), i.e.,

$$\pi^*(\tau_k) = \begin{cases} 2\left[1 - \Phi\left(\frac{z_{1-\alpha/2}}{\sqrt{\tau_k}}\right)\right], & \tau_k > 0 \\ 0, & \tau_k = 0 \end{cases} . \tag{5.22}$$

Note that $\pi^*(t)$ is an increasing function in $t$ or information time $\tau_k$ and $\pi^*(1) = \alpha$, the one-sided significance level.

As stated in Chapter 3, for the error-spending approach, the stopping boundaries are determined by

$$\Pr\left\{\cap_{j=1}^{k-1}\left[\beta_j < B(t_j) < \alpha_j\right] \cap B(t_k) \geq \alpha_k\right\} = \pi^*(\tau_k) - \pi^*(\tau_{k-1}). \tag{5.23}$$

Using (5.15), (5.23) becomes

$$\int_{\beta_1}^{\alpha_1} \cdots \int_{\beta_{i-1}}^{\alpha_{k-1}} \int_{\alpha_k}^{\infty} \frac{\exp\left(-\frac{1}{2}\sum_{i=1}^{n}\frac{(x_i - x_{i-1})^2}{t_i - t_{i-1}}\right)}{(2\pi)^{n/2}\sqrt{\Pi_{i=1}^{n}(t_i - t_{i-1})}} dx_1 \cdots dx_{k-1}dx_k$$
$$= \pi^*(\tau_k) - \pi^*(\tau_{k-1}). \tag{5.24}$$

Lan and DeMets (1983) formulated the problem without early futility stopping boundaries. Here it is generalized to the design allowing for futility stopping. Determination of the stopping boundaries $(\beta_i, \alpha_i; i = 1, ..., K)$ requires either numerical integration (Armitage, McPherson, and Rowe, 1969; Jennison and Turnbull, 2000a) or computer simulations (See Chapter 6).

The error-spending function can be any nondecreased error-spending function $\pi^*(t)$ with a range of $[0,1]$. When $\pi^*(\tau_k) = \pi^*(\tau_{k-1})$, the $k$th stage interim analysis is used for either futility stopping or modifying the design (such as its randomization), but not for efficacy stopping. Note that (5.22) is the error-spending function corresponding to the O'Brien–Fleming stopping boundaries. Other commonly used error spending functions include Pocock's $\pi^*(t) = \alpha \log[1 + (e - 1)t]$ (Kim and DeMets, 1992) and power family: $\pi^*(t) = \alpha t^\theta, \theta > 0$.

When the error-spending function $\pi^*(t)$ is prefixed, i.e., not dependent on the observed data from the trial, then the overall type-I error rate is $\Sigma_{k=1}^K \pi_k = \Sigma_{k=1}^K [\pi^*(\tau_k) - \pi^*(\tau_{k-1})] = \pi^*(1) - \pi^*(0) = \alpha$. This is true even when the number of analyses $K$ and the timing of the analyses $\tau_k$ are not predetermined. This is the most attractive feature of the error-spending function. We further illustrate the approach in the following example.

## Example 5.4   Changes in Number and Timing of Interim Analyses

An international, multicenter, randomized phase-III study to compare the test drug with a combination of drugs in patients with newly diagnosed multiple myeloma was designed using the O'Brien–Fleming spending function. The interim analysis was to be performed for 200 patients. The final analysis will be performed using 400 patients. The primary study objective is to assess the treatment difference in overall complete response rate (CR) obtained at the end of a 16-week induction phase. However, due to the complexity of the international trial, the data collection and validation became extremely challenging. It was decided that the investigator's assessment would be used because it is available much earlier than the assessment by the independent review committee (IRC)—the gold standard. However, the discrepancies between the two assessments are not known. The sponsor is concerned that if the trial is stopped based on the IDMC's recommendation, which is based on the investigator's assessment, it could be found later that the treatment difference is not significant based on the IRC's assessment. However, it is known that when the trial is stopped at the first interim analysis (IA), there will be more patients enrolled (about 300). Therefore, the sponsor decided to add a second interim analysis. The second IA is very interesting to the sponsor because if the results are significant at the first interim analysis based on investigator's assessment ($\alpha = 0.0025$), then the $p$-value based on the IRC's assessment should be somewhat close to 0.0025. With 300 patients (the exact number is based on the number of patients randomized at the first IA) at the second IA and based on the OBF spending function (5.22), the error spent on the three analyses is $\pi_1 = 2[1 - \Phi(\frac{2.240}{\sqrt{200/400}})] = 0.0016$, $\pi_2 = 2[1 - \Phi(\frac{2.240}{\sqrt{300/400}})] - 0.0016 = 0.0096 - 0.0016 = 0.008$ , and $\pi_3 = 2[1 - \Phi(2.240)] - 0.0096 = 0.025 - 0.0096 = 0.0154$. The actual $\pi_2$ should be based on the actual number of patients at the second IA.

## 5.6    Fisher–Shen Method

Fisher and Shen (Fisher, 1998; Shen and Fisher, 1999) proposed a self-designing approach for $k$-stage designs. In this method, the test statistic is defined similarly to Lehmacher–Wassmer's method, i.e., it is the weighted sums of the standardized difference $z_i$. However, the weights $w_i$ at each stage may be determined based on data from previous stages, and the number of stages $K$ does not have to be prefixed, but the condition $\Sigma_{i=1}^{K} w_i^2 = 1$ must be met. Fisher does not consider early stopping in his method. Shen and Fisher consider early futility stopping ($\alpha_1 = 0$), but do not account for its impact on type-I error; hence, it is a conservative approach.

## 5.7    Summary

In this chapter we have studied broad methods that are based on weighted inverse-normal stagewise $p$-values. The weights can be fixed such as in the GSD, the L-W method, and the Cui–Hung–Wang method, or varied depending on observed data, as in the Fisher–Shen and Lan–DeMets methods. The Cui–Hung–Wang method can be used for sample-size reestimation for a normal endpoint, and the L-W method can be used for SSR for various endpoints. The Lan–DeMets method can be used for adaptive designs with changes in the number and the timing of analyses. Fisher–Shen is a method that can be used for SSR, but it is conservative because the futility boundaries at earlier stages are not used in the construction of later stopping boundaries. Deciding which method and design are best for a trial is heavily dependent on the practical setting. Simulations should be used to assist in decision making. The SAS macros in this chapter provide powerful tools for accomplishing this goal. The electronic versions of the simulation programs can be obtained at www.statisticians.org.

## Problems

**5.1** Suppose the median times for the two treatment groups in Example 4.7 are 9 months and 12 months. Design an adaptive trial and justify the adaptive design method (MIP, MSP, MPP, MINP) and the design you have chosen.

**5.2** Use the reflection principle (Taylor and Karlin, 1998, p. 497) to prove that

$$\Pr\{M(t) \geq z,\ B(t) \leq y\} = \Pr\{B(t) \geq 2z - x\} = 1 - \Phi\left(\frac{2z - y}{\sqrt{t}}\right).$$

**5.3** The Gamler's Ruin Problem (Taylor and Karlin, 1998, p. 509)

Theorem: For a Brownian motion with drift parameter $\mu$ and variance $\sigma^2$, and $a < x < b$,

$$u(x) = \Pr\{X(T_{ab}) = b | X(0) = x\} = \frac{e^{-2\mu x/\sigma^2} - e^{-2\mu a/\sigma^2}}{e^{-2\mu b/\sigma^2} - e^{-2\mu a/\sigma^2}}, \qquad (5.25)$$

where $T_{ab}$ is a random time at which the process $X(t)$ first assumes one of the values a or b. The so-called hitting time is defined by

$$T_{ab} = \min\{t \geq 0; X(t) = a \text{ or } X(t) = b\}. \qquad (5.26)$$

It can be seen that $u(x)$ is the conditional probability of hitting threshold $b$ given the first hit occurs.

The expectation of $u(x)$ is given by

$$E[T_{ab}|X(0) = x] = \frac{1}{\mu}[u(x)(b - a) - (x - a)].$$

It is interesting to know that we cannot obtain the velocity of the Brownian motion particle by taking the derivative of $B(t)$ with respect to $t$ because $B(t)$ is continuous but not differentiable at any single point (Taylor and Karlin, 1998, p. 509). This counter-intuitive fact is difficult to comprehend.

For $\mu- > 0$, and $\sigma- > 1$, (5.25) becomes

$$u(x) = \Pr\{B(T_{ab}) = b | B(0) = x\} = \frac{x - a}{b - a}.$$

Study the possibility of using these results in adaptive design.

# Chapter 6

# Adaptive Noninferiority Design with Paired Binary Data

Noninferiority of a diagnostic test to the standard is a common issue in medical research. For instance, we may be interested in determining if a new diagnostic test is noninferior to the standard reference test because the new test might be inexpensive to the extent that some small inferior margin in sensitivity or specificity may be acceptable. Noninferiority trials are also found to be useful in clinical trials, such as image studies, where the data are collected in pairs. In such a trial sensitivity and specificity are often the two coprimary endpoints. It is usually required to demonstrate that the method is superior to the control in sensitivity and noninferior in specificity. In this chapter, we study how to design such a trial using an adaptive approach for adaptive noninferiority trial with paired binary data, including a trial example and providing the SAS program for the design simulations.

## 6.1 Noninferiority Design

As the European regulatory agency, Committee for Medicinal Products for Human Use (CHMP, 2005) stated, "Many clinical trials comparing a test product with an active comparator are designed as noninferiority trials. The term 'noninferiority' is now well established, but if taken literally could be misleading. The objective of a noninferiority trial is sometimes stated as being to demonstrate that the test product is not inferior to the comparator. However, only a superiority trial can demonstrate this. In fact a noninferiority trial aims to demonstrate that the test product is not worse than the comparator by more than a pre-specified, small amount. This amount is known as the noninferiority margin, or delta".

Until recent years, the majority of clinical trials were designed for superiority to a comparative drug (the control group). A statistic shows that
only 23% of all NDAs from 1998 to 2002 were innovative drugs, and the rest
were accounted for as "me-too" drugs (Chang, 2010). The "me-too" drugs
are judged based on noninferiority criteria. The increasing popularity of
noninferiority trials is a reflection of regulatory and industry adjustments
in response to increasing challenges in drug development.

From a methodological perspective, Brittain and Hu (2009) studied noninferiority trial design and analysis with an ordered three-level categorical
endpoint. Chan (2002) derived power and sample size formulations for
noninferiority trials using an exact method. Cook, Lee, and Li (2007)
studied noninferiority trial design for recurrent events. Kong, Kohberger,
and Koch (2004), studied noninferiority trials with correlated multiple endpoints. Rothmann et al. (2003) studied noninferiority mortality trials in
oncology. Tang and Tang (2004) studied tests of noninferiority via rate
difference for three-arm clinical trials with placebo. Wang, Chen, and Chi
(2006) studied a ratio test in active control noninferiority trials with time-
to-event endpoint. Wang, Hung, Tsong, and Cui (2001) studied group
sequential test strategies for superiority and noninferiority hypotheses in
active control clinical trials. Wiens and Heyes (2003) studied interactions
in noninferiority trials. Liu, Proschan, and Pledger (2002) investigated two
asymptotic test statistics, a Wald-type test statistic (sample-based) and a
restricted maximum likelihood estimation (RMLE-based) test statistic, to
assess noninferiority based on paired binary endpoints. They found that
the RMLE-based test controls type-I error better than the sample-based
test. Lu and Bean (1995) and Nam (1997) proposed test statistics and
sample-size determination for comparing two diagnostic methods for the
noninferiority test of sensitivity. Lu, Jin, and Genant (2003) discussed simultaneous comparisons of sensitivity and specificity. They presented three
different testing procedures and sample-size formulae for simultaneous comparison of sensitivity and specificity based on paired observations and with
known disease status. Sidik (2003) studied two exact unconditional tests
and showed that the asymptotic test is inaccurate, that is, its size exceeds
the claimed nominal level when sample sizes are small or moderately large.

There are three major sources of uncertainty about the conclusions from
a noninferiority (NI) study: (1) the uncertainty of the active-control effect
over a placebo, which is estimated from historical data; (2) the possibility
that the control effect may change over time, violating the "constancy assumption"; and (3) the risk of making a wrong decision from the test of the

noninferiority hypothesis in the NI study, i.e., the type-I error. These three uncertainties have to be considered in developing a noninferiority design method.

Most commonly used noninferiority trials are based on parallel, two-group designs. Three-group designs with a placebo may sometimes be used, but they are not very cost-effective and often face ethical challenges when including a placebo group, especially in the United States.

There are three commonly used methods of noninferiority designs: the fixed-margin method, the $\lambda$-portion method, and the synthesis method (in original and log scales). We denote the test and the active-control groups by subscripts $T$ and $C$, respectively. Where there is no confusion, the letter $T$ will also be used for test statistics. We will use the hat "^" to represent an estimate of the corresponding parameter, e.g., $\hat{\theta}$ is an estimate of $\theta$.

### 6.1.1 *Fixed-Margin Method*

The null hypothesis for the fixed-margin method can be defined as

$$H_0 : \theta_T - \theta_C - \delta_{NI} \leq 0, \tag{6.1}$$

where $\theta$ can be the mean, hazard rate, adverse event rate, recurrent events rate, or mean number of events. The constant noninferiority margin $\delta_{NI} \leq 0$ (assuming a larger value of the parameter is desirable; otherwise, $\delta_{NI}$ should be larger than zero) is usually determined based on a historical placebo-control study (see more discussions later). When $\delta_{NI} = 0$, (6.1) becomes a null hypothesis test for superiority.

The rejection of (6.1) can be expressed a simple way: The test drug $T$ is not inferior to $C$ by $\delta_{NI}$ or more.

### 6.1.2 *$\lambda$-Portion Method*

The null hypothesis for the $\lambda$-portion method is given by

$$H_0 : \theta_T - \lambda_{NI}\theta_C \leq 0, \tag{6.2}$$

where $0 < \lambda_{NI} < 1$. For the superiority test, $\lambda_{NI} = 1$.

The rejection of (6.2) can be interpreted in layman's terms: Drug $T$ is at least $100\lambda_{NI}\%$ as effective as drug $C$.

### 6.1.3    *Synthesis Method*

The null hypothesis for the synthesis method is given by

$$H_0 : \frac{\theta_T - \theta_P}{\theta_C - \theta_P} - \lambda_{NI} \leq 0. \tag{6.3}$$

Assuming we have proved $\theta_C - \theta_P > 0$, (6.3) is then equivalent to

$$H_0 : \theta_T - \theta_C + (1 - \lambda_{NI})(\theta_C - \theta_P) \leq 0, \tag{6.4}$$

where $0 < \lambda_{NI} < 1$. For the superiority test, $\lambda_{NI} = 1$.

The rejection of (6.3) can summed up in these terms: The test drug $T$ is at least $100\lambda_{NI}\%$ as effective as $C$ after subtracting the placebo effect. When $\lambda_{NI} = 0$, (6.3) represents a null hypothesis for a putative placebo-control trial.

## 6.2    Noninferiority Design with Fixed-Margin Method for Paired Data

### 6.2.1    *Classical Design*

Let $Y_1$ and $Y_2$ be, respectively, binary response variables of treatments 1 and 2 with the joint distribution $P(Y_1 = i; Y_2 = j) = p_{ij}$ for $i = 0, 1; j = 0, 1$. $\sum_{i=0}^{1} \sum_{j=0}^{1} p_{ij} = 1$. Paired data are commonly displayed in a $2 \times 2$ contingency table (Table 6.1).

Table 6.1:    Matched-Pair Data

|         | Test | | Total |
|---------|------|------|-------|
| Control | 1    | 0    |       |
| 1       | $x_{11}$ | $x_{10}$ |   |
| 0       | $x_{01}$ | $x_{00}$ |   |
| Total   |      |      | $n$   |

Nam (1997, 1998) proposed the following asymptotic test for paired data:

$$H_0 : p_{10} - p_{01} - \delta_{NI} \leq 0 \text{ vs. } H_a: H_0, \tag{6.5}$$

where $\delta_{NI} < 0$ is the noninferiority margin. The test statistic is defined as

$$Z = \frac{\hat{\varepsilon}\sqrt{n}}{\hat{\sigma}}, \tag{6.6}$$

where

$$\begin{cases} \hat{\varepsilon} = \hat{p}_{10} - \hat{p}_{01} - \delta_{NI}, \\ \hat{p}_{ij} = x_{ij}/n, \\ \hat{\sigma}^2 = 2\tilde{p}_{01} + \delta_{NI} - \delta_{NI}^2, \end{cases} \tag{6.7}$$

and $\tilde{p}_{10}$ is the restricted MLE of $p_{10}$:

$$\begin{cases} \tilde{p}_{01} = \frac{-b+\sqrt{b^2-8c}}{4}, \\ b = (2 + \hat{p}_{01} - \hat{p}_{10}) \delta_{NI} - \hat{p}_{01} - \hat{p}_{10}, \\ c = -\hat{p}_{01}\delta_{NI} (1 - \delta_{NI}). \end{cases} \tag{6.8}$$

Nam (1997) proved that $Z$ in (6.6) follows approximately the normal distribution for large $n$,

$$Z \sim N\left(\frac{\sqrt{n}\varepsilon}{\sigma}, 1\right), \tag{6.9}$$

where $\varepsilon = E(\hat{\varepsilon})$ and $\sigma = E(\hat{\sigma})$ can be obtained by replacing $\hat{p}_{ij}$ with $p_{ij}$ ($i = 0, 1; j = 0, 1$) in the corresponding expression (6.7).

The rejection rule is specified as follows (assuming a larger $\theta$ is preferred):

$$\begin{cases} \text{Reject } H_0 \text{ if } Z \geq z_{1-\alpha}, \\ \text{Accept } H_0 \text{ otherwise.} \end{cases} \tag{6.10}$$

Equivalently, we can use the confidence interval of $\varepsilon$:

$$\begin{cases} \text{Reject } H_0 \text{ if } \hat{\varepsilon} - z_{1-\alpha}\frac{\hat{\sigma}}{\sqrt{n}} \geq 0, \\ \text{Accept } H_0 \text{ otherwise.} \end{cases} \tag{6.11}$$

The power of the test statistic $T$ under a particular $H_a$ can be expressed as

$$1 - \beta = \Phi\left(\frac{\varepsilon\sqrt{n}}{\sigma} - z_{1-\alpha}\right), \tag{6.12}$$

where $\varepsilon$ and $\sigma$ are estimated by (6.7).

Solving (6.12) for the sample size, we obtain

$$n = \begin{cases} \frac{(z_{1-\alpha}+z_{1-\beta})^2\sigma^2}{\varepsilon^2}, \text{ for } \varepsilon > 0 \\ \infty, \text{ for } \varepsilon \leq 0 \end{cases}. \tag{6.13}$$

Equation (6.13) is a general sample-size formulation for a trial with a normal, binary, or survival endpoint (2007).

For the test statistic given by (6.9), the $p$-value is given by

$$p = 1 - \Phi\left(\frac{\hat{\varepsilon}\sqrt{n}}{\hat{\sigma}}\right), \qquad (6.14)$$

where $\Phi$ is the standard normal cdf.

**Remark:** A common misconception is that for an NI trial the sample-size calculation must assume $\theta_T = \theta_C$ or $p_{01} = p_{10}$, which is not true at all. One can choose an NI design because the difference $\theta_T - \theta_C$ is positive but too small for a superiority test with reasonable power or unreasonably large sample size. The treatment difference can be positive or negative depending on the particular situation. The power and sample size calculation should be based on the best knowledge about the value of $\theta_T - \theta_C$, and this knowledge should not change because of the different choice of hypothesis test. Therefore, for given values of $\theta_T - \theta_C$ and power, superiority testing always requires a larger sample size than noninferiority testing.

### 6.2.2   *Adaptive Design*

We now discuss how to incorporate Nam's (1997) formulation into group sequential and adaptive designs. Let $T_k$ be a test statistic on $p$-value scale at the $k$th stage. The stopping rules are given by

$$\begin{cases} \text{Stop for efficacy} & \text{if } T_k \leq \alpha_k, \\ \text{Stop for futility} & \text{if } T_k > \beta_k, \\ \text{Continue with adaptations if } \alpha_k < T_k \leq \beta_k, \end{cases} \qquad (6.15)$$

In a classical group sequential or adaptive design, the test statistic on $p$-value scale can be expressed as

$$T_k = 1 - \Phi\left(\sum_{i=1}^{k} w_{ki}\Phi^{-1}(1 - p_i)\right), \qquad (6.16)$$

where the weights $w_{ki}$ satisfy $\sum_{i=1}^{k} w_{ki}^2 = 1$. The weights $w_{ki}$ can be functions of the information time or sample-size fraction. For the error-spending approach, $w_{ki} = \sqrt{\frac{n_i}{\sum_{j=1}^{k} n_j}}$, $i = 1, ..., k$, $k = 1, ..., K$, where $n_i$ is the subsample size (not cumulative sample size) at stage $i$. Using the error-spending approach, the changes in the timing (information time) of the interim analyses and the total number of analyses can be changed after the initiation of the trial as long as the change is independent of treatment difference. For sample-size reestimation, we use fixed weights $w_{ki}$, i.e., the weight will not change even when the sample size is modified.

For the error-spending approach numerical integrations give the O'Brien–Fleming (OF)-like boundary, Pocock-like boundary (PF), and power-function (PF) boundary (with $\rho = 0.2$) as follows: $\alpha_1 = 0.00260$ and $\alpha_2 = 0.0240$ (OF), $\alpha_1 = 0.0147$ and $\alpha_2 = 0.0147$ (Pocock), and $\alpha_1 = 0.00625$ and $\alpha_2 = 0.02173$ (PF). These stopping boundaries will be used later in our trial example.

If we use Nam's test statistic defined by (6.6)–(6.8) for the subsample at the $i$th stage, we can then calculate the "stagewise" $p$-value for the $i$th stage based on (6.14), that is,

$$p_i = 1 - \Phi \left( \frac{\hat{\varepsilon}_i \sqrt{n_i}}{\hat{\sigma}_i} \right), \tag{6.17}$$

where $\hat{\varepsilon}_i$, $n_i$, and $\hat{\sigma}_i$ are the corresponding quantities in (6.14) but calculated based on a subsample at the $i$th stage. (6.18) is valid as long as $n_i$ is large.

## 6.3 Conditional Power and Sample-Size Reestimation

The general expression of conditional power at the interim analysis for a two-stage adaptive design can be written as (Chapter 9):

$$cP_\delta (p_1) = 1 - \Phi \left( \frac{\Phi^{-1}(1-\alpha_2) - w_1 \Phi^{-1}(1-p_1)}{w_2} - \frac{\hat{\varepsilon}_1 \sqrt{n_2}}{\hat{\sigma}_1} \right), \alpha_1 < p_1 \le \beta_1. \tag{6.18}$$

If the trial continues, i.e., $\alpha_1 < p_1 \le \beta_1$, for a given conditional power $cP$, we can solve (6.19) for the adjusted sample size for the second stage:

$$n_2 = \begin{cases} \frac{\sigma_1^2}{\varepsilon_1^2} \left( B \left( \alpha_2, z_1 \right) - \Phi^{-1} \left( 1 - cP \right) \right)^2, & \text{if } \varepsilon > 0 \\ \infty, & \text{if } \varepsilon \le 0. \end{cases} \tag{6.19}$$

## 6.4 Type-I Error Control

We have used an approximation of the normal distribution for $z$ given by (6.6) and (6.17) for the classical and adaptive designs, respectively. We want to check how well such approximations work in terms of type-I error control. Various scenarios have been checked with 1,000,000 simulation runs for each scenario. The scenarios with larger type-I errors are presented in Table 6.2 (sample size = 3000 pairs). For a classical design, we use 3000 pairs. For an adaptive design with sample-size reestimation, we use 1500 pairs for the interim analysis and the maximum sample size allowed is $N_{max} = 6000$. We can see from the Table 6.2 that type-I error is well controlled

Table 6.2:   Type-I Error Rate Control (%) against $\alpha = 2.5\%$

| Design | Proportion $p_{10}$ (%) | | | | | | | | | |
|---|---|---|---|---|---|---|---|---|---|---|
| | 0.5 | 1.0 | 2.0 | 3.0 | 4.0 | 5.0 | 10 | 20 | 30 | 50 |
| Classical Sup | 2.9 | 2.6 | 2.4 | 2.4 | 2.3 | 2.3 | 2.0 | 1.4 | 0.9 | 0.3 |
| Classical NI | 2.6 | 2.6 | 2.4 | 2.4 | 2.3 | 2.2 | 1.9 | 1.2 | 0.7 | 0.1 |
| GSD Sup | 2.9 | 2.7 | 2.5 | 2.4 | 2.3 | 2.2 | 1.9 | 1.4 | 0.9 | 0.3 |
| SSR Sup | 2.8 | 2.6 | 2.4 | 2.4 | 2.3 | 2.2 | 1.9 | 1.4 | 0.9 | 0.3 |
| SSR NI | 2.7 | 2.5 | 2.4 | 2.3 | 2.2 | 2.2 | 1.8 | 1.7 | 0.7 | 0.1 |

Note: $N = 3000$, $N_{max} = 6000$, NI margin $\delta_{NI} = -0.5p_{10}$.
For superiority design, $p_{10} = p_{01}$. SSR = Sample-size reestimation

when the proportion $p_{10} \geq 2\%$. When $p_{10} < 2\%$, there is a slight inflation of the error.

When we run the same set of simulations with a smaller sample size of 300 pairs and $N_{max} = 600$ pairs, the type-I error is far below 2.5% for all cases. For $p_{10} \geq 2\%$, smaller sample sizes give smaller error but the difference is small; for $p_{10} < 2\%$, the error is much smaller than 2.5% with 300 pairs. Therefore, we can say the method can be applied to NI adaptive designs.

## 6.5   Prostate Cancer Diagnostic Trial

### 6.5.1   *Preliminary Data for Trial Design*

The adaptive design considerations will be oriented toward comparisons of the diagnostic performance of two scanning methods, separately for sensitivity (using data from positive patients) and specificity (using data from negative patients).

The two methods (Method 1 is a good standard) for the detection of metastatic disease in a group of subjects with known prostate cancer use standardized clinical end points of documented disease including clinical outcome, serial PSA levels, contrast enhanced CT scans, and radionuclide bone scans. A small study was conducted on a group of matched patients. The sensitivity and specificity are presented in Table 6.3.

Table 6.3:   Sensitivity and Specificity

| Method | Sensitivity | Specificity |
|---|---|---|
| 1 | 63% | 80% |
| 2 | 84% | 80% |

The $2 \times 2$ table of the data for the McNemar's Test in positive patients per CT/Bone Scan is given in Table 6.4. The $2 \times 2$ table of the data for the

Table 6.4:   Positive Patients per CT/Bone Scan

|            | Method 1 | |
|------------|----------|----------|
| Method 2   | Positive | Negative |
| Positive   | 62%      | 20%      |
| Negative   | 3%       | 15%      |

Table 6.5:   Negative Patients per CT/Bone Scan

|            | Method 1 | |
|------------|----------|----------|
| Method 2   | Negative | Positive |
| Negative   | 60%      | 10%      |
| Positive   | 10%      | 20%      |

McNemar's Test in negative patients per CT/Bone Scan is given in Table 6.5.

### 6.5.2   *The Effectiveness Requirements*

The requirements for gaining the regulatory approval are defined as follows:

- Superiority on sensitivity with 10% margin (point estimate) and NI on specificity with 7.5% margin (CI); the hypothesis testing is based on the results from 2 of 3 image readers.
- Statistical methods: McNemar's test with and without cluster adjustment. However, since we don't have data about the cluster, our sample-size calculation will be based on testing without considering clustering.

The effectiveness claim will be based primarily on subject-level results, that is, a diagnosis of whether or not the patient has any evidence of metastatic prostate cancer, disregarding the number of sites of disease. The analyses of lesions will provide additional information on the ability of the diagnostic tests to determine localization and staging of the disease. For this reason, the sample size will be based on analysis results on the subject level. It is required that Method 2 has at least a 10% improvement (based on a point estimate) over Method 1 in sensitivity and is noninferior to Method 1 in specificity with a margin of 7.5%.

### 6.5.3   *Design for Sensitivity*

For the sensitivity requirement, we use group sequential design to handle the uncertain information with high power 95%. The simulation is done by setting the noninferiority margin to zero in the SAS Macro 6.1, which was also verified using the commercial software package ExpDesign Studio 5.0.

For the purpose of comparison, we first calculate the sample size required for the classical design. Given the data in Table 6.4, i.e., $p_{10} = 0.2$ and $p_{01} = 0.03$, for a 95% power at a level of significance 2.5% (one-sided), 82 pairs are required based on McNemar's test with data provided in Table 6.4.

For group sequential designs (GSD), three different error-spending functions are considered: (1) the O'Brien-Fleming-like error-spending function, (2) the power-function with $\rho = 2$, and (3) the Pocock-like error-spending function.

Given the data in Table 6.4 and a 95% power, we design the group sequential trial with one interim analysis at 50% information time. The simulation results are presented in Table 6.6. To choose an "optimal" design, we perform the following comparisons:

(1) Comparing the results from the OF and the PF designs, we can see that the latter requires a smaller expected sample size ($\bar{N}_a$), a 7.5% reduction (73 versus 67.5 pairs) because the PF design has a larger early efficacy stopping probability (ESP = 0.429) than the OF design (ESP = 0.263). The maximum sample size is almost the same for the two designs. Therefore, the PF design with $\rho = 2$ is a better design than the OF design.

(2) Comparing the results from the Pocock and PF designs, we can see that the latter requires a smaller maximum sample-size (86 versus 92) and a smaller expected sample-size (67.5 versus 63.2). We further compare the sample sizes required under other conditions, such as $H_0$.

(3) Under $H_0$: $p_{10} = p_{01} = 0.2$, the expected sample sizes are 65.3, 66.7, and 71 pairs for the OF, the PF, and the Pocock designs, respectively. The expected sample sizes under $H_0$ are thus similar for the OF and PF designs while being smaller than that for the Pocock design. The early futility stopping probabilities (EFP) are almost identical, i.e., 45% for all three designs, which deviates from the theoretical value 50% due to approximation in normality. Based on these comparisons, we believe the design with PF ($\rho = 2$) is the best design among the three. The design can save about 18% in the expected sample size from the classical design (67 versus 82 pairs).

### 6.5.4  *Design for Specificity*

For specificity, due to large uncertainty in the information (rates in Table 6.4), our design starts with a lower power 85%, then uses sample-size

Table 6.6:   Operating Characteristics of AD under $H_a$ for Sensitivity

| | $\alpha_1$ | $\alpha_2$ | ESP | Power | $\bar{N}_a$ | FSP | $\bar{N}_o$ | $N_{max}$ |
|---|---|---|---|---|---|---|---|---|
| OF | .00260 | .02400 | .263 | .95 | 73.0 | 0.45 | 65.3 | 84 |
| PF | .00625 | .02173 | .429 | .95 | 67.5 | 0.45 | 66.7 | 86 |
| Pocock | .01470 | .01470 | .625 | .95 | 63.2 | 0.45 | 71.0 | 92 |

Note: $\beta_1 = 0.5$, the proportions of shifting: $p_{10} = 0.2$, $p_{01} = 0.03$.

reestimation at interim with 50% information time and the targeted conditional power 90%.

Like the GSD for sensitivity, we start with a classical design for specificity. Given the data in Table 6.5, i.e., $p_{10} = 0.1$ and $p_{01} = 0.1$, the calculation indicates that 322 pairs are required for an 85% power at a level of significance 2.5% (one-sided) based on Nam's test (1997) and the sample-size calculation method presented earlier.

We use the same three error-spending functions for the adaptive trial for specificity: (1) OF, (2) PF with $\rho = 2$, and (3) Pocock. All designs have two stages and the interim analysis will be performed at 50% information time with a sample size of 161 pairs. The sample-size adjustment is based on a targeted conditional power of 90% and the maximum sample size $N_{max}$ is 500 pairs. In all designs we use the futility boundary $\beta_1 = 0.5$, which means approximately that if at interim analysis we observe $\hat{p}_{10} - \hat{p}_{01} - \delta_{NI} \leq 0$, we will stop the trial for futility.

The simulation results are presented in Table 6.7, where EEP and $\bar{N}_a$ are the early efficacy stopping probability and expected sample size, respectively, when $H_a$ ($p_{10} = p_{01} = 0.1$) is true.

Following the same steps for comparing different adaptive designs in sensitivity, we find the PF design is better than the OF design. To evaluate the PF design against the Pocock design, we need to perform the simulations under $H_0 : p_{10} - p_{01} - \delta_{NI} = 0$ ($p_{10} = 0.1$, $p_{01} = 0.175$ and $\delta_{NI} = 0.075$). Under this null hypothesis, the OF, PF, and Pocock designs have almost the same expected sample size ($\bar{N}_o$) 335 with futility stopping probability 47%. This is because they use the same futility boundary and same sample size at the interim analysis, while the efficacy stopping boundary has virtually no effect on sample size.

We also studied the effect of SSR. We assume there is a small difference in proportions but within the noninferiority margin: $p_{10} = 0.1$, $p_{01} = 0.11$. We want to know if the power is reasonably preserved in this case.

Table 6.7:  Operating Characteristics of Adaptive Design for Specificity

|        | $\alpha_1$ | $\alpha_2$ | $N_{max}$ | ESP  | Power | $\bar{N}_a$ | FSP  | $\bar{N}_o$ |
|--------|------------|------------|-----------|------|-------|-------------|------|-------------|
| OF     | .00260     | .02400     | 500       | .206 | .942  | 354         | 0.47 | 335         |
| PF     | .00625     | .02173     | 500       | .328 | .940  | 336         | 0.47 | 335         |
| Pocock | .01470     | .01470     | 500       | .454 | .931  | 324         | 0.47 | 335         |

The simulation results (Table 6.8) show that that GSD cannot well preserve power in this case. The effect of sample size adjustment on power is higher for the OF and PF designs than the Pocock designs because the OF and PF designs spend more alpha on stage 2. The Pocock design has already spent 50% alpha before the interim analysis; therefore, the sample-size adjustment at stage 2 has less effect on the power. Compared with the OF design with SSR, the PF design with SSR has a smaller expected sample size $\bar{N}_S$ (374 versus 386).

Table 6.8:  Power Preserved by GSD and SSR Designs for Specificity

| Boundary | Design | $\alpha_1$ | $\alpha_2$ | $N_{max}$ | $\bar{N}$ | Power |
|----------|--------|------------|------------|-----------|-----------|-------|
| OF       | GSD    | .00260     | .02400     | 322       | 299       | 0.716 |
| OF       | SSR    | .00260     | .02400     | 500       | 386       | 0.847 |
| PF       | GSD    | .00625     | .02173     | 322       | 284       | 0.705 |
| PF       | SSR    | .00625     | .02173     | 500       | 374       | 0.842 |
| Pocock   | GSD    | .01470     | .01470     | 322       | 266       | 0.659 |
| Pocock   | SSR    | .01470     | .01470     | 500       | 364       | 0.814 |

We noticed that the expected sample size under $H_0$ is high even when the null hypothesis is true. Therefore, we ran simulations with an aggressive futility boundary $\beta_1 = 0.25$ (less than original 0.5). The sample size under $H_0$ reduces from 335 to 265. However, the reduction is at the cost of power: the power is reduced from 84% to 79% when $p_{10} = 0.1$, $p_{01} = 0.11$. Therefore we still recommend using $\beta_1 = 0.5$, which means that if at interim analysis the observed difference is at the noninferiority margin, we will stop the trial for futility.

Through these comparisons, we can conclude that the PF design with SSR is most preferable for the specificity design.

## 6.5.5  *Summary of Design*

For sensitivity, 86 positive patients with one interim analysis will provide 95% power for the superiority test. The error-spending function for the stopping boundary is $\alpha t^2$, where $t$ is information time or sample-size fraction, and the futility stopping rule is $p_1 > \beta_1 = 0.5$. The design features a 43% early efficacy stopping probability if the alternative hypothesis is true and a 45% early futility stopping probability if the null hypothesis is true. The expected sample size is 68 and 67 under $H_a$ and $H_0$, respectively, an 18% savings in comparison with 82 pairs for the classical design.

For specificity, we use the two-stage design, featuring sample-size reestimation at interim analysis with 161 pairs. The sample-size reestimation will be based on a 90% conditional power with a cap of 500 pairs. The two-stage adaptive design has 94% power for the noninferiority test with an NI margin of 7.5%. The error-spending function for the stopping boundary is $\alpha t^2$, where $t$ is information time, and the futility stopping rule is $p_1 > \beta_1 = 0.5$. The design features a 33% early efficacy stopping probability when the alternative hypothesis is true, and a 47% early futility stopping probability if the null hypothesis is true. The expected sample size is 336 and 335 under $H_a$ and $H_0$, respectively, a 23% savings as compared with the classical design ($N = 438$) with the same 94% power.

Given a 95% power for the sensitivity test and a 94% power for the specificity test, which are assumed to be independent, the overall probability of getting an effectiveness claim for the diagnosis test (Method 2) is about 90%.

The stopping rules for sensitivity and specificity are the same but sample-size reestimation is allowed for the design for specificity:

If the interim $p$-value for the sensitivity (specificity) test is $p_1 \leq 0.00625$, the null hypothesis for sensitivity (specificity) will be rejected. If the $p$-value for sensitivity (specificity) test is $p_1 > 0.5$, we stop recruiting positive (negative) patients. If $0.5 \geq p_1 > 0.00625$, we continue to recruit positive (negative) patients and the sample size will be reestimated for negative patients based on a 90% conditional power. At the final analysis, if the $p$-value for the sensitivity (specificity) is $p_1 \leq 0.02173$, then the null hypothesis for sensitivity (specificity) will be rejected. In the end, if both null hypothesis tests for sensitivity and specificity are rejected, then the new diagnosis test (Method 2) will be claimed effective.

## >>SAS Macro 6.1: Adaptive Noninferiority Design with Paired Data>>

```
/* Adaptive Noninferiority Design with Paired Data */
/* Ho: p10-p01-delNI <= 0 */
/* p10 and p01 are the % of disconcordant pairs */
```

```
/* Sample size: nPairs = nPairs1 + nPairs2 from stage 1 and 2 */
/* ExpN = the expected sample size (pairs) nPairs/nRuns; */
/* nRuns = number of simulation runs */
/* alpha = one-sided significance level */
/* RejPr1 and RejPr2 = Rejection probability at stage 1 and 2 */
/* Power = probability of rejecting Ho. */
/* alpha1, alpha2=, beta1 = Stopping boundaries on p-scale. */
%Macro McNemarAD(alpha1=0.0026, alpha2=0.024, beta1=1, p10=0.125,
p01=0.125, delNI=0.1, nPairs1=154, nPairs2=154, nPairsMax=600, Tar-
getcPow=0.90, w1=0.707, w2=0.707, nRuns=1000000);
Data RnMvars;
Retain Power1 Power2 Futile nPairs;
alpha1=&alpha1; alpha2=&alpha2; beta1=&beta1;
p10=&p10; p01=&p01; delNI=&delNI;
nPairs1=&nPairs1; nPairs20=&nPairs2;
TargetcPow=&TargetcPow; nPairsMax=&nPairsMax;
nRuns=&nRuns;
w1=&w1/(&w1**2+&w2**2)**0.5; w2=&w2/(&w1**2+&w2**2)**0.5;
Power1=0; Power2=0; Futile=0; nPairs=0;
Do iRun=1 To nRuns;
nPairs=nPairs+nPairs1;
n10Stg1=RANBIN(0,nPairs1,p10);
n01Stg1=RANBIN(0,nPairs1,p01);
p10obsStg1=n10Stg1/nPairs1;
p01obsStg1=n01Stg1/nPairs1;
epsStg1=p10obsStg1-p01obsStg1-delNI;
b=(2+p01obsStg1-p10obsStg1)*delNI-p01obsStg1-p10obsStg1;
c=-p01obsStg1*delNI*(1-delNI);
p01Wave=(-b+sqrt(b*b-8*c))/4;
sigma2Stg1=2*p01Wave+delNI-delNI**2;
z1=0;
If sigma2Stg1 ^= 0 Then z1=epsStg1*Sqrt(nPairs1/sigma2Stg1);
pValue1=1-CDF('Normal',z1);
T1=pValue1;
If T1<=alpha1 Then Power1=Power1+1;
If T1>beta1 Then Futile=Futile+1;
If alpha1<T1<=beta1 Then Do;
** Sample size reestimation based on conditional power **;
Bval=(Probit(1-alpha2)-w1*Probit(1-pValue1))/w2;
```

```
nPairs2=nPairs20;
If epsStg1>0 Then
nPairs2=sigma2Stg1/epsStg1**2*(Bval-Probit(1-TargetcPow))**2;
nPairs2=Min(nPairsMax-nPairs1,nPairs2);
nPairs2=Round(Max(nPairs2, nPairs20));
n10Stg2=RANBIN(0,nPairs2,p10);
n01Stg2=RANBIN(0,nPairs2,p01);
p10obsStg2=n10Stg2/nPairs2;
p01obsStg2=n01Stg2/nPairs2;
epsStg2=p10obsStg2-p01obsStg2-delNI;
b=(2+p01obsStg2-p10obsStg2)*delNI-p01obsStg2-p10obsStg2;
c=-p01obsStg2*delNI*(1-delNI);
p01Wave=(-b+sqrt(b*b-8*c))/4;
sigma2Stg2=2*p01Wave+delNI-delNI**2;
z2=0;
If sigma2Stg2 ^=0 Then z2=epsStg2*Sqrt(nPairs2/sigma2Stg2);
pValue2=1-CDF('Normal',z2);
T2=1-CDF('NORMAL', w1*z1+w2*z2);
If T2<=alpha2 Then Power2=Power2+1;
nPairs=nPairs+nPairs2;
End;
End;
ExpN=nPairs/nRuns;
RejPr1=Power1/nRuns;
RejPr2=Power2/nRuns;
Power=RejPr1+RejPr2;
FutilePr=Futile/nRuns;
Output;
Run;
proc print data=RnMvars;
var alpha1 alpha2 beta1 nPairs1 nPairs20 nPairs2 w1 w2
TargetcPow nRuns p10 p01 FutilePr RejPr1 RejPr2 Power ExpN;
Run;
%Mend McNemarAD;
```

**<<SAS<<**

## >>SAS: Invoke SAS Macro 5.1>>

```
Title2 "Classical 1-Stage Design : Type-I erorr rate p10-p01-delNI=0";
%McNemarAD(alpha1=0.025, alpha2=0, beta1=0, p10=0.1, p01=0.175, delNI=-
0.075, nPairs1=322, nPairs2=0);
```

Title2 "PF (rho=2), beta1=0.5 with SSR (Nmax>N0)";
%McNemarAD(alpha1=0.00625, alpha2=0.02173, beta1=0.5, p10=0.1, p01=0.1,
delNI=-0.075, nPairs1=161, nPairs2=161, nPairsMax=500);
<<**SAS**<<

## 6.6   Summary

We have developed a simple method for adaptive trial design with binary
paired data. We have illustrated an application of the adaptive method for
an image study, in which both superiority in sensitivity and noninferiority
in specificity are required. Using the adaptive design, the savings in the
expected sample size is about 20%. The method can easily be used for
other cases with paired data.

**Problems**

**6.1** Prove that under the constraint $p_{10} - p_{01} - \delta_{NI} = 0$, $Z$ in (6.6) follows approximately the normal distribution for large $n$,

$$Z \sim N\left(\frac{\sqrt{n}\varepsilon}{\sigma}, 1\right),$$

where $\varepsilon = E(\hat{\varepsilon})$ and $\sigma = E(\hat{\sigma})$ can be obtained by replacing $\hat{p}_{ij}$ with $p_{ij}$ $(i = 0, 1; j = 0, 1)$ in the corresponding expression (6.7).

**6.2** Redesign the prostate cancer diagnostic trial, for the following conditions:

(1) Reduce the discordant pair for the positive patients in Table 6.4 from (20%, 3%) to (18%, 2%) and increase the harmonious pair from (62%, 15%) to (62% and 16%).

(2) Increase the discordant pairs for the negative patients in Table 6.5 from (10%, 10%) to (9%, 9%) and increase the harmonious pair from (60%, 20%) to (62% and 20%).

**6.3** Discuss other practical situations where we can apply the method discussed in this chapter.

## Chapter 7

# Adaptive Design with Incomplete Paired Data

A clinical trial design with paired data often involves missing observations. In such a case, the data from the trial become a mixture of paired and unpaired data. A commonly used approach for the analysis of the trial data is to ignore the incomplete pairs. Such a treatment of missings data is not statistically efficient. We will discuss a simple method that will allow us to use all data, including the incomplete pairs. The method is optimal in the sense that it minimizes the variance. We will show how to design classical and adaptive trials with the proposed method for different types of endpoints with superiority, noninferiority, and equivalence designs. The method can also be used for meta-analysis, in which, some trials are with paired data and some are not.

## 7.1  Introduction

Missing data are a common occurrence in scientific research and in our daily lives. In a survey, a lack of response constitutes missing data. In clinical trials, missing data can be caused by a patient's refusal to continue in a study, treatment failures, adverse events, or patient relocations. Missing data will complicate the data analysis. In many medical settings, missing data can cause difficulties in estimation and inference. In clinical trials, missing data can undermine randomization (Little, 2010). CHMP's guideline (2009) provides advices on how the presence of missing data in a confirmatory clinical trial should be addressed in a regulatory submission. It is stated that the pattern of missing data (including reasons for and timing of the missing data) observed in previous related clinical trials should be taken into account when planning a confirmatory clinical trial.

For a concise review on the topic of the missing data issue and anlaysis, see Chapter 5 in Chang's book (2011).

An example for missing in paired data could be that either baseline or postbaseline measures are missing for some patients. When multiple measures are taken from multiple locations in a body (e.g., left and right eyes), missing data often occur. In a $2 \times 2$ crossover trial, the outcomes are only present in one of the treatment periods for some patients. Case-control studies may also involve missing data. In such cases, the data from the trial become a mixture of paired and unpaired data. It is not uncommon that a meta-analysis involves a mixture of clustered and unclustered measures. Dealing with such a mixture of different data, a commonly used approach in clinical trial design and data analyses is to ignore the missing data or unpaired data. Such a treatment of data is obviously information wasting and not efficient at all. The last observation-carry-forward is often not applicable in such cases.

Recently Dittrich et al. (2012) considered the analysis of paired comparison experiments in the presence of missing responses. Their method is based on the paired comparison set of responses augmented by a set of missing data indicators for each comparison. The classical Bradley–Terry model is used for the response outcomes and a multinomial model for the missing indicators. Two missing data mechanisms—missing completely at random (MCAR) and missing not at random (MNAR)—are modeled.

In contrast, Tibeiro and Murdoch (2010) studied the analysis with incomplete paired data using Bayesian imputation, associating with a dataset concerning congenital heart disease. They used Markov chain Monte Carlo (MCMC) on a hierarchical Bayes model to estimate the underlying rates, and used correspondence analysis to study the relationships in the completed table.

## 7.2 Mixture of Paired and Unpaired Data

According to Rubin (1976) and Little and Rubin (2002), the mechanism of missingness can be classified into three different categories in terms of marginal probability distributions.

(1) If the probability of an observation being missing does not depend on observed or unobserved measurements, then the observation is classified as MCAR.

(2) If the probability of an observation being missing depends only on observed measurements, then the observation is classified as missing at

random (MAR). This assumption implies that the behavior (i.e., distribution) of the post-dropout observations can be predicted from the observed values and, therefore, that response can be estimated without bias using exclusively the observed data.

(3) When observations are neither MCAR nor MAR, they are classified as MNAR, i.e., the probability of an observation being missing depends on both observed and unobserved measurements.

Statistically, there is no way to know exactly whether missing observations are MCAR, MAR, or MNAR. However, we often believe MCAR/MAR can be a good approximation in certain situations.

Our proposed method in this paper is applicable to MCAR and MAR.

**Normal Endpoint**

Let $x_{ts} \sim N\left(\mu_t, \sigma_X^2\right)$ be the response of the $s$th subject in treatment group $t$, $s = 1, ..., n_p$ for paired data, and $s = 1, ..., n_{tu}$ for unpaired data. Assume the first $n_p$ of $x_{1i}$ and $x_{2i}$ are the paired data. For paired data, let the treatment difference $\hat{\delta}_p = \frac{1}{n_p} \sum_{i=1}^{n_p}(x_{2i} - x_{1i})$; for unpaired data, the treatment difference is estimated by $\hat{\delta}_u = \frac{1}{n_{1u}} \sum_{i=n_p+1}^{n_{1u}+n_p} x_{2i} - \frac{1}{n_{2u}} \sum_{i=n_p+1}^{n_{2u}+n_p} x_{1i}$.

We now propose the estimator for the treatment difference using a linear combination of $\delta_p$ and $\delta_u$,

$$\hat{\delta} = w_p \hat{\delta}_p + w_u \hat{\delta}_u. \tag{7.1}$$

where the prefixed weight $w_p + w_u = 1$. Assume missing data are MCAR. In such case, both estimators $\hat{\delta}_p$ and $\hat{\delta}_u$ of the treatment difference $\delta$ are unbiased. In a such case, $\hat{\delta}$ will also be an unbiased estimator of $\delta$:

$$E\hat{\delta} = w_p E\hat{\delta}_p + w_u E\hat{\delta}_u = \delta. \tag{7.2}$$

The variance of $\hat{\delta}$ is given by

$$\sigma_{\hat{\delta}}^2 = w_p^2 \sigma_{\delta_p}^2 + (1 - w_p)^2 \sigma_{\delta_u}^2. \tag{7.3}$$

The weights $w_p$ and $w_u$ can be chosen such that the variance $\sigma_{\hat{\delta}}^2$ is minimized. This can be accomplished by letting $\frac{\partial \sigma_{\hat{\delta}}^2}{\partial w_p} = 0$, which leads to

$$w_p = \frac{\sigma_{\delta_u}^2}{\sigma_{\delta_p}^2 + \sigma_{\delta_u}^2}. \tag{7.4}$$

Using the weight in (7.4), the minimum variance can be expressed as

$$\sigma_\delta^2 = \frac{\sigma_{\delta_p}^2 \sigma_{\delta_u}^2}{\sigma_{\delta_p}^2 + \sigma_{\delta_u}^2}. \tag{7.5}$$

The confidence interval constructed using this minimum variance will give the narrowest confidence interval.

For normal endpoint, denoted by $\rho$ the correlation coefficient between the matched pairs, we have

$$\sigma_{\delta_p}^2 = 2\left(1 - \rho\right) \frac{\sigma_x^2}{n_p}, \tag{7.6}$$

$$\sigma_{\delta_u}^2 = \left(\frac{1}{n_{1u}} + \frac{1}{n_{2u}}\right) \sigma_x^2. \tag{7.7}$$

Substituting (7.6) and (7.7) into (7.4) and (7.5), we obtain

$$w_p = \frac{1}{1 + 2\left(1 - \rho\right) \frac{f_{1u} f_{2u}}{f_p(f_{1u} + f_{2u})}} \tag{7.8}$$

and

$$\sigma_\delta^2 = \frac{\sigma_*^2}{n}, \tag{7.9}$$

where $n = n_p + n_{1u} + n_{2u}$, $f_p = n_p/n$, $f_{iu} = n_{iu}/n$, $(i = 1, 2)$, and the *equivalent variance* for the normal endpoint is

$$\sigma_*^2 = \frac{2\left(1 - \rho\right) \frac{1}{f_p} \left(\frac{1}{f_{1u}} + \frac{1}{f_{2u}}\right)}{2\left(1 - \rho\right) \frac{1}{f_p} + \left(\frac{1}{f_{1u}} + \frac{1}{f_{2u}}\right)} \sigma_x^2. \tag{7.10}$$

The introduction of equivalent variance will provide a simple way to design classical or adaptive trials (the details will be dicussed later with examples) to include the incomplete pairs. When $n_{1u} = n_{2u} = n_u$, the weight becomes

$$w_p = \frac{1}{1 + \left(1 - \rho\right) \frac{n_u}{n_p}}. \tag{7.11}$$

There are some special cases: (1) for paired data only, $n_u = 0$, and thus $w_p = 1$ and $w_u = 0$; (2) for independent data, $n_p = 0$, and thus $w_p = 0$ and $w_u = 1$; (3) when $\rho > 0$, $w_p > n_p/\left(n_p + n_u\right)$; when $\rho < 0$, $w_p < n_p/\left(n_p + n_u\right)$, and as $\rho \to 0$, $w_p \to n_p/\left(n_p + n_u\right)$.

Based on the derivation above, the correlation coefficient $\rho$ should be determined independent of the current data. However, if $\rho$ is (approximately) independent of $\hat{\delta}_u$ and $\hat{\delta}_p$ such as when $n$ is large, $\rho$ can be estimated from the data. The Pearson correlation coefficient is defined as

$$\hat{\rho} = \frac{\Sigma_i \left(x_{1i} - \bar{x}_1\right)\left(x_{2i} - \bar{x}_2\right)}{\sqrt{\Sigma_i \left(x_{1i} - \bar{x}_1\right)^2 \Sigma_i \left(x_{2i} - \bar{x}_2\right)^2}} \tag{7.12}$$

**Binary Endpoint**

For binary endpoint, let $x_{ts} = 1$ if subject $s$ responds to treatment $t$ and $x_{ts} = 0$ if subject $s$ does not responds to treatment $t$. Using that notation, we can write $\hat{\delta}_p = \frac{1}{n_p}\sum_{i=1}^{n_p}(x_{2i} - x_{1i})$ and $\hat{\delta}_u = \hat{\delta}_{1u} - \hat{\delta}_{2u}$ for the observed proportion (treatment) difference for paired and unpaired data, respectively. Here, $\hat{\delta}_{1u} = \frac{1}{n_{1u}}\sum_{i=n_p+1}^{n_{1u}+n_p} x_{1i}$ and $\hat{\delta}_{2u} = \frac{1}{n_{2u}}\sum_{i=n_p+1}^{n_{2u}+n_p} x_{2i}$. Thus, equations (7.1)–(7.12) are still applicable for a binary endpoint. However, the standard deviation is determined by

$$\hat{\sigma}_x^2 = \frac{1}{n_p + n_{1u}} \sum_{i=1}^{n_p+n_{1u}} (x_{1i} - \bar{x}_1)^2 + \frac{1}{n_p + n_{2u}} \sum_{i=1}^{n_p+n_{2u}} (x_{2i} - \bar{x}_2)^2. \tag{7.13}$$

The phi coefficient (mean square contingency coefficient), which is computationally equivalent to the Pearson correlation coefficient in the $2 \times 2$ case (i.e., $\hat{\rho} = \hat{\phi}$), is

$$\hat{\phi} = \frac{m_{11}m_{00} - m_{10}m_{01}}{\sqrt{\Sigma_j m_{1j}\Sigma_j m_{0j}\Sigma_i m_{i0}\Sigma_i m_{i1}}},$$

where $m_{ij}$ is the count in the $2 \times 2$ contingency table.

Alternatively, the variance for the paired mean difference is given by

$$\sigma_{\delta_p}^2 = \frac{\delta_d}{n_p}, \tag{7.14}$$

where $\delta_d$ is the proportion of discordant pairs, which can be estimated by

$$\hat{\delta}_d = \frac{1}{n_p} \sum_{i=1}^{n_p} \left[(1 - x_{2i})x_{1i} + (1 - x_{1i})x_{2i}\right]. \tag{7.15}$$

The variance for the unpaired mean difference is given by

$$\sigma_{\delta_u}^2 = \frac{\delta_{1u}\left(1 - \delta_{1u}\right)}{n_{1u}} + \frac{\delta_{2u}\left(1 - \delta_{2u}\right)}{n_{2u}}. \tag{7.16}$$

Since the correlation coefficient, $\rho$, is usually unknown, we can estimate it using data from the current experiment. However, in such a case, the weight $w_p$ is not really constant (especially when the sample size is small). We will study the impact of such approximation on the coverage probability of the confidence interval and type-I error of a hypothesis test using simulations for both normal and binary endpoints. Similar to normal endpoint, we can express the variance as

$$\sigma_\delta^2 = \frac{\sigma_*^2}{n},$$

where the "equivalent variance" $\sigma_*^2$ can be estimated by

$$\hat{\sigma}_*^2 = \frac{\frac{\hat{\delta}_d}{f_p}\left[\frac{\hat{\delta}_{1u}\left(1-\hat{\delta}_{1u}\right)}{f_{1u}} + \frac{\hat{\delta}_{2u}\left(1-\hat{\delta}_{2u}\right)}{f_{2u}}\right]}{\frac{\hat{\delta}_d}{f_p} + \frac{\hat{\delta}_{1u}\left(1-\hat{\delta}_{1u}\right)}{f_{1u}} + \frac{\hat{\delta}_{2u}\left(1-\hat{\delta}_{2u}\right)}{f_{2u}}}. \tag{7.17}$$

## 7.3 Hypothesis Test

Denote by $\delta$ the treatment different; we can write the typical hypothesis test for either normal or binary endpoint as

$$H_0 : \delta \leq 0 \text{ versus } H_a : \delta > 0, \tag{7.18}$$

and define the test statistic (for large sample size $n$) as

$$T = \frac{\hat{\delta}}{\hat{\sigma}_\delta} \sim N\left(\frac{\delta}{\sigma_\delta}, 1\right) = N\left(\frac{\delta\sqrt{n}}{\sigma_*}, 1\right). \tag{7.19}$$

When $\delta = 0$, $T$ has the standard normal distribution $T \sim N(0,1)$.

The two-sided $(1-\alpha)100\%$ confidence interval for treatment difference $\delta$ is given by

$$w_p\delta_p + (1-w_p)\delta_u \pm z_{1-\alpha/2}\frac{\sigma_*}{\sqrt{n}}, \tag{7.20}$$

where $w_p$ is given by (7.4).

This confidence interval can be used for the analysis of noninferiority trials.

## 7.4 Type-I Error Control and Coverage Probability

Because the correlation coefficient $\rho$ and variance $\sigma^2$ are usually unknown and are estimated from the current trial, we want to investigate the type-I error rate for the hypothesis test and coverage probability of the interval estimator through simulations under various combinations of different endpoints, missing correlations and sample sizes. For each scenario, we performed 100,000 simulation runs using the popular R software. The typical results are summarized in Tables 7.1, 7.2, and 7.3. The proportions of missing are presented for the scenarios of balanced and unbalanced missings.

From the simulation results, we can see that the type-I error rate and coverage probability (coverage probability = 1 - Type I error rate) are within the range of simulation error or variations for binary and normal endpoint with sample size of 500. When the sample size reduces from 100, there are negligible type-I error inflations or deflations.

Table 7.1: Normal Endpoint (Sample Size $n = 500$)

| Missings | 10%, 10% | | | 25%, 25% | | | 15%, 35% | | |
|---|---|---|---|---|---|---|---|---|---|
| $\rho$ | 0.3 | 0.5 | 0.8 | 0.3 | 0.5 | 0.8 | 0.3 | 0.5 | 0.8 |
| Type-I error | .051 | .051 | .052 | .050 | .050 | .050 | .051 | .051 | .050 |

Table 7.2: Binary Endpoint (Sample Size $n = 500$)

| Missings | 10%, 10% | | | 25%, 25% | | | 15%, 35% | | |
|---|---|---|---|---|---|---|---|---|---|
| $\rho$ | 0.3 | 0.5 | 0.8 | 0.3 | 0.5 | 0.8 | 0.3 | 0.5 | 0.8 |
| Type-I error | .050 | .051 | .049 | .051 | .051 | .052 | .051 | .050 | .051 |

Table 7.3: Binary Endpoint (Sample Size $n = 100$)

| Missings | 10%, 10% | | | 25%, 25% | | | 15%, 35% | | |
|---|---|---|---|---|---|---|---|---|---|
| $\rho$ | 0.3 | 0.5 | 0.8 | 0.3 | 0.5 | 0.8 | 0.3 | 0.5 | 0.8 |
| Type-I error | .052 | .052 | .053 | .054 | .054 | .048 | .054 | .055 | .047 |

## 7.5 Classical Trial Design

### 7.5.1 *Power and Sample Size*

If paired observations are missing, we have to replace the missing observations. Therefore, for simplicity, we assume there are no such cases.

Similar to the case when there are no imcomplete pairs, for the hypothesis test (7.18), the power for the classical design is given by

$$1 - \beta = \Phi\left(\frac{\delta}{\sigma_\delta} - z_{1-\alpha}\right).$$

The overall sample size for superiority test is given by

$$n^* = \left[ \frac{(z_{1-\alpha} + z_{1-\beta})}{\delta} \right]^2 \sigma_*^2, \tag{7.21}$$

where $\sigma_*^2$ is given in (7.10) and (7.17) for normal and binary endpoints, respectively. Such replacement of the standard deviation $\sigma$ with the equivalent standard deviation $\sigma_*$ is the key for us to use the formulations for the trials without incomplete pairs even when there are incomplete pairs. We will see such replacements in the following sections.

For normal endpoint, when $n_{1u} = n_{2u} = n_u$, then $n_p + 2n_u = n$ (total sample size) and $f_u = \frac{n_u}{n}$. Thus, from (7.10), we obtain

$$\sigma_*^2 = 2\sigma_x^2 \frac{1 - \rho}{1 - (1 + \rho)f_u}. \tag{7.22}$$

In the case in which there is no missing ($f_u = 0$), the sample size required for paired design is

$$n = \left[ \frac{(z_{1-\alpha} + z_{1-\beta})}{\delta} \right]^2 2\sigma_x^2 (1 - \rho).$$

If the incomplete pairs are ignored, the sample size required for the target power $1 - \beta$ will be inflated by a factor of $1 - 2f_u$, i.e.,

$$\tilde{n} = \frac{n}{1 - 2f_u}. \tag{7.23}$$

Since the sample size $n$ is proportional to the equivalent variance $\sigma_*^2$, the ratio of the sample size $n^*$ with missing data included, (7.21) and (7.22), to the sample size with missing data excluded, (7.23), is

$$R = \frac{n^*}{\tilde{n}} = \frac{1 - 2f_u}{1 - (1 + \rho)f_u} \tag{7.24}$$

When $\rho = 0$ (independent), $R = \frac{1-2f_u}{1-f_u}$. When $\rho \to 1$, $R \to 100\%$ and $n \to 0$. From (7.24), we can see that the relative impact ($R$) of missing data increases when the correlation coefficient ($\rho$) increases. For example, if $\rho = 0.8$ and $f_u = 0.2$ (40% missing), $R = \frac{0.6}{1-(1.8)0.2} = 93.8\%$. That is, if there are 40% incomplete pairs, the proposed method leads to a 6.2% savings in sample size in comparison to the method that ignores the incomplete pairs. For $\rho = 0.5$ and $f_u = 0.2$, $R = \frac{0.6}{1-(1.5)0.2} = 85.7\%$ and the method can have a 14.3% savings. For $\rho = 0$ and $f_u = 0.2$, $R = 75\%$ and it will have a 25% savings. For $\rho = 0.5$ and $f_u = 0.3$ (60% missing), $R = \frac{0.4}{1-(1.5)0.3} = 72.7\%$ and it can have a 27.3% savings in sample size.

### 7.5.2 *Trial Design Examples*

**Example 7.1    Superiority Trial Designs with Normal Endpoint**
The superiority test in a clinical trial is often defined as

$$H_0 : \delta \leq 0 \text{ versus } H_a : \delta > 0.$$

Assume in a $2 \times 2$ crossover trial with two treatment groups, the control and the test, there are 20% missing in the control group and 30% missing in the test group, i.e., $f_{1u} = 0.20$, $f_{2u} = 0.30$, and $f_p = 0.5$. We further assume the correlation coefficient between measurements in periods 1 and 2 is $\rho = 0.7$, the treatment difference is $\delta = 0.8$, and the standard deviation for the two treatment is $\sigma_x = 2.4$. Assuming the period, sequence and carryover effects are negligible; from (7.10), the sample size is

$$\sigma_*^2 = \frac{2\,(1 - 0.7)\,(2.4)^2}{0.5 + 2\,(1 - 0.7)\,\frac{0.2(0.3)}{0.2 + 0.3}} = 6.0.$$

Thus, the sample size for 90% power $(1 - \beta)$ and $\alpha = 2.5\%$ significance level for one-sided test is given by

$$n = \left(\frac{1.96 + 1.28}{0.8}\right)^2 6.0 = 98.$$

**Example 7.2    Noninferiority Trial Designs with Normal Endpoint**
The hypothesis for the noninferiority test (the fixed margin approach) is defined as

$$H_0 : \delta < \delta_{NI} \text{ versus } H_a : \delta \geq \delta_{NI},$$

where $\delta_{NI} < 0$ is the noninferiority margin.

Noninferiority trials have become popular in recent years, partially due to the increasing cost in drug development and great attractions to develop generic drugs after patent expiration of innovative drugs (2011). For planning such a noninferiority trial, D'Agostino (2003) suggests a list of questions to be asked, which are very helpful. Recently FDA (2011) and CHMP (2005) issued guidance on noninferiority trial. Most recently, Rothman, Owine, and Chen (2011) published an excellent book on noninferiority trial, whereas Chang (2011) gave a concise, yet comprehensive introduction.

Assume $\delta = 0$ and the noninferiority margin is $\delta_{NI} = -0.2$, but keep everything else the same as in Example 7.1. The sample size for the noninferiority trial with 90% power and one-sided $\alpha = 0.025$ can be calculated as

$$n = \frac{(z_{1-\alpha} + z_{1-\beta})^2 \sigma_*^2}{(\delta - \delta_{NI})^2} = \left(\frac{1.96 + 1.28}{0.2}\right)^2 6.0 = 1575.$$

**Example 7.3    Equivalence Trial Design with Normal Endpoint**

An equivalence test can be defined as

$$H_0 : |\delta| \geq \delta_e \text{ versus } H_a : |\delta| < \delta_e,$$

where $\delta_e$ is the equivalence margin.

The sample size for a equivalence trial design can be calculated using the approximate (conservative) formulation similar to that given by Chow, Shao, and Wang (2011):

$$n = \frac{(z_{1-\alpha} + z_{1-\beta/2})^2 \sigma_*^2}{(\delta_e - |\delta|)^2},$$

where we have replaced standard deviation $\sigma$ with our equivalent $\sigma_*$.

Using the same data as in Example 7.2, and assume the equivalence margin is $\delta_e = 0.4$, $\alpha = 0.05$, and 90% power ($\beta = 0.1$), the sample size required is

$$n = \frac{(1.645 + 1.645)^2(6.0)}{0.16} = 406$$

Suppose in the end of trial, we observed $\hat{f}_{1u} = 0.22$, $\hat{f}_{2u} = 0.28$, and $\hat{f}_p = 0.5$, $\hat{\rho} = 0.6$, $\delta_p = 0.2$, $\delta_u = 0.3$, and $\sigma_x = 2$. We can calculate the confidence interval as follows:

$$w_p = \frac{1}{1 + 2\left(1 - 0.6\right)\frac{0.22(0.28)}{0.5(0.22+0.28)}} = 0.835.$$

$$\hat{\sigma}_*^2 = \frac{2\left(1 - 0.6\right)2^2}{0.5 + 2\left(1 - 0.6\right)\frac{0.22(0.28)}{(0.22+0.28)}} = 5.35.$$

The mean difference is given by (7.1)

$$\hat{\delta} = 0.835(0.2) + (1 - 0.835)\,0.3 = 0.2165.$$

The 95% confidence interval is given by (7.20)

$$0.2165 \pm 1.96\sqrt{\frac{5.35}{406}},$$

i.e., $(-0.008, 0.441)$. Since the confidence interval is not covered completely by the equivalence lower and upper bounds $(-0.4, 0.4)$, the equivalence of treatments $A$ and $B$ cannot be claimed.

Note that equivalence studies are more often analyzed based on a log scale and 20% rule.

## Example 7.4  Superiority Trial Design with Binary Endpoint

The hypothesis for the superiority test is defined as

$$H_0 : \delta \le 0 \text{ versus } H_a : \delta > 0.$$

Assume the treatment difference in the proportion of treatment responses is $\delta_{1u} = 30\%$ and $\delta_{2u} = 45\%$. The missing proportions are $f_{1u} = f_{2u} = 0.2$, and $f_p = 1 - f_{1u} - f_{2u} = 0.6$.

If the correlation coefficient is given, e.g., $\rho = 0.777$, then the equivalent variance can be calculated from (7.10) and (7.13):

$$\sigma_*^2 = \frac{2(1-0.777)\frac{1}{0.6}\left(\frac{1}{0.2}+\frac{1}{0.2}\right)}{2(1-0.777)\frac{1}{0.6}+\left(\frac{1}{0.2}+\frac{1}{0.2}\right)}(0.3(1-0.3)+0.45(1-0.45)) = 0.316.$$

If the proportion of discordant is given, e.g., $\delta_d = 22\%$, we can calculate the equivalence variance from (7.17):

$$\sigma_*^2 = \frac{\frac{0.22}{0.6}\left(\frac{0.3(1-0.3)}{0.2}+\frac{0.45(1-0.45)}{0.2}\right)}{\frac{0.22}{0.6}+\frac{0.3(1-0.3)}{0.2}+\frac{0.45(1-0.45)}{0.2}} = 0.316.$$

Therefore, the sample size for 90% power and one-sided $\alpha = 0.025$ can be calculated as

$$n = \left(\frac{(1.96+1.28)}{0.45-0.3}\right)^2 0.316 = 147.$$

If the incomplete pairs are ignored, the sample size required would be

$$n = \left(\frac{(1.96+1.28)}{0.45-0.3}\right)^2 \frac{0.22}{0.6} = 171.$$

We can see that there is a 24 subject reduction in sample size by including incomplete pairs in the analysis.

## 7.6  Adaptive Trial Design

In the following example, we will discuss an adaptive trial design with a continuous (but not necessarily normal) endpoint. Based on the central limit theorem, the estimate $\hat{\delta}$ given by (7.1) is approximately normal distribution for a large sample size. Therefore, all the formulations for the equivalent variance and sample size from the previous sections remain valid.

### Example 7.5    A Clinical Trial of Retinal Diseases

Visual acuity (VA) is often considered an outcome measure in clinical trials of retinal diseases. Sometimes the continuous VA letter score is dichotomized based on whether or not there has been a worsening (or gain) of $\geq$ or $= 15$ letters (equivalent to $\geq$ or $= 3$ lines). A study that contrasts these two approaches was carried out by Beck et al. (2007). Here we use continuous VA for the purpose of illustration of our method.

Suppose in a single group trial, we study the effect of a clinical intervention on the vision in patients with retinal disease. The Snellen eye chart is used with 20/20 being the normal visual acuity. A score of 20/100 means one can read at 20 feet a letter that people with "normal" vision can read at 100 feet. So at 20/100, one's vision acuity is very poor. Suppose the endpoint is the change from baseline in vision acurity. In the initial group sequential design without considering missing, we use the equivalent variance, $\sigma_*^2 = 2\sigma_x^2 (1 - \rho)$. However, there could be some missing observations for the clinical endpoint, i.e., some of patients may have visional acurity score on only one eye. If such missings are observed at interim analysis, the sample size will be adjusted using the common sample-size reestimation approach as described in Chapter 6, in which the effective size (normalized treatment difference) is calculated based on the observed treatment difference and equivalent variance $\sigma_*^2$ given by (7.10).

Assume the treatment difference in visional acuity is $\delta = 0.1$ with a standard deviation $\sigma_x = 0.5$ and the correlation coefficient between baseline and post-baseline measures of same eyes, $\rho = 0.625$. For a 90% power and one-sided $\alpha = 0.025$, as a benchmark, the fixed sample-size design requires about 200 subjects.

We now compare the classical design with two different two-stage adaptive designs, one featuring sample size reestimation (SSR) with blinded data and another featuring SSR with unblinded data at the interim analysis.

We initially estimated $\sigma_* = \sqrt{2}\sigma_x\sqrt{1 - \rho} = \sqrt{2} \cdot 0.5\sqrt{1 - 0.625} = 0.433$ and treatment difference $\delta = 0.1$. The interim analysis is to performed based on 50% information (100 subjects). For the blinded SSR, the interim analysis is used for SSR only without efficacy or futility stopping.

For unblinded SSR, we use a two-stage adaptive design with O'Brien-Fleming-like error-spending function (similar to but not exactly the same as the O'Brien-Fleming stopping boundary). The $\alpha$ spent at interim and final analyses will be 0.00153 and 0.02347, respectively. The efficacy stopping boundary at $p$-value scale is 0.00153 and 0.02454 for the interim and final analyses, respectively, for rejecting the null hypothesis that there is no intervention effect.

The initial total sample size is 200, and interim analysis is performed on 100 patients' data. The maximum sample allowed is $N_{max} = 300$. The SSR is based on (4.7) (Cui, Hung, and Wang, 1999),

$$N_{new} = \begin{cases} \frac{\hat{\sigma}_*^2 \delta^2}{\hat{\delta}^2 \sigma_*^2} N, & \text{if } \hat{\delta} > 0 \\ N, & \text{if } \hat{\delta} > 0 \end{cases} \text{ for unblinded SSR,}$$

and

$$N_{new} = \frac{\hat{\sigma}_*^2}{\sigma_*^2} N \text{ for blinded SSR,}$$

where $\delta$ and $\sigma_*$ are the initial estimations and $\hat{\delta}$ and $\hat{\sigma}_*$ are the estimates from the interim analysis. The new sample size must not be less than $N$ and cannot exceed $N_{max}$. When $\hat{\delta} < 0$, no SSR will be needed, i.e., $N_{new} = N$.

Suppose that at the interim analysis, some patients have missing observations in one eye (for those who have missing endpoint measures in both eyes, we need replace just those patients). Presumably, the interim data show $f_{1u} = 0.10$, $f_{2u} = 0.15$, $f_p = 0.75$, $\hat{\sigma}_x = 0.52$, and $\hat{\rho} = 0.65$, and from (7.10), $\hat{\sigma}_* = \sigma_x \sqrt{\frac{2(1-\rho)}{2(1-\rho)\frac{f_{1u}f_{2u}}{f_{1u}+f_{2u}}+f_p}} = 0.52\sqrt{\frac{2(1-0.65)}{2(1-0.65)\frac{0.10(0.15)}{0.10+0.15}+0.75}} = 0.489$, $\hat{\delta} = 0.09$.

The simulations show that for the blinded SSR, the power for rejecting the null hypothesis is 87% with the average sample size 255, and for the unblinded SSR, the power is 89.4% with average sample size 212.

Therefore, the sample-size reestimation mechanism can protect the power when the treatment effect is lightly overestimated initially and missing data occur. The unblinded SSR works much better than the blinded SSR. If the classical design is used with 200 subjects, the power will be 74% with $\delta = 0.09$ and $\hat{\sigma}_x = 0.489$.

## >>SAS Macro 7.1: Sample-Size Reestimation Design with Incomplete Pairs>>

```
%Macro IncompletePairs(alpha1=0.00153, alpha2=0.02454, beta1=1,
sigma=0.433, NewSigma=0.489, N1=100, N2=100, Nmax = 250, u=0.1,
SSR="Blinded", nSims=100000);
Data ADIP;
Keep u sigma NewSigma alpha1 alpha2 beta1 AveN ESP FSP Power N1 N2;
```

```
alpha1=&alpha1; alpha2=&alpha2; beta1=&beta1;
sigma=&sigma; NewSigma=&NewSigma; u=&u;
N1=&N1; N2=&N2; N=N1+N2; Nmax=&Nmax;
w1 = Sqrt(N1/N); w2 = Sqrt(1-w1**2);
power = 0; AveN = 0;
FSP = 0; ESP = 0;
Do iSim = 1 To &nSims;
ThisN = 0;
uObs =Rannor(9274)*sigma/Sqrt(N1) + u;
Z1 =uObs*Sqrt(N1)/sigma;
P1 = 1 - ProbNorm(Z1);
ThisN = ThisN + N1;
* Check stopping rules;
If P1 > beta1 Then FSP = FSP + 1 / &nSims;
If P1 <= alpha1 Then ESP = ESP + 1 / &nSims;
* Blinded SSR;
If P1 > alpha1 & P1 <= beta1 Then Do;
NewN2=N2;
If &SSR="Blinded" Then * for Blinded SSR;
NewN2 = Max(N-N1,Min(Nmax-N1, (N1+N2)*(NewSigma/sigma)**2 -N1));
If &SSR="Unblinded" & uObs>0 Then * for unBlinded SSR;
NewN2 = Max(N-N1,Min(Nmax-N1,(N1+N2)*(NewSigma/sigma*u/uObs)**2-
N1));
ThisN = ThisN + NewN2;
Z2 =Rannor(9274) + u*Sqrt(NewN2)/NewSigma;
TS2 = w1*Z1 + w2*Z2;
P2 = 1 - ProbNorm(TS2);
If P2 <= alpha2 Then Power = Power + 1 / &nSims;
AveN = AveN + ThisN / &nSims;
End;
End;
Power = Power + ESP;
Output;
Run;
Proc print data=ADIP; Run;
%Mend IncompletePairs;
<<SAS<<

>>SAS>>
Title "Classical under Ha Power";
```

%IncompletePairs(alpha1=.025, alpha2=0, beta1=1, sigma=0.433, NewSigma
=0.433, N1=200, N2=0, Nmax = 200, u=0.1, SSR="Blinded", nSims=100000);
Title "Classical under H0—Type-I Error Control";
%IncompletePairs(alpha1=.025, alpha2=0, beta1=1, sigma=0.489, NewSigma
=0.489, N1=200, N2=0, Nmax = 200, u=0, SSR="Blinded", nSims=100000);
Title "Classical under Ha Power";
%IncompletePairs(alpha1=.025, alpha2=0, beta1=1, sigma=0.489, NewSigma
=0.489, N1=200, N2=0, Nmax = 200, u=0.09, SSR="Blinded");
Title "Unblinded SSR under H0—Type-I Error Control";
%IncompletePairs(alpha1=0.00153, alpha2=0.02454, beta1=1, sigma=0.433,
NewSigma=0.489, N1=100, N2=100, Nmax = 300, u=0, SSR="Unblinded");
Title "Unblinded Sample Size Reestimation";
%IncompletePairs(alpha1=.00153, alpha2=.02454, beta1=1, sigma=0.433,
NewSigma=.489, N1=100, N2=100, Nmax = 300, u=.09, SSR="Unblinded");
Title "Blinded SSR under H0—Type-I Error Control";
%IncompletePairs(alpha1=0, alpha2=.0245, beta1=1, sigma=0.433,
NewSigma=0.489, N1=100, N2=100, Nmax = 300, u=0, SSR="Blinded");
Title "Blinded Sample Size Reestimation";
%IncompletePairs(alpha1=0, alpha2=.0245, beta1=1, sigma=0.433,
NewSigma=.489, N1=100, N2=100, Nmax = 300, u=.09, SSR="Blinded");
<<**SAS**<<

## 7.7 Summary

We have utilized a simple method to effectively deal with incomplete paired
data in trial design and statistical analysis under MCAR and MAR. Instead
of completely ignoring the incomplete pairs, or using complicated methods
to implement the missing observations, our approach is straightforward
and an optimal one. The method incorporates both complete and incomplete pairs. The approximation introduced by larger sample assumption
was studied using simulations. The precision in type-I error control and
confidence interval estimation for the treatment difference are within the
acceptable range under broad practical scenarios. The applications of the
proposed methods are illustrated with four different examples, involving
superiority, equivalence, noninferiority, and adaptive trial designs.

**Problems**

**7.1** Redesign the trial in Example 7.1, assuming 30% missing in the control and 35% missing in the test group.

**7.2** Redesign the trial in Example 7.5, assuming $\rho = 0.25$ and $\delta = 0.05$.

**7.3** Redesign the trial in Example 7.4, assuming $\delta_{1u} = 25\%$ and $\delta_{2u} = 35\%$. Other specifications are kept the same.

**7.4** Discuss other practical situations with mixed paired and unpaired data, and the application of the method discussed in this chapter.

# Chapter 8

# $K$-Stage Adaptive Designs

## 8.1  Introduction

In this chapter we will present analytic, numerical, and simulation approaches to the $K$-stage design using nonparameteric stopping boundaries and the error spending approach which the latter allows for modifying the timing and number of analyses. The two methods have been implemented in SAS with MIP, MSP, MPP, and MINP. We will illustrate how to use these programs to design adaptive trials.

In a nonparametric approach, stopping boundaries are determined by the overall $\alpha$ level without specification of any function for $\pi_i$ or error-spending function. Therefore this method may not be applicable to adaptive designs with changes in the number or timing of the analyses. To allow for changes in the number and timing of interim analyses, we can prespecify discretely when the possible times are and how much error is to be spent at each interim analysis. In general, the stopping boundaries and power of a $K$-stage design can be determined using simulation or numerical integration regardless of the test statistic. Simulation is usually easier and computationally faster. Numerical integration may require dimension reductions in order to be computationally feasible.

## 8.2  Determination of Stopping Boundary

### 8.2.1  *Analytical Formulation for MSP*

The error-spending $\pi_k$ in relation to the stopping boundaries for the first two stages has been studied in Chapter 4; specifically for MSP we have

$$\pi_1 = \alpha_1 \text{ and } \pi_2 = \frac{1}{2}\left(\alpha_2 - \alpha_1\right)^2. \tag{8.1}$$

Chang (2010) provides analytical solutions for up to five-stage designs. For the third stage, we have

$$\pi_3 = \int_{\alpha_1}^{\alpha_3} \int_{\max(0,\alpha_2-p_1)}^{\alpha_3} \int_0^{\max(0,\alpha_3-p_2-p_1)} dp_3 dp_2 dp_1$$

$$= \int_{\alpha_2}^{\alpha_3} \int_0^{\alpha_3-p_1} (\alpha_3 - p_1 - p_2) dp_2 dp_1 + \int_{\alpha_1}^{\alpha_2} \int_{\alpha_2-p_1}^{\alpha_3-p_1} (\alpha_3 - p_1 - p_2) dp_2 dp_1$$

Carrying out the integration, we obtain

$$\pi_3 = \alpha_1 \alpha_2 \alpha_3 + \frac{1}{3}\alpha_2^3 + \frac{1}{6}\alpha_3^3 - \frac{1}{2}\alpha_1\alpha_2^2 - \frac{1}{2}\alpha_1\alpha_3^2 - \frac{1}{2}\alpha_2^2\alpha_3. \qquad (8.2)$$

In general, for $k$th stage, we have

$$\pi_k = \int_{\alpha_1}^{\alpha_4} \prod_{i=1}^{k-2} \left( \int_{\max(0,\alpha_{k-i}-\sum_{j=1}^{k-i-1}p_j)}^{\alpha_k} \right) \int_0^{\max(0,\alpha_k-\sum_{j=1}^{k-1}p_j)} dp_k...dp_i...dp_1.$$

$$(8.3)$$

For the fourth stage, we have (See Chang, 2010, for derivation)

$$\pi_4 = \frac{1}{8}\alpha_3^4 - \alpha_1\alpha_2\alpha_3\alpha_4 + \frac{1}{24}\alpha_4^4 - \frac{1}{3}\alpha_1\alpha_3^3 - \frac{1}{6}\alpha_1\alpha_3^3 - \frac{1}{6}\alpha_3^3\alpha_4 + \frac{1}{2}\alpha_1\alpha_2\alpha_3^2$$

$$+ \frac{1}{2}\alpha_1\alpha_2\alpha_4^2 + \frac{1}{2}\alpha_1\alpha_3^2\alpha_4 + \frac{1}{2}\alpha_2^2\alpha_3\alpha_4 - \frac{1}{4}\alpha_2^2\alpha_3^2 - \frac{1}{4}\alpha_2^2\alpha_4^2. \qquad (8.4)$$

Formulation for the fifth stage is longer, we omit it here.

We now discuss the steps to determine the stopping boundaries for $K$-stage designs:

(1) Choosing error spending $\pi_1, ..., \pi_{K-1}$, where $\sum_{k=1}^{K-1} \alpha_k < \alpha$.

(2) Calculate the error spending at the last stage: $\pi_K = \alpha - \sum_{k=1}^{K-1} \alpha_k$.

(3) Calculate the stopping boundary $\alpha_1, \alpha_2, ..., \alpha_K$, sequentially in that order.

Let's illustrate the steps with a three-stage design. Suppose the one-sided level of significance is $\alpha = 0.025$ and we want to spend less $\alpha$ at earlier stages and more on later stages. We choose $\pi_1 = 0.0025$ and $\pi_2 = 0.005$. Thus, $\pi_3 = \alpha - \pi_1 - \pi_2 = 0.0175$. Furthermore, we can obtain from (8.1) the stopping boundary $\alpha_1 = \pi_1 = 0.0025$ and $\alpha_2 = \sqrt{2\pi_2} + \alpha_1 = 0.1025$. The stopping boundary $\alpha_3$ can be solved numerically using software packages or by trial-and-error method, which is $\alpha_1 = 0.49257$ (see the first column in Table 8.1).

If we want the error-spending $\pi_1, ..., \pi_K$ to follow a certain trend (e.g., monotonic increase), we set up a so-called error-spending function $\pi^*(\tau_k)$, where $\tau_k$ is the information time or sample-size fraction at the $k$th interim

Table 8.1:   Stopping Boundaries of Three-Stage Design with MSP

| $\pi_1$ | 0.00250 | 0.00500 | 0.00250 | 0.00500 | 0.00250 | 0.00500 |
|---|---|---|---|---|---|---|
| $\pi_2$ | 0.00500 | 0.00500 | 0.00750 | 0.00750 | 0.01000 | 0.01000 |
| $\pi_3$ | 0.01750 | 0.01500 | 0.01500 | 0.01250 | 0.01250 | 0.01000 |
| $\alpha_1$ | 0.00250 | 0.00500 | 0.00250 | 0.00500 | 0.00250 | 0.00500 |
| $\alpha_2$ | 0.10250 | 0.10500 | 0.12497 | 0.12747 | 0.14392 | 0.14642 |
| $\alpha_3$ | 0.49257 | 0.47226 | 0.47833 | 0.45580 | 0.46181 | 0.43628 |

Note: One-side $\alpha = 0.025, \alpha_1 = \pi_1, \pi_3 = \alpha - \pi_1 - \pi_2$.

analysis. The commonly used error-spending functions with one-sided $\alpha$ are the O'Brien–Flemming-like error-spending function

$$\pi^*(\tau_k) = 2\left\{1 - \Phi\left(\frac{z_{1-\alpha/2}}{\sqrt{\tau_k}}\right)\right\},$$ (8.5)

the Pocock-like error-spending function

$$\pi^*(\tau_k) = \alpha \ln\left[1 + \frac{e-1}{\tau_k}\right],$$ (8.6)

and the power family,

$$\pi^*(\tau_k) = \alpha\tau_k^\gamma,$$ (8.7)

where $\gamma > 0$ is a constant.

The error-spending function $\pi^*(\tau_k)$ presents the cumulative error ($\alpha$) spent upto the information time $\tau_k$. Therefore, the error to spend at the $k$th stage with information time $\tau_k$ is determined by

$$\pi_k = \pi^*(\tau_k) - \pi^*(\tau_{k-1}).$$ (8.8)

After the error-spending $\pi_1, ..., \pi_K$ are determined, the calculations of stopping boundaries $\alpha_1, \alpha_2, ..., \alpha_K$ can be carried out sequentially as illustrated previously. For instance, suppose we decide to use the power function $\alpha\tau_k$ for the error-spending function and plan the interim analyses at the information times $\tau_1 = 1/3$ and $\tau_2 = 2/3$, and the final analysis at $\tau_3 = 1$. Puting the $\tau_k$ into (8.7), we obatin $\pi^*(\tau_1 = 1/3) = \alpha/3$, $\pi^*(\tau_1 = 2/3) = \frac{2}{3}\alpha$, and $\pi^*(\tau_1 = 1) = \alpha$. In this case, $\pi_k = \alpha/3$. In other words, we spend $\alpha$ equally over the three analyses, 30% each. The stopping boundaries based on MSP and $\alpha = 0.025$ MSP are $\alpha_1 = 0.025/3$, $\alpha_2 = 0.13743$, and $\alpha_3 = 0.41224$.

It is good to know that when the prespecified error-spending function is followed, we can change the timing and number of the interim analyses without inflating the type-I error as long as such changes are not based on

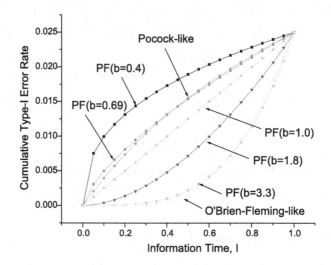

Figure 8.1:   Error-Spending Functions

treatment difference. This is the advantage when we use an error-spending function and promise the function will be followed.

### 8.2.2   *Analytical Formulation for MPP*

For MPP we have

$$\pi_1 = \alpha_1 \text{ and } \pi_2 = \alpha_2 \ln \frac{1}{\alpha_1}. \tag{8.9}$$

For the third stage, we have

$$\pi_3 = \int_{\alpha_1}^{1} \int_{\alpha_2/p_1}^{1} \int_{0}^{\alpha_3/(p_1 p_2)} dp_3 dp_2 dp_1 = \int_{\alpha_1}^{1} \int_{\alpha_2/p_1}^{1} \frac{\alpha_3}{p_1 p_2} dp_2 dp_1$$

$$= \int_{\alpha_1}^{1} \frac{\alpha_3}{p_1} (\ln p_1 - \ln \alpha_2) \, dp_1 = \alpha_3 \left[ \frac{1}{2} \ln^2 p_1 - \ln \alpha_2 \ln p_1 \right]_{\alpha_1}^{1}$$

Carrying out the integration, we obtain

$$\pi_3 = \alpha_3 \left( \ln \alpha_2 \ln \alpha_1 - \frac{1}{2} \ln^2 \alpha_1 \right). \tag{8.10}$$

For the fourth stage, we have

$$\pi_4 = \alpha_4 \left( (\ln \alpha_1 - \ln \alpha_3 - \ln \alpha_2) \ln \alpha_2 + \frac{1}{2} (\ln \alpha_3 - \ln \alpha_1) \ln \alpha_1 \right) \ln \alpha_1. \tag{8.11}$$

In general, for $k$th stage, we have

$$\pi_k = \int_{\alpha_1}^1 \int_{\alpha_2/p_1}^1 \cdots \int_{\alpha_{k-1}/(p_1 p_2 \cdots p_{k-1})}^1 \int_0^{\alpha_k/(p_1 p_2 \cdots p_{k-1})} dp_k dp_{k-1} \cdots dp_1$$

(8.12)

With (8.9) through (8.12), the stopping boundaries can be calculated similarly to the procedures in MSP.

We now use the R package for the stopping boundary and power calculations.

### 8.2.3   *Numerical Algorithm For MINP*

There are several algorithms for calculating the multivariate normal probability, which have been implemented in R packages, such as libraries "mnormt" and "mvtnorm." The following example shows how to calculate the probability

$$\Pr\left(-1 < X_1 < 1, -4 < X_2 < 4, -2 < X_3 < 2\right)$$

from multivariate normal distribution $N_3\left(0, \Sigma\right)$, where

$$\Sigma = \begin{pmatrix} 1 & 1/4 & 1/5 \\ 1/4 & 1 & 1/3 \\ 1/5 & 1/3 & 1 \end{pmatrix}$$

We can use the "mnormt" library and the following R code to get the probability:

>>**R**>>
```
library(mnormt)
mu=rep(0, 3)
s=matrix(c(1,1/4,1/5, 1/4,1,1/3, 1/5,1/3,1), 3,3)
sadmvn(lower=c(-1, -4, -2), upper=c(1, 4, 2), mu, s)
```
<<**R**<<

The output is 0.6536803 for the probability.

We now can modify this code for stopping boundary and power calculations by the following steps:

(1) Determine the error spending, $\pi_1, ..., \pi_K$, with or without using an error-spending function.

(2) Determine the stopping boundary $\alpha_1, ..., \alpha_K$ sequentially in that order using R code.

We let $\psi_k(\alpha|H_0) = \pi_k$, where $\psi_k(\alpha|H_0)$ is from (3.3), but this time we work on $Z$-scale. In addition, for simplicity and due to the nonbinding futility rule implemented currently by the FDA, in determining the efficacy stopping boundaries $\alpha_k$, we ignore all futility boundaries.

Thus after $\alpha_1, ..., \alpha_{k-1}$ are determined, the $\alpha_k$ can determined by the trial-and-error method based on the following equation:

$$\Pr(T_1 < \alpha_1, ..., T_{k-1} < \alpha_{k-1}, T_k > \alpha_k | H_0) = \pi_k. \qquad (8.13)$$

The equation says: to determine $\alpha_k$ the rejection probability at the $k$th stage when $H_0$ is true must be equal to the error spent at that stage, $\pi_k$.

From Chapter 5, we know that $z_i = \frac{1}{\sqrt{n_i}} \sum_{j=1}^{n_i} \left( y_{i_j} - x_{i_j} \right)$. For simplicity, we have assumed $\sigma = 1$ in the derivation. The test statistic at the $k$th stage is

$$T_k = \sum_{i=1}^{k} w_{ki} z_i, \qquad (8.14)$$

where the weights for the $k$th stage are $w_{ki} = \sqrt{\frac{n_i}{N_k}}$ (not the information time $\tau_i = \sqrt{\frac{n_i}{N}}$!!!) and $z_i$ is the $z$-statistic based on the subsample from the $i$th stage. For larger sample size, $z_i$ has the standard normal distribution. $T_1, ..., T_k$ have a multivariate normal distribution with mean $\mathbf{0}$ and covariance $Cov(T_k, T_m) = Cov(T_m, T_k) = \frac{\sum_{i=1}^{k} n_i}{\sum_{i=1}^{m} n_i} = \frac{N_k}{N_m} = \frac{\tau_k}{\tau_m}$, where $N_k$ and $N_m$ are the cumulative sample sizes up to the $k$th stage and $m$th stage, respectively, and $m > k$.

We are going to use a three-stage design as an example with one-sided $\alpha = 0.025$ to calculate the stopping boundaries based on (8.13) and (8.14) using $R$ programming.

(1) Suppose we choose $\pi_1 = 0.0025$, $\pi_2 = 0.005$, and $\pi_3 = 0.0175$ at information time, $\tau_1 = 1/3 = 1/3, \tau_2 = 2/3$, and $\tau_3 = 1$.

(2) $\alpha_1 = \Phi(1 - \pi_1) = \Phi(1 - 0.0025) = 2.807034$ on $z$-scale. NormalDist$(2.44) = 0.99266$, NormalInv$(1 - 0.0025; 0, 1) = 2.807$.

To calculate $\alpha_2$ we use the following $R$ code and try different values for $\alpha_2$ until the probability is very close to $\pi_2 = 0.005$. We found $\alpha_2 = 2.55453$ on the $z$-scale and $0.005316563$ on the $p$-scale.

>>**R**>>

```
library(mnormt)
mu=rep(0, 2)
alpha1=qnorm(1-0.0025); alpha2=2.55453
I1=1/3; I2=2/3; r12=I1/I2
```

```
s=matrix(c(1,r12,r12,1), 2,2)
pi2=sadmvn(lower=c(-Inf, alpha2), upper=c(alpha1, Inf), mu, s)
pScaleAlpha2=1-pnorm(alpha2)
pi2; pScaleAlpha2
```
<<R<<

(3) To calculate $\alpha_3$ we use the following $R$ code with the calculated $\alpha_1 = 2.807034$ and $\alpha_2 = 2.55453$, and try different values for $\alpha_3$ until the probability equals or is very close to $\pi_3 = 0.0175$. We found that $\alpha_3 = 2.054324$ on the $z$-scale and $0.01997217$ on the $p$-scale.

>>R>>
```
library(mnormt)
mu=rep(0, 3)
alpha1=2.807034; alpha2=2.554532; alpha3=2.054324
I1=1/3; I2=2/3; I3=1
r12=I1/I2; r13=I1/I3; r23=I2/I3
s=matrix(c(1,r12,r13, r12,1,r23, r13,r23,1), 3,3)
pi3=sadmvn(lower=c(-Inf, -Inf, alpha3), upper=c(alpha1,alpha2, Inf), mu, s)
pScaleAlpha3=1-pnorm(alpha3)
pi3; pScaleAlpha3
```
<<R<<

Finally, we have the stopping boundaries: $\alpha_1 = 2.807034$, $\alpha_2 = 2.554532$, and $\alpha_3 = 2.054324$.

For the power calculation of the two-group design with three stages, suppose mean difference is 0.1 and standard deviation $\sigma = 0.5$ and the standardized effect size $0.1/0.5 = 0.2$. We can use the following $R$ Program:

>>R>>
```
library(mnormt)
N=500
mu=0.2; mu2=rep(mu, 2); mu3=rep(mu, 3)
alpha1=2.807034-(N*I1/2)^0.5*mu
alpha2=2.554532-(N*I2/2)^0.5*mu
alpha3=2.054324-(N*I3/2)^0.5*mu
I1=1/3; I2=2/3; I3=1
r12=I1/I2; r13=I1/I3; r23=I2/I3
s2=matrix(c(1,r12, r12,1), 2,2)
s3=matrix(c(1,r12,r13, r12,1,r23, r13,r23,1), 3,3)
power1=1-pnorm(alpha1)
power2=sadmvn(lower=c(-Inf, alpha2), upper=c(alpha1,Inf), mu2, s2)
```

power3=sadmvn(lower=c(-Inf, -Inf, alpha3), upper=c(alpha1,alpha2, Inf), mu3, s3)
power=power1+power2+power3
AverageN=(power1*I1+power2*I2+power3*I3)*N
power; AverageN
<<**R**<<

From the program outputs, we know that a total sample size of $N = 600$ per group gives 86.6% power. The variables, power1 = 0.163, power2 = 0.407, and power3 = 0.296, are the rejection probabilities at stages 1, 2, and 3, respectively. The average sample size, AverageN, is 310.8 per group.

For any stage $k > 3$, similar $R$ program can be created to calculate the stopping boundaries. For power calculation of $K$-stage design, it is convenient to use Monte Carlo simulations, which are discussed next. The simulation $R$ program for the $K$-stage design is presented as *R Function D.2* in the Appendix

### 8.3   Monte Carlo Approach

#### 8.3.1   *Normal Endpoint*

SAS Macro 8.1 below can be used for simulating two-arm $K$-stage adaptive designs with normal endpoint. The SAS variables are defined as follows: **nSims** = number of simulation runs, and **Model** = adaptive design method: "MIP," "MSP," or "MPP." **nStgs** = number of stages, **ux, uy** = means for groups x and y, respectively, **NId** = noninferiority margin, and **sigma** = standard deviation. **nAdj** = "Y" to allow for sample-size adjustment; otherwise, **nAdj** = "N." **N0** = initial cumulative sample size for the final stage, $\sum_i \text{Ns}\{i\}$, and **Nmax** = maximum sample size allowed. **DuHa** = true treatment mean difference; for power calculation, **DuHa** = **uy - ux**, and for sensitivity analysis, **DuHa** $\neq$ **uy – ux**. **Ns{i}** = the $i$th stage sample-size (not cumulative one), **alpha{i}** = the efficacy stopping boundary at the $i$th stage, and **beta{i}** = the futility stopping boundary at the $i$th stage. **ESP{i}** = the efficacy stopping probability at the $i$th stage, and **FSP{i}** = the futility stopping probability at the $i$th stage. **power** = the simulated power for the trial, **Aveux** = naive mean in group x, **Aveuy** = naive mean in group y, and **AveN** = the average sample size per group.

The key algorithms for SAS Macro 8.1 are specified as follows:

(1) Take inputs: **nSims, Model, nStags, Ns{i}, alpha{i}, beta {i}, ux, uy, NId, sigma, nAdj, DuHa, Nmax, N0.**

(2) Generate stagewise means **uxObs** and **uyObs** for the two groups (not individual patient response).

(3) Compute the test statistic **TS** for either MPI, MSP, or MPP.

(4) Check if TS crosses the stopping boundary.

If the boundary is crossed, update the power and the stopping probability **ESP{i}** and/or **FSP{i}**; otherwise continue to the next stage of the trial.

(5) Loop back to step 2.

## >>SAS Macro 8.1: *K*-Stage Adaptive Designs with Normal Endpoint>>

```
%Macro NStgAdpDsgNor(nSims=1000000, Model="MIP", nStgs=3, ux=0,
uy=1, NId=0, sigma=2, nAdj="Y", DuHa=1, Nmax=200, N0=150);
DATA NStgAdpDsg; Set dInput;
KEEP power Aveux Aveuy AveN FSP1-FSP&nStgs ESP1-ESP&nStgs alpha1-
alpha&nStgs beta1-beta&nStgs;
Array Ns{&nStgs}; Array alpha{&nStgs}; Array beta{&nStgs};
Array ESP{&nStgs}; Array FSP{&nStgs};
seedx=3637; seedy=1624; nStgs=&nStgs; sigma=&sigma;
power=0; AveN=0; Aveux=0; Aveuy=0; du=abs(&uy-&ux);
cumN=0; Do i=1 To nStgs-1; cumN=cumN+Ns{i}; End;
Do i=1 To nStgs; FSP{i}=0; ESP{i}=0; End;
Do iSim=1 to &nSims;
ThisN=0; Thisux=0; Thisuy=0;
TS=0; If &Model="MPP" Then TS=1;
Do i=1 To nStgs;
uxObs=Rannor(seedx)*sigma/Sqrt(Ns{i})+&ux;
uyObs=Rannor(seedy)*sigma/Sqrt(Ns{i})+&uy;
Thisux=Thisux+uxObs*Ns{i};
Thisuy=Thisuy+uyObs*Ns{i};
ThisN=ThisN+Ns{i};
Z = (uyObs-uxObs+&NId)*Sqrt(Ns{i}/2)/sigma;
pi=1-ProbNorm(Z);
If &Model="MIP" Then TS=pi;
If &Model="MSP" Then TS=TS+pi;
If &Model="MPP" Then TS=TS*pi;
If TS>beta{i} Then Do; FSP{i}=FSP{i}+1/&nSims;
Goto Jump; End;
Else If TS<=alpha{i} then do;
Power=Power+1/&nSims; ESP{i}=ESP{i}+1/&nSims;
```

Goto Jump; End;
Else If i=1 & &Nadj="Y" Then Do;
eRatio=&DuHa/(abs(uyObs-uxObs)+0.0000001);
nFinal=min(&Nmax,max(&N0,eRatio*2*&N0));
If nStgs>1 Then Ns{nStgs}= nFinal-cumN; End;
End;
Jump:
Aveux=Aveux+Thisux/ThisN/&nSims;
Aveuy=Aveuy+Thisuy/ThisN/&nSims;
AveN=AveN+ThisN/&nSims;
End;
Output;
Run;
Proc Print; run;
%Mend NStgAdpDsgNor;
<<**SAS**<<

## Example 8.1    Three-Stage Adaptive Design

In a phase-III asthma study with two dose groups (control and active), the primary efficacy endpoint is the percent change from baseline in FEV1. The estimated FEV1 improvement from baseline is 5% and 12% for the control and active groups, respectively, with a common standard deviation of $\sigma = 22\%$.

We will discuss three-stage, group sequential designs with and without SSR using MSP. There are four simple steps to follow in order to design the trial with SAS Macro 8.1: (1) determine the stopping boundaries, (2) determine the power or sample size, (3) perform sensitivity analysis, and (4) perform estimation.

Let's first illustrate the steps using the design without SSR.

### (1) Determination of stopping boundary

Choose the number of analyses and the initial stagewise sample size and stopping boundaries alpha{i} and beta{i}. Set the null hypothesis condition (e.g., ux = 0.05, uy = 0.05). Use the following SAS macro call to calculate the power under this null condition; then adjust the value of alpha{i} and beta{i} until the power = type-I error $\alpha$.

>>**SAS**>>
Data dInput;
Array Ns{3} (100, 100, 100); Array alpha{3} (0.014,0.15,0.291);
Array beta{3} (1,1,1);

```
%NStgAdpDsgNor(Model="MSP", nStgs=3, ux=0.05, uy=0.05,
sigma=0.22, nAdj="N"); Run;
```
<<**SAS**<<

## (2) Determination of the sample size

Keep everything the same, but change the treatment effect to the alternative hypothesis. The following is the SAS macro call for the power calculation.

>>**SAS**>>
```
Data dInput;
Array Ns{3} (100, 100, 100); Array alpha{3} (0.014,0.15,0.291);
Array beta{3} (1,1,1);
%NStgAdpDsgNor(Model="MSP", nStgs=3,ux=0.05, uy=0.12,
sigma=0.22, nAdj="N"); Run;
```
<<**SAS**<<

If the power is different from the desired power, change the sample size, redetermine the stopping boundaries, and simulate the power again. The iteration process continues until the desired power is reached.

## (3) Sensitivity analysis

Because the treatment difference and its variability are not exactly known, it is necessary to run the simulation under other critical conditions, which is referred to as sensitivity analysis or risk assessment.

The example of sensitivity analysis with the control mean $u_x = 0.05$ and the test mean $u_y = 0.11$ is given by the following SAS statement.

>>**SAS**>>
```
Data dInput;
Array Ns{3} (100, 100, 100); Array alpha{3} (0.014,0.15,0.291);
Array beta{3} (1,1,1);
%NStgAdpDsgNor(Model="MSP", nStgs=3,ux=0.05, uy=0.11,
sigma=0.22, nAdj="N"); Run;
```
<<**SAS**<<

The simulation results or the operating characteristics of the design are presented in Table 8.2.

The stopping probabilities can be used to calculate the expected duration of the trial. In the current case, the conditional (on the efficacy claim)

Table 8.2:   3-Stage Design Operating Characteristics without SSR

| Case | ESP1 | ESP2 | ESP3 | FSP1 | FSP2 | FSP3 | Power | N |
|------|------|------|------|------|------|------|-------|---|
| $H_0$ | 0.014 | 0.009 | 0.002 | 0.000 | 0.500 | 0.326 | 0.025 | 246 |
| $H_a$ | 0.520 | 0.294 | 0.078 | 0.000 | 0.001 | 0.002 | 0.892 | 166 |
| $H_s$ | 0.394 | 0.293 | 0.094 | 0.000 | 0.003 | 0.008 | 0.780 | 192 |

expected trial duration is given by

$$\bar{t}_e = \sum_{i=1}^{3} ESP\{i\} \, t_i,$$

where $t_i$ is the time from the first-patient-in to the $i$th interim analysis.

The conditional (on the futility claim) expected trial duration is given by

$$\bar{t}_f = \sum_{i=1}^{3} FSP\{i\} \, t_i.$$

The unconditional expected trial duration for the trial is given by

$$\bar{t} = \sum_{i=1}^{3} \left( ESP\{i\} + FSP\{i\} \right) t_i.$$

**(4) Naive point estimations:**

The average naive point estimate can be obtained using the SAS macro. Under the null hypothesis $H_0 : u_x = u_y = 0.05$, the naive means are $\hat{u}_x = 0.0510$ and $\hat{u}_y = 0.0490$ for the control and test groups, respectively. We can see that the bias is negligible. Under the alternative $H_a: u_x = 0.05$ and $u_y = 0.12$. The naive mean estimates are $\hat{u}_x = 0.0462$ and $\hat{u}_y = 0.1240$. Under $H_s: u_x = 0.05$ and $u_y = 0.11$, the naive means are $\hat{u}_x = 0.0460$ and $\hat{u}_y = 0.1141$ for the two groups.

Similarly, for a three-stage design with SSR using MSP, the SAS macro calls for the design are given as follows.

**(1) Determine the stopping boundaries**

Using the following SAS macro call to determine the stopping boundaries.

>>**SAS**>>

```
Data dInput;
Array Ns{3} (100, 100, 100); Array alpha{3} (0.014,0.15,0.291);
Array beta{3} (1,1,1);
%NStgAdpDsgNor( Model="MSP", nStgs=3,ux=0.05, uy=0.05,
```

sigma=0.22, nAdj="Y", Nmax=500, N0=300);
<<**SAS**<<

By trial-and-error method, we can find that the stopping boundaries are virtually the same as those without SSR.

**(2) Determine sample size**

Use the following SAS macro call to determine the sample size required for the desired power.

>>**SAS**>>
Data dInput;
Array Ns{3} (100, 100, 100); Array alpha{3} (0.014,0.15,0.291);
Array beta{3} (1,1,1);
%NStgAdpDsgNor(Model="MSP", nStgs=3,ux=0.05, uy=0.12,
sigma=0.22, nAdj="Y", Nmax=500, N0=300);
<<**SAS**<<

**(3) Sensitivity assessment**

Use the following SAS call for the sensitivity analysis.

>>**SAS**>>
Data dInput;
Array Ns{3} (100, 100, 100); Array alpha{3} (0.014,0.15,0.291);
Array beta{3} (1,1,1);
%NStgAdpDsgNor(Model="MSP", nStgs=3,ux=0.05, uy=0.11,
sigma=0.22, nAdj="Y", Nmax=500, N0=300);
<<**SAS**<<

**(4) Operating characteristics**

The operating characteristics are summarized in Table 8.3.

Table 8.3: 3-Stage Design Operating Characteristics with SSR

| Case | ESP1 | ESP2 | ESP3 | FSP1 | FSP2 | FSP3 | Power | N |
|------|------|------|------|------|------|------|-------|---|
| $H_0$ | .014 | .009 | .002 | .000 | .500 | .326 | .025 | 342 |
| $H_a$ | .520 | .294 | .100 | .000 | .001 | .000 | .914 | 204 |
| $H_s$ | .394 | .292 | .137 | .000 | .003 | .001 | .823 | 254 |

Note that the operating characteristics are virtually the same under $H_0$, with or without SSR ($N_{max} = 500$). The sample adjustment is performed at the first interim analysis. Under $H_s$ (ux = 5% vs. uy = 11%), the power increases by 4.3% (from 78% to 82.3%) with SSR compared to without SSR.

**Naive point estimations:**

The naive mean estimates are $(\hat{u}_x = 0.0521,\ \hat{u}_y = 0.0480)$ under $H_0$, $(\hat{u}_x = 0.0455, \hat{u}_y = 0.1247)$ under $H_a$, and $(\hat{u}_x = 0.0450,\ \hat{u}_y = 0.1150)$ under $H_s$. These numbers indicate the magnitude of the potential bias caused by an adaptive design.

### 8.3.2  *Binary Endpoint*

SAS Macro 8.2 below can be used for two-arm, $N$-stage adaptive designs with binary endpoints. The SAS variables are defined as follows: **nSims** = number of simulation runs, and **Model** = adaptive design method: "MIP," "MSP," or "MPP." **nStgs** = number of stages, **Px, Py** = response rates for groups x and y, respectively. **NId** = noninferiority margin, and **sigma** = standard deviation. **nAdj** = "Y" to allow for sample-size adjustment; otherwise, **nAdj** = "N." **N0** = initial sample size for the final stage, and **Nmax** = maximum sample size allowed. **DuHa** = treatment difference; for power calculation, **DuHa** = **Py** – **Px**, and for sensitivity analysis, **DuHa** $\neq$ **Py** – **Px**. **Ns{i}** = the $i$th stage sample size (not cumulative one), **alpha{i}** = the efficacy stopping boundary at the $i$th stage, and **beta{i}** = the futility stopping boundary at the $i$th stage. **ESP{i}** = the efficacy stopping probability at the $i$th stage, and **FSP{i}** = the futility stopping probability at the $i$th stage. **power** = the simulated power for the trial, **AvePx** = naive average response rate in group x, **AvePy** = naive average response rate in group y, and **AveN** = the average sample size per group.

The key algorithms for SAS Macro 8.2 are specified as follows:

(1) Take inputs: **nSims, Model, nStags, Ns{i}, alpha{i}, beta {i}, Px, Py, NId, nAdj, DuHa, Nmax, N0.**

(2) Generate stagewise response rates **PxObs** and **PyObs** for the two groups.

(3) Compute the test statistic **TS** for MPI, MSP, or MPP.

(4) Check if **TS** crosses the stopping boundary.

If the boundary is crossed, update the power and the stopping probability **ESP{i}** or **FSP{i}**; otherwise continue to the next stage of the trial.

(5) Loop back to step 2.

**>>SAS Macro 8.2: *K*-Stage Adaptive Designs with Binary Endpoint>>**

%Macro NStgAdpDsgBin(nSims=1000000, Model="MIP", nStgs=3, Px=0, Py=1, NId=0, nAdj="Y", DuHa=1, Nmax=200, N0=150);

```
DATA NStgAdpDsg; Set dInput;
KEEP power AvePx AvePy AveN FSP1-FSP&nStgs ESP1-ESP&nStgs alpha1-
alpha&nStgs beta1-beta&nStgs;
Array Ns{&nStgs}; Array alpha{&nStgs}; Array beta{&nStgs};
Array ESP{&nStgs}; Array FSP{&nStgs};
seedx=3637; seedy=1624; nStgs=&nStgs; Px=&Px; Py=&Py;
power=0; AveN=0; AvePx=0; AvePy=0; cumN=0;
Do i=1 To nStgs-1; cumN=cumN+Ns{i}; End;
Do i=1 To nStgs; FSP{i}=0; ESP{i}=0; End;
Do iSim=1 to &nSims;
ThisN=0; ThisPx=0; ThisPy=0;
TS=0; If &Model="MPP" Then TS=1;
ThisN=0;
Do i=1 To nStgs;
PxObs=RanBin(seedx,Ns(i),Px)/Ns(i);
PyObs=RanBin(seedy,Ns(i),Py)/Ns(i);
ThisPx=ThisPx+PxObs*Ns(i);
ThisPy=ThisPy+PyObs*Ns(i);
ThisN=ThisN+Ns{i};
sigma=((PxObs*(1-PxObs)+PyObs*(1-PyObs))/2)**0.5;
Z = (PyObs-PxObs+&NId)*Sqrt(Ns{i}/2)/sigma;
pi=1-ProbNorm(Z);
If &Model="MIP" Then TS=pi;
If &Model="MSP" Then TS=TS+pi;
If &Model="MPP" Then TS=TS*pi;
If TS>beta{i} Then Do; FSP{i}=FSP{i}+1/&nSims;
Goto Jump; End;
Else If TS<=alpha{i} then do;
Power=Power+1/&nSims; ESP{i}=ESP{i}+1/&nSims;
Goto Jump; End;
Else If i=1 & &Nadj="Y" Then Do;
eRatio=&DuHa/(abs(PyObs-PxObs)+0.0000001);
nFinal=round(min(&Nmax,max(&N0,eRatio*2*&N0)));
If nStgs>1 Then Ns{nStgs}= nFinal-cumN; End;
End;
Jump:
AvePx=AvePx+ThisPx/ThisN/&nSims;
AvePy=AvePy+ThisPy/ThisN/&nSims;
AveN=AveN+ThisN/&nSims;
```

Eend;
Output;
Run;
Proc print; Run;
%Mend NStgAdpDsgBin;
<<**SAS**<<

### Example 8.2    Four-Stage Adaptive Design

A phase-III trial is to be designed for patients with acute ischemic stroke of recent onset. The composite endpoint (death and MI) is the primary endpoint and the event rate is 14% for the control group and 12% for the test group. The sample size for a classical design is 5937 per group, which will provide 90% power at a one-sided alpha = 0.025.

For illustration purpose, we choose a four-stage design with and without SSR using MSP. Again, there are four simple steps to follow in order to design the trial with this SAS macro: (1) determine the stopping boundaries, (2) determine the power or sample size, (3) perform sensitivity analysis, and (4) perform estimation.

Let's first discuss the design without SSR.

### (1) Determination of stopping boundaries

Choose the number of analyses and the initial stagewise sample size, and stopping boundaries **alpha{i}** and **beta{i}**. Set the null hypothesis condition (e.g., Px = 0.14, Py = 0.14) and repeat the simulation using the following SAS macro call with different values of alpha{i} and beta{i} until the simulated power = type-I error $\alpha$.

>>**SAS**>>
Data dInput;
Array Ns{4} (1500, 1500, 1500, 1500); Array beta{4} (1,1,1,1);
Array alpha{4} (0.002,0.0011,0.0003, 0.00011);
%NStgAdpDsgBin(Model="MPP", nStgs=4, Px=0.14, Py=0.14, DuHa=0.02,
Nmax=10000, N0=6000); Run;
<<**SAS**<<

### (2) Determination of  sample-size

Keep everything the same, but change the treatment effect to the alternative hypothesis; then submit the following SAS statement to obtain the power.

>>**SAS**>>
Data dInput;

Array Ns{4} (1500, 1500, 1500, 1500);  Array beta{4} (1,1,1,1);
Array alpha{4} (0.002, 0.0011, 0.0003, 0.00011);
%NStgAdpDsgBin(Model = "MPP", nStgs=4, Px=0.12, Py=0.14, DuHa=0.02,
Nmax=10000, N0=6000); Run;
<<**SAS**<<

### (3) Operating characteristics
The operating characteristics are summarized in Table 8.4.

Table 8.4:  4-Stage Design Operating Characteristics without SSR

| Case | ESP1 | ESP2 | ESP3 | ESP4 | Power | N | $\bar{u}_x$ | $\bar{u}_y$ |
|------|------|------|------|------|-------|---|------|------|
| $H_0$ | .002 | .007 | .007 | .009 | .025 | 5959 | .140 | .140 |
| $H_a$ | .105 | .333 | .249 | .168 | .855 | 4155 | .119 | .141 |

### (4) Naive point estimations:
The naive point estimates $\hat{u}_x$ and $\hat{u}_y$ are also presented in Table 8.4.

We now follow the same steps to simulate the designs with sample-size adjustment.

### (1) Determination of stopping boundaries
Repeatedly submit the following SAS macro call with different values of alpha{i} and beta{i} to determine the stopping boundaries:

>>**SAS**>>
Data dInput;
Array Ns{4} (1500, 1500, 1500, 1500); Array beta{4} (1,1,1,1);
Array alpha{4} (0.002,0.0011,0.0003, 0.00011);
%NStgAdpDsgBin(Model="MPP", nStgs=4, Px=0.14, Py=0.14, nAdj="Y",
DuHa=0.02, Nmax=10000, N0=6000); Run;
<<**SAS**<<

### (2) Determine sample size
Use the following SAS macro call to determine the sample size required for the desired power.

>>**SAS**>>
Data dInput;
Array Ns{4} (1500, 1500, 1500, 1500); Array beta{4} (1,1,1,1);
Array alpha{4} (0.002,0.0011,0.0003, 0.00011);
%NStgAdpDsgBin( Model="MPP", nStgs=4, Px=0.12, Py=0.14, nAdj="Y",
DuHa=0.02, Nmax=10000, N0=6000); Run;
<<**SAS**<<

### (3) Operating Characteristics

The operating characteristics are presented in Table 8.5. The power increases from 85.5% to 97.1% due to SSR.

Table 8.5:    4-Stage Design Operating Characteristics with SSR

| Case | ESP1 | ESP2 | ESP3 | ESP4 | Power | N | $\bar{u}_x$ | $\bar{u}_y$ |
|------|------|------|------|------|-------|------|------|------|
| Ho | .002 | .007 | .007 | .009 | .025 | 9824 | .140 | .140 |
| Ha | .105 | 0.333 | .249 | .284 | .971 | 5374 | .118 | .142 |

### 8.3.3    *Survival Endpoint*

SAS Macro 8.3 below can be used for two-arm $K$-stage adaptive designs with binary, normal, or survival endpoints. The SAS variables are defined as follows: **nSims** = number of simulation runs, **nStgs** = number of stages, and **ux**, **uy** = means, response rates, or hazard rate for groups x and y, respectively, depending on the endpoint; **NId** = noninferiority margin; and **sigma** = standard deviation. **nAdj** = "Y" to allow for sample-size adjustment, otherwise, **nAdj** = "N", **N0** = initial cumulative sample size for the final stage, and **Nmax** = maximum sample size allowed. **DuHa** = treatment difference; for power calculation **DuHa = uy – ux**; for sensitivity analysis, **DuHa ≠ uy – ux**. **tAcr** = uniform accrural duration, **tStd** = trial duration, and   **Ns{i}** =   the $i$th stage sample size (not cumulative one). **alpha{i}** = the efficacy stopping boundary at the $i$th stage, **beta{i}** = the futility stopping boundary at the $i$th stage. **ESP{i}** = the efficacy stopping probability at the $i$th stage, and **FSP{i}** = the futility stopping probability at the $i$th stage. **power** = the simulated power for the trial, **Avewx** = average response in group x, **Avewy** = average response in group y, and **AveN** = the average sample size per group. **EP** = "normal," "binary," or "survival." **Model** is for the methods, which can be MIP, MSP, MPP, WZ, or UWZ. WZ is for the inverse-normal method with constant weights and UWZ is for the inverse-normal method with information time as the weights.

The key algorithms for SAS Macro 8.3 are specified as follows:

(1) Take inputs: **nSims, Model, nStags, Ns{i}, alpha{i}, beta {i}, ux, uy, NId, sigma, nAdj, DuHa, Nmax, N0, tAcr,** and **tStd.**

(2) Compute "standard deviation" sigma based on different endpoints.

(3) Generate stagewise response **uxObs**, and **uyObs** for the two groups.

(3) Compute the test statistic **TS** for MPI, MSP, MPP, WZ, and UWZ.

(4) Check if **TS** crosses the stopping boundary.

If the boundary is crossed, update the power and the stopping probability **ESP{i}** or **FSP{i};** otherwise continue to the next stage of the trial.

(5) Loop back to step 2.

## >>SAS Macro 8.3: *K*-Stage Adaptive Designs with Various Endpoints>>

```
%Macro TwoArmNStgAdpDsg(nSims=100000, nStgs=3, ux=0, uy=1, NId=0,
EP="normal", Model="MSP", nAdj="N", DuHa=1, Nmax=300, N0=100,
sigma=2, tAcr=10, tStd=24);
DATA NStgAdpDsg; Set dInput;
KEEP power Aveux Aveuy AveN FSP1-FSP&nStgs ESP1-ESP&nStgs alpha1-
alpha&nStgs beta1-beta&nStgs;
Array Ns{&nStgs}; Array alpha{&nStgs}; Array beta{&nStgs};
Array ESP{&nStgs}; Array FSP{&nStgs}; Array Ws{&nStgs};
Array sumWs{&nStgs}; Array TSc{&nStgs};
seedx=3637; seedy=1624; Model=&Model; nStgs=&nStgs;
sigma=&sigma; power=0; AveN=0; Aveux=0; Aveuy=0;
cumN=0; Do i=1 To nStgs-1; cumN=cumN+Ns{i}; End;
Do k=1 To nStgs;
sumWs{k}=0;
Do i=1 To k;  sumWs{k}=sumWs{k}+Ws{i}**2;  End;
sumWs{k}=Sqrt(sumWs{k});
End;
* Calcate the standard deviation, sigma for different endpoints *;
u=(&ux+&uy)/2;
If &EP="normal" Then sigma=&sigma;
If &EP="binary" Then sigma=(u*(1-u))**0.5;
If &EP="survival" Then do;
expud=exp(-u*&tStd);
sigma=u*(1+expud*(1-exp(u*&tAcr))/(&tAcr*u))**(-0.5); End;
Do i=1 To nStgs; FSP{i}=0; ESP{i}=0; End;
Do iSim=1 to &nSims;
ThisN=0; Thisux=0; Thisuy=0;
Do i=1 To nStgs; TSc{i}=0; End;
TS=0; If &Model="MPP" Then TS=1;
Do i=1 To nStgs;
uxObs=Rannor(seedx)*sigma/Sqrt(Ns{i})+&ux;
uyObs=Rannor(seedy)*sigma/Sqrt(Ns{i})+&uy;
Thisux=Thisux+uxObs*Ns{i};
Thisuy=Thisuy+uyObs*Ns{i};
```

```
ThisN=ThisN+Ns{i};
TS0 = (uyObs-uxObs+&NId)*Sqrt(Ns{i}/2)/sigma;
If Model="MIP" Then TS=1-ProbNorm(TS0);
If Model="MSP" Then TS=TS+(1-ProbNorm(TS0));
If Model="MPP" Then TS=TS*(1-ProbNorm(TS0));
If Model="WZ" Then Do;
Do k=i to nStgs;
TSc{k}=TSc{k}+Ws{i}/sumWs{k}*TS0;
End;
TS=1-ProbNorm(TSc{i});
End;
If Model="UWZ" Then Do;
TS0=((Thisuy-Thisux)/ThisN+&NId)*Sqrt(ThisN/2)/sigma;
TS=1-ProbNorm(TS0);
End;
If TS>beta{i} Then Do; FSP{i}=FSP{i}+1/&nSims;
Goto Jump; End;
Else If TS<=alpha{i} then do;
Power=Power+1/&nSims; ESP{i}=ESP{i}+1/&nSims;
Goto Jump; End;
Else If i=1 & &Nadj="Y" Then Do;
eRatio=&DuHa/(abs(uyObs-uxObs)+0.0000001);
nFinal=min(&Nmax,max(&N0,eRatio*2*&N0));
If nStgs>1 Then Ns{nStgs}= nFinal-cumN; End;
End;
Jump:
Aveux=Aveux+Thisux/ThisN/&nSims;
Aveuy=Aveuy+Thisuy/ThisN/&nSims;
AveN=AveN+ThisN/&nSims;
End;
Output;
Run;
Proc Print; Run;
%Mend TwoArmNStgAdpDsg;
```
<<**SAS**<<

## Example 8.3    Adaptive Design with Survival Endpoint

Consider a two-arm comparative oncology trial comparing a test drug to an active control with respect to the primary efficacy endpoint, time to disease progression (TTP). Based on data from previous studies, the median

TTP is estimated to be 10 months (hazard rate = 0.0693) for the control group and 13 months (hazard rate = 0.0533) for the test group. Assume that there is a uniform enrollment with an accrual period of 10 months and that the total study duration is expected to be 24 months. Sample-size calculation will be performed under the assumption of an exponential survival distribution.

To do the simulation, choose the number of analyses ($K = 3$), the initial stagewise sample size, and stopping boundaries alpha{i} and beta{i}. Define the null hypothesis condition (e.g., ux = 0.0693, uy = 0.0693). Similar to the steps in the previous two examples with normal and binary endpoints, there are four simple steps to follow in order to design the trial with this SAS macro: (1) determine the stopping boundaries, (2) determine the power or sample-size, (3) perform sensitivity analysis, and (4) perform estimation. The corresponding SAS macro calls are presented as follows:

### (1) Determination of stopping boundary

Use the following SAS macro call as an example to determine the stopping boundaries.

>>**SAS**>>

```
Data dInput;
Array Ns{3} (150, 150, 150); Array alpha{3} (0.002,0.01,0.02);
Array beta{3} (1,1,0.02); Array Ws{3} (1,1,1);
%TwoArmNStgAdpDsg(nStgs=3,ux=0.0693,     uy=0.0693,     EP="survival",
Model="WZ", tAcr=10, tStd=24); Run;
```

<<**SAS**<<

### (2) Determination of sample size

Keep everything the same, but change the treatment effect to the alternative hypothesis. Use the following SAS macro call to obtain the power.

>>**SAS**>>

```
Data dInput;
Array Ns{3} (150, 150, 150); Array alpha{3} (0.002,0.01,0.02);
Array beta{3} (1,1,0.02); Array Ws{3} (1,1,1);
%TwoArmNStgAdpDsg(nStgs=3,  ux=0.0533,  uy=0.0693,  EP="survival",
Model="WZ", tAcr=10, tStd=24); Run;
```

<<**SAS**<<

## (3) Sensitivity analysis

Use the following SAS macro call as an example for the sensitivity analysis.

>>**SAS**>>

Data dInput;

Array Ns{3} (150, 150, 150); Array alpha{3} (0.002,0.01,0.02);

Array beta{3} (1,1,0.02); Array Ws{3} (1,1,1);

%TwoArmNStgAdpDsg(nStgs=3,    ux=0.0533,    uy=0.066,    EP="survival",

Model="WZ", tAcr=10, tStd=24); Run;

<<**SAS**<<

## (4) Operating characteristics

The operating characteristics are summarized in Table 8.6.

Table 8.6:   Two-Arm Design Operating Characteristics without Adjustment

| Case | ESP1 | ESP2 | ESP3 | Power | N | $\bar{u}_x$ | $\bar{u}_y$ |
|------|------|------|------|-------|-----|------|------|
| Ho | .002 | .009 | .014 | .025 | 448 | .069 | .069 |
| Ha | .155 | .474 | .259 | .888 | 332 | .052 | .070 |
| Hs | .085 | .345 | .297 | .727 | 373 | .053 | .067 |

Similarly, for the design with sample-size adjustment, the stopping boundaries, the initial sample-size determination, and the sensitivity analysis can be carried out using the SAS macro calls as described below:

## (1) Determination of Stopping Boundaries

Use the following SAS macro call as an example to determine the stopping boundaries.

>>**SAS**>>

Data dInput;

Array Ns{3} (150, 150, 150); Array alpha{3} (0.002,0.0075,0.02);

Array beta{3} (1,1,0.02); Array Ws{3} (1,1,1);

%TwoArmNStgAdpDsg(nStgs=3,    ux=0.0693,    uy=0.0693,    EP="survival",

Model="UWZ",   Nadj="Y",   DuHa=0.016,   Nmax=600,   N0=450,   tAcr=10,

tStd=24);

<<**SAS**<<

## (2) Determination of sample-size

Keep everything the same, but change the treatment effect to the alternative hypothesis. Use the following SAS macro call to obtain the power.

>>**SAS**>>

Data dInput;

Array Ns{3} (150, 150, 150); Array alpha{3} (0.002,0.0075,0.02);

Array beta{3} (1,1,0.02); Array Ws{3} (1,1,1);

%TwoArmNStgAdpDsg(nStgs=3,ux=0.0533,   uy=0.0693,   EP="survival",

Model="UWZ", Nadj="Y", DuHa=0.016,   Nmax=600, N0=450, tAcr=10,

tStd=24);

<<**SAS**<<

### (3) Sensitivity analysis

Use the following SAS macro call as an example for the sensitivity analysis.

>>**SAS**>>

Data dInput;

Array Ns{3} (150, 150, 150); Array alpha{3} (0.002,0.0075,0.02);

Array beta{3} (1,1,0.02); Array Ws{3} (1,1,1);

%TwoArmNStgAdpDsg(nStgs=3,ux=0.0533,   uy=0.066,   EP="survival",

Model="UWZ", Nadj="Y", DuHa=0.016,   Nmax=600, N0=450, tAcr=10,

tStd=24);

<<**SAS**<<

### (4) Operating characteristics

The operating characteristics are summarized in Table 8.7.

Table 8.7:   Two-Arm Operating Characteristics with SSR

| Case | ESP1 | ESP2 | ESP3 | Power | N | $\bar{u}_x$ | $\bar{u}_y$ |
|------|------|------|------|-------|-----|------|------|
| Ho | .002 | .007 | .016 | .025 | 597 | .069 | .069 |
| Ha | .155 | .435 | .366 | .956 | 400 | .052 | .070 |
| Hs | .085 | .306 | .449 | .840 | 470 | .052 | .067 |

## 8.4   Summary

In this chapter we have demonstrated how to implement adaptive design with more than two stages using different approaches, and we provided the SAS macros and *R* functions. We have shown step by step how to use these computer programs to conduct trial designs. In determining the appropriate adaptive design, it is important to conduct sensitivity analyses and compare operating characteristics among different designs. In contrast to the simulation method, we will introduce you to the recursive adaptive design methods in Chapter 10, where you will find many closed forms for $K$-stage adaptive designs. However, before that we will discuss another interesting method used mainly for two-stage designs: the conditional error function method.

**Problems**

**8.1** If the test statistic at stage $k$ is defined as the average of the stage-wise $p$-values, i.e., $T_k = \frac{1}{k} \sum_{i=1}^{k} p_i$, derive the similar expressions for $\pi_1$, $\pi_2$, $\pi_3$, and $\pi_4$ as in (8.1) through (8.4).

**8.2** SAS Macro 8.1 is based on the randomly degenerated mean responses for individual groups. Modify the macro such that it is based on the randomly generated individual patient response, instead of mean responses; then compare the results from the two different approaches for small sample-size trials.

**8.3** Assuming the standard deviation $\sigma = 25\%$ in Example 8.1, redesign the trial and justify your choice of method (MSP, MPP, or MINP) and type of stopping boundary.

# Chapter 9

# Conditional Error Function Method and Conditional Power

In this chapter, we are going to discuss the so-called conditional error function method (CEFM), used mainly for two-stage designs. Researchers of this method include Proschan and Hunsberger (1995), Liu and Chi (2001), Müller and Schäfer (2001), and Denne (2001), among others. We will use the conditional error function method to easily derive the stopping boundary formulations for two general $p$-value combination methods.

## 9.1 Proschan–Hunsberger Method

Proschan and Hunsberger (1995) proposed a conditional error function method for two-stage design. Here we modify the Proschan–Hunsberger method slightly to fit different types of endpoints by using inverse-normal transformation $z_k = \Phi^{-1}(1 - p_k)$ and $p_k = 1 - \Phi(z_k)$, where $p_k$ is the stagewise $p$-value based on a subsample from stage $k$.

Let the test statistics for the first stage (sample-size $n_1$) and second stage (sample-size $n_2$) be

$$T_1 = p_1 \tag{9.1}$$

and

$$T_2 = 1 - \Phi\left(w_1\Phi^{-1}(1 - p_1) + w_2\,\Phi^{-1}(1 - p_2)\right), \tag{9.2}$$

respectively.

The stopping rules are given by

$$\begin{cases} \text{If } T_k \leq \alpha_k, \ (k = 1, 2), \ \text{stop and reject } H_0 \\ \text{If } T_k > \beta_k, \ (k = 1, 2), \ \text{stop and accept } H_0 \\ \text{Otherwise} \qquad\qquad\quad \text{continue,} \end{cases} \tag{9.3}$$

where $\alpha_2 = \beta_2$.

Assume that $T_1$ has the standard normal distribution under the null hypothesis. Let $A(p_1)$ be the conditional probability of making type-I error at the second stage given $T_1 = p_1$. Notice that $p_1$ is uniformly distributed over $[0,1]$; a level $\alpha$ test requires

$$\alpha = \alpha_1 + \int_{\alpha_1}^{\beta_1} A(p_1) \, dp_1, \tag{9.4}$$

where $A(p_1)$ is called the conditional error function on a $p$-scale, which is similar to the conditional error function on a $z$-scale given by Proschan and Hunsberger (1995). The conditional error function can be any nondecreasing function $0 \le A(p_1) \le 1$ as far as type-I error is concerned.

Proschan and Hunsberger (1995) suggest the circular conditional error function:

$$A(p_1) = 1 - \Phi(\sqrt{[\Phi^{-1}(1 - \alpha_1)]^2 - [\Phi^{-1}(1 - p_1)]^2}), \quad \alpha_1 < p_1 \le \beta_1. \tag{9.5}$$

Let $\beta_1 = \alpha_2$. For a given $\alpha$ and a predetermined $\alpha_1$, $\beta_1$ can be calculated numerically by substituting (9.5) into (9.4). For example, with a one-sided $\alpha = 0.025$, and $\alpha_1 = 0.0147$, $\beta_1$ will be 0.174.

The stopping boundaries are derived for a classical group sequential design, i.e., no other adaptations such as sample-size reestimation. With sample-size modification, the stopping boundaries are still valid if the weight $w_k$ (9.2) is prefixed. However, if the sample size at the second stage is dependent on the data from the first stage and the weights in (9.2) are not constant, e.g., $w_i = \sqrt{n_i/(n_1 + n_2)}$, $(i = 1, 2)$, the stopping boundaries determined using the above method are not valid anymore. In such cases, Proschan and Hunsberger (1995) suggest modifying $\alpha_2$ but leaving the conditional error function $A(p_1)$ unchanged, and consequently the test is still a level $\alpha$ test.

To determine $\alpha_2$, let's first derive the conditional power and conditional error function.

Let $cP_\delta(n_2, \alpha_2|p_1)$ be the conditional power $\Pr(T_2 \le \alpha_2|p_1, \delta)$, where $\delta$ is the effect size or treatment. Assuming a large sample-size and known variance $\sigma^2$, we can obtain conditional power (see Section 9.4):

$$cP_\delta(n_2, \alpha_2|p_1) = 1 - \Phi\left[\frac{\Phi^{-1}(1 - \alpha) - w_2\Phi^{-1}(1 - p_1)}{w_1} - \frac{\delta}{\sigma}\sqrt{\frac{n_2}{2}}\right], \tag{9.6}$$

where $w_1^2 + w_2^2 = 1$. For a given $\alpha_1$ and $\beta_1$, the conditional type-I error can be obtained by letting $\delta = 0$ in (9.6):

$$A(p_1) = 1 - \Phi \left[ \frac{\Phi^{-1}(1 - \alpha_2) - w_2 \Phi^{-1}(1 - p_1)}{w_1} \right]. \tag{9.7}$$

Because $A(p_1)$ is the same with or without SSR, it can be obtained through the procedure described for no SSR; then solve (9.7) for $\alpha_2$:

$$\alpha_2 = \frac{\sqrt{n_1} \Phi^{-1}(1 - p_1) + \sqrt{n_2} \Phi^{-1}(1 - A(p_1))}{\sqrt{n_1 + n_2}}. \tag{9.8}$$

Note that we have used the equation $w_i = \sqrt{n_i/(n_1 + n_2)}$. From (9.6) and (9.7), we can obtain the conditional power

$$cP_\delta(n_2, z_c|p_1) = 1 - \Phi \left( \Phi^{-1}(1 - A(p_1)) - \frac{\delta}{\sigma} \sqrt{\frac{n_2}{2}} \right). \tag{9.9}$$

To achieve a target conditional power $cP$, the sample-size required can be obtained by solving (9.9) for $n_2$:

$$n_2 = \frac{2\sigma^2}{\delta^2} \left[ \Phi^{-1}(1 - A(p_1)) - \Phi^{-1}(1 - cP) \right]^2. \tag{9.10}$$

Note that for constant conditional error, $A(p_1) = c$, where $c$ is a constant, (9.5) leads to $\alpha = \alpha_1 + c(\beta_1 - \alpha_1)$. Therefore, the constant conditional error approach is equivalent to MIP.

## Example 9.1    Adaptive Design for Coronary Heart Disease Trial

Suppose we are interested in a clinical trial in patients with coronary heart disease that compares a cholesterol-reducing drug to a placebo with respect to angiographic changes from baseline to end of study (Proschan and Hunsberger, 1995). The coronary arteries are first divided into segments; for each segment the difference in minimum lumen diameter from baseline to end of study is computed, and the average difference over all segments of a patient is the outcome measure. It is not known what constitutes a minimum clinically relevant change, but another similar study showed an effect size of about one third of the observed standard deviation. The sample size required for 90% power to detect a similar effect size is about 190 patients per group. It has been predetermined that the circular conditional error function will be used with one interim analysis based on evaluations of 95 patients in each arm. If $z_1 > 2.27$ ($p_1 < 0.0116$), the trial will be stopped for efficacy. If $z_1 < 0$ ($p_1 > 0.5$) at the interim analysis, the trial will be stopped for futility. If $0 \leq z_1 < 2.27$ ($0.0116 < p_1 \leq 0.5$), the trial will proceed to the second stage. Suppose after the interim analysis, the z-score $z_1 = 1.5$ ($p_1 = 0.0668$). The corresponding effect size ($\delta/\sigma$) is about 0.218. The conditional error is $A(0.0668) = 0.0436$ which is obtained from (9.7) with $w_1 = w_2 = \sqrt{0.5}$ and $\alpha_2 = 0.0116$. To have 80% conditional power under the empirically estimated treatment effect, the newly estimated sample size for the second stage is 274/group from (9.10).

## 9.2 Denne Method

Denne (2001) developed a new procedure for SSR at an interim analysis. Instead of keeping the conditional error ($\int_{\alpha_1}^{\beta_1} A(p_1) dp_1$) constant when making an adaptation, the Denne method ensures that the conditional error function $A(p_1)$ remains unchanged.

Let $w_{01}$, $w_{02}$, and $\alpha_{02}$ be weights and the final stopping boundary before sample-size modification; let $w_1$, $w_2$, and $\alpha_2$ be weights and the final stopping boundary after sample-size modification. To control overall $\alpha$, the stopping boundary $\alpha_2$ is adjusted such that $A(p_1)$ is unchanged:

$$\frac{\Phi^{-1}(1 - \alpha_{02}) - w_{02}\Phi^{-1}(1 - p_1)}{w_{01}} = \frac{\Phi^{-1}(1 - \alpha_2) - w_2\Phi^{-1}(1 - p_1)}{w_1},$$

(9.11)

where $w_{0i} = \sqrt{n_{0i}/(n_{01} + n_{02})}$ and $\tilde{w}_i = \sqrt{n_i/(n_1 + n_2)}$; $n_{0i}$ and $n_i$ are the subsample size at the $i$th stage before and after sample-size modification ($n_{01} = n_1$).

Equation (9.11) can be solved for $\alpha_2$:

$$\alpha_2 = 1 - \Phi\left[\frac{w_1}{w_{01}}\left\{\Phi^{-1}(1 - \alpha_{02}) - w_{02}\Phi^{-1}(1 - p_1)\right\} + w_2\Phi^{-1}(1 - p_1)\right].$$

(9.12)

Denne also stated that we can first modify the sample size based on the estimated variance at the first stage before unblinding the data, without modifying the stopping boundary. In such cases, the subsample size $n_2$ is the sample size after modification based on blinded data.

Note that Denne's method is originally based on a $z$-scale; hence, the stopping boundary is given by

$$c_2 = \frac{w_1}{w_{01}}\{c_{02} - w_{02}z_1\} + w_2z_1,$$

(9.13)

where $c_{02}$ and $c_2$ are the original and modified final stopping boundaries.

## 9.3 Müller–Schäfer Method

The procedure developed by Müller and Schäfer (2001) is based on calculating conditional rejection error probabilities for classical group sequential designs with any number of stages. The conditional rejection error probability is the probability that the null hypothesis will be rejected at a future stage of the design, given the value of the test statistic at an interim analysis, if the null hypothesis is true. Thereby, every choice of $n$-stage group sequential boundaries in the usual model of a Brownian motion process implicitly defines a conditional error function from which the type-I error risk for the rest of the trial after the interim analysis can be obtained (Müller and Schäfer, 2004). The Müller–Schäfer procedure can be viewed as a special case of the general concept developed by Müller and Schäfer (2004) applied to conventional group sequential designs in the Brownian motion model at the predetermined time points of the interim analyses. Müller and Schäfer (2001) showed, by combining the method with the product of $p$-values and the method with Brownian motion, how one could make any data dependent change in an ongoing adaptive trial and still preserve the overall type-I error. To achieve this, all one need do is preserve the conditional type-I error of the remaining portion of the trial. The conditional error usually can be calculated in real time for a given observed treatment difference.

We will discuss the trial examples of Müller–Schäfer in Chapter 10 as special cases of recursive two-stage adaptive designs.

In the next section, we will compare different methods based on their conditional error and conditional power functions.

## 9.4 Extension of Conditional Error Approach

Using conditional error approach, we can easily develop closed forms of stopping boundaries for two-stage adaptive designs with various test statistics. Let's denote the test statistic by $T(p_1, p_2)$ for the second stage and the rejection rule by $T(p_1, p_2) \leq \alpha_2$. On the stopping boundary at the second stage, $T(p_1, p_2) = \alpha_2$, from which we can solve for $p_2(p_1, \alpha_2)$. Under the null condition, $p_2 = p_2(p_1, \alpha_2)$ is the conditional error function. We will discuss two general forms of test statistics, MLPP (method based on a linear combination of power function of $p$-values) and MPPP (method based on the production of power function of $p$-values).

The test statistic for MLPP is defined as

$$\begin{cases} T_1 = p_1, \\ T_2 = w_1 p_1 + w_2 p_2^v, \end{cases} \tag{9.14}$$

To determine the stopping boundary, we let $T_2 = \alpha_2$ in (9.14), which leads to the conditional error under $H_0$

$$p_2 | H_0 = \begin{cases} \left[ \frac{1}{w_2} (\alpha_2 - w_1 p_1) \right]^{1/v}, & \text{if } p_1 \leq \frac{\alpha_2}{w_1}, \\ 0, & \text{otherwise} \end{cases} \tag{9.15}$$

where $v > 0$, $w_1 > 0$, $w_2 > 0$, and preferably $w_1 + w_2 = 1$. The conditional error indicates that when $p_1 \geq \min(1, \alpha_2/w_1)$, the trial should stop at the interim since in this case we will never be able to reject the null hypothesis. Therefore, the futility boundary should meet the criterion: $\beta_1 \leq \alpha_2/w_1$.

From (9.4) we know that to control error rate at $\alpha$ level, it is required that

$$\alpha = \alpha_1 + \int_{\alpha_1}^{\beta_1} \left[ \frac{1}{w_2} (\alpha_2 - w_1 p_1) \right]^{1/v} dp_1$$

Carrying out the integration, we obtain

$$\alpha = \alpha_1 + \frac{1}{w_1 w_2^{1/v}} \frac{1}{1 + 1/v} \left[ (\alpha_2 - w_1 \alpha_1)^{(1+1/v)} - (\alpha_2 - w_1 \beta_1)^{(1+1/v)} \right], \tag{9.16}$$

where $\alpha_1 < \beta_1 \leq \alpha_2/w_1$. For nonbinding futility rule, we can let $\beta_1 = \alpha_2/w_1$, thus (9.16) reduces to

$$\alpha = \alpha_1 + \frac{1}{w_1 w_2^{1/v}} \frac{1}{1 + 1/v} \left[ (\alpha_2 - w_1 \alpha_1)^{(1+1/v)} \right]. \tag{9.17}$$

Solving for $\alpha_2$, we have

$$\alpha_2 = w_1 \alpha_1 + \left[ (\alpha - \alpha_1) w_1 w_2^{1/v} (1 + 1/v) \right]^{\frac{v}{1+v}}. \tag{9.18}$$

To be effective in SSR design, various weights can be chosen. For $v = 1$, we have

$$\begin{cases} T_1 = p_1, \\ T_2 = w_1 p_1 + w_2 p_2. \end{cases} \tag{9.19}$$

When $w_1 = w_2 = 1$ and $v = 1$, MLPP reduces to MSP. For $w_1 = w_2 = 0.5$, we obtain

$$\alpha_2 = \frac{\alpha_1}{2} + \frac{1}{2}\left[(\alpha - a_1)\frac{1+v}{v}\right]^{\frac{v}{1+v}}. \tag{9.20}$$

For $w_1 = w_2 = 0.5$ and $v = 1$, we have the method based mean $p$-values (MMP).

For MLPP with $w_1 = 1/3, w_2 = 2/3$ and $v = 5$, the test statistic is

$$\begin{cases} T_1 = p_1, \\ T_2 = \frac{1}{3}p_1 + \frac{2}{3}p_2^5 \end{cases}. \tag{9.21}$$

Some examples of stopping boundaries are presented in Tables 9.1 and 9.2.

Table 9.1:  Stopping Boundaries with MMP $(w_1 = w_2 = 1/2)$

| $\alpha_1$ | 0.00000 | 0.00250 | 0.00500 | 0.00750 | 0.01000 | 0.01250 | 0.01500 |
|---|---|---|---|---|---|---|---|
| $\alpha_2$ | 0.11180 | 0.10732 | 0.10250 | 0.09729 | 0.09160 | 0.08531 | 0.07821 |

Table 9.2:  Stopping Boundaries with MLP $(w_1 = 1/3, w_2 = 2/3)$

| $\alpha_1$ | 0.00000 | 0.00250 | 0.00500 | 0.00750 | 0.01000 | 0.01250 | 0.01500 |
|---|---|---|---|---|---|---|---|
| $\alpha_2$ | 0.10541 | 0.10083 | 0.09595 | 0.09069 | 0.08498 | 0.07870 | 0.07167 |

We now discuss the second class of test statistic (MPPP):

$$\begin{cases} T_1 = p_1 \\ T_2 = p_1 p_2^v \end{cases}, \tag{9.22}$$

where $v > 1$ and $0 \leq T_2 \leq 1$. The intersect $a_0 = +\infty$. Substitute $p_2 = \left(\frac{\alpha_2}{p_1}\right)^{\frac{1}{v}}$ into (9.4), we can obtain

$$\alpha = \alpha_1 + \int_{\alpha_1}^{\beta_1} \left(\frac{\alpha_2}{p_1}\right)^{\frac{1}{v}} dp_1, \tag{9.23}$$

$$\alpha = \alpha_1 + \frac{1}{1 - 1/v}\alpha_2^{\frac{1}{v}}\left[\beta_1^{(1-1/v)} - \alpha_1^{(1-1/v)}\right]. \tag{9.24}$$

With nonbinding futility rule, $\beta_1 = 1$, (9.24) becomes

$$\alpha = \alpha_1 + \frac{1}{1 - 1/v}\alpha_2^{\frac{1}{v}}\left[1 - \alpha_1^{(1-1/v)}\right] \tag{9.25}$$

Solving for $\alpha_2$ we obtain

$$\alpha_2 = \left[\frac{(\alpha - \alpha_1)(1 - 1/v)}{1 - \alpha_1^{(1-1/v)}}\right]^v. \tag{9.26}$$

Table 9.3 shows examples of stopping boundaries for MPPP with $v = 1.5$.

Table 9.3: Example Stopping Boundaries with MPPP ($v = 1.5$)

| $\alpha_1$ | 0.0025 | 0.0050 | 0.0075 | 0.0100 | 0.0125 | 0.0150 |
|---|---|---|---|---|---|---|
| $\alpha_2 \, (\times 10^{-4})$ | 8.0837 | 7.2116 | 6.1771 | 5.0877 | 3.9968 | 2.9431 |

The conditional error functions and stopping boundaries are summarized in Tables 9.4 and 9.5, respectively.

Table 9.4:  Conditional Error Functions (under $H_0$)

| Method | Test Statistic at Stage 2 $T_2(p_1, p_2)$ | Conditional Error Function $A(p_1)$ | Intersect $\alpha_0$ |
|---|---|---|---|
| MSP | $p_1 + p_2$ | $\max(0, \alpha_2 - p_1)$ | $p_1 = \alpha_2$ |
| MLP | $w_1 p_1 + w_2 p_2$ | $\max\left\{0, \frac{1}{w_2}(\alpha_2 - w_1 p_1)\right\}$ | $p_1 = \frac{\alpha_2}{w_1}$ |
| MLPP | $w_1 p_1 + w_2 p_2^v$ | $\max\left\{0, \frac{1}{w_2}(\alpha_2 - w_1 p_1)\right\}^{\frac{1}{v}}$ | $p_1 = \frac{\alpha_2}{w_1}$ |
| MPP | $p_1 p_2$ | $\frac{\alpha_2}{p_1}$ | $p_1 = +\infty$ |
| MPPP | $p_1 p_2^v$ | $\left(\frac{\alpha_2}{p_1}\right)^{\frac{1}{v}}$ | $p_1 = +\infty$ |
| MINP | $\sum_{i=1}^{2} w_i \Phi^{-1}(1 - p_i)$ | $1 - \Phi\left(\frac{\Phi^{-1}(1-\alpha_2) - w_1 \Phi^{-1}(1-p_1)}{w_2}\right)$ | |

Note: for MINP $w_1^2 + w_2^2 = 1$, for others $w_1 + w_2 = 1$.

Table 9.5:  Stopping Boundaries without Futility Binding

| Method | Test Statistic at Stage 2 $T_2(p_1, p_2)$ | Stopping Boundary $\alpha_2$ (no futility binding) |
|---|---|---|
| MSP | $p_1 + p_2$ | $\alpha_2 = \alpha_1 + \sqrt{2(\alpha - \alpha_1)}$ |
| MLP | $w_1 p_1 + w_2 p_2$ | $\alpha_2 = w_1^* \alpha_1 + \sqrt{2 w_1 w_2 (\alpha - \alpha_1)}.$ |
| MLPP | $w_1 p_1 + w_2 p_2^v$ | $\alpha_2 = w_1 \alpha_1 + \left[w_1 w_2^{1/v} \frac{1+v}{v}(\alpha - \alpha_1)\right]^{\frac{v}{1+v}}.$ |
| MPP | $p_1 p_2$ | $\alpha_2 = \frac{1}{\ln \alpha_1}(\alpha_1 - \alpha)$ |
| MPPP | $p_1 p_2^v$ | $\alpha_2 = \left[\frac{(\alpha - \alpha_1)(1 - 1/v)}{1 - \alpha_1^{(1-1/v)}}\right]^v$ |

The efficacy boundary $\alpha_2$ is usually a constant, but it can be a function of $p_1$. To visualize the differences of various methods (MIP, MSP, MPP, and MINP), the stopping boundaries at the second stage are plotted for the same stopping boundaries ($\alpha_1 = 0.005$, $\beta_1 = 0.25$) at the first stage (Figure 9.1). We can see that MPP and MINP are similar. MSP and MIP has some constraints on the consistency of the results from the different stages. In other words, when $p_1$ and $p_2$ are very different, the statistical significance can not be declared using MSP or MIP. On the other hand, if $p_1 = 0.006$ and $p_2 = 0.6$ (100 times difference! The fact of one-sided $p_2 = 0.6$ indicates the wrong direction of the treatment effect!), the null $H_0$ will still be rejected using MPP.

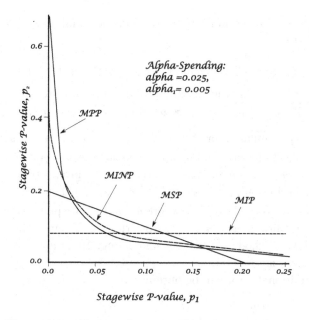

Figure 9.1: Various Stopping Boundaries at Stage 2

## 9.5 Conditional Power

The term *conditional power* is the probability of rejecting the null hypothesis in the remaining part of a trial, given the interim data that fall between the efficacy and futility stopping boundaries. Conditional power is a very useful operating characteristic for adaptive designs. It can be used for the interim decision making and to make comparisons among different designs and statistical methods. Because the stopping boundaries for most existing methods are based on either a $z$-scale or a $p$-scale, for the purpose of later comparisons, we will convert them all to $p$-scale using the following simple transformation: $p_k = 1 - \Phi(z_k)$. Inversely, we have $z_k = \Phi^{-1}(1 - p_k)$, where $z_k$ is the $z$-score from the subsample, which has an asymptotically normal distribution with $N(\delta/se\left(\hat{\delta}_2\right), 1)$ under the alternative hypothesis, where $\hat{\delta}_2$ is an estimation of treatment difference in the second stage and $se\left(\hat{\delta}_2\right) = \sqrt{\frac{2\hat{\sigma}^2}{n_2}} \approx \sqrt{\frac{2\sigma^2}{n_2}}$. To derive the conditional power, we express the criterion for rejecting $H_0$ as

$$z_2 \geq B(\alpha_2, p_1). \qquad (9.27)$$

From (9.14), we can immediately obtain the conditional probability at the second stage:

$$cP_\delta(p_1) = 1 - \Phi\left(B(\alpha_2, p_1) - \frac{\delta}{\sigma}\sqrt{\frac{n_2}{2}}\right), \alpha_1 < p_1 \leq \beta_1. \qquad (9.28)$$

For Fisher's combination method, the rejection criterion for the second stage is $p_1 p_2 \leq \alpha_2$, i.e., $z_2 \geq \Phi^{-1}\left(1 - \frac{\alpha_2}{p_1}\right)$. Therefore, $B(\alpha_2, p_1) = \Phi^{-1}\left(1 - \frac{\alpha_2}{p_1}\right)$. Similarly, for the method based on the sum of stagewise $p$-values, the rejection criterion for the second stage is $p_1 + p_2 \leq \alpha_2$, i.e., $z_2 = B(\alpha_2, p_1) = \Phi^{-1}(1 - \max(0, \alpha_2 - p_1))$. For the inverse-normal method, the rejection criterion for the second stage is $w_1 z_1 + w_2 z_2 \geq \Phi^{-1}(1 - \alpha_2)$, i.e., $z_2 \geq \frac{\Phi^{-1}(1-\alpha_2)-w_1\Phi^{-1}(1-p_1)}{w_2}$, where $w_1$ and $w_2$ are prefixed weights satisfying the condition: $w_1^2 + w_2^2 = 1$. Note that the group sequential design and the CHW method (Cui, Hung, and Wang, 1999) are special cases of the inverse-normal method.

The conditional error can be obtained by setting $\delta = 0$ in (9.28):

$$A(p_1) = 1 - \Phi(B(\alpha_2, p_1)), \alpha_1 < p_1 \leq \beta_1, \qquad (9.29)$$

and the functions $B(\alpha_2, z_1)$ are summarized in Table 9.8 for different design methods.

Substituting (9.29) into (9.4), we can obtain the following formulation for determining the stopping boundaries for various designs:

$$\alpha = \alpha_1 + \int_{\alpha_1}^{\beta_1} 1 - \Phi(B(\alpha_2, p_1)) \, dp_1. \qquad (9.30)$$

If the trial continues, i.e., $\alpha_1 < p_1 \leq \beta_1$, for given conditional power $cP$, we can solve (9.26) for the adjusted sample-size for the second stage:

$$n_2 = \frac{2\sigma^2}{\delta^2}\left(B(\alpha_2, z_1) - \Phi^{-1}(1 - cP)\right)^2. \qquad (9.31)$$

Table 9.6:   *B*-Function for Conditional Power and Sample-Size Reestimation

| Method | Test Statistic at Stage 2 | Function $B(\alpha_1, p_1)$ |
|---|---|---|
| MSP | $p_1+p_2$ | $\Phi^{-1}(1-\max(0,\alpha_2-p_1))$ |
| MLP | $w_1p_1+w_2p_2$ | $\Phi^{-1}\left(1-\max\left\{0,\frac{1}{w_2}(\alpha_2-w_1p_1)\right\}\right)$ |
| MLPP | $w_1p_1+w_2p_2^v$ | $\Phi^{-1}\left(1-\max\left\{0,\frac{1}{w_2}(\alpha_2-w_1p_1)\right\}^{\frac{1}{v}}\right)$ |
| MPP | $p_1p_2$ | $\Phi^{-1}\left(1-\frac{\alpha_2}{p_1}\right)$ |
| MPPP | $p_1p_2^v$ | $\Phi^{-1}\left(1-\left(\frac{\alpha_2}{p_1}\right)^{\frac{1}{v}}\right)$ |
| MINP | $\sum_{i=1}^2 w_i\Phi^{-1}(1-p_i)$ | $\frac{1}{w_2}\left(\Phi^{-1}(1-\alpha_2)-w_1\Phi^{-1}(1-p_1)\right)$ |

Note: For MINP $w_1^2+w_2^2=1$, for others $w_1+w_2=1$.

For $K$-stage design with MINP, the condtional power at stage $k$ can be expressed as (Jennison and Turnbull, 2000b):

$$cP_\delta(k) = \Phi\left(\frac{Z_k\sqrt{I_k}-z_{1-\alpha}\sqrt{I_K}+(I_K-I_k)\delta}{\sqrt{I_K-I_k}}\right), k=1,...,K-1, \qquad (9.32)$$

where information level

$$I_k = \left(\frac{\sigma_A^2}{n_{Ak}}+\frac{\sigma_B^2}{n_{Bk}}\right)^{-1}.$$

Here $n_{Ak}$ and $n_{Bk}$ are cumulative sizes in treatment groups $A$ and $B$.

The Bayesian preditive power at stage $k$ is given by

$$P_\delta(k) = \Phi\left(\frac{Z_k\sqrt{I_k}-z_{1-\alpha}\sqrt{I_K}}{\sqrt{I_K-I_k}}\right), k=1,...,K-1, \qquad (9.33)$$

For convenience, the conditional power (9.28) is implemented in SAS Macro 9.1 below. The SAS variables are defined as follows: the endpoint **EP** = "normal" or "binary"; **ux** and **uy** = the responses (means or proportions) for the two groups, respectively, **sigma** = standard deviation for the normal endpoint; **Model** ="MIP," "MSP," "MPP," or "MINP" for the four methods in Table 9.6; **alpha2** = the efficacy boundary at the second stage; **cPower** = the conditional power; **p1** = the stagewise $p$-value at the first stage; **w1** and **w2** = weights for Lehmacher–Wassmer method; and **n2** = sample size per group for the second stage.

## >>SAS Macro 9.1:   Conditional Power>>

```
%Macro ConPower(EP="normal", Model="MSP", alpha2=0.205, ux=0.2,
uy=0.4, sigma=1, n2=100, p1=0.8, w1=1, w2=1);
** cPower=Two-stage conditional power. eSize=delta/sigma;
data cPower;
a2=&alpha2; Model=&Model;
```

```
u=(&ux+&uy)/2;
w1=&w1/sqrt(&w1**2+&w2**2);
w2=&w2/sqrt(&w1**2+&w2**2);
If &EP="normal" Then sigma=&sigma;
If &EP="binary" Then sigma=(u*(1-u))**0.5;
eSize=(&uy-&ux)/sigma;
If Model="MIP" Then BFun=Probit(1-a2);
If Model="MSP" Then BFun=Probit(1-max(0.0000001,a2-&p1));
If Model="MPP" Then BFun=Probit(1-a2/&p1);
If Model="MINP" Then BFun=(Probit(1-a2)- w1*Probit(1-&p1))/w2;
cPower=1-ProbNorm(BFun-eSize*sqrt(&n2/2));
Run;
Proc Print data=cPower; Run;
%Mend ConPower;
```
<<**SAS**<<

An example of determining the sample size based on conditional power using SAS Macro 9.1 is given below.

<<**SAS**<<
```
%ConPower(EP="binary", Model="MSP", alpha2=0.2050, ux=0.2, uy=0.4,
n2=100, p1=0.1);
%ConPower(EP="binary", Model="MIP", alpha2=0.0201, ux=0.2, uy=0.4,
n2=100, p1=0.1);
%ConPower(EP="binary", Model="MPP", alpha2=0.0043, ux=0.2, uy=0.4,
n2=100, p1=0.1);
%ConPower(EP="binary", Model="MINP", alpha2=0.0226, ux=0.2, uy=0.4,
n2=100, p1=0.1, w1=1, w2=1);
%ConPower(EP="normal", Model="MSP", alpha2=0.2050, ux=0.2, uy=0.4,
sigma=1, n2=200, p1=0.1);
%ConPower(EP="normal", Model="MIP", alpha2=0.0201, ux=0.2, uy=0.4,
sigma=1, n2=200, p1=0.1);
%ConPower(EP="normal", Model="MPP", alpha2=0.0043, ux=0.2, uy=0.4,
sigma=1, n2=200, p1=0.1);
%ConPower(EP="normal", Model="MINP", alpha2=0.0226, ux=0.2, uy=0.4,
sigma=1, n2=200, p1=0.1, w1=1, w2=1);
```
<<**SAS**<<

The results with a nonbinding futility boundary are presented in Table 9.7. We can see that MSP produces the highest power. It is important to know that in adaptive design, conditional power is more important than

Table 9.7:  Comparisons of Conditional Powers $cP$

|  | Endpoint | MSP | MIP | MPP | MINP |
|---|---|---|---|---|---|
| $\alpha_2$ |  | 0.2050 | 0.0210 | 0.0043 | 0.0226 |
| $cP$ (n = 100) | binary | 0.967 | 0.850 | 0.915 | 0.938 |
| $cP$ (n = 200) | normal | 0.772 | 0.479 | 0.611 | 0.673 |

Note: $\alpha_1 = 0.005$, $\beta_1 = 0.25$, and $p_1 = 0.01$.

unconditional power.

The sample size required at the second stage based on the conditional power (9.28) is below implemented in SAS Macro 9.2. The SAS variables are defined as follows: **nAdjModel** = "MIP," "MSP," "MPP," or "MINP" for the four methods in Table 9.6: **alpha2** = the efficacy boundary at the second stage; **eSize** = standard effect size; **cPower** = the conditional power; **p1** = the stagewise $p$-value at the first stage; **w1** and **w2** = weights for Lehmacher–Wassmer method; and **n2New** = new sample size required for the second stage to achieve the desired conditional power.

>>**SAS Macro 9.2:   Sample Size Based on Conditional Power**>>
```
%Macro nByCPower(nAdjModel, alpha2, eSize, cPower, p1, w1, w2, n2New);
a2=&alpha2;
If &nAdjModel="MIP" Then BFun=Probit(1-a2);
If &nAdjModel="MSP" Then BFun=Probit(1-max(0.0000001,a2-&p1));
If &nAdjModel="MPP" Then BFun=Probit(1-a2/&p1);
If &nAdjModel="MINP" Then
BFun=(Probit(1-a2)- &w1*Probit(1-&p1))/&w2;
&n2New=2*((BFun-Probit(1-&cPower))/&eSize)**2; *n per group;
%Mend nByCPower;
```
<<**SAS**<<

An example of determining the sample size based on conditional power using SAS Macro 9.2 is given below.

>>**SAS**>>
```
Data cPow; keep n2New;
%nByCPower("MSP", 0.1840, 0.21, 0.8, 0.0311, 0.707, 0.707, n2New);
Run;
Proc Print; Run;
```
<<**SAS**<<

Based on the SAS output, the new sample size required for the second stage is 158 per group.

## 9.6    Adaptive Futility Design

### 9.6.1    *Utilization of an Early Futility Boundary*

In a trial with an early futility boundary, theoretically the final alpha for claiming statistic significance should increase. This may cause concern on the part of regulatory bodies, as the current practice is that the futility boundaries are not strictly followed by the sponsors, and therefore, the futility boundary should not be used to determine the later stopping boundaries. However, this is not very reasonable in the sense that we punish someone for others not following the rules. A more reasonable approach is that if the futility boundaries were actually followed, then the stopping boundaries with futility boundaries considered can be used. If the futility boundaries were not followed, i.e., the trial was continued even though it had crossed the futilities boundaries, then the early futility boundary cannot be considered in constructing the later stopping boundaries. For example, in a two-stage trial with MSP, the stopping boundaries in a two-stage design are $\alpha_1 = 0.0025$, $\beta_1 = 0.15$, $\alpha_2 = 0.2288$. Suppose the stagewise $p$-value from the first stage was $p_1 = 0.1$, and the trial was continued to the second stage. Therefore, the futility boundary has been followed, and the final stopping boundary should be $\alpha_2 = 0.2288$. On the other hand, if $p_1 = 0.2$, and the trial was continued, the futility boundary has been violated. Therefore, the final stopping boundary should be $\alpha_2 = 0.2146$ (corresponding to $\alpha_1 = 0.0025$, $\beta_1 = 1$), instead of 0.2288.

Note that MIP uses the early stopping boundary to construct the later stopping boundaries; this is different from traditional separate trials.

### 9.6.2    *Design with a Futility Index*

During any interim analysis, we should always perform futility checking and ask the question: Is it better to start a new trial than to continue the current one? When the conditional power is less than the power of the new trial with a sample size equal to the adjusted sample size for the current trial, it is better to start a new trial, theoretically. In other words, if the conditional power $cP_{\delta_1}(n_2)$ is less than the unconditional power $p_{\delta_1}(n_2)$, where $n_2$ is the sample size for the second stage, then statistically, it is better to start a new trial. Alternatively, we can use a predetermined futility boundary to prevent the trial from continuing to the second stage when the conditional power is lower or the futility index is high.

## 9.7 Summary

Conditional error function methods allow for a broad selection of conditional error functions $A(p_1)$, as long as they are monotonic in the stagewise $p$-value $p_1$ and bound by $[0,1]$. The selection of different $A(p_1)$ implies using different weights for the data from the two stages. The CEFM requires keeping the conditional error unchanged when we make adaptations to the trial. The Muller–Schafer and Denne methods are special methods, i.e., they keep the conditional function unchanged after adaptations. In other words, we ensure the condition $A^*(p_1) = A(p_1)$ given the observed stagewise $p$-value $p_1$ regardless of an adaptation, where $A(p_1)$ and $A^*(p_1)$ are the conditional error functions before and after the adaptation. The difference between the Müller–Schäfer and the Denne methods is that Denne uses a particular $A(p_1)$ to obtain the closed form solution, while Müller and Shäfer consider a more general situation and emphasize that the $A(p_1)$ needs to be calculated only for the observed $p_1$ through simulations, and determination of the stopping boundaries afterwards is based on the condition $A^*(p_1) = A(p_1)$. They also stress that this concept can be recursively used in a trial. We will discuss recursive approaches in the next chapter.

In this chapter, we have also discussed the conditional power for different designs. The conditional power can be used to compare different methods, and for the purpose of trial monitoring. When we force the treatment effect to zero, the conditional power function becomes the conditional error function, which allows for comparisons between different methods from the conditional error point of view.

**Problems**

**9.1** Derive the conditional power for the two-stage adaptive design (see Problem 4.2) with the test statistic:

$$T_k = \frac{1}{k} \sum_{i=1}^{k} p_i \text{ for k = 1 and 2,}$$

where $p_i$ is the stagewise $p$-value based on subsample from the $i$th stage.

**9.2** Derive conditional power formulations for the three-stage designs with MSP and MPP.

**9.3** Prove conditional power formulation (9.32).

# Chapter 10

# Recursive Adaptive Design

In this chapter, we will study the so-called recursive two-stage adaptive design (RTAD; Chang, 2006). The recursive approach provides closed forms for stopping boundaries and adjusted $p$-values for any $K$-stage design and avoids any numerical integration; at the same time it allows for a broad range of adaptations such as SSR, dropping losers, and changing the number and timing of analyses without specification of an error-spending function. The key ideas of the RTAD are (1) a $K$-stage design ($K > 1$) can be constructed using recursive two-stage designs, (2) the conditional error principle ensures that the recursive process will not inflate type-I error, and (3) the closed form solutions are obtained through recursively utilizing the two-stage design solutions for stopping boundary, adjusted $p$-value, and conditional power. In this approach, the trial is designed one step ahead at every interim analysis.

We will first introduce the concept of p-clud in Section 10.1 and review the two-stage approaches: MSP, MPP, and MINP in Section 10.2. In Section 10.2, we introduce the error-spending principle, from which we derive the conditional error principle. The latter is a key element for deriving the recursive formula for the RTAD in Section 10.4. A clinical trial application of RTAD is also presented in Section 10.4. In Sections 10.5 and 10.6, we will introduce two other adaptive methods for $K$-stage adaptive designs proposed by Müller and Shäfer (2004) and by Brannath, Posch, and Bauer (2002). Section 10.7 is a summary and discussion.

## 10.1   p-clud Distribution

The methods discussed in this chapter will assume the condition of p-clud (Brannath et al., 2002).

**Definition 10.1 p-clud**: $p$-values $p_1$ and $p_2$ are p-clud if the distribution of $p$-value $p_1$ and the conditional distribution of $p_2$ given $p_1$ are stochastically larger than or equal to the uniform distribution on $[0,1]$, i.e.,

$$\Pr_{H_0}(p_1 \leq \alpha) \leq \alpha \text{ and } \Pr_{H_0}(p_2 \leq \alpha|p_1) \leq \alpha, \forall \alpha \in [0,1]. \qquad (10.1)$$

It is usually assumed that the $p$-values $p_1$ and $p_2$ are stochastically independent under $H_0$. Although stochastically independent sample units are recruited at the two stages, this is not necessarily the case. For example, assume that rank tests are used at the two stages. The discrete distribution of $p_2$ under the null hypothesis may depend on $p_1$ via a sample-size reassessment rule: The experimenter may choose $n_2$ depending on the value observed for $p_1$. However, $p_2$ is still p-clud (Brannath et al., 2002). But, when $p_1$ and $p_2$ are independent and uniformly distributed on $[0,1]$, the level $\alpha$ is exhausted in (10.1).

We now study the distribution of stagewise $p$-values under the null hypothesis.

Let $X$ be a continuous random variable with probability density function $f_x(x)$, $F_X(x)$ be the cdf, and $Y = g(X)$. $X = \eta(Y) = g^{-1}(Y)$ are monotonic increasing functions, where $x$ is a realization of $X$ and $y$ is a realization of $Y$.

The pdf of $Y$ is given by (Kokoska and Zwillinger, 2000, p.40)

$$f_Y(y) = f_X(\eta(y))\eta'(y), \ g'(x) \neq 0. \qquad (10.2)$$

From (10.2), we have

$$F_Y(y) = \int_{-\infty}^{Y} f_Y(x)\,dx = \int_{-\infty}^{Y} f_X(\eta(x))\eta'(x)\,dx$$

$$= \int_{-\infty}^{\eta(y)} f_X(\eta(x))\,d\eta(x).$$

Therefore,

$$F_Y(y) = F_X(\eta(y)). \qquad (10.3)$$

Now let $X$ be the test statistic for testing $H_0 : \delta = 0$ against the alternative $H_a : \delta > 0$. Let $(-\infty, y)$ be the rejection region, and $g(y) = F_Y(y|\delta)$, i.e., the $p$-value ($p$-value is reviewed as a function of critical point $y$), then $\eta(y) = F_Y^{-1}(y|\delta)$. Substituting this into (10.3), we obtain

$$F_Y(y) = F_X(F_Y^{-1}(y|\delta)). \qquad (10.4)$$

Notice that under the null hypothesis, $F_Y^{-1}(y|\delta = 0) = F_X^{-1}(y)$, Equation (10.4) becomes

$$F_Y(y) = F_X\left(F_X^{-1}(y)\right) = y, \tag{10.5}$$

which implies that $Y$ is uniformly distributed on [0,1].

## 10.2  Error-Spending and Conditional Error Principles

We are going to formally introduce the so-called error-spending principle, from which we derive the second useful principle: the conditional error principle. The latter will be used to construct the recursive two-stage adaptive designs in the next section. The error-spending principle has been implicitly used from time to time (Lan and DeMets, 1983). The conditional error principle also appears informally in a different form (Müller and Shäfer, 2001).

In an initial $K$-stage adaptive trial for testing the global null hypothesis $H_0 : \cap_{j=1}^K H_{0j}$, where $H_{0j}$ is the null hypothesis at the $j$th stage, the type-I error control requirement can be expressed as

$$\alpha = \pi_1 + \dots + \pi_k + \pi_{k+1} + \dots + \pi_K, \tag{10.6}$$

where $\pi_i$ is $\alpha$ spent at the $i$th stage in the initial design of an adaptive trial.

Now assume that after the $k$th interim analysis, adaptations are made that result in changes to stagewise hypotheses and error spending after the $k$th stage. We denote $H_{0i}^*$ and $\pi_i^*$ $(i = k + 1, ..., K^*)$ as the new hypotheses and the new error spending, respectively, where $K^*$ is the new total number of analyses. The overall $\alpha$-control becomes

$$\alpha = \pi_1 + \dots + \pi_k + \pi_{k+1}^* + \dots + \pi_{K^*}^*. \tag{10.7}$$

From (10.7), the unconditional error rate after the $k$th stage can be expressed as

$$\alpha - \sum_{j=1}^k \pi_j = \sum_{j=k+1}^K \pi_j = \int_{\alpha_k}^{\beta_k} A(p_k)\, dp_k. \tag{10.8}$$

Similarly, from (10.8), the unconditional error rate after the $k$th stage can be expressed as

$$\alpha - \sum_{j=1}^k \pi_j = \sum_{j=k+1}^{K^*} \pi_j^* = \int_{\alpha_k}^{\beta_k} A^*(p_k)\, dp_k, \tag{10.9}$$

where $A(p_k)$ and $A^*(p_k)$ are called conditional error functions (under the global null hypothesis). $\alpha_k$ and $\beta_k$ are constants. Comparing (10.8) and (10.9), we immediately have the following error-spending principle.

**Error-spending principle:** In an adaptive trial, if an adaptation at the $k$th stage ensures the invariance of unconditional error, i.e.,

$$\int_{\alpha_k}^{\beta_k} A(p_k)\,dp_k = \int_{\alpha_k}^{\beta_k} A^*(p_k)\,dp_k, \qquad (10.10)$$

then the overall $\alpha$ is controlled under the global null hypothesis:

$$H_0: \left(\cap_{j=1}^{k} H_{0j}\right) \cap \left(\cap_{j=k+1}^{K^*} H_{0j}^*\right). \qquad (10.11)$$

The principle (10.10) is very general. The commonly used error-spending approach (Lan and DeMets, 1983) is a special form of the error-spending principle, which requires prespecification of the unconditional error as a function of information time. The conditional error method (Proschan and Hunsberger, 1995) is a special use of the error-spending principle for two-stage designs. Importantly, if we let $A(p_k) = A^*(p_k)$, then (10.10) holds and the overall $\alpha$ is controlled. Therefore, we can formally introduce the following principle.

**Conditional error principle:** In an adaptive trial, if an adaptation at the $k$th stage ensures the invariance of conditional error, i.e.,

$$A^*(p_k) = A(p_k), \qquad (10.12)$$

then the overall $\alpha$ is controlled under the global null hypothesis (10.11).

The conditional error principle allows changes in the total number of analyses, the timing of analyses, randomization, hypothesis changes, etc. in adaptive trials. The principle proposed by Müller and Shäfer (2001) is the applied Brownian model at predefined time points of the interim analyses (Müller and Shäfer, 2004). Müller and Shäfer extend their principle and allow for changes in the timing of an interim analysis. They did not explicitly specify the condition (10.11). The significance of (10.12) is that it provides a simple but very general way to control $\alpha$ by simulating the conditional error on flying; at same time, it allows for different adaptations. (10.12) tells us that one can make any adaptation as long as the conditional error is unchanged. Equation (10.12) can be used repeatedly, meaning that one can apply adaptations as many times as one wants as long as the conditional error rate remains unchanged at each stage.

The conditional error function for MPP, MSP, MMP, MLPP, MPPP, and MINP can be obtained by substituting $\delta = 0$ into the conditional power formula, as summarized in Table 9.6 and listed below:

$$A(p_1) = \frac{\alpha_2}{p_1}, \ \alpha_1 < p_1 \leq \beta_1 \text{ for MPP} \tag{10.13}$$

$$A(p_1) = \alpha_2 - p_1, \ \alpha_1 < p_1 \leq \beta_1 \text{ for MSP} \tag{10.14}$$

and

$$P_c(p_1, \delta) = 1 - \Phi\left(\frac{z_{1-\alpha_2} - w_1 z_{1-p_1}}{w_2}\right), \alpha_1 < p_1 \leq \beta_1 \text{ for MINP} \tag{10.15}$$

## 10.3   Recursive Two-Stage Design

We can see that the conditional error principle allows for a broad range of adaptations without inflating the alpha, but the calculation of conditional error usually requires computer simulations as indicated by Müller and Shäfer (2001). In this section, we will derive a closed form solution for a $K$-stage design that allows for a broad range of adaptations by recursively using the conditional error principle and two-stage formula for the conditional error, stopping boundary, adjusted $p$-value, and confidence interval. Naturally, this method is called recursive two-stage adaptive design (RTAD).

First, let's explain the concept and mechanics of the recursive two-stage design. Suppose we want to design an adaptive trial, but we may not know how many stages and what allowable adaptations will be best to meet the trial objectives. We start with a two-stage design. At the interim analysis (IA), we can make adaptations including SSR, increasing the number of analyses, etc., but we don't want to fully specify the rules. To meet the requirement, we can make the "short-term" plan by adding one more analysis into the design. Now the trial became a 3-stage adaptive design. However, instead of constructing a statistical method based on a 3-stage design, we view this 3-stage design as a stagnation of 2 two-stage designs. In other words, stages 1 and 2 are considered the first two-stage design, and stages 2 and 3 are viewed as the second two-stage design. In general, the $k$th and $(k+1)$th stages are considered to be the $k$th two-stage design. Each new two-stage design is tested at a different level of $\alpha$ that is equal to the newly calculated conditional error rate (Figure 10.1).

In what follows, we will derive the formulation for recursive two-stage adaptive design based on MSP and MPP. The reason we can derive the

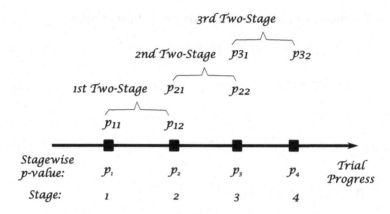

Figure 10.1:   Recursive Two-Stage Adaptive Design

closed form is that we have the explicit forms of the conditional error probability and stopping boundaries for two-stage designs.

### 10.3.1   *Sum of Stagewise p-values*

Suppose at a typical stage $i$, we decide to increase the number of stages in addition to other adaptations. The test statistic for the $i$th two-stage design is defined as

$$\left\{ \begin{array}{ll} T_{i1} = p_{i1} & \text{for stage 1,} \\ T_{i2} = p_{i1} + p_{i2} & \text{for stage 2,} \end{array} \right. \tag{10.16}$$

where $p_{i1} = p_i$ and $p_{i2} = p_{i+1}$, $p_i$ is the naive stagewise $p$-value based on the subsample from the $i$th stage. Note that $p_{i1}$ and $p_{i2}$ are mutually independent and uniformly distributed over $[0, 1]$ under $H_0$.

If $p_{i1} > \beta_{i1}$, stop the trial and accept $H_0$; if $p_{i1} \leq \alpha_{i1}$, stop the trial and reject $H_0$; if $\alpha_{i1} < p_{i1} \leq \beta_{i1}$, the trial continues and we can either go with the previous plan with the stopping boundary $\alpha_{i2}$ for the final stage with or without sample-size adjustment or plan the next "two-stage" design. Based on the conditional error principle, the new two-stage design should be tested at level $A(p_{i1})$, where $A(p_{i1})$ is the conditional error rate at the $i$th stage. From (10.14), we can obtain the conditional error rate at the $i$th IA (we always choose $\beta_{i1} \leq \alpha_{i2}$):

$$A(p_{i1}) = \alpha_{i2} - p_{i1}, \alpha_{i1} < p_{i1} \leq \beta_{i1}. \tag{10.17}$$

The stopping boundaries are determined for the new two-stage design by

$$A\left(p_{i1}\right) = \alpha_{i+1,1} + \alpha_{i+1,2}(\beta_{i+1,1} - \alpha_{i+1,1}) - \frac{1}{2}(\beta_{i+1,1}^2 - \alpha_{i+1,1}^2), \ i = 0, 1, \ldots \tag{10.18}$$

where for convenience, we define $A\left(p_{01}\right) = \alpha$. We can predetermine $\beta_{i+1,1}$ and $\alpha_{i+1,1}$, then the third value is given by

$$\alpha_{i+1,2} = \frac{A\left(p_{i1}\right) + \frac{1}{2}(\beta_{i+1,1}^2 - \alpha_{i+1,1}^2) - \alpha_{i+1,1}}{\beta_{i+1,1} - \alpha_{i+1,1}}. \tag{10.19}$$

Conditional power is similar to (9.15), but replaces $\alpha_2$ with $\alpha_{i2}$ and $p_1$ with $p_{i1}$; that is,

$$P_c\left(p_{i1}, \delta\right) = 1 - \Phi\left(\Phi^{-1}\left(1 - \alpha_{i2} + p_{i1}\right) - \frac{\delta}{\sigma}\sqrt{\frac{n_{i2}}{2}}\right), \ \alpha_{i1} < p_{i1} \le \beta_{i1}. \tag{10.20}$$

The sample size based on the target conditional power $P_c$ is given by

$$n_{i2} = \left[\frac{\sqrt{2}\sigma}{\delta}\left(\Phi^{-1}\left(1 - \alpha_{i2} + p_{i1}\right) - \Phi^{-1}\left(1 - P_c\right)\right)\right]^2. \tag{10.21}$$

### 10.3.2 *Product of Stagewise p-values*

For a test statistic based on the product of stagewise $p$-values,

$$\begin{cases} T_{i1} = p_{i1} & \text{for stage 1,} \\ T_{i2} = p_{i1}p_{i2} & \text{for stage 2.} \end{cases} \tag{10.23}$$

Similar to (10.13), the conditional error rate at the $i$th IA is given by

$$A\left(p_{i1}\right) = 1 - \frac{\alpha_{i2}}{p_{i1}}, \ \alpha_{i1} < p_{i1} \le \beta_{i1}. \tag{10.24}$$

If $p_{i1} > \beta_{i1}$, stop the trial and accept $H_0$; if $p_{i1} \le \alpha_{i1}$, stop the trial and reject $H_0$; if $\alpha_{i1} < p_{i1} \le \beta_{i1}$, the trial continues and we can either go with the previous plan with the stopping boundary $\alpha_{i2}$ for the final stage or plan the next "two-stage" design at level $A\left(p_{i1}\right)$. For the next two-stage design, we can predetermine $\beta_{i+1,1}$ and $\alpha_{i+1,1}$, then the third value is given by

$$\alpha_{i+1,2} = \frac{A\left(p_{i1}\right) - \alpha_{i+1,1}}{\ln\beta_{i+1,1} - \ln\alpha_{i+1,1}}. \tag{10.25}$$

### 10.3.3　*Inverse-Normal Stagewise p-values*

For the method based on inverse-normal stagewise $p$-value (MINP),

$$\begin{cases} T_{i1} = 1 - z_{1-p_{i1}} & \text{for stage 1,} \\ T_{i2} = 1 - \Phi\left(w_1 z_{1-p_{i1}} + w_2 z_{1-p_{i2}}\right) & \text{for stage 2.} \end{cases} \tag{10.27}$$

Similar to (10.27), the conditional error rate at the $i$th IA is given by

$$A\left(p_{i1}\right) = 1 - \Phi\left(\frac{z_{1-\alpha_{i2}} - w_1 z_{1-p_{i1}}}{w_2}\right),\ \alpha_{i1} < p_{i1} \le \beta_{i1}. \tag{10.28}$$

If $p_{i1} > \beta_{i1}$, stop the trial and accept $H_0$; if $p_{i1} \le \alpha_{i1}$, stop the trial and reject $H_0$; if $\alpha_{i1} < p_{i1} \le \beta_{i1}$, the trial continues and we can either go with the previous plan with the stopping boundary $\alpha_{i2}$ for the final stage or plan the next "two-stage" design at level $A\left(p_{i1}\right)$. Again the stop boundaries can be determined through simulations using SAS Macro 5.1.

### 10.3.4　*Application Example*

**Example 10.1　Recursive Two-Stage Adaptive Design**

For an adaptive design, the conditional power is often more important than the unconditional power because the sample size can be adjusted to reach the desired (conditional) power. In other words, we can design a trial with low power, but allow for SSR later. A recursive two-stage design is ideal for this kind of adaptive design.

Suppose we are planning an early acute coronary syndrome trial with a composite endpoint of a 30-day death or myocardial infarction. The event rate is 11% for the control group and 13% for the test group. A classical two-group design requires 5546/group to have 90% power at a significance level of 2.5% (one-sided test). However, the estimation of 11% is an approximation. To reduce the risk, interim analyses are considered. In case there is a very small treatment difference, the trial will allow for early stopping; if the effect size is moderate we increase the sample size; if the effect size is large, we want to have a chance to make an earlier efficacy claim. Consider the uncertainty of the recruitment rate and inflexibility of the IDMC board's schedule. The information times for interim analyses may deviate from the plan. One way to deal with this is to use the error-spending approach to adjust the stagewise alpha according to the information time. However, the error-spending approach requires predetermination of the error-spending function, which may lead to undesirable operating characteristics. Therefore, it is desirable to have the flexibility to adjust both the timing and the error-spending independently. We are going to illustrate how to use the recursive two-stage design to accomplish this.

We think that 2 interim analyses and one final analysis will be a reasonable way of reducing risk and potentially shortening the time to market. Also, this plan is operationally feasible. Therefore, we start the first two-stage design with 4000 patients per group; the first stage will have 2000 patients per group. The first interim analysis is used to adjust the sample size and assess futility stopping, but not efficacy stopping. The algorithm for SSR does not have to be specified at this moment. We use MSP with stopping boundaries: one-sided $\alpha_{11} = 0$ and $\beta_{11} = 0.2$; then $\alpha_{12} = 0.2250$ is calculated from (10.19). The power of rejecting the null hypothesis of no treatment effect at the interim analysis is zero and about 78% at the second stage. This power is calculated approximately from a classical design with 4000/group. The exact power can be calculated using simulation, but we don't have to do that because the conditional power is more important and can be easily calculated using (10.20) at the time of the interim analysis.

At the first IA, suppose we observe event rates $r_1 = 0.129$ and $r_2 = 0.114$ for the control and test groups, respectively. We estimate a treatment difference $\hat{\delta} = r_1 - r_2 = 0.015$, and standard deviation $\hat{\sigma} = \sqrt{[r_1(1 - r_1) + r_2(1 - r_2)]/2} = 0.3266$. The chi-square test statistic or equivalently, the $z$-score is $z_1 = \frac{\delta}{\hat{\sigma}}\sqrt{n_1/2} = 1.452$ and the corresponding adjusted one-sided $p$-value $p_{11} = 1 - \Phi(1.452) = 0.0732 < \beta_{11}$. Therefore, the trial should continue. We assume that $\delta = \hat{\delta}$, $\sigma = \hat{\sigma}$. To reach a conditional power of $P_c = 90\%$, the sample size is calculated from (10.20), i.e.,

$$
n_{12} = \left[ \frac{\sqrt{2}\sigma}{\delta} \left( \Phi^{-1}(1 - \alpha_{12} + p_{11}) - \Phi^{-1}(1 - P_c) \right) \right]^2
$$

$$
= \left[ \frac{0.3266\sqrt{2}}{0.015} \left( \Phi^{-1}(1 - 0.225 + 0.0732) - \Phi^{-1}(1 - 0.9) \right) \right]^2
$$

$$
= [30.792 (1.0287 + 1.2814)]^2
$$

$$
= 5060.
$$

We don't want to simply increase the sample size and delay the analysis because timing is so important in this trial. Therefore, we construct the second two-stage design as specified below:

(1) Calculate the conditional error using (10.17): $A\left(p_{11}\right) = \alpha_{12} - p_{11} = 0.225 - 0.0732 = 0.1518$;

(2) Choose $\alpha_{21} = 0.1$ and $\beta_{21} = 0.4$, (10.18) can be written as

$$0.1518 = 0.1 + \alpha_{22}(0.4 - 0.1) - \frac{1}{2}\left(0.4^2 - 0.1^2\right).$$

Solving it for $\alpha_{22}$, we obtain $\alpha_{22} = 0.42267$.

(3) Select $n_{21} = 2000/\text{group}$ and $n_{22} = 3000/\text{group}$ for the second two-stage design. Note that $\alpha_{21}$ and $n_{21}$ are chosen such that the conditional power (assume $\delta = \hat{\delta} = 0.015$) for rejecting $H_0$ at the second IA (i.e., the first stage of the second two-stage design) is reasonably high, specifically,

$$P_c\left(p_{11}, \delta\right) = 1 - \Phi\left(\Phi^{-1}\left(1 - \alpha_{12} + p_{11}\right) - \frac{\delta}{\sigma}\sqrt{\frac{n_{12}}{2}}\right)$$

$$= 1 - \Phi\left(1.0287 - \frac{0.015}{0.3266}\sqrt{\frac{2000}{2}}\right)$$

$$= 1 - \Phi\left(-0.42367\right) = 66.41\%.$$

The sample size $n_{22}$ is not important at all because we can either change it later or add a new two-stage design. Suppose at the second IA, the event rate is $r_1 = 0.129$ and $r_2 = 0.116$. The stagewise $p$-value $p_{21} = p_2 = 1 - \Phi(\frac{0.013}{0.3278}\sqrt{\frac{2000}{2}}) = 0.1049 > \alpha_{21} = 0.1$ and $H_0$ should not be rejected.

We may be curious about the classical design with the same data. In fact, if we pool 4000 subjects per group from stages 1 and 2 to calculate the $p$-value, as a classical design the one-sided $p$-value will be equal to $\Phi(-\frac{(0.015+0.013)/2}{\sqrt{(0.3266^2+0.3278^2)/2}}\sqrt{\frac{4000}{2}}) = \Phi(-1.9135) > 0.0278 > \alpha = 0.025$. Therefore, the classical design would fail to reject the null.

We now construct the third two-stage design:

(1) Calculate the conditional error using (10.47): $A\left(p_{21}\right) = \alpha_{22} - p_{21} = 0.42267 - 0.1049 = 0.31777$;

(2) Choose $\alpha_{31} = 0.2$ and $\beta_{31} = 0.6$,

$$0.31777 = 0.2 + \alpha_{32}(0.6 - 0.2) - \frac{1}{2}\left(0.6^2 - 0.2^2\right).$$

Solving it, we have $\alpha_{32} = 0.69443$.

(3) Select $n_{31} = 2000/\text{group}$ and $n_{23} = 2000/\text{group}$ for the second two-stage design. Assuming the true parameters are the estimates from the pooled data: $\delta = (0.015 + 0.013)/2 = 0.014$ and $\sigma =$

$\sqrt{(0.3266^2 + 0.3278^2)/2} = 0.3272$. The conditional power is calculated as

$$P_c(p_{21}, \delta) = 1 - \Phi\left(\Phi^{-1}(1 - \alpha_{22} + p_{21}) - \frac{\delta}{\sigma}\sqrt{\frac{n_{23}}{2}}\right)$$

$$= 1 - \Phi\left(0.783\,4 - \frac{0.014}{0.3272}\sqrt{\frac{2000}{2}}\right)$$

$$= 71.55\%.$$

Suppose at the first stage IA of the third two-stage design (i.e., the third stage), the event rate again is $r_1 = 0.129$ and $r_2 = 0.116$. The stagewise $p$-value $p_{31} = p_3 = 1 - \Phi\left(\frac{0.013}{0.3278}\sqrt{\frac{2000}{2}}\right) = 0.1049 < \alpha_{31} = 0.2$, and $H_0$ is rejected.

Note if we reestimate the sample size for the second stage with a little bit higher conditional power, say, 67.7% instead of 66.4%, the required sample size is $n_{21} = 2100$, $p_{21} = 0.0994 < \alpha_{21}$, and the $H_0$ would be rejected at the second stage.

The summary of the recursive design is presented in Table 10.1.

Table 10.1: Summary of the Recursive Two-Stage Design

| $\alpha_{11}$ | $\beta_{11}$ | $\alpha_{12}$ | $\alpha_{21}$ | $\beta_{21}$ | $\alpha_{22}$ | $\alpha_{31}$ | $\beta_{31}$ | $\alpha_{32}$ |
|---|---|---|---|---|---|---|---|---|
| 0 | 0.200 | 0.225 | 0.100 | 0.400 | 0.423 | 0.200 | 0.600 | 0.694 |
| $r_1$ | $r_2$ | $\sigma$ | $r_1$ | $r_2$ | $\sigma$ | $r_1$ | $r_2$ | $\sigma$ |
| 0.129 | 0.114 | 0.327 | 0.129 | 0.116 | 0.328 | 0.129 | 0.116 | 0.328 |
| $z_{1-p_{11}}$ | $p_{11}$ | $\alpha$ | $z_{1-p_{21}}$ | $p_{21}$ | $A(p_{11})$ | $z_{1-p_{31}}$ | $p_{31}$ | $A(p_{21})$ |
| 1.452 | 0.073 | 0.025 | 1.029 | 0.105 | 0.152 | 1.029 | 0.105 | 0.312 |

## 10.4  Recursive Combination Tests

In this section we will discuss the recursive combination tests proposed by Brannath, Posch, and Bauer (2002). Assume $p_1$ and $p_2$ are independent and uniformly distributed random variables on $[0, 1]$ or p-clud.

For two-stage designs, if $p_1 < \alpha_1$, reject the null; if $p_1 \geq \beta_1$, accept the null; if $\alpha_1 < p_1 \leq \beta_1$, the trial continues to the second stage. At the second stage if $C(p_1, p_2) \leq c$, reject the null; otherwise accept the null. The combination $C(p_1, p_2)$ can be many different forms. To exclude nonstochastic curtailing, we assume $c < \alpha_1$; otherwise, for $\alpha_1 < p_1 \leq c$, the null hypothesis could be rejected without a second sample, although no formal stopping condition applies.

The level $\alpha$ test requires:

$$\alpha_1 + \int_{\alpha_1}^{\beta_1} \int_0^1 \mathbf{1}_{[C(x,y)\leq c]} dy dx = \alpha, \qquad (10.29)$$

where $\mathbf{1}_{[C(x,y)\leq c]}$ equals 1 if $C(x,y) \leq c$ and 0 otherwise.

For multiple-stage adaptive design, Brannath, Posch, and Bauer (2002) define a $p$-value for the combination test by

$$q(p_1, p_2) \begin{cases} p_1 & \text{if } p_1 \leq \alpha_1 \text{ or } p_1 > \beta_1, \\ \alpha_1 + \int_{\alpha_1}^{\beta_1} \int_0^1 \mathbf{1}_{[C(x,y)\leq c]} dy dx & \text{otherwise.} \end{cases} \qquad (10.30)$$

For Fisher combination, $C(p_1, p_2) = p_1 p_2$, the level $\alpha$ test requirement (10.29) becomes

$$c = \frac{\alpha - \alpha_1}{\ln \beta_1 - \ln \alpha_1}. \qquad (10.31)$$

Carrying out the integration in (10.30), we obtain

$$q(p_1, p_2) \begin{cases} p_1 & \text{if } p_1 \leq \alpha_1 \text{ or } p_1 > \beta_1, \\ \alpha_1 + p_1 p_2 (\ln \beta_1 - \ln \alpha_1) & \text{if } p_1 \in (\alpha_1, \beta_1] \text{ and } p_1 p_2 \leq \alpha_1, \\ p_1 p_2 + p_1 p_2 [\ln \beta_1 - \ln(p_1 p_2)] & \text{if } p_1 \in (\alpha_1, \beta_1] \text{ and } p_1 p_2 > \alpha_1. \end{cases} \qquad (10.32)$$

The trial design is extended two-stage by two-stage until we don't want to extend any more. Let's denote the stopping boundaries by $\alpha_{i1}$, $\beta_{i1}$, and $c_i$ for the $i$th two-stage design, and the combination test $p$-value for the $i$th two-stage design as $q_i(p_i, p_{i+1})$ for $i = 1, ..., K-1$, where $K$ is the final stage, then the overall $p$-value can be obtained through recursion:

$$p = q_1(p_1, q_2(p_2, q_3(...q_{K-1}(p_{K-1}, q_K)))). \qquad (10.33)$$

Brannath, Posch, and Bauer stated the decision roles as: we reject the null $H_0$, if and only if $p \leq \alpha$.

(Question for readers: Assume $K = 5$. How can we make a decision based on (10.33) at the third stage before we know $K = 5$? Equation (10.29) implies that stopping will be based on the boundaries ($\alpha_1$ and $\beta_1$), is it consistent with the stopping rule based on (10.33) if we know $K = 5$?)

The critical value can be expressed for the $i$th two-stage design as

$$c_i = \frac{c_{i-1} - \alpha_{i1}}{\ln \beta_{i1} - \ln \alpha_{i1}}, \qquad (10.34)$$

where $c_0 = \alpha$.

To plan the next two-stage design, the conditional error has to be calculated by

$$A_{i+1}(p_i) = \frac{c_i}{p_i}, \tag{10.35}$$

where $A_1(\cdot) = \alpha$.

## Example 10.2  Application of Recursive Combination Method

Brannath et al. (2002) illustrate the recursive combination test method for the hypothesis $H_0 : \mu \leq 0$ against $H_a : \mu > 0$, where $\mu$ is the mean of a normally distributed random variable with known variance $\sigma^2 = 1$. For the classical design, a sample size 144 will provide 85% power to detect an effect size of 0.25 at a one-sided level of 0.025. To use the recursive approach, the first interim is planned based on 48 patients with efficacy boundary $\alpha_{11} = 0.0102$ and futility boundary $\beta_{11} = 0.5$. This leads to the critical value $c_1 = 0.0038$ from Equation (10.34).

Assume we get the stagewise $p$-value $p_1 = p_{11} = 0.199$ for the first stage, which satisfies $\beta_{11} > p_1 > \alpha_{11}$; thus, the trial continues. The value of the conditional error function $A_2(p_1) = \frac{c_1}{p_1} = 0.0191$. The sample size required for the second stage to achieve a conditional power of 0.8 is as large as 136. We decide to perform a second interim analysis after the next 68 sample units. Because the estimated mean, $\hat{\delta}_1 = \Phi^{-1}(1 - p_1)/\sqrt{n_1} = 0.122$, is not too promising, the option of stopping for futility is also taken for the second interim analysis with $a_{21} = 0.00955$ and $\beta_{21} = 0.5$. The critical value $c_2 = 0.00241$ from Equation (10.34). Suppose we obtain the stagewise value $p_2 = p_{21} = 0.0284$ and the trial continues based on the stopping boundaries $\alpha_{21}$ and $\beta_{21}$. The mean estimated from the pooled samples 1 and 2 is 0.186. The conditional error is $A_3(p_2) = \frac{c_2}{p_2} = 0.0850$. The sample size $n_3 = 68$ will provide the conditional power 0.075 for the third stage given an effect size of 0.25. We now decide not to extend any further. Assume we now observe the stagewise $p$-value $p_3 = 0.00781$. The overall $p$-value can be calculated using Equation (10.29) as follows:

$$q_2(p_2, p_3) = 0.00955 + 0.0284(0.00781)\ln\frac{0.5}{0.00955} = 0.0104.$$

$$p = q_1(p_1, q_2) = 0.0102 + 0.199(0.0104)\ln\frac{0.5}{0.0102} = 0.0183.$$

Because the overall $p$-value $p < \alpha = 0.025$, we can reject the null hypothesis.

$$p_i(\delta_0) = 1 - \Phi\left((\bar{X}_i - \delta_0)\sqrt{n_i}\right). \tag{10.36}$$

The computation of the confidence bounds can be pursued as follows:

(1) Based on observed data, calculate sample mean $\bar{X}_i$ for the $i$th sub-sample.

(2) Select a value for $\delta_0$ to calculate stagewise $p_i$ using (10.35).

(3) Calculate overall $p$-value using (10.33).

(4) Go back to step 2 using a different $\delta_o$ until the overall $p$-value equals $\alpha$. This $\delta_0$ is the CI bound.

For Example 10.2, Brannath et al. (2002) calculate the 97.5% CI to be 0.0135, and the 95% CI bound 0.0446. The 50% CI is 0.1835 and gives a median unbiased point estimate for the effect size. As a comparison, the average of all the observations obtained up to the third stage equals 0.2255.

Note that when adjusting $\delta_0$, the rejection of $H_0$ could occur earlier than it was actually rejected. Brannath et al. (2002) didn't discuss this situation. For more details on estimations after adaptive designs, see, e.g., Posch et al. (2005).

## 10.5 Decision Function Method

Müller and Schäfer (2004) generalize their early work (2001; Chapter 7) to arbitrary decision function. Their early method is based on conditional rejection probability (CRP) or more precisely on the conditional error principle, i.e., we can redesign the trial at any interim analysis as long as we keep the conditional error unchanged. Their derivation is based on the discretized Brownian motion and includes the conventional group sequential designs in Brownian motion model at the prespecified time points of the interim analysis as a special case.

We now discuss the generalization of the method. Let $X = (X_1, ..., X_k)$ denote the data collected during the experiment. Define a *decision function* $\varphi(X) = \varphi(X_1, ..., X_k) \in [0,1]$, which can be a test statistic. At the end of the experiment the null hypothesis $H_0$ will be maintained if $\varphi(X) = 0$ or rejected if $\varphi(X) = 1$ is realized. For other values of $\varphi(X)$, the decision is based on a random experiment, i.e., throwing a biased coin with rejection probability given by the realized value of $\varphi(X)$. Müller and Schäfer realize that in clinical trials the decision based on the result of throwing a coin is problematic and suggest in the final analysis the nonrandomized modification of the decision function, in which $H_0$ will be accepted if $\varphi(X) < 1$ is realized.

We partition the $X$ into two parts at the time of the $j$th interim analysis: the observed dataset $X_L$ and the planned future data $X_U$, $X_L \cup X_U = X$ and $X_L \cap X_U = \phi$. Define the conditional expectation of decision function as

$$\varepsilon_\theta\left(x_L\right) = E_\theta\left\{\varphi\left(X_L, X_U\right) | X_L = x_L\right\} \text{ for } \forall\theta \in H_0. \tag{10.37}$$

The generalized method can be simply described as follows: At any interim analysis, the trial can be redesigned with any decision function at an interim analysis as long as we keep the expected conditional decision function unchanged. The redesign procedure can be recursively applied.

## 10.6 Summary and Discussion

Based on the conditional error principle and closed form solutions for two-stage design, the RTAD approach provides an integrated process of design, monitoring, and analysis. RTAD allows trials to be designed stage by stage. At each stage, the conditional power is calculated, which is typical for monitoring, and further design can be based on this conditional power. During the redesign, information within and outside of this trial can be used. To select an optimal design for the remainder of the study at interim analysis, one can use the conditional power or utility functions. The method is applicable for general $K$-stage adaptive designs that allow for a very broad range of adaptations. The stopping boundary determination and the adjusted $p$-value calculation are straightforward with the closed forms, and no software is required.

One should be aware that every adaptive design method requires prespecification of certain aspect(s). The classical group sequential method specifies the number and timing of the analyses. The error-spending method allows for changes in the number and timing of the analyses but requires prespecification of the error-spending function. The conditional error function method prespecifies the conditional error function. The RTAD requires the prespecification that the conditional error rate will be retained at each stage based on the observed data. It is important to know that the flexibility of this method does not mean that you can design the first interim analysis arbitrarily. In fact, careful thinking and planning are required for the initial design. Spending too much alpha at the first stage means that one has less alpha to spend at later stages, which could limit the design's ability to have good operating characteristics. Also, changing the hypothesis during a trial should be done with great caution, because it could lead to a very different clinical implication.

RTAD can also be useful in many situations. For example, it is usually unrealistic to plan many interim analyses at design stage to deal with all possible scenarios. Therefore, there are opportunities (e.g., safety concern, unexpected slow enrollment) for adding new interim analyses, changing the total number and the timing of the coming analyses after a trial is initiated, and adjusting sample size. In these situations, RTAD is very suitable.

In addition to RTAD, we have also briefly introduced two other recursive approaches, but the computations for those methods are not as simple as RTAD.

## Problems

**10.1** Describe how to use a recursive two-stage adaptive design with MSP for the trial in Example 8.1, assuming the $p$-value at the first interim is between efficacy and futility stopping boundaries.

**10.2** Describe how to use a recursive two-stage adaptive design with MPP for the trial in Example 8.1, assuming the $p$-value at the first interim is between efficacy and futility stopping boundaries.

**10.3** Describe how to use a recursive two-stage adaptive design with MINP for the trial in Example 8.1, assuming the $p$-value at the first interim is between efficacy and futility stopping boundaries.

# Chapter 11

# Unblinded Sample-Size Reestimation Design

## 11.1 Opportunity

Despite a great effort, we often face a high degree of uncertainty about parameters when designing a trial or justifying the sample size at the design stage. This could involve the initial estimates of within- or between-patient variation, a control group event rate for a binary outcome, the treatment effect desired to be detected, the recruiting pattern, or patient compliance, all of which affect the ability of the trial to address its primary objective (Shih, 2001). This uncertainty can also include the correlation between the measures (if a repeated measure model is used) or among different variables (multiple endpoints, covariates). If a small uncertainty of prior information exists, a classical design can be applied. However, when the uncertainty is greater, a classical design with a fixed sample size is inappropriate. Instead, it is desirable to have a trial design that allows for reestimation of sample size in the middle of the trial based on unblinded data. Several different algorithms have been proposed for sample-size reestimation, including the conditional power approach and Cui–Hung–Wang's approach based on the ratio of observed effect size versus expected effect size.

In this chapter, we will evaluate the performance of different sample-size modification methods. Operationally, it is a concern that sample-size reestimation will release the unblinded efficacy data to the general public prematurely. Using a discrete function for sample-size reestimation is suggested, so that the exact effect size would not be revealed. We will study the impact on efficiency of this information-mask approach. The adjusted $p$-value, the point estimate, and confidence interval calculation will also be discussed.

It is important to differentiate the two different properties: those at the design stage and those at the interim analyses. For example, power is an interesting property at the design stage, but at the time of interim analysis, power has little value, and the conditional power is of great concern. From a statistical point of view, most adaptive design methods do not require a prespecification of sample-size adjustment rules at the design stage. How to adjust the sample size can be determined right after the interim analysis.

Later in the chapter, we'll give two examples using SSR: a myocardial infarction prevention trial and a noninferior adaptive trial with Farrington–Manning margin. Summaries and discussions will be presented in the last section.

## 11.2  Adaptation Rules

There are many possible rules for sample-size adjustment. Here we will discuss only two types of adjustments: (1) sample-size adjustment based on the effect-size ratio between the initial estimate and the observed estimate, and (2) sample-size adjustment based on conditional power.

### 11.2.1  *Adjustment Based on Effect-Size Ratio*

The formation for sample-size adjustment based on the ratio of the initial estimate of effect size $(E_0)$ to the observed effect size $(E)$ is given by

$$N = \left| \frac{E_0}{E} \right|^a N_0, \tag{11.1}$$

where $N$ is the newly estimated sample size per group, $N_0$ is the initial sample size per group which can be estimated from a classical design, and $a > 0$ is a constant, and

$$E = \frac{\hat{\eta}_{i2} - \hat{\eta}_{i1}}{\hat{\sigma}_i}. \tag{11.2}$$

With a large sample assumption, the common variance for the two treatment groups is given by (see Chapter 2)

$$\hat{\sigma}_i^2 = \begin{cases} \hat{\sigma}_i^2 & \text{for normal endpoint,} \\ \bar{\eta}_i(1 - \bar{\eta}_i) & \text{for binary endpoint,} \\ \bar{\eta}_i^2 \left[ 1 - \frac{e^{\bar{\eta}_i T_0} - 1}{T_0 \bar{\eta}_i e^{\bar{\eta}_i T_s}} \right]^{-1} & \text{for survival endpoint,} \end{cases} \tag{11.3}$$

where $\bar{\eta}_i = \frac{\hat{\eta}_{i1} + \hat{\eta}_{i2}}{2}$ and the logrank test is assumed to be used for the survival analysis. Note that the standard deviations for proportion and survival have several versions. There are usually slight differences in the resulting sample size or power among the different versions.

The sample-size adjustment in (11.1) should have additional constraints: (1) it should be smaller than $N_{\max}$ (due to financial and or other constraints) and greater than or equal to $N_{\min}$ (the sample size for the interim analysis) and (2) if $E$ and $E_0$ have different signs at the interim analysis, no adjustment should be made.

To avoid numerical overflow when $E = 0$, the actual algorithm implemented in SAS macros in this chapter is

$$N = min \left\{ N_{max},\, max \left( N_0,\, \frac{E_0}{abs(E) + 0.0000001} N_0 \right) \right\}. \qquad (11.4)$$

## 11.2.2 Adjustment Based on Conditional Power

For an SSR design, the conditional power is more important than the power. The conditional power for a two-stage design is given by (Chapter 9)

$$cP = 1 - \Phi \left( B\left( \alpha_2, p_1 \right) - \frac{\delta}{\sigma} \sqrt{\frac{n_2}{2}} \right),\ \alpha_1 < p_1 \le \beta_1,$$

where the B-function $B\left( \alpha_2, p_1 \right)$ is given in Table (9.6). The formulation for the new sample size for a two-stage design is discussed in Chapter 9 and given by

$$n_2 = \frac{2\sigma^2}{\delta^2} \left[ B\left( \alpha_2, p_1 \right) - \Phi^{-1}\left( 1 - cP \right) \right]^2, \qquad (11.5)$$

where $cP$ is the target conditional power. The actual algorithm implemented in SAS Macro 11.2 is

$$n_2 = \begin{cases} max \left\{ N_{2\min},\, \frac{2\sigma^2}{\delta^2} \left[ B\left( \alpha_2, p_1 \right) - \Phi^{-1}\left( 1 - cP \right) \right]^2 \right\} & \text{If } \alpha_1 < p_1 < \beta_1 \\ 0, & \text{otherwise,} \end{cases}$$
$$(11.6)$$

where $\delta = \left( \mu_2 - \mu_1 \right)/\sigma$, $n_2$ is the sample size per group at stage 2 with a minimum of $N_{2\min}$. Assume a known $\sigma$.

For a $K$-stage design, (11.5) is an approximation. Suppose we are interested only in the case where SSR takes place only at the first interim analysis, and the sample-size change affects only the last stage sample size.

Note that (11.4) allows only a sample-size increase from $N_0$, but (11.6) allows both an increase and decrease in sample size. The futility boundary is suggested because (1) a certain small $\delta_1$ will virtually never lead to statistical significance at the final analysis, and (2) a small $\hat{\delta}$ at the final analysis will be clinically unjustifiable; therefore, adding a futility boundary could be cost-saving.

## 11.3    Stopping Boundaries for SSR

When the sample size at the second-stage change is based on $p_1$ from the first stage, will the stopping boundaries derive from group sequential design in Chapters 4 and 5 still be valid? In previous chapters, we have used the same stopping boundaries for SSR design without discussing it. Now it is time for us to look into the question.

For MINP, $T_2 = \sqrt{\tau_1}z_1 + \sqrt{1-\tau_1}z_2$, where the information time $\tau_1 = n_1/N$, under $H_0$, $z_1$ and $z_2$ are iid from $N(0,1)$, which seems to imply that sample-size modification will not affect the stopping boundaries because a linear combination of normal variables is a normal distribution. However, since $\tau_1$ is a function of sample size and sample-size adjustment is depdendent on $z_1$ or $p_1$, $T_2$ is no longer a linear combination of two indenpendent standard normal distributions. As a result, the stopping boundaries from GSD have to be changed in order to control the type-I error.

For MSP, MLP, MMSv, MPP, MPPv, the conditional distribution of $p_2$ given be $p_1$ must be uniformly distribution in [0,1] or p-clud under the null hypothesis $H_0$. We can easily check this condition. If $p_2 = 1 - \Phi\left(\bar{X}_2\sqrt{\frac{n_2}{\sigma}}\right)$, the second stage mean $\bar{X}_2$ is independent of $p_1$ but the sample size at the second stage $n_2$ is a function of $p_1$. Therefore, when $p_1$ and $p_2$ are independent and uniformly distributed in [0,1] for the sequential design without sample-size reestimation, they are not independent anymore when the sample $n_2$ is adjusted based on $p_1$ directly or indirectly and we cannot guarantee the two p-values are p-clud. Fortunately, when the null hypothesis is true and regardless of sample size $n_2$, $p_2$ is uniformly distributed in [0,1] or p-clud because $\bar{X}_2\sqrt{\frac{n_2}{\sigma}}$ has the standard normal distribution regardless of sample size $n_2$ as long as $H_0$ is true. As a result, the stopping boundaries discussed in previous chapters can be used for MSP, MLP, MMSv, MPP, MPPv. For MINP, the weights $w_{ki}$ must be fixed or have flexible information time and follow a predetermined error-spending function; otherwise the same stopping boundary for GSD cannot be used for SSR design.

## 11.4    Basic Considerations in Designing SSR Trial

Suppose the trial study team estimates the treatment effect of a test drug over the control is $\delta = \mu_T - \mu_C = 0.85$ with a common standard deviation $\sigma_T = \sigma_C = 3$. For 90% power at one-sided $\alpha = 0.025$, the sample size required for a classical two-group design is $n = 262$ per group. But the estimation of effect size is inaccurate, and the treatment difference might be as low as 0.7 or as high as 1.0. If the effect size $\delta = 0.7$, the power will drop to 76% with sample size 262 per group. The sponsor is willing to increase to the maximum sample of 400 per group if the treatment difference is lower. If $\delta = 0.7$, the sample size 400/group will provide 91% power for the fixed sample-size design. However, the problem is that if a sample size 400 used, when $\delta = 1$, it will provide more than 99% power, which is considered unnecessarily high and the unnecessary larger sample size will prolong the trial duration and potentially delay the delivery of effective drug to the patients. Moreover, if the drug is ineffective the larger trial may lead to exposure of a larger patient population to a potential harmful compound. Therefore, it is not a wise decision to commit a trial with a fixed sample size of 400. If the sample size can be adjusted automatically as the effective size changes, that will solve the problem. This is essentially the motivation behind the sample-size reestimation. As we have discussed in previous chapters, there are several adaptive methods we can use, including MINP, MSP, MLPP, MPP, and MPPP among others. In what follows, we will compare various methods, evaluate their operating characteristics, and make recommendations. In all these simulations, we start with sample size $n_0 = 262$/group with interim sample size $n_1 = 131$ per group and the maximum sample size $N_{\max} = 400$ per group.

We have evaluated the expected sample size and power for $\delta = 0.7, 0.85$, and 1.0 using a BF-like conservative stopping boundary with $\alpha_1 = 0.0025$ and more aggressive stopping boundary with $\alpha_1 = 0.01$ (Tables 11.1 through 11.3). We also include the early stopping probability (ESP) in the evaluation since it is an indicator for the expected duration of the trial. A large ESP implies a short trial duration. For $\alpha_1 = 0.0025$, the stopping boundaries $\alpha_2$ for the methods (MINP, MINP$_2$, MPP, MSP, and MLP) are 0.024, 0.024, 0.00375534, 0.21463, and 0.06389, respectively. The early stopping probabilities are ESP = 0.178, 0.305, and 0.457, for $\delta = 0.7$, $\delta = 0.85$, and $\delta = 1.0$, respectively. For $\alpha_1 = 0.01$, the stopping boundaries $\alpha_2$ for the methods (MINP, MINP$_2$, MPP, MSP, and MLP) are 0.0188, 0.0188, 0.0032572, 0.18321, and 0.052962, respectively. The early stopping probabilities are ESP = 0.331, 0.487, and 0.646 for $\delta = 0.7$, $\delta = 0.85$, and $\delta = 1.0$, respectively.

From Table 11.1 we can see that for a lower $\alpha_1$ (e.g., 0.0025) MINP performs well in comparison with other methods. On the other hand, from Table 11.2 we can see that for a higher $\alpha_1$ (e.g., 0.01), MINP$_2$ performs better. If we are also concerned that the drug may not be effective at all,

Table 11.1:   Comparisons of Adaptive Design Methods ($\alpha_1 = 0.0025$)

| Methods | $\delta = 0.7$ | | $\delta = 0.85$ | | $\delta = 1.0$ | |
|---|---|---|---|---|---|---|
| | Ave. N | Power | Ave. N | Power | Ave. N | Power |
| MINP | 304.6 | 0.875 | 266.4 | 0.963 | 229.1 | 0.991 |
| MINP$_2$ | 312.8 | 0.873 | 274.8 | 0.957 | 235.1 | 0.988 |
| MPP | 310.0 | 0.874 | 271.4 | 0.961 | 232.8 | 0.992 |
| MSP | 266.6 | 0.787 | 248.3 | 0.902 | 220.8 | 0.961 |
| MLP | 324.1 | 0.845 | 289.3 | 0.939 | 248.2 | 0.978 |

Note: MLP: $w_1 = 0.1, w_2 = 0.9$; MINP$_2$ : $w_1 = 0.5, w_2 = 0.866$

Table 11.2:   Comparisons of Adaptive Design Methods ($\alpha_1 = 0.01$)

| Methods | $\delta = 0.7$ | | $\delta = 0.85$ | | $\delta = 1.0$ | |
|---|---|---|---|---|---|---|
| | Ave. N | Power | Ave. N | Power | Ave. N | Power |
| MINP | 287.9 | 0.865 | 246.5 | 0.960 | 207.3 | 0.992 |
| MINP$_2$ | 296.2 | 0.880 | 253.5 | 0.967 | 213.6 | 0.993 |
| MPP | 291.8 | 0.867 | 249.7 | 0.962 | 210.0 | 0.992 |
| MSP | 244.9 | 0.775 | 223.9 | 0.898 | 197.5 | 0.958 |
| MLP | 299.4 | 0.864 | 261.8 | 0.959 | 221.8 | 0.990 |

Note: MLP: $w_1 = 0.1, w_2 = 0.9$; MINP$_2$ : $w_1 = 0.5, w_2 = 0.866$

Table 11.3:   Comparisons of Adaptive Design Methods with ($\beta_1 = 0.15$)

| Methods | $\delta = 0.7$ | | $\delta = 0.85$ | | $\delta = 1.0$ | |
|---|---|---|---|---|---|---|
| | Ave. N | Power | Ave. N | Power | Ave. N | Power |
| MINP | 251.4 | 0.747 | 238.7 | 0.876 | 216.2 | 0.946 |
| MINP$_2$ | 259.8 | 0.725 | 246.5 | 0.864 | 222.2 | 0.941 |
| MPP | 256.4 | 0.739 | 243.8 | 0.876 | 233.1 | 0.993 |
| MSP | 266.2 | 0.786 | 247.7 | 0.902 | 220.9 | 0.961 |
| MLP | 324.0 | 0.847 | 288.7 | 0.938 | 248.6 | 0.978 |

Note: MLP: $w_1 = 0.1, w_2 = 0.9$; MINP$_2$ : $w_1 = 0.5, w_2 = 0.866$; $\alpha_1 = .0025$

we should check even lower effect size, e.g., $\delta = 0.5$ or $\delta = 0$. In such case, adding a futility boundary will be cost-effective. For example, using futility boundary $\beta_1 = 0.15$ (two-sided test $\beta_1$ 0.3), the simulation results are presented in Table 11.3, We can see that in order to save sample size when $H_0$ is true, the performance of MINP, MINP2 and MPP is worsening under $H_a$, but MSP and MLP are virtually the same as the designs without futility boundary under $H_a$. This is because for MSP the futility boundary $\beta_1 = \alpha_2$ is automatically built into the method. Similarly, the futility boundary $\beta_1 = \alpha_2/w_1$ has already been built into the MLP as discussed in Chapter 9.

Information time is also a factor, but we like to leave the question to the reader. The SAS macro to generate the results from Table11.1 through Table11.3 is presented in SAS Macro 11.1.

## >>SAS Macro 11.1: Two-Stage Sample-Size Reestimation>>

```
%Macro nByCPower(Model, a2, eSize, TargCPow, p1, w1, w2, v, n2, n2New,
cPower);
* It is required that the futiltiy boundary b1<=a2/w1;
* Target conditional powr: TargCPow;
If &Model="MIP" Then BFun=Probit(1-&a2);
If &Model="MLPP" Then
BFun=Probit(1-(max(0.00000001,(1/&w2)*(&a2-&w1*&p1)))**(1/&v));
If &Model="MPPP" | Model="MPP" Then
BFun=Probit(1-(&a2/&p1)**(1/&v));
If &Model="MINP" Then
BFun=(Probit(1-&a2)- &w1*Probit(1-&p1))/&w2;
&n2New=2*((BFun-Probit(1-&TargCPow))/&eSize)**2; *n per group;
&cPower=1-ProbNorm(BFun-eSize*sqrt(&n2/2));
%Mend nByCPowerUB;
%Macro SSR2Stage(nSims=1000000, Model="MINP", w1=0.5, w2=0.5, v=1.2,
alpha=0.025, beta=0.2, sigma=2, ux=0, uy=1, nInterim=50, Nmax=100,
N0=100, cPower=0.9, nAdj="Y", alpha1=0.01, beta1=0.15, alpha2=0.1871);
* Require uy>ux v>=1;
Data MINP; Keep Model uy FSP ESP AveN N0 Nmax Power TargCPow nClassic
alpha1 alpha2 beta1 n2New cPower;
alpha=&alpha; Nmax=&Nmax; Model=&model; w1=&w1; w2=&w2; v=&v;
ux=&ux; uy=&uy; sigma=&sigma;
alpha1=&alpha1; alpha2=&alpha2; beta1=&beta1; TargCPow=&cPower;
N1=&nInterim; N0=&N0;
* Calcualte the stopping boundaries without the futility binding rule;
If Model="MPP" Then
alpha2=(alpha-alpha1)/log(1/alpha1);
If Model="MPPP" Then
alpha2=((alpha-alpha1)*(1-1/v)/(1-alpha1**(1-1/v)))**v;
If Model="MLPP" Then do;
alpha2=w1*alpha1+((alpha-alpha1)*w1*w2**(1/v)*(1+1/v))**(v/(1+v));
beta1=alpha2/w1;
End;
If uy^=ux Then
nClassic=Round(2*((Probit(1-alpha)+Probit(1-&beta))/abs(uy-
ux)*sigma)**2);
FSP=0; ESP=0; AveN=0; Power=0;
Do isim=1 To &nSims;
```

```
nFinal=N1;
ux1 = Rannor(0)*sigma/Sqrt(N1)+ux;
uy1 = Rannor(0)*sigma/Sqrt(N1)+uy;
z1 = (uy1-ux1)*Sqrt(N1)/2**0.5/sigma;
p1=1-ProbNorm(z1);
If p1>beta1 Then FSP=FSP+1/&nSims;
If p1<=alpha1 Then Do;
Power=Power+1/&nSims; ESP=ESP+1/&nSims;
End;
If alpha1<p1<=beta1 Then Do;
nFinal=N0;
eSize=(uy1-ux1)/sigma;
If &nAdj="Y" Then Do;
n2=n0-n1;
%nByCPower(Model, alpha2, eSize, TargCPow, p1, w1, w2, v, n2, n2New,
cPower);
nFinal=min(max(n2New+N1,N0),Nmax); ;
End;
ux2 = Rannor(0)*sigma/Sqrt(nFinal-N1)+ux ;
uy2 = Rannor(0)*sigma/Sqrt(nFinal-N1)+uy;
z2 = (uy2-ux2)*Sqrt(nFinal-N1)/2**0.5/sigma;
p2=1-ProbNorm(z2);
If Model="MINP" Then
T2=1-ProbNorm((w1*z1+w2*z2)/Sqrt(w1*w1+w2*w2));
If Model="MLPP" Then T2=w1*p1+w2*p2**v;
If Model="MPPP" | Model="MPP" Then T2=p1*p2**v;
If .<T2<=alpha2 Then Power=Power+1/&nSims;
End;
AveN=AveN+nFinal/&nSims;
End;
Output;
Run;
Proc Print Data=MINP; Run;
%Mend SSR2Stage;
```
<<**SAS**<<

The following SAS code is typical an SAS macro calls.

>>**SAS: Invoke SAS Macro 11.1**>>

```
Title2 "MINP fixed weight w1=0.5, w2=0.86603";
%SSR2Stage(nSims=1000000, Model="MINP", w1=0.5, w2= 0.86603, v=1, al-
```

pha=0.025, beta=0.1, sigma=3, ux=0, uy=0.7, nInterim=131, Nmax=400, N0=262, cPower=0.9, nAdj="Y", alpha1=0.0025, beta1=0.15, alpha2=0.024);
%SSR2Stage(nSims=100000,
Model="MLPP", w1=0.1,w2=0.9, v=1, alpha=0.025, beta=0.1, sigma=3, ux=0, uy=0.7, nInterim=131, Nmax=400, N0=262, cPower=0.9, nAdj="Y", alpha1=0.0025, beta1=0.15, alpha2=0.084983);
<<SAS<<

## 11.5  SAS Macros for Sample-Size Reestimation

SAS Macro 11.2 below is developed to simulate a two-arm, $K$-stage adaptive design with a normal, binary, or survival endpoint using "MIP," "MSP," "MPP," or "MINP." The sample-size adjustment is based on the conditional power method (11.6) for a two-stage design or (11.4) for $K$-stage design $(K > 2)$. The sample-size adjustment is allowed only at the first interim analysis, and the sample-size adjustment affects only the final stage-wise sample size. **ux** and **uy** = the means, response rates, or hazard rates for the two groups, and **Ns{k}** = sample-size in group x at stage $k$. The random increment in sample-size of **nMinIcr** is added for the information mask, **nMinIcr** = minimum sample-size increment in group x for the conditional power approach only, **n2new** = the re-estimated sample-size for group x at the second stage, and **eSize** = the standardized effect size. **nSims** = number of simulation runs, **nStgs** = number of stages, **alpha0** = overall $\alpha$, and **EP** = "normal", "binary", or "survival". **Model** = "MIP", "MSP", "MPP", or "LW"; **nAdj** = "N" for the case without SSR; **nAdj** = "Y" for the case with SSR. **cPower** = target conditional power, **ux** and **uy** = the true treatment effects of the two groups. **DuHa** = estimated treatment difference, **Nmax** = the maximum sample-size allowed for group x, **N2min** = minimum sample size (not cumulative) in group x for stage 2, **sigma** = standard deviation for normal endpoint, **tAcr** = accrual time, **tStd** = study duration, and **power** = initial target power for the trial, **nRatio** = the sample size ratio of group y to group x for an imbalanced design. **NIType** = "FIXED" for noninferiority design with a fixed NI margin and **NIType** = "PCT" for noninferiority design with Farrington-Manning NI margin, **NId** = NI margin. **Aveux**, **Aveuy**, and **AveN** = average simulated responses (mean, proportion, or hazard rate) and sample size, **FSP{i}** = futility stopping probability at the $i$th stage, **ESP{i}** = efficacy stopping probability at the $i$th stage, and **alpha{i}** and **beta{i}** = efficacy and futility stopping boundaries at the $i$th stage.

## >>SAS Macro 11.2:    *K*-Stage Adaptive Design with Sample-Size Reestimation>>

```
%Macro nByCPowerUB(nAdjModel, a2, eSize, cPower, p1, w1, w2, n2New);
If &nAdjModel="MIP" Then BFun=Probit(1-&a2);
If &nAdjModel="MSP" Then BFun=Probit(1-max(0.0000001,&a2-&p1));
If &nAdjModel="MPP" Then BFun=Probit(1-&a2/&p1);
If &nAdjModel="MINP" Then BFun=(Probit(1-&a2)- &w1*Probit(1-&p1))/
&w2;
&n2New=2*((BFun-Probit(1-&cPower))/&eSize)**2; *n for group 1;
%Mend nByCPowerUB;
%Macro TwoArmNStgAdpDsg(nSims=1000000, nStgs=2,ux=0, uy=1,
NId=0, NItype="FIXED", EP="normal", Model="MSP",
nAdj="Y", cPower=0.9, DuHa=1, Nmax=300, N2min = 150,
nMinIcr=1, sigma=3, tAcr=10, tStd=24, nRatio=1);
DATA NStgAdpDsg; Set dInput;
KEEP Model power Aveux Aveuy AveTotalN FSP1-FSP&nStgs ESP1-
ESP&nStgs;
Array Ns{&nStgs}; Array alpha{&nStgs}; Array beta{&nStgs};
Array ESP{&nStgs}; Array FSP{&nStgs}; Array Ws{&nStgs};
Array sumWs{&nStgs}; Array TSc{&nStgs};
Model=&Model; cPower=&cPower;
nRatio=&nRatio; NId=&NId; NItype=&NItype; N2min=&N2min;
nStgs=&nStgs; sigma=&sigma; power=0; AveTotalN=0; Aveux=0; Aveuy=0;
cumN=0; Do i=1 To nStgs-1; cumN=cumN+Ns{i}; End;
N0=CumN+Ns{nStgs};
Do k=1 To nStgs;
sumWs{k}=0; Do i=1 To k; sumWs{k}=sumWs{k}+Ws{i}**2; End;
sumWs{k}=sqrt(sumWs{k});
End;
* Calcate the standard deviation, sigma for different endpoints *;
If &EP="normal" Then Do sigmax=&sigma; sigmay=&sigma; End;
If &EP="binary" Then Do
sigmax=Sqrt(&ux*(1-&ux)); sigmay=Sqrt(&uy*(1-&uy));
End;
If &EP="survival" Then Do
sigmax=&ux*(1+exp(-&ux*&tStd)*(1-exp(&ux*&tAcr))/(&tAcr*&ux))**(-
0.5);
sigmay=&uy*(1+exp(-&uy*&tStd)*(1-exp(&uy*&tAcr))/(&tAcr*&uy))**(-
0.5);
```

```
End;
If NItype="PCT" Then sigmax=(1-NId)*sigmax;
Do i=1 To nStgs; FSP{i}=0; ESP{i}=0; End;
Do iSim=1 to &nSims;
ThisNx=0; ThisNy=0; Thisux=0; Thisuy=0;
Do i=1 To nStgs; TSc{i}=0; End;
TS=0; If &Model="MPP" Then TS=1;
Do i=1 To nStgs;
uxObs=Rannor(746)*sigmax/sqrt(Ns{i})+&ux;
uyObs=Rannor(874)*sigmay/sqrt(nRatio*Ns{i})+&uy;
Thisux=Thisux+uxObs*Ns{i};
Thisuy=Thisuy+uyObs*nRatio*Ns{i};
If NItype="PCT" Then NId=uxObs*&NId;
ThisNx=ThisNx+Ns{i};
ThisNy=ThisNy+Ns{i}*nRatio;
StdErr=(sigmax**2/Ns{i}+sigmay**2/(nRatio*Ns{i}))**0.5;
TS0 = (uyObs-uxObs+NId)/StdErr;
If Model="MIP" Then TS=1-ProbNorm(TS0);
If Model="MSP" Then TS=TS+(1-ProbNorm(TS0));
If Model="MPP" Then TS=TS*(1-ProbNorm(TS0));
If Model="MINP" Then Do;
Do k=i to nStgs; TSc{k}=TSc{k}+Ws{i}/sumWs{k}*TS0; End;
TS=1-ProbNorm(TSc{i});
End;
If TS>beta{i} Then Do; FSP{i}=FSP{i}+1/&nSims; Goto Jump; End;
Else If TS<=alpha{i} then do;
Power=Power+1/&nSims; ESP{i}=ESP{i}+1/&nSims; Goto Jump; End;
Else If nStgs>1 & i=1 & &Nadj="Y" Then Do;
eSize=&DuHa/(abs(uyObs-uxObs)+0.0000001);
nFinal=min(&Nmax, max(N0,eSize*Abs(eSize)*N0));
If nStgs=2 Then do;
*eSize=(uyObs-uxObs+NId)/((sigmax+sigmay)*sqrt(0.5+0.5/nRatio));
 eSize=(uyObs-uxObs+NId)/Sqrt(0.5*sigmax**2+0.5*sigmay**2/nRatio);
%nByCPowerUB(Model, alpha{2}, eSize, cPower, TS, ws{1}, ws{2}, n2New);
*Force a minimum n increment for info mask;
nFinal=Round(min(&Nmax,ns{1}+n2New+&nMinIcr/2), &nMinIcr);
nFinal=max(N2min+Ns{1},nFinal);
End;
If nStgs>1 Then Ns{nStgs}= max(1,nFinal-cumN);
```

End;
End;
Jump:
Aveux=Aveux+Thisux/ThisNx/&nSims;
Aveuy=Aveuy+Thisuy/ThisNy/&nSims;
AveTotalN=AveTotalN+(ThisNx+ThisNy)/&nSims;
End;
Output;
Run;
Proc Print; Run;
%Mend TwoArmNStgAdpDsg;
<<**SAS**<<

Note that SAS Macro 11.2 actually includes two macros: nByCPowerUB and TwoArmNStgAdpDsg; the latter calls the former.

## 11.6    Power Comparisions in Promising-Zone

Chen, DeMets, and Lan (2004) proposed the "Promising-Zone" method. We know that MINP using the fixed weights usually takes the square-root of the information time at the interim analysis with the original final sample size $N_0$ as the denominator, i.e., $\tau_0 = \frac{n_1}{N_0}$.

$$T_2 = \max \sqrt{\tau_0} z_1 + \sqrt{1 - \tau_0} z_2. \tag{11.7}$$

Note that $T_2$ has a normal distribution, but when it is conditionally on the second stage, $T_2 | (\alpha_1 < t_1 < \beta_1)$ is no longer a normal distribution.

The weighted $Z$-statistic approach (11.7) is flexible in that the decision to increase the sample size and the magnitude of sample-size increment are not mandated by prespecified rules. However, some researchers prefer using an equal weight for each patient ("one patient one vote"). For this reason, Chen, DeMets, and Lan (2004) proposed a conservative test statistic:

$$\begin{cases} T_1 = z_1 \\ T_2 = \max \left\{ \sqrt{\frac{n_1}{N_0}} z_1 + \sqrt{\frac{N_0 - n_1}{N_0}} z_2, \sqrt{\frac{n_1}{N}} z_1 + \sqrt{\frac{N - n_1}{N}} z_2 \right\} \end{cases}, \tag{11.8}$$

where $z_1$ and $z_2$ are the usual $Z$-statistic based on the subsamples from stages 1 and 2, respectively. $n_1$ is the sample size at the interim analysis, $N_0$ is the original final sample size and $N$ is the new final sample size after adjustment based on the interim analysis.

In my view, the "one patient one vote" policy for the test statistic at the second stage only is not justified because the patients from the first stage $(T_1)$ have potentially two opportunities to "vote" in the decision making (rejecting or not rejecting the $H_0$), one at the interim analysis and the other at the final analysis, while patients from the second stage have at most one time to "vote" when the trial continues to the second stage. For this reason, the second stage patients should be given more weight. Furthermore, the weighting is less important in hypothesis testing than in estimation, even though they are somewhat related. Using this modified test statistic, the authors prove that when the conditional probability with original sample size is larger than 50%, then adjusted sample size, i.e., increasing the sample size when the unblinded interim result is promising will not inflate the type-I error rate and therefore no statistical adjustment is necessary. The unblinded interim result is considered promising if the conditional power is greater than 50% or, equivalently, the sample size increment needed to achieve a desired power does not exceed an upper bound.

Following Chen's idea of promising zone, we are going to make comparisons between different methods for SSR at the promising zone. To accomplish this, we add a futility boundary at the first stage in the two-stage design to stop the trial when the observed treatment effect is much smaller than expected. In other words, we want to effectively put resources on the drug candidates that are likely effective or that might fail marginally at the final analysis with the original sample size, based the information seen at the interim analysis.

Mehta and Pocock (2011) proposed another Promising-Zone method, in which they define the promising zone as the interim $p$-value $p_1$ between 0.1587 ($z_1 = 1.206$) and 0.0213 ($z_1 = 2.027$). This is because when one-sided $p$-value $p_1$ is larger but close to 0.1 at the interim analysis with information time $\tau = 0.5$, the trial is likely to marginally fail to reject $H_0$ at the final analysis with $p$-value around 0.06 to 0.15. Those drug candidates are likely clinically effective, thus we want to "save" those trials to show statistical significance by increasing the sample size. If the $p_1$ is, say, larger than 0.2 (0.4 for two-sided $p$-value), we will stop the trial earlier at the first stage. Therefore, we recommend the following approach: combine the futility boundary with the upper bound of the promising zone and recommend using $\beta_1 = 0.2$ for the one-sided $p$-value at the interim analysis with information time 0.5. The following comparisons are based on this concept of promising zone.

We now use SAS Macro 11.2 to study the operating characteristics of various sample-size reestimation methods for two-stage adaptive designs. The nonbinding futility rule is currently adopted by the regulatory bodies, based on which the futility boundaries don't have to be followed. Therefore, the earlier futility boundaries cannot be considered in constructing later stopping boundaries. For this reason, it is important to study the performance of different methods with nonbinding futility boundaries. We will compare the power and sample sizes among different methods. The scenarios considered are (1) the trial has a futility boundary, and (2) the sample size increases discretely for information mask. For each of the scenarios, we simulate the classical and adaptive designs using the following three different methods: MSP, MPP, and MINP. The simulations are performed for a normal endpoint with a means $u_A = 0$ for the control group and $u_B = 1$ for the test group, and a common standard deviation of $\sigma = 3$.

The results in Tables 11.4 and 11.5 are generated using the following typical SAS macro calls. $\bar{N}$ is the average total sample size from the simulations, and $\bar{u}_A$ and $\bar{u}_B$ are the average means in group A and group B from the simulations. Each scenario has 1,000,000 simulation runs. ESP1 in the output is the early stopping probability at the first stage.

>>**SAS**>>

Data dInput;
Array Ns{2} (80, 80); Array alpha{2} (0.005,0.205); Array beta{2} (0.20, 0.205); Array Ws{2} (1,1);
%TwoArmNStgAdpDsg(ux=0, uy=0, Model="MSP", cPower=0.9, DuHa=1.25, Nmax=200, N2min=0, nMinIcr=1, sigma=3); Run;


Data dInput;
Array Ns{2} (80, 80); Array alpha{2} (0.005,0.205); Array beta{2} (0.20, 0.205); Array Ws{2} (1,1);
%TwoArmNStgAdpDsg(ux=0, uy=1, Model="MSP", cPower=0.9, DuHa=1.25, Nmax=200, N2min=0, nMinIcr=20, sigma=3); Run;


Data dInput;
Array Ns{2} (80, 80); Array alpha{2} (0.005,0.0038); Array beta{2} (0.20, 0.0038); Array Ws{2} (1,1);
%TwoArmNStgAdpDsg(ux=0, uy=1, Model="MPP", cPower=0.9, DuHa=1.25, Nmax=200, N2min=0, nMinIcr=1, sigma=3); Run;

Data dInput;
Array Ns{2} (80, 80); Array alpha{2} (0.005,0.0226); Array beta{2} (0.20, 0.0226); Array Ws{2} (0.7071,0.7071);
%TwoArmNStgAdpDsg(ux=0, uy=1, Model="MINP", cPower=0.9, DuHa=1.25, Nmax=200, N2min=0, nMinIcr=20, sigma=3); Run;
<<**SAS**<<

## Scenario 1: Effect of Early Stopping Boundary

Assume the effect size is $1/3$ in a two-group adaptive design with SSR. Let's use $\alpha_1 = 0.005$, $\beta_1 = 0.2$, $\alpha_2 = 0.205$, and $N_1 = 80$. Note that when $p_1 > \beta_1 = 0.205$, there is no possibility of rejecting the null hypothesis at the second stage for MSP. The maximum sample size $N_{max}$ is 200 per group. Table 11.4 gives a quick comparison of different methods, where $\bar{N}_o$ is the expected sample-size under the null and $\bar{N}_a$ is the expected sample-size under the alternative. All designs have a 90% target conditional power. Overall, MSP design performs better than other designs under the null and alternative conditions; MPP and MINP perform equally well.

Table 11.4: Comparisons of Adaptive Methods

| Method | $\alpha_2$ | $N_o$ | $N_a$ | Power |
|---|---|---|---|---|
| Classical | .0250 | 284 | 284 | 80.0% |
| MSP | .2050 | 204 | 276 | 83.5% |
| MPP | .0038 | 204 | 266 | 81.5% |
| MINP | .0226 | 204 | 268 | 82.7% |

Note: $\alpha_1 = 0.005$, $\beta_1 = 0.2$, effect size $=1/3$.

## Scenario 2: Discrete SSR for Information Mask

To study the impact of the discrete SSR, we study the minimum sample-size increment from 1, 20, and 40 per group. The simulation results are presented in Table 11.5. We can see that the discretization of sample-size increment has a small impact on the power and sample size for the adaptive designs. Using a larger minimal increase will not only help mask the treatment difference, but also increase the effectiveness of SSR.

Table 11.5: Summary of Comparisons with Lower Initial Power

| | $\Delta N_{min} = 1$ | | $\Delta N_{min} = 20$ | | $\Delta N_{min} = 40$ | |
|---|---|---|---|---|---|---|
| Method | $\bar{N}$ | Power | N | Power | N | Power |
| MSP | 276 | 83.5% | 281 | 84.1% | 286 | 84.5% |
| MPP | 266 | 81.5% | 271 | 82.1% | 276 | 82.7% |
| MINP | 268 | 82.7% | 273 | 83.3% | 278 | 83.8% |

Note: Note: $\alpha_1 = 0.005$, $\beta_1 = 0.2$, effect size $=1/3$

Note that comparison based on power is not the best way to judge adaptive designs. The power depends on many different things: (1) the unknown true treatment difference $\delta$, (2) the sample size at stage 1, and (3) the rule for SSR. Because $\delta$ is an unknown, we may use Bayesian prior distribution $\pi(\delta)$ (Chapter 21). Note that there are two types of conditional power we have considered: (1) conditioning on $p_1$ and (2) conditioning on $p_1$ and $\delta = \hat{\delta}_1$. The former is what we are really interested in, while the latter is just an estimation of the former. Just as with conditional power, there are two types of power: (1) the power depending on true $\delta$ and (2) the power depending on $\hat{\delta}$ that is estimated at the initial design. Therefore, we should not make general conclusions regarding which method is better based only on the power.

### Scenario 3: Comparison of Conditional Power

As stated earlier, for adaptive design, conditional power is often a better measure than power regarding the efficiency. The difference in conditional power between different methods is dependent on the stagewise $p$-value from the first stage. From Tables 11.6 and 11.7 and Figure 11.1, it can be seen that conditional power for MSP is uniformly higher for $p_1$ around 0.1 than the other two methods. Therefore, if you believe that $p_1$ is somewhere between (0.005, 0.18), then MSP is much more efficient than MPP and MINP or MINP; otherwise, MPP and MINP are better.

Table 11.6:   Conditional Power as Function of $N_2$

| Method | $\alpha_2$ | $N_2 = 100$ Power | $N_2 = 200$ Power | $N_2 = 300$ Power | $N_2 = 400$ Power |
|--------|-----------|---------|---------|---------|---------|
| MSP | .21463 | 0.584 | 0.788 | 0.894 | 0.948 |
| MPP | .00375 | 0.357 | 0.567 | 0.748 | 0.853 |
| MINP | .02400 | 0.460 | 0.686 | 0.825 | 0.906 |

Note: $\alpha_1 = 0.0025$. $p_1 = 0.1$, effect size = 0.2, no futility binding.

An example of SAS macro calls for generating the results in Table 11.6 is presented in the following.

>>**SAS**>>
%ConPower(EP="normal", Model="MSP", alpha2=.21463, ux=0.2, uy=0.4, sigma=1, n2=200, p1=0.1);
%ConPower(EP="normal", Model="MPP", alpha2=.00375, ux=0.2, uy=0.4, sigma=1, n2=200, p1=0.1);
%ConPower(EP="normal", Model="MINP", alpha2=.02400, ux=0.2, uy=0.4, sigma=1, n2=200, p1=0.1, w1=1, w2=1);
<<**SAS**<<

Table 11.7:   Conditional Powers as Function of $p_1$

| Method | | | | $p_1$ | | |
|--------|-------|-------|-------|-------|-------|-------|
| | 0.010 | 0.050 | 0.100 | 0.150 | 0.180 | 0.220 |
| | | | | Power | | |
| MSP | 0.880 | 0.847 | 0.788 | 0.685 | 0.572 | 0.044 |
| MPP | 0.954 | 0.712 | 0.567 | 0.516 | 0.485 | 0.453 |
| LW | 0.937 | 0.802 | 0.686 | 0.595 | 0.547 | 0.490 |

Note: $\alpha_1 = 0.0025$. $N_2 = 200$, effect size $= 0.2$, no futility binding.

The differences in conditional power among the three methods are presented in Figure 11.1.

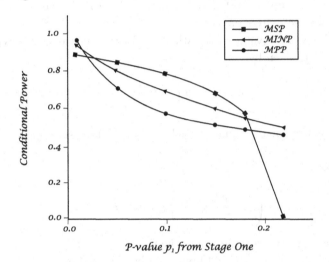

Figure 11.1:   Conditional Power versus $p$-value from Stage 1

## 11.7   Analysis of Design with Sample-Size Adjustment

### 11.7.1   *Adjusted p-value*

We recommend the $p$-value that has been discussed in Chapters 4 and 5. For MSP, we use

$$p(t;k) = \begin{cases} t, & k = 1 \\ \alpha_1 + \frac{1}{2}(t - \alpha_1)^2, & k = 2 \text{ and } \alpha_1 < t \le \beta_1 \\ \alpha_1 + t(\beta_1 - \alpha_1) - \frac{1}{2}(\beta_1^2 - \alpha_1^2), & k = 2 \text{ and } \beta_1 < t \le \alpha_1 + 1 \\ t + t\beta_1 - \frac{1}{2}t^2 - \frac{1}{2}\beta_1^2 - \frac{1}{2}, & k = 2 \text{ and } t > \alpha_1 + 1 \end{cases}$$

$$(11.9)$$

For MPP, we use

$$p(t; k) = \begin{cases} t, & k = 1, \\ \alpha_1 + t \ln \frac{\beta_1}{\alpha_1}, & k = 2 . \end{cases} \tag{11.10}$$

For MINP, we use simulations to determine the adjusted $p$-value.

### 11.7.2    *Confidence Interval*

From the duality of the confidence and hypothesis test, we know that a $100(1 - \alpha)\%$ CI consists all $\delta_0$ such that the null hypothesis $H_0 : \delta \leq \delta_0$ is not rejected at any stage before stage $K_s$, where $K_s$ is the stage at which the trial was actually stopped.

The stagewise $p$-value at the $i$th stage for the one-sided null hypothesis $H_0 : \delta \leq \delta_0$ is given by

$$p_i = 1 - \Phi\left(\frac{\hat{\delta}_i - \delta_0}{\sigma}\sqrt{\frac{n_i}{2}}\right), \tag{11.11}$$

where $\hat{\delta}_i$ is the naive estimate based on the $i$th stage subsample.

Therefore, for MSP, the stagewise CI limits can be obtained by solving (11.11) for $\delta_{\alpha_k}$:

$$\sum_{i=1}^{k}\left[1 - \Phi\left(\frac{\hat{\delta}_i - \delta_{\alpha_k}}{\sigma}\sqrt{\frac{n_i}{2}}\right)\right] = \alpha_k, \ k = 1, ..., K_s, \tag{11.12}$$

where stage $K_s$ is the stage where the trial was actually stopped.

For MPP, the stagewise CI limits can be obtained by solving (11.11) for $\delta_{\alpha_k}$:

$$\prod_{i=1}^{k}\left[1 - \Phi\left(\frac{\hat{\delta}_i - \delta_{\alpha_k}}{\sigma}\sqrt{\frac{n_i}{2}}\right)\right] = \alpha_k, \ k = 1, ..., K_s. \tag{11.13}$$

For MINP, the stagewise CI limits can be obtained by solving (11.12) for $\delta_{\alpha_k}$:

$$\sum_{i=1}^{k} w_{ki}\left(\frac{\hat{\delta}_i - \delta_{\alpha_k}}{\sigma}\sqrt{\frac{n_i}{2}}\right) = \alpha_k, \ k = 1, ..., K_s, \tag{11.14}$$

where $w_{ki}$ are predetermined weights satisfying $\sum_{i=1}^{k} w_{ki}^2 = 1$.

The $100(1 - \alpha)\%$ confidence limit $\delta_{0\,\text{min}}$ is given by

$$\delta_{0\,\text{min}} = \max\left\{\delta_{\alpha_1}, ..., \delta_{\alpha_{K_s}}\right\}. \tag{11.15}$$

Equation (11.15) is also an adjusted $100(1 - \sum_{i=1}^{K_s} \pi_i)\%$ CI (see Chapter 27).

Note that (11.14) reduces to the classical CI when $K = 1$. Equation (11.14) can be solved analytically. For example, for the second stage, we have

$$\delta_{\alpha_2} = \frac{w_{k1}\sqrt{n_1}\hat{\delta}_1 + w_{k2}\sqrt{n_2}\hat{\delta}_2 - \sqrt{2}\sigma z_{1-\alpha_2}}{w_{k1}\sqrt{n_1} + w_{k2}\sqrt{n_2}}. \tag{11.16}$$

So far, we have not considered the futility boundaries in constructing CI.

### 11.7.3 *Adjusted Point Estimates*

**Design without Possible Early Stopping**

When there is no early stopping, e.g., the interim analysis is for SSR only, then the unbiased estimate can be easily found (Brannath, Koenig, and Bauer, 2006; Liu, Proschan, and Pledger 2002; and Proschan, 2003). For example, the following weighted stagewise estimate is unbiased:

$$\hat{\delta}_u = \sum_{i=1}^{K} \omega_i \hat{\delta}_i, \tag{11.17}$$

where $\hat{\delta}_i$ is the naive estimate based on the $i$th stage subsample, e.g., mean difference or response rate difference between the two groups. Note that $E(\delta_i) = \delta$ $(i = 1, ..., K)$; hence, for any predetermined constant weights $\omega_i$, satisfying $\sum_{i=1}^{K} \omega_i = 1$ will provide a unbiased estimate. However, for consistency with the CI, the weight should be carefully chosen. If the SSR trial only allows for sample-size increase such that the final sample size is between the initial sample size $N_0$ and the maximum sample size $N_{\max}$, then the following weights might be a good choice for the two-stage SSR design:

$$\omega_1 = \frac{2n_1}{N_0 + N_{\max}}, \quad \omega_2 = 1 - \omega_1. \tag{11.18}$$

**Design with Possible Early Stopping**

If symmetric stopping boundaries are used, an unbiased point estimate for a two-stage design is given by

$$\hat{\delta}_u = \frac{w_1\sqrt{n_1}\hat{\delta}_1 + w_2\sqrt{n_2}\hat{\delta}_2}{w_1\sqrt{n_1} + w_2\sqrt{n_2}}, \tag{11.19}$$

where $w_i$ are predetermined constants, which are suggested to be $w_1 = \sqrt{\frac{n_1}{n_1+n_{02}}}$ and $w_2 = \sqrt{\frac{n_{02}}{n_1+n_{02}}}$. Here $n_{02}$ is the initial sample size for the second stage (Lawrence and Hung, 2003).

For a general adaptive design, there is an absolute minimum sample size $n_{\min}$ required regardless of the adaptations. We can use the first $n_{\min}$ patients per group to construct an unbiased point estimate:

$$\hat{\delta}_u = \sum_{i=1}^{n_{\min}} \frac{x_{Bi}}{n_i} - \sum_{i=1}^{n_{\min}} \frac{x_{Ai}}{n_i}, \qquad (11.20)$$

where $x_{Ai}$ and $x_{Bi}$ are the observed responses of the $i$th patient in groups A and B, respectively.

Equation (11.20) is difficult to justify: Why are only the first $n_{\min}$ patients' outcomes considered? If we believe bias is not the only issue in drug development, we should balance the bias and interpretability of the results. There will be a more in-depth discussion in Chapter 27.

Using an estimate that has a median equal to $\delta$ independently from the adaptation (Brannath, Koenig and Bauer, 2002; Cheng and Shen, 2004; Lawrence and Hung, 2003; and Proschan, 2003) has also been suggested.

For a design featuring early stopping, (11.19) is an unbiased median, but the mean bias and variance of $\hat{\delta}_u$ depend on the adaptation rule.

The maximum bias for a two-stage adaptive design with early stopping and SSR is bound by

$$0.4\frac{\sigma}{\sqrt{n_1}}\frac{N_{\max} - n_1}{N_{\max}} = \frac{0.4\sigma}{\sqrt{n_1}}\frac{r_{\max} - 1}{r_{\max}} < \frac{0.4\sigma}{\sqrt{n_1}}, \qquad (11.21)$$

where $N_{\max}$ is the maximum sample size per group and $r_{\max} = N_{\max}/n_1$.

An interesting method to obtain an unbiased estimate is to recruit at least two more patients for each stage $i > k$ when the trial is stopped at the $k$th stage due to efficacy or futility such that we use (11.17) and (11.18). However, the extra patients enrolled will not be used for the hypothesis test. When the trial stops at the first stage, there could be a consistency issue between point estimation and hypothesis test.

## 11.8   Trial Examples

### Example 11.1   Myocardial Infarction Prevention Trial

This example is based on the case presented by Cui, Hung, and Wang (1999). In a phase-III, two-arm trial to evaluate the effect of a new drug on the prevention of myocardial infarction in patients undergoing coronary artery bypass graft surgery, a sample size of 300 patients per group will provide 95% power to detect a 50% reduction in incidence from 22% to 11% at the one-sided significance level $\alpha = 0.025$. Although the sponsor is confident about the incidence of 22% in the control group, the sponsor is not that sure about the 11% incidence rate in the test group.

Because of the wide range of the estimated incidence rate in the test group, the sponsor felt uncomfortable choosing a fixed sample size. A fixed sample size can be either too small for a small effect size or too large for a large effect size. Therefore, an adaptive design with SSR is used. Further, assume a safety requirement for a minimum number of patients to be treated that precludes interim efficacy stopping. Therefore, an adaptive trial with futility stopping and SSR is chosen.

Suppose we decide to use MSP for a two-stage adaptive design featuring sample-size reestimation. The conditional power approach (11.5) will be used for sample-size adjustment based on the results of interim, which is scheduled when efficacy assessments have been completed for 50% of the patients. The stopping rules are (1) at stage 1, stop for futility if the stagewise $p$-value $p_1 > \beta_1$ and stop for efficacy if $p_1 \leq \alpha_1$ and (2) at the final stage, if $p_1 + p_2 \leq \alpha_2$, claim efficacy; otherwise, claim futility. The designs with and without SSR will be evaluated using stopping boundaries: $\alpha_1 = 0$, $\beta_1 = 0.2$, $\alpha_2 = 0.225$. The upper limit of the sample size is $N_{\max} = 500$ per group. The SAS macro calls for the simulations are shown as follows.

>>**SAS**>>

```
Title "Example 11.1";
Data dInput;
Array Ns{2} (150, 150); Array alpha{2} (0,0.225);
Array beta{2} (0.2,0.225); Array Ws{2} (1,1);
%TwoArmNStgAdpDsg(nStgs=2,      ux=0.11,      uy=0.22,      EP="binary",
Model="MSP", Nadj="N");
%TwoArmNStgAdpDsg(nStgs=2, ux=0.11, uy=0.22,
EP="binary",   Model="MSP",   Nadj="Y",   cPower=0.95,   DuHa=0.11,
Nmax=500, N2min=150, nMinIcr=50);
%TwoArmNStgAdpDsg(nStgs=2,      ux=0.14,      uy=0.22,      EP="binary",
Model="MSP", Nadj="N");
%TwoArmNStgAdpDsg(nStgs=2,      ux=0.14,      uy=0.22,      EP="binary",
Model="MSP", Nadj="Y", cPower=0.95, DuHa=0.11, Nmax=500, N2min=150,
nMinIcr=50);
%TwoArmNStgAdpDsg(nStgs=2,      ux=0.22,      uy=0.22,      EP="binary",
Model="MSP", Nadj="N");
```

238 *Adaptive Design Theory and Implementation*

%TwoArmNStgAdpDsg(nStgs=2,     ux=0.22,     uy=0.22,     EP="binary",
Model="MSP", Nadj="Y", cPower=0.95, DuHa=0.11, Nmax=500, N2min=150,
nMinIcr=50);
Run;
<<**SAS**<<

The simulation results are presented in Table 11.8. From the simulation results, there are noticeable features of adaptive designs:

(1) For the GSD with futility boundary $\beta_1 = 0.2$ without SSR, there is a reduction in sample size under $H_0$ as compared to the classical design, but a decrease in power as compared to the classical design, as well.

(2) For the designs with SSR, the power and sample size increase when the treatment effect is overestimated.

Table 11.8:   Comparison of Adaptive Designs

| Design | \multicolumn{5}{c}{Event Rate in the Test Group $P_T$} | | | | |
| | 0.110 | | 0.14 | | 0.22 |
| | $N_a$ | Power (%) | $N_a$ | Power (%) | $N_o$ |
|---|---|---|---|---|---|
| Classical | 600 | 94.2 | 600 | 72.3 | 600 |
| GSD | 588 | 92.0 | 550 | 67.0 | 360 |
| SSR | 928 | 95.8 | 874 | 80.0 | 440 |

Note: $\alpha_1 = 0$, $\beta_1 = 0.2$, $N_{\max} = 500$/group, target $cP = 0.95$.

Based on the simulation results, we suggest using the adaptive design with SSR. We promise that if the trial stops at the first stage, two more patients will be enrolled for the estimation. Therefore we can use (11.17) and (11.18).

Regardless of whether the trial is stopped at the first stage or the second stage, we have two stagewise naive estimates, $\hat{\delta}_1$ and $\hat{\delta}_2$. Suppose an interim analysis is performed with 150 patients per group. The observed event rates are 0.22 and 0.165 for the control and test groups, respectively. The $p$-value can be calculated using the chi-square test or, equivalently, $p_1 = 1 - \Phi\left(\frac{(0.22-0.165)\sqrt{150}}{\sqrt{0.31}}\right) = 1 - \Phi(1.2111) = 0.1129 < \beta_1 = 0.2$. Therefore, the trial proceeds to the second stage with a newly estimated sample size per group for the second stage $n_2 = N_{\max} - n_1 = 650$ for a target conditional power of 90% with effect size of 0.14. This sample size is considered too big due to financial consideration. $n_2 = 400$ is finally used, which provides about 78% conditional power. Suppose the observed event rates for stage 2 are 0.22 and 0.175 for the control and test groups, respectively; the stagewise $p$-value is $p_2 = 1 - \Phi\left(\frac{(0.22-0.175)\sqrt{400}}{\sqrt{0.316}}\right) = 1 - \Phi(1.6011) = 0.0547$. Therefore, the test statistic $t = p_1 + p_2 = 0.1676 < \alpha_2 = 0.225$, and the null hypothesis is rejected.

The adjusted $p$-value is calculated from (11.9):

$$p_{adj} = \alpha_1 + t(\beta_1 - \alpha_1) - \frac{1}{2}(\beta_1^2 - \alpha_1^2)$$

$$= 0.1676(0.2) - \frac{1}{2}(0.2^2) = 0.0135.$$

The confidence limit is calculated using (11.12). It is obvious that $\delta_{\alpha_1} = -\infty$. To obtain $\delta_{\alpha_2}$, we need to solve the following equation:

$$2 - \Phi\left(\frac{(0.055 - \delta_{\alpha_2})\sqrt{150}}{\sqrt{0.31}}\right) - \Phi\left(\frac{(0.045 - \delta_{\alpha_2})\sqrt{400}}{\sqrt{0.316}}\right) = 0.225. \quad (11.22)$$

Using the trial-and-error method in (11.22), we obtain $\delta_{\alpha_2} = 0.007$. Therefore, the confidence limit is given by $\delta_{0\,\min} = 0.007$.

The adjusted estimate of treatment difference in event rate can be obtained from (11.19) with $w_i = \sqrt{0.5}$:

$$\delta_u = \frac{0.055\sqrt{0.5}\sqrt{150} + 0.045\sqrt{0.5}\sqrt{400}}{\sqrt{0.5}\sqrt{150} + \sqrt{0.5}\sqrt{400}} = 0.0488.$$

The unbiased estimate of treatment difference in event rate can be obtained from (11.17) with $w_1 = \frac{2(150)}{300+550} = \frac{6}{17}$ and $w_2 = 11/17$ from (11.18):

$$\delta_u = \frac{6(0.055)}{17} + \frac{11(0.045)}{17} = 0.0485.$$

The naive estimate is given by

$$\hat{\delta} = \frac{150(0.055)}{550} + \frac{400(0.045)}{550} = 0.0477$$

In summary, the test drug has about a 4.8% reduction in event rate with a one-sided 97.5% confidence limit of 0.7%. The adjusted $p$-value (one-sided) is 0.0135. So far the binding futility boundaries are used.

Note that the actual trial was designed without SSR. The sponsor asked for SSR at interim analysis, and was rejected by the FDA. The trial eventually failed to demonstrate statistical significance.

## Example 11.2   Adaptive Design with Farrington-Manning NI Margin

There are two ways to define the noninferiority margin: (1) a pre-fixed noninferiority (NI) margin and (2) a noninferiority margin that is proportional to the effect of the active control group, i.e., the Farrington–Manning noninferiority margin. The former has been discussed in Chapter 2. We now discuss the latter. The Farrington–Manning noninferiority test was proposed for a classical design with a binary endpoint (Farrington and Manning, 1990), but can be extended to adaptive designs with different endpoints, in which the null hypothesis can be defined as $H_0 : u_t - (1 - \delta_{NI}) u_c \leq 0$, where $0 < \delta_{NI} < 1$ and $u_t$ and $u_c$ are the responses (mean, proportion, median survival time) for test and control groups, respectively. The test statistic is defined as

$$T_k = \frac{u_t - (1 - \delta_{NI}) u_c}{\sqrt{\sigma_t^2/n_t + (1 - \delta_{NI})\sigma_c^2/n_c}}, \qquad (11.23)$$

where $n_t$ and $n_c$ and the sample sizes for the test and control groups, respectively, and where $\sigma_t^2 = var\,(u_t)$ and $\sigma_c^2 = var\,(u_c)$ are given by Table 2.1 and (11.3) for a large sample. It is important to know that there is a variance reduction in comparison with the prefixed NI margin approach, in which the variance is $\sigma_t^2 + \sigma_c^2$ instead of $\sigma_t^2 + (1 - \delta_{NI})^2\sigma_c^2$. Therefore, the Farrington–Manning test is usually much more powerful than the fixed margin approach. SAS Macro 11.2 provides the capability for simulating both NI test methods with either balanced or imbalanced designs.

## 11.9  Summary and Discussion

In this chapter, we have studied the different SSR approaches, in which we have combined the general adaptive design methods (MSP, MPP, and MINP/LW) with two sample-size adjustment rules given in (11.4) and (11.6). We have compared the performances of different approaches using the simulations. You can use SAS Macro 11.1 or the R program in Appendix D to conduct your own simulations. In fact, it is strongly suggested that you do so before selecting a design. Here is a summary of what we have studied in this chapter:

(1) Futility stopping can reduce the sample size when the null is true. The futility boundary is suggested because in the case of a very small effect size, to continue the trial would require an unrealistically large sample size, and an increased sample size to $N_{max}$ still may not have enough power.

(2) From an $\alpha$-control point of view, for the methods in this chapter (MSP, MPP, and L-W), the algorithm for sample-size adjustment does not have to be predetermined; instead, it can be determined after we observed the results from the interim analysis.

(3) It might be a concern if the sample size is based on a predetermined algorithm, IDMC's determination of the new sample size will actually require the disclosure of the efficacy information for the trial. There are at least two approaches to handle this: (a) use a discrete increment of sample size or (2) set a target conditional power, and let the IDMC choose the new sample-size approximation for the conditional power with consideration of other factors.

(4) Unbiased estimates (point and confidence interval) can be obtained by using the fixed weight method, but interpretation may be difficult. In addition to the unbiased estimate, report the unbiased estimate with a bias assessment at the true mean = naive estimate.

(6) Power is an estimation, made at the initial design stage, of the probability of rejecting the null hypothesis. Therefore, it is less important when the sample size can be adjusted at the interim analysis (IA). In other words, the initial total sample size is irrelevant to the final sample size (it is only relevant for budgeting and operational planning), but the sample size at the first stage is relevant.

(7) For adaptive designs, the conditional power is more important than the unconditional power. MSP often shows superior over other methods. The nonbinding futility rule is currently adopted by regulatory bodies. With nonbinding futility boundaries, MSP is often superior over other methods.

It is interesting to know that increasing sample size when the unblinded interim result is promising will not inflate the type-I error rate. The unblinded interim result is considered promising if the conditional power is greater than 50% or, equivalently, the sample-size increment needed to achieve a desired power does not exceed an upper bound (Chen, DeMets, and Lan, 2004).

There are other practical issues, e.g., what if the stagewise $p_1$ and $p_2$ are very different? Does this inconsistency cause any concern? If the answer is "yes," then should we check this consistency for a classical design too? MSP emphasizes the consistency, but MPP and MINP do not. More discussions on the controversial issues will be presented in Chapter 29.

Finally, it is interesting to know that a group sequential design with early stopping is a specific use of discrete functions of sample-size reestimation. Menon and Chang (2012) studied the optimization of sample size reestimation using simulations. Hung and Wang (2012) studied the sample size adaptation in fixed-dose combination drug trial.

**Problems**

**11.1** Use MPP and MINP to redesign the trial in Example 11.1.

**11.2** Study noninferiority adaptive designs with both prefixed noninferiority margin and Farrington–Manning margin and compare the results using both MSP and MINP.

**11.3** Use SAS or R to develop a simulation program for a $K$-stage adaptive design with SSR. The sample-size reestimation should be based on the conditional power given in (9.32) for MINP.

# Chapter 12

# Blinded and Semi-Blinded
# Sample-Size Reestimation Design

## 12.1 Introduction

Wittes and Brittain (1990) and Gould and Shih (1992, 1998) discussed methods of blinded SSR. In contrast to unblinded SSR, blinded SSR assumes that the actually realized effect size estimate is not revealed through unblinding the treatment code. In blinded sample-size reestimation, interim data are used without unblinding treatment assignment to provide an updated estimate of a nuisance parameter in order to update the sample size for the trial based on the estimate. Nuisance parameters mentioned in this context are usually the variance for continuous outcomes. Wittes et al. (1999) and Zucker et al. (1999) investigated the performance of various blinded and unblinded SSR methods by simulation. They observed some slight type-I error violations in cases with small sample size. Kieser and Friede (2003) and Friede and Kieser (2006) suggested a method of blinded sample size. Blinded sample reestimation is generally well accepted by regulators (ICH, 1999).

Theoretically, MSP, MPP, MLP, and MINP can all be used for blinded SSR using the same stopping boundaries as those for unblinded SSR. It seems there is a common perception that pooled data analysis will not reveal the treatment difference. However, this is not true. There are several ways to estimate the treatment difference without unblinding the treatment code. We will discuss those methods for our SSR.

In the chapter, we will discuss the Max-Info design, which make SSR based on the estimation of the nuisance parameter $\sigma_0$. We will also discuss how to estimate the treatment difference without unblinding the data and incorporating such estimation into SSR design. These blinded (or semi-blinded) SSR methods and an unblinding SSR method will be compared though computer simulations.

## 12.2 Maximum Information Design

In clinical trials, the sample size is determined by a clinically meaningful difference and information on the variability of the primary endpoint. Due to lack of knowledge of the new treatment, estimates of the variability for the primary endpoint are often not precise. As a result, the initially planned sample size may turn out to be inappropriate and need to be adjusted at interim analysis to ensure the power if the observed variability of the accumulated response on the primary endpoint is very different from that used at the planning stage. To maintain the maximum integrity of the trial, it is suggested that sample-size reestimation be performed without unblinding the treatment codes if the study is to be conducted in a double-blind fashion. Procedures have been proposed for adjusting the sample size during the course of the trial without unblinding and altering the significance level (Gould, 1992; Gould and Shih, 1992). Proschan (2005) gives an excellent review on early research on two-stage SSR designs. A simple approach to dealing with nuisance parameter $\sigma_0$ is to use the maximum information design. The idea behind this approach is that recruitment continues until the prespecified information level ($I = N/(2\hat{\sigma}_0^2) = I_{\max}$) is reached. For a given sample size, the information level is reduced when the observed variance increases. The sample size per group for the two-group parallel design can be written in this familiar form:

$$N = \frac{2\hat{\sigma}_0^2}{\delta^2}(z_{1-\alpha} + z_{1-\beta})^2, \qquad (12.1)$$

where $\delta$ is treatment difference and $\hat{\sigma}_0$ is the observed common standard deviation.

Since the variance from the pooled data is (we will provide the proof later)

$$\sigma^2 = \sigma_0^2 + \left(\frac{\delta}{2}\right)^2, \qquad (12.2)$$

where is the $\sigma_0^2$ common variance for the two group, which can be estimated for each group and averaged.

If we know (e.g., from a Phase-II single-arm trial) $\sigma_0^2$, we then know or at least can estimate the treatment difference $\delta$ from (12.2). From (12.1) and (12.2), we can see that

$$N = 2\left(\frac{\sigma^2}{\delta^2} - \frac{1}{4}\right)(z_{1-\alpha} + z_{1-\beta})^2. \qquad (12.3)$$

Practically, we use the approximation

$$N = 2\frac{\sigma^2}{\delta^2}(z_{1-\alpha} + z_{1-\beta})^2 \qquad (12.4)$$

for simplicity. If we use the initial estimate $\delta_0$ and the new blinded estimate $\hat{\sigma}^2$ at the interim analysis in (12.4), we can obtain

$$N = 2\frac{\hat{\sigma}^2}{\delta_0^2}(z_{1-\alpha} + z_{1-\beta})^2. \qquad (12.5)$$

We can use simulations to evaluate the performance of (12.1) and (12.5).

## 12.3 Distribution-Informed Design

### 12.3.1 *Mean Difference Estimated from Blinded Data*

We know that *variance* is the second central moment of a distribution, which measures the variability of the data. *Skewness* is the third central moment, measuring the asymmetry of the distribution. For normal distribution the skewness is zero because of the symmetrical distribution. *Kurtosis* (standardized) is the forth central moment, measuring the flatness of the distribution. For normal distribution, the kurtosis is 3 (the standardized kurtosis is 0). In general, the $n$th central moment of a random variable $X$ is defined as the expectation of $(X - \mu)^n$, where $\mu$ is the population mean. These moments, despite their simplicity, can be very useful. For example, many people think that in principle we cannot precisely estimate the treatment difference between the test drug and placebo based on the lumped (treatment blinded) data. But that is not exactly true. The treatment difference can be calculated without separating the two treatment groups. This is because data from the mixture of two different normal distributions (not the distribution of sum of two normal variables) will have two modes if the difference between the two means is sufficiently large and a single mode if the two means are the same or close to each other (Figure 12.1). Moreover, the mean difference is reflected in the variance and kurtosis. Let's discuss how we can calculate the mean difference from the pooled data.

Suppose we have two equally sized groups of patients, treated with either placebo or the test drug. Assume the treatment effects are normally distributed with means $\mu_1$ and $\mu_2$, i.e., $X \sim N(\mu_1, \sigma_0^2)$ and $Y \sim N(\mu_2, \sigma_0^2)$, respectively. The variance of the mixed distribution is

$$\sigma^2 = \sigma_0^2 + \left(\frac{\delta}{2}\right)^2, \qquad (12.6)$$

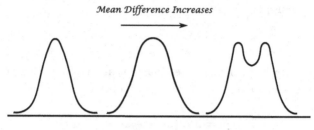

*Mixed Distribution of Two Normal Variables*

Figure 12.1:   Mixed Distribution Changes as the Means Change

where $\delta$ is the treatment difference; that is, $\delta = |\mu_2 - \mu_1|$. This formulation implies that the variance calculated from the pooled data is $\frac{\delta^2}{2}$ larger than the variance calculated for each group separately. If $\sigma_0^2$ is known (e.g., from previous single-group trials), then $\delta$ can be estimated based on (12.6); that is, $\hat{\delta} = 2\sqrt{\hat{\sigma}^2 - \sigma_0^2}$. But $\sigma_0^2$ is usually an unknown. Fortunately, because the kurtosis $\kappa$ of the mixed normal distribution is

$$\kappa = \frac{1}{\sigma^4}\left(3\sigma_0^4 + 6\sigma_0^2\left(\frac{\delta}{2}\right)^2 + \left(\frac{\delta}{2}\right)^4\right), \tag{12.7}$$

we can use (12.6) and (12.7) to solve for $\delta$ and $\sigma^2$; that is,

$$\begin{cases} \delta = 2\sigma \left(\frac{3-\kappa}{2}\right)^{1/4} \\ \sigma_0^2 = \sigma^2 \left(1 - \sqrt{\frac{3-\kappa}{2}}\right) \end{cases}. \tag{12.8}$$

The $\sigma$ and $\kappa$ can be estimated or calculated from the pooled data, and thus, the $\delta$ is estimated; that is,

$$\hat{\delta} = 2\hat{\sigma}\left(\frac{3 - \hat{\kappa}}{2}\right)^{1/4}. \tag{12.9}$$

The accuracy of the calculated $\delta$ will depend on the accuracy of the calculated $\sigma^2$ and $\kappa$, which in turn depend on the actual treatment difference and the sample size.

For convenience, we call (12.9) the $\sigma$-$\kappa$ method. Note that because $\hat{\kappa}$ is estimate, it can be larger than 3; therefore, there can be no solution for $\hat{\delta}$. A solution is to force a positive value:

$$\hat{\delta} = 2\hat{\sigma}\max\left(0, \frac{3 - \hat{\kappa}}{2}\right)^{1/4}. \tag{12.10}$$

Clearly, this estimator will be positively biased. The smaller the $\delta$, the larger the bias will be. Also, a smaller sample size $n$ will lead to more bias. Since when $\delta$ is overestimated, $\sigma^2$ will be underestimated, both of them will lead to an underestimated sample size.

The SAS code for generating the mixture of two normal distributions is presented in the following:

>>**SAS**>>
Title "Histogram of mixed normal distribution";
Data MixedNorm;
u=3; nSims=1000000;
Do i=1 To nSims; x = Rannor(0); output; x = Rannor(0)+u; output; End; run;
Proc Univariate nonprint; histogram x / midpoints=-1 to 7 by 0.1; run;
<<**SAS**<<

## 12.3.2  Mean Difference: Unequal Variance

Let's study a more general case when the variances and sample sizes are different in the two groups. Let the mixed distribution be

$$f(x) = \sum_{i=1}^{K} w_i f_i\left(x; \mu_i, \sigma_i^2\right), \tag{12.11}$$

where the constant weight $w_i > 0$ and $\sum_{i=1}^{K} w_i = 1$. For normal distribution

$$f_i\left(x; \mu_i, \sigma_i^2\right) = \frac{1}{\sqrt{2\pi}\sigma_i} \exp\left(-\frac{(x - \mu_i)^2}{2\sigma_i^2}\right), \tag{12.12}$$

and the mean of the mixed distribution is

$$\mu = E(X) = \sum_{i=1}^{K} w_i \mu_i, \tag{12.13}$$

$$\sigma^2 = E(X - \mu)^2 = \sum_{i=1}^{K} w_i\left(\sigma_i^2 + \mu_i^2\right) - \mu^2. \tag{12.14}$$

For a two-group design $K = 2$ and sample size $n$, $|\mu_i - \mu| = \delta/2$, where $\delta = |\mu_2 - \mu_1|$; thus,

$$\sigma^2 = \left(w_1\sigma_1^2 + w_2\sigma_2^2\right) + w_1 w_2 \delta^2. \tag{12.15}$$

For equal variance $\sigma_1^2 = \sigma_2^2 = \sigma_0^2$, we have

$$\sigma^2 = \sigma_0^2 + w_1 w_2 \delta^2. \tag{12.16}$$

The normalized skewness of the mixed distribution is (Casella and Berger, 2001; and Wang, 2001, 2006)

$$\gamma = \frac{1}{\sigma^3} E \left( X - \mu \right)^3 = \frac{1}{\sigma^3} \sum_{i=1}^{K} w_i \left( \mu_i - \mu \right) \left[ 3\sigma_i^2 + \left( \mu_i - \mu \right)^2 \right]. \tag{12.17}$$

The normalized kurtosis is

$$\kappa = \frac{1}{\sigma^4} E \left( X - \mu \right)^4 = \frac{1}{\sigma^4} \sum_{i=1}^{K} w_i \left[ 3\sigma_i^4 + 6 \left( \mu_i - \mu \right)^2 \sigma_i^2 + \left( \mu_i - \mu \right)^4 \right]. \tag{12.18}$$

For a two-group design with randomization ratio $w_1 : w_2$, we have

$$\kappa = \frac{1}{\sigma^4} \left( 3 \left( w_1 \sigma_1^4 + w_2 \sigma_2^4 \right) + 6 \left( \frac{\delta}{2} \right)^2 \left( w_1 \sigma_1^2 + w_2 \sigma_2^2 \right) + \left( \frac{\delta}{2} \right)^4 \right). \tag{12.19}$$

For equal variance $\sigma_1^2 = \sigma_2^2 = \sigma_0^2$, we further simplify it to:

$$\kappa = \frac{1}{\sigma^4} \left( 3\sigma_0^4 + 6\delta^2 \sigma_0^2 + \left( \frac{\delta}{2} \right)^4 \right). \tag{12.20}$$

Solving (12.16) for $\sigma_0^2$, we obtain

$$\sigma_0^2 = \sigma^2 - w_1 w_2 \delta^2. \tag{12.21}$$

Substituting (12.21) into (12.20), then solving it for $\delta^2$, we have

$$\delta^2 = \frac{4\sigma^2 \left( -3 + 12 w_1 w_2 - \sqrt{6 + \kappa - 24\kappa w_1 w_2 + 48\kappa w_1^2 w_2^2} \right)}{1 - 24 w_1 w_2 + 48 w_1^2 w_2^2}, \tag{12.22}$$

where $0.05 \leq w_1 \leq 0.95$ to avoid the denominator being zero.

Equation (12.22) can be used to estimate the treatment difference in unbalanced design with randomization ratio $w_1 : w_2$. When $w_1 = w_2 = 0.5$, (12.22) reduces to (12.8). To estimate $\delta$, we use the estimate $\hat{\sigma}^2 = \sum_{i=1}^{n} \left( X_i - \bar{X} \right)^2 / n$ and $\hat{\kappa} = \frac{1}{\hat{\sigma}^4} \sum_{i=1}^{n} \left( X_i - \bar{X} \right)^4 / n$ to replace $\sigma^2$ and $\kappa$ in (12.22).

### 12.3.3 *Rate Difference*

Since for large (very large) sample size, the binomial distribution can be approximated by a normal distribution, it seems that in theory the results in the previous section can also be used for a binary endpoint. But a further investigation indicates that it is not true. This is because the covariance between treatment difference $\delta = p_2 - p_1$ and the pooled rate $p$ (Proschan, 2005) is

$$
\begin{aligned}
cov\left(\hat{p}, \hat{\delta}\right) &= cov\left(\frac{n_1 \hat{p}_1 + n_2 \hat{p}_2}{n_1 + n_2}, \hat{p}_2 - \hat{p}_1\right) \\
&= \frac{n_1 var(\hat{p}_1) - n_2 var(\hat{p}_2)}{n_1 + n_2} \\
&= \frac{p_1 (1 - p_1) - p_2 (1 - p_2)}{n_1 + n_2},
\end{aligned}
$$

which is general not zero unless $p_1 = p_2$, but it becomes zero when the sample size approaches infinity. In other words, $\hat{p}$ and $\hat{\delta}$ are asymptotically independent even when $p_1 \neq p_2$. Here is a dilemma: On one hand, to use (12.9) for estimate treatment difference for binary endpoint, we have to use normal approximation, which require a larger $n$. On the other hand, when $n$ gets larger, the correlation between $\hat{p}$ and $\hat{\delta}$ diminishes, which means that the lumped rate $p$ (and variance $p(1-p)/n$ ) will not provide any information about treatment difference $\delta$.

### 12.3.4 *Semi-Blinded Method*

This method is based on $m$ stages or interim analyses; each subsample has $2n_0$ observations. Let $x_{ji} \sim N\left(\mu_1, \sigma_1^2\right)$ and $y_{ji} \sim N\left(\mu_2, \sigma_2^2\right)$, $(i = 1, ..., 2n_0;$ $j = 1, ..., m)$ be the observations from the mixed distribution (12.11) with $K = 2$ and $w_1 = w_2$. The mixture of the two normal distributions has a mean $\mu = (\mu_1 + \mu_2)/2$ and variance

$$
\sigma^2 = \frac{1}{2}\left(\sigma_1^2 + \sigma_2^2\right) + \left(\frac{\delta}{2}\right)^2. \tag{12.23}
$$

Let $n = 2m \cdot n_0$ be the total number of subjects. With $n_0$ in each group, $\bar{x}_j = \frac{1}{n_0}\sum_{i=1}^{n_0} x_{ji} \sim N\left(\mu_1, \frac{\sigma_1^2}{n_0}\right)$ and $\bar{y}_j = \frac{1}{n_0}\sum_{i=1}^{n_0} y_{ji} \sim N\left(\mu_2, \frac{\sigma_2^2}{n_0}\right)$. Note that without unblinding the data, $\bar{x}_j$ and $\bar{y}_j$ are not observable. What is observable without unblinding is the average $\bar{Z}_j = \frac{\bar{x}_j + \bar{y}_j}{2}$. $\bar{Z}_j$ has the normal distribution with mean $\mu$ and variance

$$
\sigma_{\bar{z}}^2 = \frac{1}{4n_0}\left(\sigma_1^2 + \sigma_2^2\right). \tag{12.24}
$$

Solving the equation system (12.23) and (12.24) for $\delta^2$, we obtain

$$\delta^2 = 4(\sigma^2 - 2n_0\sigma_{\bar{z}}^2), \qquad (12.25)$$

where $\sigma^2$ and $\sigma_{\bar{z}}^2$ can be estimated by

$$\hat{\sigma}^2 = \frac{1}{n}\sum_{j=1}^{m}\sum_{i=1}^{n_0}\left(x_{ji}^2 + y_{ji}^2\right) - \bar{z}^2, \qquad (12.26)$$

$$\hat{\sigma}_{\bar{z}}^2 = \frac{1}{m}\sum_{j=1}^{m} z_j^2 - \bar{z}^2. \qquad (12.27)$$

From (12.27), we know that the variance of $\hat{\sigma}_{\bar{z}}^2$, $\text{var}(\hat{\sigma}_{\bar{z}}^2)$, is proportional to $1/m$. Therefore, to reduce $\text{var}(\hat{\sigma}_{\bar{z}}^2)$, we should maximum $m$; that is, taking $m = n$ and $n_0 = 1$, as such, (12.25) reduces to

$$\delta = 2\sqrt{\sigma^2 - 2\sigma_{\bar{z}}^2}. \qquad (12.28)$$

### 12.3.5  *Simulation Comparison*

We use simulations to compare the sample size required by different methods (unblinded MLE, blinded $\sigma - \kappa$ method, and semi-blinded method) to achieve a precision of $\sigma_{\hat{\delta}} = 0.05$ for the mean difference. Given means from the two groups are normally distributed with the common standard of 1, the MLE of mean difference $\hat{\delta}$ has a standard deviation of $\sigma_{\hat{\delta}}^2 = \frac{2}{n}$. Therefore, for the unblinded MLE $\hat{\delta}$ with $\sigma_{\hat{\delta}} = 0.05$, the sample size is $2/\sigma_{\hat{\delta}}^2 = 800$.

SAS Macro 12.1 is used to generate the results in Table 12.1.

Table 12.1:   Sample Size per Group Required ($\sigma - \kappa$ Method)

| $\delta$ | 0.2 | 0.3 | 0.4 | 0.5 | 1 | 2 | 3 | 5 | $\infty$ |
|---|---|---|---|---|---|---|---|---|---|
| $\hat{\delta}_{BL}$ | 0.20 | 0.30 | 0.40 | 0.50 | 1.00 | 2.00 | 3.00 | 5.00 | |
| $N$ | | | | 3,000,000 | 85000 | 4600 | 2100 | 1700 | 800 |

Note: Precision $\sigma_{\hat{\delta}} = 0.05$.

>>**SAS Macro 12.1: Blinded** $\sigma - \kappa$ **Method for Mean Difference**>>

%Macro KSigma(MeanDiff=3, N=2100, nSims=1000);
Title "Blinded Treatment Estimation Using Variance and Kurtosis";
Data MixedNorm;

```
Keep N uxhat Sigma2 Kurtosis PctUnestimable MeanDiff MLE MeanDiffBlind
Bias;
Array x{500000}; Array y{500000};
MeanDiff=&MeanDiff; N=&N;
Unestimable=0;
Do isim=1 To &nSims;
uxhat=0; Kurtosis=0; Sigma2=0;
Do i=1 To N;
x(i) = Rannor(0);
if ranuni(0)>0.5 then x(i) = x(i)+MeanDiff;
uxhat=uxhat+x(i)/N;
End;
Do i=1 To N;
Sigma2=Sigma2+(x(i)-uxhat)**2/N;
Kurtosis=Kurtosis+(x(i)-uxhat)**4/N;
End;
Kurtosis=Kurtosis/(sigma2**2); * Standardize it;
If 3-Kurtosis<0 Then Unestimable=Unestimable+1;
Else delta=sqrt(sigma2)*((3-Kurtosis)/2)**0.25;
MLE=2*uxhat;
MeanDiffBlind=2*delta;
Bias=MeanDiffBlind-MeanDiff;
PctUnestimable=Unestimable/nSims;
Output;
End;
Run;
Proc means data=MixedNorm; Run;
%Mend KSigma;
%KSigma(MeanDiff=3, N=2100, nSims=1000);
```
<<**SAS**<<

The SAS macro can be invoked by the following typical code.

>>**SAS**>>
```
%Macro KSigma(MeanDiff=3, N=2100, nSims=1000);
```
<<**SAS**<<

SAS Macro 12.2 is used to generate the results in Table 12.2.

Table 12.2:  Sample Size per Group Required (Semi-Blinded Method)

| $\delta$ | 0.2 | 0.3 | 0.4 | 0.5 | 1 | 2 | 3 | 5 | $\infty$ |
|---|---|---|---|---|---|---|---|---|---|
| $\hat{\delta}_{BL}$ | 0.20 | 0.30 | 0.40 | 0.50 | 1.00 | 2.00 | 3.00 | 5.00 | |
| $N$ | 44000 | 20000 | 12000 | 7000 | 2400 | 1200 | 980 | 850 | 800 |

Note: Precision $\sigma_{\hat{\delta}} = 0.05$.

## >>SAS Macro 12.2: Semi-Blinded Method for Mean Difference>>

```
%Macro SemiBlinded(MeanDiff=0.5, N=10000, nSims=1000);
Title "Mean Diffeence Estimation Using Semi-blinded Method";
Data MixedNorm;
Keep N MeanDiff PctUnestimables UnblindEstimate BlindEstimate Disagree
BiasBlind BiasUnblind ;
Array means(1000000);
MeanDiff=&MeanDiff; * True trt difference;
N=&N; * Sample size per group;
nSims=&nSims; * The number of simulation runs;
m=N;
n0=round(N/m); * m set of samples, each with n0 subjects per group;
Unestimable=0;
Do isim=1 To nSims;
sigma2=0; Sigma2mean=0; mean=0; UnblindEstimate=0;
Do j=1 To m;
means(j)=0;
Do i=1 To n0;
x = Rannor(0);
y = Rannor(0)+MeanDiff;
UnblindEstimate=UnblindEstimate+(y-x)/(n0*m); *If unblind;
means(j)=means(j)+(x+y)/(2*n0);
sigma2=sigma2+(x*x+y*y)/(2*n0*m);
End;
mean=mean+means(j)/m;
sigma2Mean=Sigma2Mean+means(j)*means(j)/m;
End;
sigma2=sigma2-mean**2;
sigma2Mean=Sigma2Mean-mean**2;
If 2*n0*Sigma2Mean>sigma2 Then Unestimable=Unestimable+1;
Else BlindEstimate=2*sqrt(sigma2-2*n0*Sigma2Mean);
Disagree=abs(BlindEstimate-UnblindEstimate);
```

BiasBlind=BlindEstimate-MeanDiff;
BiasUnblind=UnblindEstimate-MeanDiff;
Output;
End;
PctUnestimables=Unestimable/nSims; output;
Run;
Proc Means Data=MixedNorm;run;
Proc Univariate data=MixedNorm noprint;
histogram BiasBlind/ midpoints=-0.5 to 0.5 by 0.02;
Run;
Proc Gplot Data=MixedNorm;
Plot UnblindEstimate*blindEstimate;
Run;
Mend SemiBlinded;
<<**SAS**<<

A typical SAS code to invoke the SAS macro follows:

>>**SAS**>>
%SemiBlinded(MeanDiff=0.5, N=10000, nSims=1000);
<<**SAS**<<

## 12.4 Operating Characteristics of Sample-Size Reestimation

We are comparing the three different methods for blinded SSR design. The blinded SSR designs are characterized by the FDA as a well-understood adaptive design (AD) in the AD guidance (FDA, 2010), which can be understood as no alpha adjustment is required.

To implement the variance-kurtosis ($\sigma$-$\kappa$) method for SSR based on conditional power, we need the expression for the standardized effect size, which can be obtained from (12.8). That is,

$$\begin{cases} \frac{\hat{\delta}}{\hat{\sigma}_0} = \frac{2\left(\frac{3-\kappa}{2}\right)^{1/4}}{\sqrt{1-\sqrt{\frac{3-\kappa}{2}}}}, & \text{if } 1 < \kappa \le 3, \\ \frac{\hat{\delta}}{\hat{\sigma}_0} \approx \frac{\delta_0}{\hat{\sigma}}, & \text{otherwise.} \end{cases} \qquad (12.29)$$

where $\delta_0$ is the initial estimation of treatment difference in the classical design. Logically, since the observations have already occurred at interim, the formulation for the new sample size for a two-stage design should be similar to those in Chapter 11, that is,

$$n_2 = 2 \left( \frac{\hat{\sigma}_0}{\hat{\delta}} \right)^2 \left[ \frac{1}{\sqrt{1 - w_1^2}} (z_{1-\alpha} - w_1 z_{1-p_1}) - z_{1-cP} \right]^2, \qquad (12.30)$$

where $w_1 = \sqrt{\frac{n_1}{N_0}}$. Equation (12.30) gives the approximate target conditional power $cP$.

Since the estimates of $\delta$ and $\sigma_0$ from $\sigma - \kappa$ method are very poor unless the sample size is huge, we simply use $\delta_0$ to replace $\hat{\delta}$ and $\sigma$ to replace $\sigma_0$ in (12.30) with $w_1 = w_2 = \sqrt{1/2}$; that is,

$$n_2 = 2 \left( \frac{\hat{\sigma}}{\delta_0} \right)^2 \left[ \sqrt{2} z_{1-\alpha} - z_{1-p_1} - z_{1-cP} \right]^2. \qquad (12.31)$$

For convenience we call SSR based on (12.31) the $\sigma$-$cP$ method (variance–conditional power method).

Table 12.3:   Comparisons of SSR Methods

| | | | $\delta = 0.7$ | | $\delta = 0.85$ | | | | $\delta = 1.0$ | |
| | | | $\sigma = 3$ | | $\sigma = 3$ | | $\sigma = 4$ | | $\sigma = 3$ | |
| | $\alpha$ | $\bar{N}_{H_0}$ | N | Pow | N | Pow | N | Pow | N | Pow |
|---|---|---|---|---|---|---|---|---|---|---|
| Classical | .0250 | 262 | 262 | .760 | 262 | .900 | 262 | .680 | 262 | .968 |
| Max-Info | .0270 | 266 | 263 | .777 | 262 | .910 | 445 | .893 | 261 | .972 |
| $\sigma$-$cP$ | .0314 | 414 | 285 | .857 | 262 | .948 | 393 | .893 | 244 | .984 |
| $\sigma$-$\kappa$ | .0316 | 414 | 285 | .858 | 261 | .946 | 393 | .893 | 244 | .984 |
| MINP | .0275 | 304 | 288 | .793 | 262 | .888 | 298 | .730 | 233 | .943 |

Note: $\alpha = 0.025$, $N_{max} = 500$/group. cPower = 90%. $w_1 = w_2$, infotime = 0.5. $N_0$ for × 256 (Max-Info), 220 for × ($\sigma$-$cP$ and $\sigma$-$\kappa$), 130 for × (MINP without early stopping)

We have implemented (SAS Macro 12.3) the Max-Info method, the $\sigma$-$cP$ method, and the $\sigma$-$\kappa$ method for blinded SSR and the MINP with fixed weights for unblinded SSR. In initial design we believe the treatment effect is $\delta = 0.85$ and variance $\sigma^2 = 3^2$, which might be right or wrong. We will compare their operating characteristics under four different scenarios: (1) the true treatment effect $\delta = 0.85$ and variance $\sigma^2 = 3^2$, (2) the true $\delta = 0.85$ but $\sigma^2 = 4^2$, (3) the true $\delta = 0.7$ and $\sigma^2 = 3^2$, and (4) $\delta = 1.0$ and $\sigma^2 = 3^2$ (see Table 12.3).

For the purpose of comparison, we have chosen a different initial final sample size $n_0$ for different SSR methods such that the average sample size for all the methods is the same as that in the classical design, i.e., $\bar{N} = 262$ when $\delta = 0.85$ and $\sigma = 3$. The simulation results show how different designs behave when the actual situation deviates from the assumptions. We can see clearly the following:

(1) For classical design, when $\delta = 0.85$ and $\sigma = 3$, $N = 262$ will provide 90% power, but when actual $\sigma$ is 4, the power drops to 68%. If $\sigma = 3$ is estimated correctly but the treatment difference is actually lower, say, 0.7, the power drops to 76%. On the other hand, if $\delta$ is actually higher at 1, the power is 96.8%.

(2) The $\sigma - cP$ design and $\sigma - \kappa$ are virtually identical. Therefore, we will only discuss the $\sigma - cP$ design. We can see the power of the design is robust against changes of the treatment difference and the variance. When $\sigma$ is underestimated (actual $\sigma = 4$ but estimated 3), the sample size is adjusted automatically to preserve the power ($\bar{N} = 393$, power $= 0.893$). When $\delta$ and $\sigma$ are estimated correctly, the $\sigma - cP$ design has much higher power than the classical design with the sample size (94.8% versus 90%). When $\delta$ is overestimated (actual $\delta = 0.7$, but estimated 0.85), the sample size increases automatically to remain a high power ($\bar{N} = 285$, power $= 0.857$)—an unexpected but truly desirable mechanism. When $\delta$ is underestimated (actual $\delta = 1$ but estimated 0.85), the expected sample size remains lower than the classical design (244 versus 262), but the power is higher than that for the classical design (0.984 versus 0.968). The disadvantage of the $\sigma - cP$ design is that when $H_0$ is true, the sample size will increase dramatically from 262 in the classical design to 414 per group. There is also a slight $\alpha$-inflation of 0.0314 from the target 0.025.

(3) The Max-Info design performs worse than the $\sigma - cP$ design in all cases. As expected, the Max-Info design fails to adjust the sample size appropriately when the actual treatment difference ($\delta = 0.7$) is smaller than the estimated ($\delta = 0.85$).

(4) The unblinded SSR (MINP) can well preserve the power when the actual $\delta$ is smaller (or $\sigma$ is bigger) than expected. Its performances are not as good as the $\sigma - cP$ design in all the cases except under $H_0$. This is somewhat surprising. When $H_0$ is true, the expected sample size is smaller with MINP SSR than with the $\sigma - cP$ design.

(5) There is some $\alpha$-inflation due to a small sample size. Such inflation will still exist when the sample size increases due to a smaller $\delta_0$. This $\alpha$-inflation is probably due to the lumped variance that contains information about treatment difference.

We now can conclude that the blinded $\sigma - cP$ and $\sigma - \kappa$ methods are generally better designs under $H_a$ than the unblinded MINP for SSR. However, under $H_0$, MINP with fixed weights performs better than the

$\sigma - cP$ and $\sigma - \kappa$ methods in terms of sample size required. For this reason, it is reasonable to combine the blinded and unblinded methods for designing an efficient SSR trial. In other words, we use unblinded data to facilitate the futility stopping at the interim when the observed data do not show promising results so that the sample size will reduced under $H_0$, but when the data pass the futility boundary checking, we use the blinded $\sigma - cP$ method for SSR. We will present the encouraging simulation results in the next section. But for now let present the SAS macro for generating the results in Table 12.3.

In SAS Macro 12.3, **ux** and **uy** are the true treatment difference, while **delta0** is estimated treatment difference at the design stage. The **sigma** is the true standard deviation. Other variables are self-explanatory.

>>**SAS Macro 12.3: Blinded and Unblinded Sample Size Reestimation**>>

```
%Macro  SSR2Stage(nSims=1000000,  w1=0.7071,  alpha=0.025,  sigma=2,
delta0=0.85, ux=0, uy=1, nInterim=50, Nmax=100, N0=100, cPower=0.9,
nAdj="Y", SSRMethod="Kurt-Sigma", Weight="Fixed");
Data MINP;
Keep ux0 uy0 AveN N0 Nmax Power sigma SSRMethod Weight;
alpha=&alpha;   Nmax=&Nmax;   ux0=&ux;   uy0=&uy;   sigma=&sigma;
delta0=&delta0;
SSRMethod=&SSRMethod; Weight=&Weight;
N1=&nInterim; N0=&N0; w1=&w1; w2=sqrt(1-w1**2);
AveN=0; Power=0;
Do isim=1 To &nSims;
nFinal=N0; u1=0; u2=0; u3=0; u4=0; TrtDiff=0; ux=0; uy=0;
Do i=1 To N1;
ux1 = Rannor(0)*sigma+ux0;
uy1 = Rannor(0)*sigma+uy0;
ux=ux+ux1/N1;
uy=uy+uy1/N1;
u1=u1+(ux1+uy1)/(2*N1);
u2=u2+(ux1**2+uy1**2)/(2*N1);
u3=u3+(ux1**3+uy1**3)/(2*N1);
u4=u4+(ux1**4+uy1**4)/(2*N1);
End;
Sigma2=u2-ux**2-uy**2;
z1 = (uy-ux)*Sqrt(N1/2/sigma2);
p1=max(1-ProbNorm(z1), 0.00000001); *For numerical stability;
```

```
/* Variance-Kurtosis method for trt difference estimation */
Kurtosis=u4-3*u1**4-4*u3*u1+6*u2*u1**2;
If u2>u1**2 Then eSize=delta0/sqrt(u2-u1**2);
If SSRMethod="Unblind" Then eSize=(uy-ux)/sqrt(sigma2);
If 3>Kurtosis>1 and SSRMethod="Kurt-Sigma" Then
eSize=(2*((3-Kurtosis)/2)**0.25)/Sqrt(1-Sqrt((3-Kurtosis)/2));
/* End of Variance-Kurtosis method */
If &nAdj="Y" and eSize>0 Then Do;
BFun=(Probit(1-&alpha)- w1*Probit(1-p1))/w2;
nFinal=N1+2*((BFun-Probit(1-&cPower))/eSize)**2;
If SSRMethod="Max-Info" Then
nFinal=2*Sigma2/delta0**2*(Probit(1-&alpha)+Probit( &cPower))**2;
*Max-Info Design;
nFinal=Round(min(max(nFinal,N0),Nmax));  * make sure N0  <=Nfinal<=
Nmax;
End;
N2=nFinal-N1;
ux=0; uy=0; u2=0;
Do i=1 To N2;
ux2 = Rannor(0)*sigma+ux0 ;
uy2 = Rannor(0)*sigma+uy0;
ux=ux+ux2/N2;
uy=uy+uy2/N2;
u2=u2+(ux2**2+uy2**2)/(2*N2);
End;
Sigma2=u2-ux**2-uy**2;
z2 = (uy-ux)*Sqrt(N2/2/sigma2);
p2=1-ProbNorm(z2);
If &Weight="InfoTime" Then w1=sqrt(N1/nFinal);
w2=sqrt(1-w1**2);
T2=1-ProbNorm(w1*z1+w2*z2);
If .<T2<=alpha Then Power=Power+1/&nSims;
AveN=AveN+nFinal/&nSims;
End;
Output;
Run;
Proc Print Data=MINP; Run;
%Mend SSR2Stage;
```

<<**SAS**<<

A typical macro call follows.

**>>SAS: Invoke SAS Macro 12.3>>**

%SSR2Stage(alpha=0.023, sigma=3, ux=0, uy=0.85, nInterim=110,
Nmax=500, N0=220, cPower=0.9, nAdj="Y", Weight="InfoTime");
%SSR2Stage(alpha=0.023, sigma=4, ux=0, uy=0.85, nInterim=110, Nmax=500,
N0=220, cPower=0.9, nAdj="Y", SSRMethod="Max-Info", Weight=
"InfoTime");
%SSR2Stage(w1=0.7071, alpha=0.024, sigma=3, ux=0, uy=0.7, nInterim=65,
Nmax=500, N0=130, cPower=0.9, nAdj="Y", SSRMethod="Unblind");
**<<SAS<<**

## 12.5    Mixed-Method for Sample-Size Reestimation Design

As we have just discussed, we want to improve the blinded $\sigma - cP$ SSR method by adding a futility boundary, hoping that it will dramatically reduced the sample size under $H_0$ and only slightly reduce the power under $H_a$. We cannot use a very aggressive futility boundary if we want to preserve the power; hence, we choose $\beta_1 = 0.5$. In other words, if the one-sided $p$-value at the interim analysis is larger than 0.5, the trial will stop due to futility. The simulation results (mixed versus $\sigma - cP$) show that the average sample size under $H_0$ is lowered from 3550 ($\sigma - cP$ method without futility stopping) to 1999 (labeled mixed), while there is only mild/moderate reduction in sample size and power under $H_a$.

According to current practice, we can use the same stopping boundaries as for the standard group sequential design since our SSR does not depend on the unblinded data and the futility boundary will further reduce the type-I error. However, simulation results show there are some type-I error inflations; therefore, we adjust the rejection criterion to $p < 0.022$ (instead of $p < 0.025$) for mixed method (labeled mixed[2]). With this adjustment, the mixed method still performs very well (see Table 12.4).

Here is the SAS macro for the simulation results in Table 12.4. In SAS Macro 12.4, **ux** and **uy** are the true treatment differences, while **delta0** is estimated treatment difference at the design stage. The **sigma** is the true standard deviation. Other variables are self-explanatory.

**>>SAS Macro 12.4:    Sample-Size Reestimation with Mixed Methods>>**

%Macro SSR2StageMixed(nSims=1000000, alpha=0.025, sigma=2, delta0=0.85,
ux=0, uy=1, nInterim=50, Nmax=100, N0=100, cPower=0.9, beta1=0.3);

Table 12.4:  Comparisons of SSR Mixed Methods

|  |  |  | $\delta = 0.25$ | | $\delta = 0.3$ | | | | $\delta = 0.35$ | |
|  |  |  | $\sigma = 3$ | | $\sigma = 3$ | | $\sigma = 4$ | | $\sigma = 3$ | |
|  | $\alpha$ | $\bar{N}_{H_0}$ | N | Pow | N | Pow | N | Pow | N | Pow |
|---|---|---|---|---|---|---|---|---|---|---|
| Classical | .0250 | 2101 | 2101 | .771 | 2101 | .900 | 2101 | .681 | 2101 | .966 |
| $\sigma$-$cP$ | .0309 | 3550 | 2303 | .862 | 2112 | .945 | 2998 | .878 | 1996 | .981 |
| Mixed | .0288 | 1999 | 2187 | .831 | 2069 | .929 | 2823 | .839 | 1968 | .974 |
| Mixed$^2$ | .0247 | 2038 | 2232 | .825 | 2105 | .927 | 2881 | .834 | 1995 | .972 |

Note: $\alpha = 0.025$, $N_{max} = 4000$/group. $N_1 = 900$, $N_0 = 1800$. cPower= 90%.
$\sigma$-$cP$: $\beta_1 = 1$; mixed $\sigma$-$cP$: $\beta_1 = 0.5$; mixed$^2$: adjust $\alpha$ to 0.022.

```
Data MINP;
Keep ux0 uy0 AveN N0 Nmax Power sigma delta0;
alpha=&alpha; beta1=&beta1; Nmax=&Nmax; ux0=&ux; uy0=&uy;
sigma=&sigma; delta0=&delta0; N1=&nInterim; N0=&N0;
AveN=0; Power=0;
Do isim=1 To &nSims;
nFinal=N1; u1=0; u2=0; ux=0; uy=0;
Do i=1 To N1;
ux1 = Rannor(0)*sigma+ux0;
uy1 = Rannor(0)*sigma+uy0;
ux=ux+ux1/N1; uy=uy+uy1/N1;
u1=u1+(ux1+uy1)/(2*N1);
u2=u2+(ux1**2+uy1**2)/(2*N1);
End;
sigma2Blind=u2-u1**2;
sigma2=u2-ux**2-uy**2;
z1 = (uy-ux)*Sqrt(N1/2/sigma2);
p1=Max(1-ProbNorm(z1), 0.00000001); *For numerical stability;
If p1>&beta1 Then Goto Futile;
If sigma2Blind>0 Then eSize=delta0/sqrt(sigma2Blind);
BFun=sqrt(2)*Probit(1-&alpha)- Probit(1-p1);
nFinal=N1+2*((BFun-Probit(1-&cPower))/eSize)**2;
*Enforce N0<=Nfinal<=Nmax;
nFinal=Round(min(max(nFinal,N0),Nmax));
N2=nFinal-N1;
ux=0; uy=0; u2=0;
Do i=1 To N2;
ux2 = Rannor(0)*sigma+ux0 ;
uy2 = Rannor(0)*sigma+uy0;
ux=ux+ux2/N2; uy=uy+uy2/N2;
```

```
u2=u2+(ux2**2+uy2**2)/(2*N2);
End;
w1=Sqrt(N1/nFinal);
w2=Sqrt(1-w1**2);
sigma2=u2-ux**2-uy**2;
z2 = (uy-ux)*Sqrt(N2/2/sigma2);
p2=1-ProbNorm(z2);
T2=1-ProbNorm(w1*z1+w2*z2);
If .<T2<=alpha Then Power=Power+1/&nSims;
Futile:
AveN=AveN+nFinal/&nSims;
End;
Output;
Run;
Proc Print Data=MINP; Run;
%Mend SSR2StageMixed;
```
<<**SAS**<<

SAS Macros 12.4 can be invoked using the following SAS code.

>>**SAS: Invoke SAS Macro 12.4**>>
```
%SSR2StageMixed(nSims=100000, alpha=0.025, sigma=3, delta0=0.3, ux=0,
uy=0, nInterim=900, Nmax=4000, N0=1800, cPower=0.9, beta1=1);
%SSR2StageMixed(nSims=100000, alpha=0.025, sigma=3, delta0=0.3, ux=0,
uy=0, nInterim=900, Nmax=4000, N0=1800, cPower=0.9, beta1=0.5);
%SSR2StageMixed(nSims=100000, alpha=0.022, sigma=3, delta0=0.3, ux=0,
uy=0, nInterim=900, Nmax=4000, N0=1800, cPower=0.9, beta1=0.5);
%SSR2StageMixed(nSims=100000, alpha=0.025, sigma=3, delta0=0.3, ux=0,
uy=0.25, nInterim=900, Nmax=4000, N0=1800, cPower=0.9, beta1=1);
%SSR2StageMixed(nSims=100000, alpha=0.025, sigma=3, delta0=0.3, ux=0,
uy=0.25, nInterim=900, Nmax=4000, N0=1800, cPower=0.9, beta1=0.5);
%SSR2StageMixed(nSims=100000, alpha=0.022, sigma=3, delta0=0.3, ux=0,
uy=0.25, nInterim=900, Nmax=4000, N0=1800, cPower=0.9, beta1=0.5);
```
<<**SAS**<<

## 12.6 Revealing Treatment Difference via Stratified Randomization

Shih and Zhao (1997) proposed a blinded sample-size reestimation method. The key in their method is to use different randomization ratios in different strata and to use the responses in the strata to estimate the treatment effect and variance of each treatment.

Suppose in a clinical trial with two treatment groups 1 and 2, and two strata, $A$ and $B$ according to the baseline covariates. The randomization in stratum $A$ is $\pi : (1 - \pi)$, while in stratum $B$, the randomization ratio is switched. In other words, in stratum $A$, patients are randomly allocated to treatment group $i = 1$ with probability $\pi$ and to treatment group $i = 2$ with probability $1 - \pi$. In stratum $B$, patients are randomly allocated to treatment group $i = 1$ with probability $1 - \pi$ and to treatment group $i = 2$ with probability $\pi$. The overall balance of the treatment allocation is preserved. Here $\pi \neq 0.5$, otherwise it defeats the purpose of stratification. Denote the expected response rates to treatments 1 and 2 by $\theta_1$ and $\theta_2$, and the expected responses in strata $A$ and $B$ by $\theta_A$ and $\theta_B$, respectively. In follows that we have the identities

$$\theta_A = \pi\theta_1 + (1 - \pi)\theta_2 \tag{12.32}$$
$$\theta_B = (1 - \pi)\theta_1 + \pi\theta_2.$$

Solving (12.32) for $\theta_1$ and $\theta_2$, we have

$$\theta_1 = \frac{\pi\theta_A - (1 - \pi)\theta_B}{2\pi - 1} \tag{12.33}$$
$$\theta_2 = \frac{\pi\theta_B - (1 - \pi)\theta_A}{2\pi - 1},$$

where $\pi \neq 0.5$.

Equation (12.33) gives the unbiased estimators of the true event rates for the treatment groups, being weighted averages of the pooled rates from the two strata. The treatment difference can be expressed as

$$\theta_2 - \theta_1 = \frac{\theta_B - \theta_A}{2\pi - 1}. \tag{12.34}$$

Suppose we want to conduct an interim analysis based on data of $n_1$ subjects per group. We estimate the treatment effects $\hat{\theta}_1$ and $\hat{\theta}_2$ based on the blinded (treatment pooled) estimates $\hat{\theta}_A$ and $\hat{\theta}_B$ in the two strata. The two estimates can be used for sample-size reestimation. Note that the covariance matrix of $\hat{\theta}_1$ and $\hat{\theta}_2$ can be obtained as follows:

$$cov\begin{pmatrix} \hat{\theta}_1 \\ \hat{\theta}_2 \end{pmatrix} = \frac{1}{(2\pi - 1)^2} \begin{bmatrix} \pi & \pi - 1 \\ \pi - 1 & \pi \end{bmatrix} \begin{bmatrix} \sigma_{\theta_1}^2 & 0 \\ 0 & \sigma_{\theta_2}^2 \end{bmatrix} \begin{bmatrix} \pi & \pi - 1 \\ 1 - \pi & \pi \end{bmatrix}$$

$$= \frac{1}{(2\pi - 1)^2} \begin{bmatrix} \pi^2 \sigma_{\theta_1}^2 + (\pi - 1)^2 \sigma_{\theta_2}^2 & \pi(\pi - 1)\left(\sigma_{\theta_1}^2 + \sigma_{\theta_2}^2\right) \\ \pi(\pi - 1)\left(\sigma_{\theta_1}^2 + \sigma_{\theta_2}^2\right) & \pi^2 \sigma_{\theta_2}^2 + (\pi - 1)^2 \sigma_{\theta_1}^2 \end{bmatrix},$$

$$(12.35)$$

where $\sigma_{\theta_k}^2 = var\left(\hat{\theta}_k\right) = \frac{\theta_k(1-\theta_k)}{n_k}$ and $n_k$ is the number of patients in stratum $k$; $k = A, B$. Thus, we obtain the variance of the estimated treatment effect: $var\left(\hat{\theta}_1 - \hat{\theta}_2\right) = var\left(\hat{\theta}_1\right) + var\left(\hat{\theta}_2\right) - cov\left(\hat{\theta}_1, \hat{\theta}_2\right)$. That is,

$$\hat{\sigma}_{\hat{\theta}_1 - \hat{\theta}_2}^2 = var\left(\hat{\theta}_1 - \hat{\theta}_2\right) = \frac{1}{(2\pi - 1)^2}\left(\frac{\theta_A(1 - \theta_A)}{n_A} + \frac{\theta_B(1 - \theta_B)}{n_B}\right),$$

$$(12.36)$$

which is estimable by substitution of $\theta_k$ with $\hat{\theta}_k$ for stratum $k = A$ and $B$.

We can see that the variance of the estimated treatment effect with blinded data is inflated by the stratification factor $(2\pi - 1)^2$. Thus to improve the efficiency, Shih and Zhao (1997) suggest choosing a $\pi$ closer to 0 or 1, e.g., 0.2. However, a larger imbalanced design can also be a problem for the final analysis, i.e., lost efficiency/power for the hypothesis test and practically, an imbalanced design may impair the safety evaluation when one group does not have enough patients. The imbalanced stratified randomization can also cause a problem when there is an interaction between treatment and stratum. Noting that $\theta_B - \theta_A = (1 - 2\pi)\delta$ and, thus, setting $\pi = 0.2$ is to allow 0.6 times of the treatment effect being shown by the strata.

With the estimate of treatment difference and variance from the interim data, Shih and Zhao (1997) reestimate the sample size based on the classical design without stratification, pretending no observations have been collected yet. That is, the sample size per group is given by:

$$N = \frac{n_1 \hat{\sigma}_{\hat{\theta}_1 - \hat{\theta}_2}^2}{\hat{\theta}^2}(z_{1-\alpha} + z_{1-\beta})^2. \qquad (12.37)$$

Logically, since the observations have already occurred at interim, the formulation for the new sample size per group for a two-stage design should be similar to those in Chapter 11, that is,

$$n_2 = \frac{n_1 \hat{\sigma}_{\hat{\theta}_1 - \hat{\theta}_2}^2}{\hat{\theta}^2}\left[B(\alpha, p_1) - \Phi^{-1}(1 - cP)\right]^2, \qquad (12.38)$$

where the $B$-function $B(\alpha_2, p_1)$ is given in Table (9.6). The conditional power for a two-stage design is given by (Chapter 11)

$$cP = 1 - \Phi\left(B(\alpha, p_1) - \frac{\delta}{\sigma}\sqrt{\frac{n_2}{2}}\right), \alpha_1 < p_1 \leq \beta_1. \qquad (12.39)$$

Note that in (12.38) and (12.39), $\alpha$ is used instead of a smaller value $\alpha_2$ due to the penalty for the potential early efficacy stopping in an unblinding SSR design.

It is interesting to noticing that the Shih–Zhao method actually does "unblind" the treatment group. Paradoxically, if the treatment is estimated as well as MLE, then the type-I error will be inflated. If such an estimate is not accurate, then it may not help SSR.

We have implemented the Shih–Zhao method in SAS Macro 12.5.

**>>SAS Macro 12.5: Sample-Size Reestimation with Shih–Zhao Method>>**

```
%Macro SSR2StageBin(nSims=1000000, alpha=0.025, px=0.3, py=0.5, pi=0.3,
N1A=110, N1B=110, N0=220, Nmax=500, cPower=0.9, beta1=0.3);
Data MINP;
Keep px py pi alpha N1A N1B N0 Nmax AveN Nmax cPower Power;
alpha=&alpha; Nmax=&Nmax; pi=&pi; px=&px; py=&py;
N0=&N0; N1A=&N1A; N1B=&N1B; cPower=&cPower;
N1=(N1A+N1B)/2; AveN=0; Power=0;
Do isim=1 To &nSims;
nFinal=N0;
uxA = RANBIN(0,Round(N1A*pi),px);
uyA = RANBIN(0,Round(N1A*(1-pi)),py);
uyB = RANBIN(0,Round(N1B*pi),py);
uxB = RANBIN(0,Round(N1B*(1-pi)),px);
uA = (uxA+uyA)/N1A;
uB = (uyB+uxB)/N1B;
TrtDiffBlind=(uB-uA)/(2*pi-1);
uy=(uyA+uyB)/(Round(N1A*(1-pi))+Round(N1B*pi));
ux=(uxA+uxB)/(Round(N1B*(1-pi))+Round(N1A*pi));
TrtDiffUnblind=py-px;
sigma2=(uA*(1-uA)/n1A+uB*(1-uB)/n1B)/(2*pi-1)**2*N1;
If TrtDiffBlind>0 Then
nFinal=Sigma2/TrtDiffBlind**2*(Probit(1-&alpha)+Probit(&cPower))**2;
nFinal=Round(Min(Nmax,Max(N0,nFinal)));
N2=nFinal-N1;
ux = (RANBIN(0,N2,px)+uxA+uxB)/nFinal;
```

```
uy = (RANBIN(0,N2,py)+uyA+uyB)/nFinal;
Sigma2=(ux*(1-ux)+uy*(1-uy))/nFinal;
z = (uy-ux)/Sqrt(sigma2);
p=1-ProbNorm(z);
If .<p<=alpha Then Power=Power+1/&nSims;
AveN=AveN+nFinal/&nSims;
End;
Output;
Run;
Proc Print Data=MINP; Run;
%Mend SSR2StageBin;
```
<<**SAS**<<

## Example 12.1 Blinded Sample-Size Reestimation for Binary Endpoint

The Shih–Zhao method is not efficient for SSR. For example, given the response rates 0.3 and 0.4 for the two groups and a sample size of 476 per group, the classical design has 90% power. With Shih–Zhao's method, assume the two strata have an equal size and blinded interim analysis conducted when 50% of patients are enrolled (238 in each of the stratum), and the randomization ratio is $\pi = 0.3 : 1-\pi = 0.7$. With the maximum sample size 800 per group, the SSR design will have 95% power with an average sample size of 670. When the actual rates are 0.3 and 0.38, the design will provide 85% power with average sample size of 686 per group. However, for 85% power, the classical design requires only 628 per group for the rates 0.3 versus 0.38. We can use the following SAS code to invoke the macro.

>>**SAS**>>

```
Title "Type-I Error Check for Shih–Zhao's method";
%SSR2StageBin(nSims=1000000,  alpha=0.025,  px=0.3,  py=0.3,  pi=0.3,
N1A=238, N1B=238, N0=476, Nmax=800, cPower=0.9);
Title "Power of Shih–Zhao's method with rates 0.3 and 0.4";
%SSR2StageBin(nSims=100000,  alpha=0.025,  px=0.3,  py=0.4,  pi=0.3,
N1A=238, N1B=238, N0=476, Nmax=800, cPower=0.9);
Title "Power of Shih–Zhao's method with rates 0.3 and 0.38";
%SSR2StageBin(nSims=100000,  alpha=0.025,  px=0.3,  py=0.38,  pi=0.3,
N1A=238, N1B=238, N0=476, Nmax=800, cPower=0.9);
```
<<**SAS**<<

The Shih–Zhao method can also be similarly applied to a normal endpoint or other types of endpoints (Problem 12.4).

## 12.7 Summary

We have studied the distribution of the pooled data without unblinding the treatment code and discussed several methods to estimate the treatment effect without unblinding. However, such estimates are generally not accurate with a sample size commonly used in clinical trials. Unless the sample size is 10 to 1000 times bigger than we usually have in clinical trial, the treatment effect is virtually unknown with pooled data analysis. We then studied the blinded and semi-blinded sample-size reestimation methods and compared them with unblinded sample-size reestimation method. Through simulations, we conclude that the blinded SSR method, i.e., the $\sigma - cP$ method, is usually more powerful than the unblinded MINP when the test drug is effective. However, when the test drug is not effective, i.e., $H_0$ is true, the expected sample size with the $\sigma - cP$ method is very large. To overcome the problem, we have proposed the mixed method for SSR, which basically is the $\sigma - cP$ method featuring a futility boundary to reduce the expected sample size under $H_0$. The simulations show that the mixed method is a very effective tool for SSR design, better than all the blinded and unblinded SSR methods. We highly recommend the mixed approach in practice. As there is a slight inflation of type-I error with the mixed method (not related to the unblinding at all), we can use a smaller $\alpha$ to control the type-I error.

**Problems**

**12.1** For the mixed normal distribution, prove (12.13), (12.14), (12.17), and (12.18).

**12.2** Using variance and kurtosis of a mixed normal distribution, we have obtained the estimation for the treatment difference as shown in (12.8). Derive the formulation for the mean treatment difference using the mean absolute deviation (MD) and other moments of the mixed distribution.

**12.3** Implement the Shih-Zhao method for blind estimate of mean difference and SSR using SAS or R, and study the operating characteristics.

Chapter 13

# Adaptive Design with Coprimary Endpoints

In a clinical trial with multiple coprimary endpoints, the efficacy requirement is defined as meeting two or more endpoints simultaneously. Therefore, in an adaptive design of multiple endpoint trial, we have to deal with the multiplicity due to multiple endpoints and multiple analyses at different times. We will use mathematical induction to prove that the stopping boundaries from group sequential stopping boundaries with a single endpoint can be use directly without inflation or deflation the type-I error. We will also derive the formulations for conditional power and power for group sequential design with multiple endpoints, which is an extension of the conditional power for single endpoint developed by Lan and Wittes (1988). The extension of the method to sample-size reestimation design is also provided with illustrative examples (Cheng, 2014; Cheng, Menon, and Chang, 2014).

## 13.1 Introduction

In the case of diseases of unknown etiology, where no clinical consensus has been reached on the single most important clinical efficacy endpoint, coprimary endpoints may be used. When diseases manifest themselves in multidimensional ways, drug effectiveness is often characterized by the use of composite endpoints, global disease scores, or the disease activity index (DAI). When a composite primary efficacy endpoint is used, we are often interested in the particular aspect or endpoint where the drug has demonstrated benefits. An ICH guideline (European Medicines Agency, 2007) suggests: "If a single primary variable cannot be selected from multiple measurements associated with the primary objective, another useful strategy is to integrate or combine the multiple measurements into a single or 'composite' variable, using a predefined algorithm.... This approach addresses the multiplicity problem without requiring adjustment to the type-I error." For some indications, such as oncology, it is difficult to use a gold standard endpoint, such as survival, as the primary endpoint because it requires a longer follow-up time and because patients switch treatments after disease progression. Instead, a surrogate endpoint, such as time-to-progression, might be chosen as the primary endpoint with other supporting efficacy evidence, such as infection rate. Huque and Röhmel (2010) provide an excellent overview of multiplicity problems in clinical trials from the regulatory perspective. Following are some motivating examples.

Hypotheses related to multiple coprimary endpoints, which are defined as the efficacy of the test drug in a clinical trial that need to declare the significance on more than one endpoint simultaneously, have received a lot of attention in recent years (Meyerson et al., 2007). These problems are also called the reverse multiplicity problems. There are several diseases and therapeutic areas in which the regulatory agencies need the treatment to demonstrate statistical significance on multiple coprimary endpoints. Some examples of diseases where at least two primary endpoints may be of interest are (1) migraine which is accompanied by nausea and photophobia, (2) Alzheimer's disease which is assessed by Alzheimer's disease assessment scale–cognitive and clinician interview–based impression of change, (3) multiple sclerosis, which is measured by relapse rate at 1 year and disability at 2 years, and (4) osteoarthritis which is evaluated by pain, patient global assessment, and quality of life. Hence, an efficacy in these diseases is evaluated with multiple endpoints. The study power may be considerably reduced in comparison with a single-endpoint problem, depending on the correlation(s) among the endpoints.

Consider that $X_1, X_2, ..., X_N$ are independent random vectors drawn from the multivariate normal distribution with $d$ dimensions $N_d(\boldsymbol{\mu}_d, \boldsymbol{\Sigma})$, where $\boldsymbol{\mu}_d = (\mu_1, \mu_2, ..., \mu_d)'$. Without loss of generality, let $\boldsymbol{\Sigma} = (1 - \rho)\boldsymbol{I}_d + \rho \boldsymbol{J}_d$. In this case, the covariance matrix of $\boldsymbol{X}$ and the correlation matrix are identical. We are interested in the following hypothesis:

$$H_0 : \mu_j \leq 0 \text{ for at least one } j \in (1, 2, ..., d) \tag{13.1}$$
$$H_a : \mu_j > 0 \text{ for all } j \in (1, 2, ..., d).$$

Equivalently we can write the hypothesis test as

$$H_0 : \cup_{j=1}^d H_{0j} \text{ versus } H_a : \cap_{j=1}^d H_{aj}, \tag{13.2}$$

where $H_{0j} : \mu_j \leq 0$ and $H_{aj} : \mu_j > 0$. The test statistics for these individual endpoints are defined in a usual way: $Z_{Nj} = \sum_{i=1}^N X_{ij}/\sqrt{N}$. We reject

$H_{0j}$ if $Z_{Nj} \geq c$, the common critical value for all endpoints. Therefore, we reject (13.2) and, furthermore, reject (13.1) if $Z_{Nj} \geq c$ for all $j$. It is straightforward to prove that for $\forall j$ and $k$, where $j, k = 1, 2, ..., d$, the covariance/correlation between the test statistics is the same as the covariance/correlation between the endpoints, i.e., $Corr(Z_{Nj}, Z_{Nk}) = \rho$ for $j \neq k$.

In general, it is more difficult to achieve significance simultaneously with the increase in the number of multiple endpoints. The regulatory agencies may require a treatment to demonstrate statistically significant effect on multiple endpoints, each at the one-sided 2.5% level. It is a conservative test since the overall type-I error can be smaller than 2.5%. Chuang-Stein et al. (2007) introduced the concept of the average type-I error approach to adjust for the significance level. They assumed that parameters of effect sizes are uniformly distributed over the restricted null space and averaged the power function under the uniform distribution of the region of the restricted null space. In this case, the local significance level can be inflated more than 2.5% but still control the average type-I error at the desired significance level. Thus, this method does not strictly control the overall type-I error.

Some methods for the calculation of the power and determining the sample size in clinical trials with more than one primary endpoint have been developed and published in the research literature. Xiong et al. (2005) introduced a formula to calculate the power with bivariate normal coprimary endpoints with known variance–covariance matrix. Sozu et al. (2006) extended it to include unknown variance–covariance matrix using the Wishart distribution. Sozu, Sugimoto, and Hamasaki (2010) proposed the closed form solution for the calculation of power and sample size with multiple coprimary binary endpoints. Sozu, Sugimoto, and Hamasaki (2011) provided the formulae to calculate power and sample size for some situations in superiority trials.

For two-stage adaptive designs with coprimary endpoint problems, we will discuss stopping boundary determination, and the power and the conditional power calculations. We will show that the stopping boundaries for study with a single endpoint can be used for multiple coprimary endpoints and such method is $\alpha$-exaustive. Therefore, the method is neither a conservative nor unconservative approach.

## 13.2 Group Sequential Design with Multiple Coprimary Endpoints

To introduce the group sequential design of clinical trials with multiple coprimary endpoints, we start from the simplest case, that a study is one-arm and two-stage $(K = 2)$ with two $(d = 2)$ coprimary normal endpoints with known covariance matrix, which is the same as the correlation matrix. Consider $X_1, X_2, ..., X_N$ are independent random vectors drawn from the multivariate normal distribution with 2 dimensions, $N(\boldsymbol{\mu}_2, \boldsymbol{\Sigma})$, where $\boldsymbol{\mu}_2 = (\mu_1, \mu_2)'$ and $\boldsymbol{\Sigma} = \begin{pmatrix} 1 & \rho \\ \rho & 1 \end{pmatrix}$.

In this case, the covariance matrix of $X$ is the same as the correlation matrix. We are interested in the following hypothesis:

$$H_0 : \mu_1 \leq 0 \text{ or } \mu_2 \leq 0 \tag{13.3}$$
$$H_a : \mu_1 > 0 \text{ and } \mu_2 > 0.$$

Let the information time $\tau = n/N$. The stopping rules for the two-stage design are

(1) At Stage 1, if $Z_1(\tau) \geq z_{1-\alpha_1}$ and $Z_2(\tau) \geq z_{1-\alpha_1}$ stop, reject $H_0$; otherwise, continue the study.
(2) At the final stage, if $Z_1(1) \geq z_{1-\alpha_2}$ and $Z_2(1) \geq z_{1-\alpha_2}$ stop, reject $H_0$; otherwise, stop and don't reject $H_0$.

Here $Z_j(\tau)$ and $Z_j(1)$ are the interim and final $Z$ statistics, respectively, for the $j$th endpoint, and $Z_{1-\alpha_1}$, $Z_{1-\alpha_2}$ and $Z_{\alpha_2}$ are the stopping criterion for the two stages. The joint distribution of the test statistics of two endpoints and at two stages is

$$\begin{pmatrix} Z_1(\tau) \\ Z_2(\tau) \\ Z_1(1) \\ Z_2(1) \end{pmatrix} \sim N_4 \left( \begin{pmatrix} \sqrt{n}\mu_1 \\ \sqrt{n}\mu_2 \\ \sqrt{N}\mu_1 \\ \sqrt{N}\mu_2 \end{pmatrix}, \begin{pmatrix} 1 & \rho & \sqrt{\tau} & \sqrt{\tau}\rho \\ \rho & 1 & \sqrt{\tau}\rho & \sqrt{\tau} \\ \sqrt{\tau} & \sqrt{\tau}\rho & 1 & \rho \\ \sqrt{\tau}\rho & \sqrt{\tau} & \rho & 1 \end{pmatrix} \right). \tag{13.4}$$

The power function of the hypothesis test in Equation (13.3) is

$$P((Z_1(\tau) > z_{1-\alpha_1} \cap Z_2(\tau) > z_{1-\alpha_1}) \cup (Z_1(1) > z_{1-\alpha_2} \cap Z_2(1) > z_{1-\alpha_2})|\boldsymbol{\mu}). \tag{13.5}$$

## 13.3   Stopping Boundaries

Controlling the overall type-I error of the group sequential design with multiple coprimary endpoints is not easy. It is known that the type-I error rate can be inflated due to performing the test at multiple interim looks. However, at each interim analysis, the coprimary endpoint test causes the drop of power in comparison with a single endpoint test. It is the combination of a multiplicity and reverse multiplicity problem.

The errors spent at different stages are given by

$$\pi_1 = P\left(\boldsymbol{Z}\left(\tau_1\right) \geq z_{1-a_1} | H_0\right) \tag{13.6}$$

$$\pi_2 = P\left(\boldsymbol{Z}\left(\tau_2\right) \geq z_{-1a_2} \cap \boldsymbol{Z}\left(\tau_1\right) \not\geq z_{1-a_1} | H_0\right)$$

$$\vdots$$

$$\pi_k = P\left(\boldsymbol{Z}\left(\tau_k\right) \geq z_{1-a_k} \cap_{i=1}^{k-1} \boldsymbol{Z}\left(\tau_i\right) \not\geq z_{1-a_i} | H_0\right)$$

and the cumulative error up to the $k$th stage is $\pi_k^* = \sum_{i=1}^{k} \pi_i$. The type-I error control requires $\sup_{\mu \in H_0} \pi_K^* \leq \alpha$ (the nominal level). The question is: When or under which conflagration of the individual hypotheses $H_{0i}$ does the maximum type I error rate occur? The following theorem will give a simple answer to the question.

**Theorem 13.1** $\pi_K^*$ *reaches the maximum value when one element of $\boldsymbol{\mu}_d$ is 0 while the other elements are $+\infty$.*

This theorem implies that the stopping boundaries of the multiple coprimary endpoints will be the same as the stopping boundaries for the single endpoint. Thus, even in the case of coprimary endpoints, one can use the stopping rules of the single endpoint!

**Proof.** First, we provide the conditional Brownian distribution $B\left(\tau_i\right) | B\left(\tau_{i-1}\right)$:

$$B\left(\tau_i\right) | B\left(\tau_{i-1}\right) \sim N_d \left(B\left(\tau_{i-1}\right) + \mu_d \sqrt{N}\left(\tau_i - \tau_{i-1}\right), \left(\tau_i - \tau_{i-1}\right)\Sigma\right) \tag{13.7}$$

We prove Theorem 1 by mathematical induction. We denote $b_{\alpha_i} = z_{a_i}\sqrt{\tau_i}$. For $K = 2$,

$$\begin{aligned}
\pi_2^* &= \pi_1 + \pi_2 \\
&= \pi_1^* + \Pr\{B\left(\tau_2\right) > b_{\alpha_2} \cap B\left(\tau_1\right) \not\geq b_{\alpha_1} | H_0\} \\
&= \pi_1^* + \Pr\{B\left(\tau_2\right) > b_{\alpha_2} \cap B\left(\tau_1\right) \not\geq b_{\alpha_1}, H_0\}\left(1 - \pi_1^*\right) \\
&\quad \pi_1^* + \gamma_2\left(1 - \pi_1^*\right),
\end{aligned}$$

where $\gamma_2 = \Pr\{B\left(\tau_2\right) > b_{\alpha_2} | B\left(\tau_1\right) \not\geq b_{\alpha_1}, H_0\}$. From Equation (13.7), it is easy to verify that $\gamma_2$ reaches the maximum at $\mu_{d,0}$ in the $H_0$ domain when one element of $\mu_d$ is 0, while the others are $+\infty$. To simplify, let $\mu_{d,0} = (0, +\infty, ..., +\infty)$. Also $\pi_1^*$ reaches the maximum at $\mu_{d,0}$. Note that $0 < \pi_1^*, \gamma_2 < 1$. $\pi_2$ is monotonically increasing as $\pi_1^*$ and $\gamma_2$ increase when

$0 < \pi_1, \gamma_2 < 1$, since $\frac{\partial \pi_2^*}{\partial \pi_1^*} = 1 - \gamma_2 > 0$ and $\frac{\partial \pi_2^*}{\partial \gamma_2^*} = 1 - \pi_1^* > 0$. Therefore, $\pi_2^*$ reaches the maximum value when both $\pi_1^*$ and $\gamma_2$ reach the maximum value.

Assuming that the theorem holds for $K = N$, i.e., $\pi_N^*$ reaches the maximum at $\mu_{p,0}$, for $K = N + 1$, we have

$$
\begin{aligned}
\pi_{N+1}^* &= \pi_N^* + \pi_{N+1} \\
&= \pi_N^* + \Pr\left\{ B\left(\tau_{N+1}\right) > b_{\alpha_{N+1}} \cap_{i=1}^{N} B\left(\tau_i\right) \not> b_{\alpha_i} | H_0 \right\} \\
&= \pi_N^* + \gamma_{N+1} \left(1 - \pi_N^*\right),
\end{aligned}
$$

where $\gamma_{N+1} = \pi_N^* + \Pr\left\{ B\left(\tau_{N+1}\right) > b_{\alpha_{N+1}} | \cap_{i=1}^{N} B\left(\tau_i\right) \not> b_{\alpha_i}, H_0 \right\}$. From Equation (13.7), $\gamma_{N+1}$ achieves the maximum at $\mu_{p,0}$. $\pi_{N+1}^*$ reaches the maximum value at $\mu_{p,0}$ by using a similar argument where $K = 2$. Thus, the theorem is proved.        $\square$

## 13.4    Examples of Coprimary Endpoint Design

Consider a two-stage $(K = 2)$ clinical trial with an interim analysis planned at information time $\tau = 0.5$ and using the O'Brien–Fleming stopping boundaries (see Chapter 5); that is, the rejection boundaries are $z_{1-\alpha_1} = 2.80$ and $z_{1-\alpha_2} = 1.98$ at a one-sided level of significance $\alpha = 0.025$.

When the alternative of the hypothesis (13.3) is true, the examples of power computed from (13.5) with information time $\tau = 0.5$ are shown in Table 13.1.

Table 13.1:   Overall Power

| Correlation | −0.8 | −0.5 | −0.2 | 0 | 0.2 | 0.5 | 0.8 |
|---|---|---|---|---|---|---|---|
| Overall Power | 0.59 | 0.60 | 0.62 | 0.64 | 0.65 | 0.68 | 0.73 |

Note: Power for each individual endpoint = 80%.

For example, if we want to detect the effect size of 0.2 for each of the two normally distributed endpoints, 197 samples are needed for 80% power for each of the two endpoints. Using the group sequential design discussed above, the power with different correlations between endpoints is shown in Table 13.1. If the endpoints are more positively correlated, the overall power is higher.

Table 13.2 shows the maximum sample size needed to reach the overall 80% power if we want to detect the effect size 0.2 for both endpoints. From Table 13.2, we can also see that considering the correlation between the endpoints can gain the power. From the distribution in (13.4), we can see the maximum sample size required depends on the information $\tau$, the choice of the stopping boundaries, the designed parameters including $\mu$ and $\Sigma$, and the desired levels of $\alpha$ and $\beta$. It is hard to give a closed form solution. The numbers in Table 13.2 are from the numerical integration based on the R code below.

Table 13.2:  Maximum Sample Size with Overall Power 80%

| Correlation | 0 | 0.2 | 0.5 | 0.8 |
|---|---|---|---|---|
| Maximum $N$ Required | 260 | 256 | 248 | 231 |

Note: One-sided $\alpha = 0.025$, $\tau = 0.5$.

The $R$-function for generating a typical result in Tables 13.1 and 13.2 is presented in the following.

**>>R Function 13.1:    Power of Two Coprimary Endpoints>>**

```
library(mnormt)
Power=function (n, tau, mu1, mu2, rho, za1, za2)
{
u1=sqrt(n*tau)*mu1; u2=sqrt(n)*mu2
r12=rho; r13=sqrt(tau); r14=r12*r13
r23=r14; r24=r13; r34=r12
s1=matrix(c(1,r12, r12,1), 2,2)
s2=matrix(c(1,r12,r13, r14, r12,1, r23, r24, r13, r23,1, r34, r14, r24, r34, 1), 4,4)
power1=sadmvn(lower=c(za1,za1), upper=c(Inf, Inf), rep(u1,2), s1)
power2=sadmvn(lower=c(za2,za2), upper=c(Inf, Inf), rep(u2,2), s1)
powerOverlap=sadmvn(lower=c(za1, za1, za2, za2), upper=rep(Inf, 4), c(u1, u1, u2, u2), s2)
power=power1+power2-powerOverlap
return (power)
}
```
**<<R<<**

To invoke the function, we can, for example, use the following line of code.

**>>R>>**
```
Power(n=197, tau=0.5, mu1=0.2, mu2=0.2, rho=0.5, za1=2.8, za2=1.98)
```
**<<R<<**

Note that if we use the *pmvnorm* function instead of the *sadmvn* function in $R$, the results will be slightly different due to numerical errors.

## 13.5 Simulation of Group Sequential Trial with Coprimary Endpoints

In Section 13.4, we use numerical integration to obtain the power for classical design with fixed sample size. For adaptive design, it is convenient to use simulation to determine the sample size or power. Here is the R-function for designing the two-group, two-endpoint, two-stage group sequential designs.

**>>R Function 13.2: Power of Two Coprimary Endpoints by Simulation>>**

```
## Two-group, two-endpoint with two-stage design
## muij: standardized means of j endpoint in group i
## rho: the true correlation between the two endpoints
## c1 and c2 are the stopping boundaries
## N: maximum sample size per group
library(mvtnorm)
power=function(mu11,mu12, mu21, mu22,rho,tau,c1,c2,N,rep=10000)
{
rej=rep(0,rep)
for (i in 1:rep)
{
n=round(N*tau)
varcov=matrix(c(1,rho,rho,1),2,2)
trtStg1=rmvnorm(n,mean=c(mu11,mu12), sigma=varcov)
ctStg1 =rmvnorm(n,mean=c(mu21,mu22), sigma=varcov)
t11=t.test(trtStg1[,1],ctStg1[,1])$statistic
t12=t.test(trtStg1[,2],ctStg1[,2])$statistic
trtStg2=rmvnorm(N-n, mean=c(mu11,mu12), sigma=varcov)
ctStg2 =rmvnorm(N-n, mean=c(mu21,mu22), sigma=varcov)
trt1=c(trtStg1[,1], trtStg2[,1]); trt2=c(trtStg1[,2], trtStg2[,2])
ct1 =c(ctStg1[,1], ctStg2[,1]); ct2 =c(ctStg1[,2], ctStg2[,2])
t21=t.test(trt1,ct1)$statistic; t22=t.test(trt2,ct2)$statistic
rej[i]=(t11>c1 & t12>c1) | (t21>c2 & t22>c2)
}
return (mean(rej))
}
```
**<<R<<**

**Example 13.1   Power and Sample Size for Two-Arm Trial with Coprimary Endpoints**

Suppose in a clinical trial, the standardized responses (mean divided by the standard deviation) for the two coprimary endpoints are estimated to be 0.2 and 0.25 for the test group and 0.005 and 0.015 for the control group. The correlation between the two endpoints is estimated to be $\rho = 0.25$. We use a two-stage group sequential design with O'Brien–Fleming boundary for efficacy stopping. The interim analysis will be performed at information time $\tau = 0.5$. To calculate the sample size for 90% overall power, we can invoke the $R$-function with different sample size $N$ until the power is close to 90%. It turns out that $N$ is 584 per group.

>>R>>
power(mu11=0.2,mu12=0.25, mu21=0.005, mu22=0.015, rho=0.25, tau=0.5, c1=2.80, c2=1.98, N=584, rep=10000)
<<R<<

## 13.6   Conditional Power and Sample Size Reestimation

Table 13.3 (Cheng, 2014; Cheng et al. 2014) provides the results of overall conditional power (CP), when the conditional power of each subhypothesis test achieves 85%, controlling each single test at one-sided 2.5%. From Table 13.3, we observe that there are two main factors affecting the overall CP: the correlation between each pair of endpoints and number of coprimary endpoints. Controlling the test to achieve a conditional power of 85% on every single endpoint, we can see with increase of the correlation, the overall CP increases as well. With the number of coprimary endpoints increasing, the overall CP decreases.

Table 13.3:   Overall Conditional Power

| Correlation | Number of Coprimary Endpoints | | | | |
|---|---|---|---|---|---|
| | 2 | 3 | 4 | 5 | 9 |
| 0 | 0.73 | 0.61 | 0.52 | 0.44 | 0.23 |
| 0.2 | 0.74 | 0.65 | 0.58 | 0.51 | 0.35 |
| 0.5 | 0.76 | 0.70 | 0.65 | 0.61 | 0.51 |
| 0.8 | 0.79 | 0.76 | 0.73 | 0.72 | 0.66 |
| 1.0 | 0.85 | 0.85 | 0.85 | 0.85 | 0.85 |

Note: Marginal 85% conditional power, $\alpha = 0.025$

In this section, a fixed-weight sample-size reestimation method for coprimary endpoints based on the conditional power will be introduced. In the case of testing the location of the mean of a normal population $N(\mu, \sigma^2)$, assume the variance is known with $\sigma = 1$. Consider the two-stage design ($K = 2$) and denote $N_0$ as the designed maximum sample size needed. The test statistic at the final stage can be decomposed as

$$Z = \sqrt{\tau}Z_1 + \sqrt{1-\tau}Z_2 = \sqrt{\frac{n}{N_0}}Z_1 + \sqrt{\frac{N_0-n}{N_0}}\frac{\sum_{i=n+1}^{N_0}X_i}{N_0-n}. \qquad (13.8)$$

The test statistic can be considered as the sum of the test statistics before and after the interim analysis by multiplying weights $\sqrt{\tau}$ and $\sqrt{1-\tau}$. At the interim analysis, $Z_1$ is observed and fixed. Assume the sample size is adjusted from $N_0$ to $N$ ($N$ can increase or decrease). The modified fixed-weight test statistic is

$$U = \sqrt{\frac{n}{N_0}}Z_1 + \sqrt{\frac{N_0-n}{N_0}}\frac{\sum_{i=n+1}^{N}X_i}{N-n}. \qquad (13.9)$$

Still consider the example of hypothesis (13.1) with $d = 2$ coprimary endpoints and $K = 2$ stage design. The test statistic vector can be decomposed to

$$Z = \sqrt{\tau}\frac{\sum_{i=1}^{n}X_i}{\sqrt{n}} + \sqrt{1-\tau}Z_{1-\tau} \qquad (13.10)$$

$$= \sqrt{\tau}\frac{\sum_{i=1}^{n}X_i}{\sqrt{n}} + \sqrt{1-\tau}\frac{\sum_{i=n+1}^{N_0}X_i}{\sqrt{n}},$$

where $\tau = n/N_0$. Denote $N$ the total sample size after adjustment, the weighted $Z$-statistic with the fixed weights, which is denoted by $U$, is

$$U = \sqrt{\tau}Z_\tau + \sqrt{1-\tau}\frac{\sum_{i=n+1}^{N}X_i}{\sqrt{N-n}}, \qquad (13.11)$$

where $U = (U_1, U_2)$. Note that $N - n$ is the sample size needed for the second stage of the study. Denote it as $n_2$. We have

$$Cov\,(U_1, U_2 | Z_\tau) = Cov\left(\sqrt{1-\tau}\frac{\sum_{i=n+1}^{N}X_{i1}}{\sqrt{N-n}}, \sqrt{1-\tau}\frac{\sum_{i=n+1}^{N}X_{i2}}{\sqrt{N-n}}\right)$$

$$= (1-\tau)\rho. \qquad (13.12)$$

To control the type-I error rate at the worst case, consider $\boldsymbol{\mu}_0 = (0, +\infty)'$. In this case, we need to consider only the endpoint 1 (EP1) as it can always declare the significance for the endpoint 2 (EP2). Cui et al. (1999) showed that for the single endpoint, when $\mu = 0$, $U_1 | Z_1, \tau$ follows a normal distribution with

$$E(U_1|Z_{1,\tau}) = \sqrt{\tau}Z_{1,\tau}, \tag{13.13}$$
$$Var(U_1|Z_{1,\tau}) = 1 - \tau.$$

Thus $U_1|Z_{1,\tau}$ and $Z_1|Z_{1,\tau}$ will have the same distribution. It follows that $(Z_{1,\tau}, U_\tau)$ and $(Z_{1,\tau}, Z_1)$ have the same distribution. Therefore,

$$P_{\mu_0}(\mathbf{Z}_\tau > c_1 \cup \mathbf{U} > c_2) = P_{\mu_0}(\mathbf{Z}_\tau > c_1 \cup \mathbf{Z} > c_2).$$

And it follows that the maximum type-I error rate will be preserved.

Let the conditional power be the target conditional power, $1 - \beta_0$. We have:

$$\Pr\left(\sqrt{\tau}\mathbf{Z}_\tau + \sqrt{1-\tau}\frac{\Sigma_{i=n+1}^{N}\mathbf{X}_i}{\sqrt{n_2}} > z_{\alpha_2}|\hat{\boldsymbol{\mu}}, \rho = \hat{\rho}\right) = 1 - \beta_0. \tag{13.14}$$

Rewriting (13.14), we can get

$$\Pr\left(\frac{\Sigma_{i=n+1}^{N}\mathbf{X}_i}{\sqrt{n_2}} > \frac{z_{\alpha_2} - \sqrt{\tau}\mathbf{Z}_\tau}{1-\tau}|\hat{\boldsymbol{\mu}}, \rho = \hat{\rho}\right) = 1 - \beta_0. \tag{13.15}$$

Note that

$$\frac{\Sigma_{i=n+1}^{N}\mathbf{X}_i}{\sqrt{n_2}}|\left(\hat{\boldsymbol{\mu}} = \frac{\Sigma_{i=1}^{N}\mathbf{X}_i}{n}, \rho = \hat{\rho}\right) \sim N_2\left(\begin{pmatrix}\sqrt{n_2}\hat{\mu}_1 \\ \sqrt{n_2}\hat{\mu}_2\end{pmatrix}, \begin{pmatrix}1 & \hat{\rho} \\ \hat{\rho} & 1\end{pmatrix}\right). \tag{13.16}$$

By combining (13.15) with (13.16), the $n_2$ can be solved using the numerical integration.

## Example 13.2   Conditional Power and Sample-Size Reestimation in Single/Paired Group Trial with Coprimary Endpoints

Consider a one-arm two-stage study with two coprimary endpoints, EP1 and EP2. If we want to detect the effect size of 0.2 for both endpoints with the common standard deviation of 1 and designed correlation of 0, with O'Brien–Fleming stopping boundaries ($z_{1-\alpha_1} = 2.8$ and $z_{1-\alpha_2} = 1.98$), a sample of 260 subjects is needed to reach 80% power. At interim analysis, $\tau = 0.5$, $n = 130$, assume the observed means are $\hat{\mu}_1 = 0.1333$ and $\hat{\mu}_2 = 0.1605$. Thus, $Z_1(0.5) = \hat{\mu}_1\sqrt{n} = 0.1333\sqrt{130} = 1.52 < z_{1-\alpha_1}$ and $Z_2(0.5) = 1.83 < z_{1-\alpha_1}$; the trial will continue to the second stage. Suppose the correlation calculated from the interim data is $\hat{\rho} = 0.35$. If we keep the original sample size for the second stage, i.e., $n_2 = 130$, then the overall conditional power is only 31%. To retain the conditional power 80%, $n_2 = 414$ subjects are needed (see the R programs below).

Based on (13.15) and (13.16), the calculation of the conditional power or new sample size is implemented in *R*-function 13.3.

**>>R Function 13.3: Overall Conditional Power for One-Group Design with Two Coprimary Endpoints>>**

```
#Conditional power for one-arm, two-stage design with two primary endpoints
#mu1, mu2, rho: estimated from the interim analysis.
#n1: interim sample size
#za2: critical value at stage 2
library(mnormt)
cPowerOneArm=function(mu1, mu2, n1, n2, rho, tau, za2)
{
Z1t=sqrt(n1)*mu1; Z2t=sqrt(n1)*mu2
mean= c(sqrt(n2)*mu1,sqrt(n2)*mu2)
s=matrix(c(1,rho, rho,1), 2,2)
c1=(za2-sqrt(tau)*Z1t)/(1-tau)
c2=(za2-sqrt(tau)*Z2t)/(1-tau)
return (sadmvn(lower=c(c1,c2), upper=c(Inf, Inf), mean, s))
}
```
**<<R<<**

To generate the results mentioned in the previous example, the following code can be used.

**>>R>>**
```
cPowerOneArm(mu1=0.1333, mu2=0.1605, n1=130, n2=130, rho=0.35, tau=0.5,
za2=1.98)
cPowerOneArm(mu1=0.1333, mu2=0.1605, n1=130, n2=414, rho=0.35, tau=0.5,
za2=1.98)
```
**<<R<<**

The conditional power can also be obtained through simulations. The simulation program can be modified from *R*-function 13.2 by letting the first stage data equal the observed data instead of the simulated data.

In phase-III clinical trials, there are two-group more often designs than single-group designs. For a two-group design, we can use *R*-function 13.4 below. See Example 13.3.

## Example 13.3 Conditional Power for Two-Group Design with Two Coprimary Endpoints

Consider a two-group (the test and the control), two-stage study with two coprimary endpoints, EP1 and EP2. We want to detect the treatment differences $\mu_1 = 0.32$ and $\mu_2 = 0.4$ in the two endpoints, respectively. The common standard deviations of the two treatment groups are $\sigma_1 = 2$ and $\sigma_2 = 1.8$ for the two endpoints, respectively. The designed correlation between the two endpoints is conservatively set to 0 at the design stage. With O'Brien–Fleming stopping boundaries ($z_{1-\alpha_1} = 2.8$ and $z_{1-\alpha_2} = 1.98$), a sample of 680 subjects is required to reach the power of 80%. At interim analysis, $\tau = 0.5$, $n = 340$, assume the observed means of EP1 and EP2 are $\hat{\mu}_1 = 0.28$ and $\hat{\mu}_2 = 0.35$ with the common standard deviations of $\hat{\sigma}_1 = 1.9$ and $\hat{\sigma}_2 = 2.2$ for EP1 and EP2, respectively. Thus, we obtain $Z_1(0.5) = \left(\hat{\mu}_1\sqrt{n/2}/\hat{\sigma}_1\right) = 0.28\sqrt{340/2}/1.9 = 1.9214 < z_{1-\alpha_1}$ and $Z_2(0.5) = \left(\hat{\mu}_2\sqrt{n/2}/\hat{\sigma}_2\right) = 0.35\sqrt{340/2}/2.2 = 2.0743 < z_{1-\alpha_1}$; the trial will continue to the second stage. Suppose the correlation calculated from the interim data is $\hat{\rho} = 0.3$. If we keep the original sample size for the second stage, i.e., $n_2 = 340$, then the overall conditional power is only 66.5%. To retain the conditional power 80%, $n_2 = 482$ subjects per group are needed (see the $R$ programs below). Note that we use mu1 $= \hat{\delta}_1$ and mu2 $= \hat{\delta}_2$ when we invoke the $R$-function. One may be curious about the conditional power when the observed data at the interim analysis are identical to the assumptions made at the design stage, that is, $\hat{\mu}_1 = \mu_1 = 0.32$, $\hat{\mu}_2 = \mu_2 = 0.4$, $\hat{\sigma}_1 = \sigma_1 = 2$, $\hat{\sigma}_2 = \sigma_2 = 1$, and $n_2 = 340$. The conditional power is 86%, larger than the unconditional power 80% at design stage. This is logical, because the data from the first stage are given, which reduces the variability of the trial data at the final analysis and O'Brien–Fleming boundary is very conservative, and spends a very small $\alpha$ at the first stage.

## >>R Function 13.4: Overall Conditional Power for Two-Group Design with Two Coprimary Endpoints>>

```
#Conditional power for two-group design, two-stage design with two primary
endpoints
#mu1, sigma1, mu2, sigma2, rho: the interim estimates
#n1: interim sample size per group
#za2: critical value at stage 2
library(mnormt)
cPowerTwoArms=function(mu1, sigma1, mu2, sigma2, n1, n2, rho, tau, za2)
{
delta1=mu1/sqrt(2)/sigma1; delta2=mu2/sqrt(2)/sigma2
Z1t=sqrt(n1)*delta1; Z2t=sqrt(n1)*delta2
mean= c(sqrt(n2)*delta1,sqrt(n2)*delta2)
```

```
s=matrix(c(1,rho, rho,1), 2,2)
c1=(za2-sqrt(tau)*Z1t)/(1-tau); c2=(za2-sqrt(tau)*Z2t)/(1-tau)
return (sadmvn(lower=c(c1,c2), upper=c(Inf, Inf), mean, s))
}
```
<<**R**<<

To invoke the function for the Example 13.3, we can use the following code.

>>**R**>>
```
cPowerTwoArms(mu1=0.28, sigma1=1.9, mu2=0.35, sigma2=2.2, n1=340,
n2=340, rho=0.3, tau=0.5, za2=1.98)
cPowerTwoArms(mu1=0.28, sigma1=1.9, mu2=0.35, sigma2=2.2, n1=340,
n2=482, rho=0.3, tau=0.5, za2=1.98)
cPowerTwoArms(mu1=0.32, sigma1=2, mu2=0.4, sigma2=1.8, n1=340, n2=340,
rho=0.3, tau=0.5, za2=1.98)
```
<<**R**<<

## 13.7 Summary

We have discussed the design and statistical monitoring methods for the clinical trials with coprimary endpoints. It has been proved that the stopping boundaries of the GSD with coprimary endpoints are the same for a trial with a single endpoint. However, the power calculation is different and depends on the correlations among the endpoints (or the test statistics for the coprimary endpoints). It has been shown that the method gains power when considering the correlation among the endpoints over the method in which multiple coprimary endpoints are considered as independent. Furthermore, the power increases as the correlation among endpoints increases and the number of endpoints decreases. The design is $\alpha$-exhaustive, that is, the familywise type-I error is strongly controlled. The methods discussed in this chapter can be extended to continuous–binary endpoints. The key step is to evaluate the covariance between a continuous random variable and a binary random variable.

## Problems

**13.1** Derive the joint distribution of the test statistics with three coprimary endpoints (see Equation 13.4) and power (see Equation 13.5).

**13.2** Implement the formulations obtained from Problem 13.1 using R or SAS for determining the stopping boundaries (see R-functions 13.1 and 13.2).

**13.3** Develop an SAS or R-program to calculate (simulate) the sample size required for the overall power of the hypothesis testing with three coprimary endpoints.

**13.4** Suppose in a two-group trial design, the responses of the primary endpoint are 0.7 for the test group and 0.4 for the control group; determine the sample sizes required for two and three coprimary endpoints.

# Chapter 14

# Multiple-Endpoint Adaptive Design

Multiple-endpoint problems can arise in many different situations. For instance, when there is a single primary efficacy endpoint with one or more secondary endpoints, we try to claim the drug effect on primary and secondary endpoints; when there are two endpoints, at least one needs to be statistically significant to claim efficacy of the test drug; in a clinical trial we can use a surrogate endpoint for an accelerated approval and a clinically important endpoint for a full approval. In this chapter, we will first review the single-stage and stepwise methods in classical designs, then discuss multiple-endpoint issues in adaptive designs. We will use trial examples to give step by step instructions.

## 14.1  Multiple-Testing Taxonomy

Let $H_{0i}$ $(i = 1, ..., K)$ be the null hypotheses of interest in an experiment. There are at least three different types of global multiple-hypotheses testing that can be performed.

**(1) Union-Intersection Testing**

$$H_0 : \cap_{i=1}^{K} H_{0i} \text{ versus } H_a : \bar{H}_0. \tag{14.1}$$

In this setting, if any $H_{0i}$ is rejected, the global null hypothesis $H_0$ is rejected. For union-intersection testing, if the global testing has a size of $\alpha$, then this has to be adjusted to a smaller value for testing each individual $H_{io}$, called the local significance level.

**Example 14.1   A Union-Intersection Test**

In a typical dose-finding trial, patients are randomly assigned to one of several $(K)$ parallel dose levels or a placebo. The goal is to find out if there is a drug effect and which dose(s) has the effect. In such a trial,

$H_{0i}$ will represent the null hypothesis that the $i$th dose level has no effect in comparison with the placebo. The goal of the dose-finding trial can be formulated in terms of hypothesis testing (14.1).

**(2) Intersection-Union Testing**

$$H_0 : \cup_{i=1}^{K} H_{0i} \text{ versus } H_a : \bar{H}_0. \tag{14.2}$$

In this setting, if and only if all $H_{0i}$ $(i = 1, ..., K)$ are rejected is the global null hypothesis $H_0$ rejected. For intersection-union testing, the global $\alpha$ will apply to each individual $H_{io}$ testing.

**Example 14.2    Intersection-Union Test with Alzheimer's Trial**

Alzheimer's trials in mild to moderate disease generally include ADAS Cog and CIBIC (Clinician's Interview Based Impression of Change) endpoints as coprimaries. The ADAS Cog endpoint measures patients' cognitive functions, while the CIBIC endpoint measures patients' deficits in activities of daily living. For proving a claim of a clinically meaningful treatment benefit for this disease, it is generally required to demonstrate statistically significant treatment benefit on each of these two primary endpoints (called coprimary endpoints). If we denote $H_{01}$ as the null hypothesis of no effect in terms of the ADAS Cog and $H_{02}$ as the null hypothesis of no effect in terms of CIBIC, then the hypothesis testing for the efficacy claim in the clinical trial can be expressed as (14.2).

**(3) Union-Intersection Mixture Testing**

This is a mixture of (1) and (2), for example,

$$H_0 : \cap_{i=1}^{K} H_{0i}^* \text{ versus } H_a : \bar{H}_0, \tag{14.3}$$

where $H_{0i}^* = \cup_{j=1}^{K_i} H_{0ij}$.

**Example 14.3    Union-Intersection Mixture Testing**

This example is a combination of Example 14.1 and Example 14.2. Suppose this dose-finding trial has $K = 2$ dose levels and a placebo. For each dose level, the efficacy claim is based on the coprimary endpoints, ADAS Cog and CIBIC. Let $H_{0i1}$ and $H_{0i2}$ be the null hypotheses for the two primary endpoints for the $i$th dose level. Rejection of $H_{0i}^*$ will lead to an efficacy claim for the $i$th dose in terms of the two coprimary endpoints. Then, the efficacy claim in this trial can be postulated in terms of hypothesis test (14.3).

## Familywise Error Rate

Familywise Error Rate (FWER) is the maximum (sup) probability of falsely rejecting $H_0$ under all possible null hypothesis configurations:

$$FWER = \sup_{H_0} P \text{ (rejecting } H_0). \tag{14.4}$$

The strong FWER $\alpha$ control requires that

$$FWER = \sup_{H_0} P \text{ (rejecting } H_0) \leq \alpha. \tag{14.5}$$

On the other hand, the weak FWER control requires only $\alpha$ control under the global null hypothesis. We will focus on the strong FWER control for the rest of this chapter.

*Local alpha:* A local alpha is the type-I error rate (often called the size of a local test) allowed for individual $H_{0i}$ testing. In most hypothesis test procedures, the local $\alpha$ is numerically different from (smaller than) the global (familywise) $\alpha$ to avoid FWER inflation. Without the adjusted local $\alpha$, FWER inflation usually increases as the number of tests in the family increases.

Suppose we have two primary endpoints in a two-arm, active-control, randomized trial. The efficacy of the drug will be claimed as long as one of the endpoints is statistically significant at level $\alpha$. In such a scenario, the FWER will be inflated. The level of inflation is dependent on the correlation between the two test statistics (Table 14.1). The maximum error rate inflation occurs when the endpoints are independent. If the two endpoints are perfectly correlated, there is no alpha inflation. For a correlation as high as 0.75, the inflation is still larger than 0.08 for a level 0.05 test. Hence, to control the overall $\alpha$, an alpha adjustment is required for each test. Similarly, to study how alpha inflation is related to the number of analyses, simulations are conducted for the two independent endpoints, $A$ and $B$. The results are presented in Table 14.2. We can see that alpha is inflated from 0.05 to 0.226 with five analyses and to 0.401 with ten analyses.

Table 14.1: Error Inflation Due to Correlations between Endpoints

| Level $\alpha_A$ | Level $\alpha_B$ | Correlation $R_{AB}$ | FWER |
|---|---|---|---|
| | | 0 | 0.098 |
| | | 0.25 | 0.097 |
| 0.05 | 0.05 | 0.50 | 0.093 |
| | | 0.75 | 0.083 |
| | | 1.00 | 0.050 |

Note: $\alpha_A = \alpha$ for endpoint $A$, $\alpha_A = \alpha$ for endpoint $B$.

Table 14.2:    Error Inflation Due to Different Numbers of Endpoints

| Level $\alpha_A$ | Level $\alpha_B$ | Number of analyses | FWER |
|---|---|---|---|
| | | 1 | 0.050 |
| | | 2 | 0.098 |
| 0.05 | 0.05 | 3 | 0.143 |
| | | 5 | 0.226 |
| | | 10 | 0.401 |

*Closed family:* A closed family is one for which any subset intersection hypothesis involving members of the testing family is also a member of the family. For example, a closed family of three hypotheses $H_1$, $H_2$, $H_3$ has a total of seven members, listed as follows: $H_1$, $H_2$, $H_3$, $H_1 \cap H_2$, $H_2 \cap H_3$, $H_1 \cap H_3$, $H_1 \cap H_2 \cap H_3$.

*Closure principle:* This was developed by Marcus et al. (1976). This principle asserts that one can ensure strong control of FWER and coherence (see below) at the same time by conducting the following procedure. Test every member of the closed family using a local $\alpha$-level test (here, $\alpha$ refers to the comparison-wise error rate, not the FWER). A hypothesis can be rejected provided (1) its corresponding test was significant at the $\alpha$-level, and (2) every other hypothesis in the family implies it has also been rejected by its corresponding $\alpha$-level test.

*Closed testing procedure:* A test procedure is said to be closed if and only if the rejection of a particular univariate null hypothesis at an $\alpha$-level of significance implies the rejection of all higher-level (multivariate) null hypotheses containing the univariate null hypothesis at the same $\alpha$-level. The procedure can be described as follows (Bretz et al., 2006):

(1) Define a set of elementary hypotheses, $H_1; ...; H_K$, of interest.
(2) Construct all possible $m > K$ intersection hypotheses, $H_I = \cap H_i$, $I \subseteq \{1, ..., K\}$.
(3) For each of the $m$ hypotheses find a suitable local $\alpha$-level test.
(4) Reject $H_i$ at FWER $\alpha$ if all hypotheses $H_I$ with $i \in I$ are rejected, each at the (local) $\alpha$-level.

This procedure is not often used directly in practice. However, the closure principle has been used to derive many useful test procedures, such as those of Holm (1979), Hochberg (1988), Hommel (1988), and gatekeeping procedures.

$\alpha$-*exhaustive procedure:* If $P$ (Reject $H_I$) $= \alpha$ for every intersection hypothesis $H_I, I \subseteq \{1, ..., K\}$, the test procedure is $\alpha$-exhaustive.

*Partition principle:* This is similar to the closed testing procedure with strong control over the familywise $\alpha$-level for the null hypotheses. The partition principle allows for test procedures that are formed by partitioning the parameter space into disjointed partitions with some logical ordering. Tests of the hypotheses are carried out sequentially at different partition steps. The process of testing stops upon failure to reject a given null hypothesis for predetermined partition steps (Dmitrienko et al., 2010, pp. 45–46; Hsu, 1996). We will discuss this more later in this chapter.

*Coherence* and *consonance* are two interesting concepts in closed testing procedures. *Coherence* means that if hypothesis $H$ implies $H^*$, then whenever $H$ is retained, so must be $H^*$. *Consonance* means that whenever $H$ is rejected, at least one of its components is rejected, too. Coherence is a necessary property of closed test procedures; consonance is desirable but not necessary. A procedure can be coherent but not consonant because of asymmetry in the hypothesis testing paradigm. When $H$ is rejected, we conclude that it is false. However, when $H$ is retained, we do not conclude that it is true; rather, we say that there is not sufficient evidence to reject it. Multiple comparison procedures that satisfy the closure principle are always coherent but not necessarily consonant (Westfall et al., 1999).

## Adjusted $p$-value

The adjusted $p$-value for a hypothesis test is defined as the smallest significance level at which one would reject the hypothesis using the multiple-testing procedure (Westfall and Young, 1993). If $p_I$ denotes the $p$-value for testing intersection hypothesis $H_I$, the adjusted $p$-value for $H_{0i}$ is given by

$$p_i^{adj} = \max_{I:i \in I} p_I. \tag{14.6}$$

If $p_i^{adj} \leq \alpha$, $H_{0i}$ is rejected.

## Simultaneous confidence interval

It is well known that a two-sided $(1-\alpha)\%$ confidence interval for parameter $\theta$ consists of all parameter values for which the hypothesis $H_0 : \theta = 0$ is retained at level $\alpha$. This concept can be applied to multiple-parameter problems to form a confidence set or a simultaneous confidence interval.

## 14.2   Multiple-Testing Approaches

### 14.2.1   *Single-Step Procedures*

The commonly used single-stage procedures include the Sidak (1967) method, the simple Bonferroni method, the Simes–Bonferroni method (Global test; Simes, 1986), and Dunnett's test (1955) for all active arms against the control arm. In the single-step procedure, to control the FWER, the unadjusted $p$-values are compared against the adjusted alpha to make the decision to reject or not reject the corresponding null hypothesis. Alternatively, we can use the adjusted $p$-values to compare against the original $\alpha$ for decision making.

**Sidak Method**

The Sidak method is derived from the simple fact that the probability of rejecting at least one null hypothesis is equal to $1 - Pr$(all null hypotheses are correct). To control the FWER, the adjusted alpha $\alpha_k$ for the null hypothesis $H_{0k}$ ($k = 1, ..., K$) can be found by solving the following equation:

$$\alpha = 1 - \left(1 - \alpha_k\right)^K. \tag{14.7}$$

Therefore, the adjusted alpha is given by

$$\alpha_k = 1 - \left(1 - \alpha\right)^{1/K}. \tag{14.8}$$

If the $p$-value is less than or equal to $\alpha_k$, reject $H_{0k}$. Alternatively we can calculate the adjusted $p$-value:

$$\tilde{p}_k = 1 - \left(1 - p_k\right)^K. \tag{14.9}$$

If the adjusted $p$-value $\tilde{p}_k$ is less than or equal to $\alpha$, then reject $H_{0k}$.

**Bonferroni Method**

The simple Bonferroni method is a simplification of the Sidak method that uses the Bonferroni inequality:

$$P(\cup_{k=1}^{K} H_k) \leq \sum_{k=1}^{K} P(H_k). \tag{14.10}$$

Based on (14.10), we can conservatively use the adjusted alpha,

$$\alpha_k = \frac{\alpha}{K}, \tag{14.11}$$

and the adjusted $p$-value,

$$\tilde{p}_k = K p_k.$$

This is a very conservative approach without consideration of any correlations among $p$-values.

The alpha doesn't have to be split equally among all tests. We can use the so-called weighted Bonferroni tests, for which the adjusted alpha and $p$-value are given by

$$\alpha_k = w_k \alpha \text{ and } \tilde{p}_k = \frac{p_k}{w_k}, \quad (14.12)$$

where the weight $w_k \geq 0$ and $\sum_{k=1}^{K} w_k = 1$. The weight $w_k$ can be determined based on the clinical importance of the $k$th hypothesis or the power of the $k$th hypothesis test.

## Simes Global Testing Method

The Simes–Bonferroni method is a global test in which the type-I error rate is controlled for the global null hypothesis (14.1). We reject the null hypothesis $H_0$ if

$$p_{(k)} \leq \frac{k\alpha}{K} \text{ for at least one } i = 1, ..., K, \quad (14.13)$$

where $p_{(1)} < ... < p_{(K)}$ are the ordered $p$-values.

The adjusted $p$-value is given by

$$\tilde{p} = \max_{k \in \{1, ..., K\}} \left\{ \frac{K}{k} p_{(k)} \right\}. \quad (14.14)$$

If $\tilde{p} \leq \alpha$, the global null hypothesis (14.1) is rejected.

## Dunnett's Method

Dunnett's method can be used for multiple comparisons of active groups against a common control group, which is often done in clinical trials with multiple parallel groups. Let $n_0$ and $n_i$ $(i = 1, ..., K)$ be the sample sizes for the control and the $i$th dose group; the test statistic (one-sided) is given by (Westfall et al., 1999, p. 77)

$$T = \max_{i} \frac{\bar{y}_i - \bar{y}_0}{\sigma \sqrt{1/n_i + 1/n_0}}. \quad (14.15)$$

The multivariate $t$-distribution of $T$ in (14.15) is called one-sided Dunnett distribution with $v = \sum_{i=1}^{K+1} (n_i - 1)$ degrees of freedom. The cdf is defined by

$$F(x|K, v) = P(T \leq x). \quad (14.16)$$

The calculation of (14.16) requires numerical integrations (Hochberg and Tamhane, 1987, p. 141). Tabulation of the critical values is available from the book by Kanji (2006) and in software such as SAS.

The adjusted $p$-value corresponding to $t_i$ is given by

$$\tilde{p}_i = 1 - F\left(t_i | K, v\right). \tag{14.17}$$

If $\tilde{p}_i < \alpha$, $H_i$ is rejected, $i = 1, ..., K$.

**Fisher-Combination Test**

To test the global null hypothesis $H_0 = \cap_{i=1}^{K} H_{0i}$, we can use the so-called Fisher combination statistic,

$$\chi^2 = -2 \sum_{i=1}^{K} \ln\left(p_i\right), \tag{14.18}$$

where $p_i$ is the $p$-value for testing $H_{0i}$. When $H_{0i}$ is true, $p_i$ is uniformly distributed over [0,1]. Furthermore, if the $p_i$ $(i = 1, ..., K)$ are independent, the test statistic $\chi^2$ is distributed as a chi-square statistic with $2K$ degrees of freedom. Thus, $H_0$ is rejected if $\chi^2 \geq \chi^2_{2K, 1-\alpha}$. Note that if the $p_i$ are not independent or $H_0$ is not true (e.g., one of the $H_{0i}$ is not true), then $\chi^2$ is not necessarily a chi-square distribution.

## 14.2.2    *Stepwise Procedures*

Stepwise procedures are different from single-step procedures in the sense that a stepwise procedure must follow a specific order to test each hypothesis. In general, stepwise procedures are more powerful than single-step procedures. There are three categories of stepwise procedures which are dependent on how the stepwise tests proceed: stepup, stepdown, and fixed-sequence procedures. The commonly used stepwise procedures include the Bonferroni–Holm stepdown method (Holm, 1979), the Sidak–Holm stepdown method (Westfall et al., 1999, p. 31), Hommel's procedure (Hommel 1988), Hochberg's stepup method (Hochberg, 1990), Rom's method (Rom, 1990), and the sequential test with fixed sequences (Westfall et al., 1999).

**Stepdown Procedure**

A stepdown procedure starts with the most significant $p$-value and ends with the least significant. In this procedure, the $p$-values are arranged in ascending order,

$$p_{(1)} \leq p_{(2)} \leq \cdots \leq p_{(K)}, \tag{14.19}$$

with the corresponding hypotheses

$$H_{(1)}, H_{(2)}, ..., H_{(K)}.$$

The test proceeds from $H_{(1)}$ to $H_{(K)}$. If $p_{(k)} > C_k \alpha$ $(k = 1, ..., K)$, retain all $H_{(i)}$ $(i \geq k)$; otherwise, reject $H_{(k)}$ and continue to test $H_{(k+1)}$. The critical values $C_k$ are different for different procedures.

The adjusted $p$-values are

$$\begin{cases} \tilde{p}_1 = C_1 p_{(1)}, \\ \tilde{p}_k = \max\left(\tilde{p}_{k-1}, C_k p_{(k)}\right), \; k = 2, ..., n. \end{cases} \tag{14.20}$$

Therefore, an alternative test procedure is to compare the adjusted $p$-values against the unadjusted $\alpha$. After adjusting $p$-values, one can test the hypotheses in any order.

## Stepup Procedure

A stepup procedure starts with the least significant $p$-value and ends with the most significant $p$-value. The procedure proceeds from $H_{(K)}$ to $H_{(1)}$. If, $P_{(k)} \leq C_k \alpha$ $(k = 1, ..., K)$, reject all $H_{(i)}$ $(i \leq k)$; otherwise, retain $H_{(k)}$ and continue to test $H_{(k-1)}$. The critical values $C_k$ for the Hochberg stepup procedure are $C_k = K - k + 1$ $(k = 1, .., K)$.

The adjusted $p$-values are

$$\begin{cases} \tilde{p}_K = C_K p_{(K)}, \\ \tilde{p}_k = \min\left(\tilde{p}_{k+1}, C_k p_{(k)}\right), \; k = K - 1, ..., 1. \end{cases} \tag{14.21}$$

Therefore, an alternative test procedure is to compare the adjusted $p$-values against the unadjusted $\alpha$.

The Hochberg stepup method does not control the FWER for all correlations, but it is a little conservative when $p$-values are independent (Westfall et al., 1999, p. 33). The Rom method (1990) controls $\alpha$ exactly for independent $p$-values. However, the calculation of $C_k$ is complicated.

## Fixed-Sequence Test

This procedure is a stepdown procedure with the order of hypotheses predetermined:

$$H_1, H_2, ..., H_K.$$

The test proceeds from $H_1$ to $H_K$. If $p_k > \alpha$ $(k = 1, ..., K)$, retain all $H_i$ $(i \geq k)$. Otherwise, reject $H_k$ and continue to test $H_{k+1}$.

The adjusted $p$-values are given by

$$\tilde{p}_k = \max\left(p_1, ..., p_k\right), \; k = 1, .., K. \tag{14.22}$$

The sequence of the tests can be based on the importance of hypotheses or the power of the tests. Note that if the previous test is not significant, the next test will not proceed even if its $p$-value is extremely small.

**Dunnett Stepdown Procedure**

A commonly used stepdown procedure is the Dunnett stepdown procedure. The adjusted $p$-values are formulated as follows. First, $p$-values are arranged in a descending order,

$$t_{(1)} \geq t_{(2)} \geq \dots \geq t_{(K)},$$

with the corresponding hypotheses

$$H_{(1)}, H_{(2)}, \dots, H_{(K)}.$$

Based on (14.16), we calculate $p_k^* = 1 - F\left(t_{(k)} | K - k + 1, v\right)$, where the second argument in $F(\cdot)$ is $K - k + 1$ instead of $K$ as in the single-step Dunnett test. The adjusted $p$-values are then calculated as follows:

$$\tilde{p}_k = \begin{cases} p_1^* & \text{if } k = 1, \\ \max\left(\tilde{p}_{k-1}, p_k^*\right) & \text{if } k = 2, \dots, K. \end{cases} \tag{14.23}$$

The decision rule can be specified as: if $\tilde{p}_k < \alpha$, reject $H_{(k)}$.

**Holm Stepdown Procedure**

Suppose there are $K$ hypothesis tests $H_i$ ($i = 1, \dots, K$). The Holm stepdown procedure (Holm 1979; Dmitrienko et al., 2010) can be outlined as follows:

Step 1. If $p_{(1)} \leq \alpha/K$, reject $H_{(1)}$ and go to the next step; otherwise, retain all hypotheses and stop.

Step $i$ ($i = 2, \dots, K - 1$). If $p_{(i)} \leq \alpha/(K - i + 1)$, reject $H_{(i)}$ and go to the next step; otherwise, retain $H_{(i)}, \dots, H_{(K)}$ and stop.

Step $K$. If $p_{(K)} \leq \alpha$, reject $H_{(K)}$; otherwise, retain $H_{(K)}$.

The adjusted $p$-values are given by

$$\tilde{p}_k = \begin{cases} p_{(K)} & \text{if } k = K \\ \min\left(\tilde{p}_{k+1}, (K - k + 1)\, p_{k+1}\right) & \text{if } k = K - 1, \dots, 1. \end{cases} \tag{14.24}$$

**Shaffer Procedure**

(Shaffer 1986; Dmitrienko et al., 2010) uses logical dependencies between the hypotheses to improve the Holm procedure. The dependency means that the truth of certain hypotheses implies the truth of other hypotheses. To illustrate, suppose a trial with four dose levels and a placebo group has a treatment mean $\mu_i$ for the $i$th group ($i = 0$ for the placebo). If the null hypotheses under consideration are $H_{ij}{:}\mu_i = \mu_j$, then $H_{12}$ and $H_{13}$ imply $H_{23}$. The steps of the Shaffer procedure are similar to those for the Holm procedure, but replacing the divisors $(K - i + 1)$ by $k_i$. Here $k_i$ is the maximum number of hypotheses $H_{(i)}, ..., H_{(K)}$ that can be simultaneously true, given that $H_{(1)}, ..., H_{(i-1)}$ are false. Thus, at the $i$th step, reject $H_{(i)}$ if

$$p_{(j)} \leq \frac{\alpha}{k_j}, \; j = 1, ..., i. \tag{14.25}$$

As an example, for the five-group dose-response study, there can be $k_1 = \binom{5}{2} = 10$ pairwise comparisons (the same as for the Holm procedure). After $H_{(1)}$ is rejected, there are $k_2 = \binom{4}{2} = 6$ possible pairwise comparisons (compared to $K - i + 1 = 9$ in the Holm procedure).

**Fallback Procedure**

The Holm procedure is based on a data-driven order of testing, while the fixed-sequence procedure is based on a prefixed order of testing. A compromise between them is the so-called fallback procedure. The fallback procedure was introduced by Wiens (2003) and was further studied by Wiens and Dmitrienko (2005) and Hommel and Bretz (2008). The test procedure can be outlined as follows:

Suppose hypotheses $H_i$ ($i = 1, ..., K$) are ordered according to (14.22). We allocate the overall error rate $\alpha$ among the hypotheses according to their weights $w_i$, where $w_i \geq 0$ and $\sum_i w_i = 1$. For the fixed-sequence test, $w_1 = 1$ and $w_2 = ... = w_K = 0$.

(1) Test $H_1$ at $\alpha_1 = \alpha w_1$. If $p_1 \leq \alpha_1$, reject this hypothesis; otherwise, retain it. Go to the next step.

(2) Test $H_i$ at $\alpha_i = \alpha_{i-1} + \alpha w_i$ ($i = 2, ..., K - 1$) if $H_{i-1}$ is rejected and at $\alpha_i = \alpha w_i$ if $H_{i-1}$ is retained. If $p_i \leq \alpha_i$, reject $H_i$; otherwise, retain it. Go to the next step.

(3) Test $H_K$ at $\alpha_K = \alpha_{K-1} + \alpha w_K$ if $H_{K-1}$ is rejected and at $\alpha_K = \alpha w_K$ if $H_{K-1}$ is retained. If $p_K \leq \alpha_K$, reject $H_K$; otherwise, retain it.

**Example 14.4   Multiple Testing for Dose-Finding Trial**

Suppose that a dose-finding trial has been conducted to compare low ($L$), medium ($M$), and high ($H$) doses of a new antihypertension drug. The primary efficacy variable is diastolic blood pressure (DBP). The mean reduction in DBP is denoted by $\mu_P$, $\mu_L$, $\mu_M$, and $\mu_H$ for the placebo, and low, medium, and high doses, respectively. The global null hypothesis of equality, $\mu_P = \mu_L = \mu_M = \mu_H$, can be tested using an F-test from a model such as analysis of covariance (ANCOVA). However, for strong FWER control, this $F$-test is not sufficient. We illustrate how to apply various multiple-testing procedures to this problem. One is interested in three pairwise comparisons (one for each dose) against a placebo ($P$) with null hypotheses: $H_1 : \mu_P = \mu_L$, $H_2 : \mu_P = \mu_M$, and $H_3 : \mu_P = \mu_H$.

Denote the $p$-values for these tests by $p_1, p_2$, and $p_3$, respectively. A one-sided significance level $\alpha$ of 2.5% is used for the trial.

In the following methods or procedures (1) to (8), we assume $p_1 = 0.009$, $p_2 = 0.0085$, and $p_3 = 0.008$.

### (1) Weighted Bonferroni Procedure

Suppose we suspect the high dose may be more toxic than the low dose. Unless the high dose is more efficacious than the low dose, we will choose the low dose as the target dose. For this reason, we want to spend more alpha in the low-dose comparison than in the high-dose comparison. Specifically, we choose one-sided significance levels $\alpha_1 = 0.01$, $\alpha_2 = 0.008$, and $\alpha_3 = 0.007$ $(\alpha_1 + \alpha_2 + \alpha_3 = \alpha)$, which will be used to compare $p_1$, $p_2$, and $p_3$, respectively, for rejecting or accepting the corresponding hypotheses. Since $p_1 = 0.009 < \alpha_1$, $p_2 = 0.0085 > \alpha_2$, and $p_3 = 0.008 > \alpha_3$, we will reject $H_1$ but accept $H_2$ and $H_3$.

### (2) Simes-Bonferroni Method

We first order the $p$-values: $p_{(1)} = p_3 < p_{(2)} = p_2 < p_{(3)} = p_1$; the adjusted $p$-values calculated from (14.14) are $\tilde{p} = \max\{\frac{3}{1}p_{(1)} = 0.024, \frac{3}{2}p_{(2)} = 0.01275, \frac{3}{3}p_{(3)} = 0.009\} = 0.024 < \alpha$. Therefore, the global hypotheses $(\mu_P = \mu_L = \mu_M = \mu_H)$ are rejected, and we conclude that one or more dose levels are effective, but the testing procedure has not indicated which one.

### (3) Fisher Combination Method

This method usually requires independent $p$-values; otherwise, the test may be on the conservative or liberal side. However, for illustrating the calculation procedure, let's pretend the $p$-values are independent. From (14.18), we can calculate the chi-square value: $\chi^2 = -2\ln((0.009)(0.0085)(0.008)) = 28.62$ with 6 degrees of freedom. The corresponding $p$-value is $0.0001 < \alpha$. Thus, the global null hypothesis is rejected.

### (4) Fixed-Sequence Procedure

Suppose we have fixed the test sequence as $H_3, H_2, H_1$ before we see the data. Since $p_3 < \alpha$, we reject $H_3$ and continue to test $H_2$. Because $p_2 < \alpha$, we reject $H_2$ and continue to test $H_1$. Since $p_1 < \alpha$, we reject $H_1$.

### (5) Holm Procedure

Since $p_{(1)} = p_3 = 0.008 < \alpha/K = 0.025/3$, reject $H_3$ and continue to test $H_2$. Because $p_{(2)} = p_2 = 0.0085 < \alpha/(K-2+1) = 0.025/2 = 0.0125$, reject $H_2$ and continue to test $H_1$. Since $p_1 = 0.009 < \alpha/(K-3+1) = 0.025$, $H_1$ is rejected.

### (6) Shaffer Procedure

Since $p_{(1)} = p_3 = 0.008 < \alpha/k_1 = 0.025/3$, reject $H_3$. After $H_3$ is rejected, $H_1$ and $H_2$ can be simultaneously true, but $k_2 = 2$ and $p_{(2)} = p_2 = 0.0085 < \alpha/k_2 = 0.025/2 = 0.0125$, so reject $H_2$. We have only $H_1$ left, and thus $k_3 = 1$ and $p_1 = 0.009 < \alpha/(K - 3 + 1) = 0.025$; $H_1$ is rejected. We can see that in this case the Holm and Shaffer procedures are equivalent. This is because we are not interested in the other possible comparisons: $\mu_1$ versus $\mu_2$, $\mu_2$ versus $\mu_3$, and $\mu_3$ versus $\mu_1$.

**(7) Fallback Procedure**

Choose equal weights $w_i = 1/K = 1/3$. $\alpha_1 = \alpha/3 = 0.00833$, $\alpha_2 = \alpha_1 + \alpha/3 = 0.0167$, and $\alpha_3 = \alpha_2 + \alpha/3 = \alpha = 0.025$. Since $p_1 = 0.009 > \alpha_1$, $p_2 = 0.0085 < \alpha_2$, and $p_3 = 0.008 < \alpha_3$, $H_1$ is retained but $H_2$ and $H_3$ are rejected.

**(8) Hochberg Stepup Procedure**

Since $p_{(3)} = 0.009 < \alpha = 0.025$, we reject all three hypotheses, $H_1$, $H_2$, and $H_3$. The adjusted $p$-values $\tilde{p}_1$, $\tilde{p}_2$, and $\tilde{p}_3$ can be calculated using (14.21).

**(9) Dunnett's Procedure**

Suppose the adjusted $p$-values calculated from (14.17) (requiring a software package) are $\tilde{p}_1 = 0.027 > \alpha$, $\tilde{p}_2 = 0.021 < \alpha$, and $\tilde{p}_3 = 0.019 < \alpha$. Then, we reject $H_2$ and $H_3$ but retain $H_1$.

**(10) Dunnett's Stepdown Procedure**

Suppose the test statistics $t_{(1)} = t_3 > t_{(2)} = t_2 > t_{(3)} = t_1$ for the three hypotheses $H_3, H_2$, and $H_1$. Assume that the $p$-values are $p_1^* = 0.019$, $p_2^* = 0.018$, and $p_3^* = 0.0245$ for the hypotheses $H_{(1)} = H_3, H_{(2)} = H_2$, and $H_{(3)} = H_1$, respectively. The adjusted $p$-values can be calculated from (14.23): $\tilde{p}_1 = p_1^* = 0.019 < \alpha$, $\tilde{p}_2 = \max(\tilde{p}_1, p_2^*) = 0.019 < \alpha$, $\tilde{p}_3 = \max(\tilde{p}_2, p_1^*) = 0.0245 < \alpha$. Then, we reject $H_3, H_2$, and $H_1$.

### 14.2.3 Common Gatekeeper Procedure

The gatekeeper procedure (Dmitrienko et al., 2005, pp. 106–127) is an extension of the fixed-sequence method. The method is motivated by the following hypothesis-testing problems in clinical trials. (1) Benefit of secondary endpoints can be claimed in the drug label only if the primary endpoint is statistically significant. (2) If there are coprimary endpoints (multiple primary endpoints), secondary endpoints can be claimed only if one of the primary endpoints is statistically significant. (3) In multiple-endpoint problems, the endpoints can be grouped based on their clinical importance.

Suppose there are $K$ null hypotheses to test. We group them into $m$ families. Each family is a composite of hypotheses. The null hypotheses in the $i$th $(i = 1, ..., m_i)$ family are denoted by either a serial gatekeeper

$$F_i = H_{i1} \cup H_{i2} \cup ... \cup H_{im_i} \qquad (14.26)$$

or a parallel gatekeeper

$$F_i = H_{i1} \cap H_{i2} \cap ... \cap H_{im_i}. \qquad (14.27)$$

The hypothesis test proceeds from the first family, $F_1$, to the last family, $F_m$. To test $F_i$ $(i = 2, ..., m)$, the test procedure has to pass $i - 1$ previous gatekeepers, i.e., reject all $F_k$ $(k = 1, ..., i - 1)$ at the predetermined level of significance $\alpha$.

For a parallel gatekeeper we can either weakly or strongly control the familywise type-I error. For a serial gatekeeper, we always strongly control the familywise error. The serial gatekeeping procedure is straightforward: test each family of null hypotheses sequentially at a level $\alpha$ with any strong $\alpha$-control method.

The stepwise procedure of parallel gatekeeping proposed by Dmitrienko and Tamhane (2007) can be described as follows: The procedure is built around the concept of a rejection gain factor. At the $k$th stage, the significance test is performed at the $\rho_k \alpha$ level, $k = 1, 2, ..., m$, where $\alpha$ is the FWER, and the rejection gain factor, $0 \leq \rho_k \leq 1$ (with $\rho_1 = 1$), depends on the number and importance of the hypotheses rejected at the earlier stages.

The stepwise parallel gatekeeping procedure for testing the null hypotheses in $F_1, ..., F_m$ can be performed as follows:

(1) Family $F_k$, $k = 1, ..., m - 1$: Test the null hypotheses using the Bonferroni test at the $\rho_k \alpha$ level.
(2) Family $F_m$: Test the null hypotheses using the weighted Holm test at the $\rho_m \alpha$ level.

The rejection gain factors $\rho_i$ are given by

$$\rho_1 = 1, \ \rho_k = \prod_{i=1}^{k-1} \left( \sum_{j=1}^{m_i} r_{ij} w_{ij} \right), \ k = 2, ..., m, \qquad (14.28)$$

where the weights $w_{ij} \geq 0$ with $\sum_{j=1}^{n_i} w_{ij} = 1$ represent the importance of the null hypotheses in $F_i$, and $r_{ij} = 1$ if $H_{ij}$ is rejected and 0 otherwise. For equally weighted hypotheses ($w_{ij} = 1/m_i$), the formula for $\rho_k$ reduces to

$$\rho_k = \prod_{i=1}^{k-1} \left( \frac{r_i}{m_i} \right), k = 2, ..., m, \qquad (14.29)$$

where $r_i = \sum_j r_{ij}$ is the number of rejected hypotheses in $F_i$. Thus, $\rho_k$ is the product of the proportions of previously rejected hypotheses in $F_1$ through $F_{k-1}$.

The modified adjusted $p$-value for $H_{ij}$, $i = 2, ..., m$, is given by $p_{ij}^* = \tilde{p}_{ij}/\rho_i$, where $\tilde{p}_{ij}$ is the usual adjusted $p$-value produced by the multiple tests within $F_i$. Inferences in $F_2, ..., F_m$ can be performed by $p_{ij}^*$ to the prespecified FWER, $\alpha$.

## Example 14.5    Multiple Testing for Primary and Secondary Endpoints

This example was given by Dmitrienko and Tamhane (2007). The trial was designed to compare a single dose of an experimental drug with a placebo. Two families of endpoints were considered in this trial. $F_1$ consisted of two hypotheses related to the primary endpoints, P1 (lung function) and P2 (mortality), and $F_2$ consisted of two hypotheses related to the secondary endpoints, S1 (ICU-free days) and S2 (quality of life). The raw $p$-values $p_{ij}$ for the endpoints P1, P2, S1, and S2 are 0.048, 0.003, 0.026, and 0.002, respectively. $F_1$ was chosen as a parallel gatekeeper. P1 was deemed more important than P2 in $F_1$ with weights $w_{11} = 0.9$ and $w_{12} = 0.1$, respectively; S1 and S2 were considered equally important with weight $w_{21} = w_{22} = 0.5$. The FWER is to be controlled at $\alpha = 0.05$.

To apply the stepwise parallel gatekeeping procedure, one first considers the adjusted $p$-values produced by the weighted Bonferroni test and the Holm test for the null hypotheses in $F_1$ and $F_2$, respectively. The adjusted $p$-values $\tilde{p}_{ij}$ for the endpoints P1, P2, S1, and S2 are $0.048/0.9 = 0.053$ (the weighted Bonferroni test), $0.003/0.1 = 0.03$ (the weighted Bonferroni test), $0.026$ (the Holm test), and $0.002 \times 2 = 0.004$, respectively. Next, since $\rho_1 = 1$, the primary hypotheses are tested at the full $\alpha = 0.05$ level. The P2 comparison is significant at this level, whereas the P1 comparison is not. Therefore, the rejection gain factor for the secondary family based on (14.31) is $\rho_2 = w_{12} = 0.1$, and the adjusted $p$-values for S1 and S2 are $0.026/\rho_2 = 0.260$ and $0.004/\rho_2 = 0.040$, respectively. It is clear that only the hypothesis concerning S2 is rejected.

### 14.2.4   Tree Gatekeeping Procedure

The tree gatekeeping procedure (TGP) is a stepwise procedure that combines the characteristics of both the parallel and series gatekeeping methods. For each individual hypothesis $H_{ij}$ in family $F_i$, where $i = 2, ..., m$, $j = 1, ..., n_i$, we define two associated hypothesis sets: the serial rejection set, $R_{ij}^S$, and the parallel rejection set, $R_{ij}^P$. These sets consist of some hypotheses from $F_1, ..., F_{i-1}$; at least one of them is nonempty. Without loss of generality, we assume $R_{ij}^S$ and $R_{ij}^P$ do not overlap.

Dmitrienko et al. (2007) developed Bonferroni-based and resampling-based tree gatekeeping procedures. The Bonferroni-based tree-gatekeeping procedure is described as follows.

Let $H$ be any nonempty intersection of the hypotheses $H_{ij}$ and let $w_{ij}(H)$ be the weight assigned to the hypothesis $H_{ij} \in H$. From (14.14), we know that the Bonferroni (adjusted) $p$-value for testing $H$ is given by $p(H) = \min_{i,j}\{\frac{p_{ij}}{w_{ij}(H)}\}$. Because there can be more than one $H$ that includes each $H_{ij}$, we need to further adjust the $p$-value $p(H)$. The multiplicity-adjusted $p$-value for the null hypothesis $H_{ij}$ is defined as $\tilde{p}_{ij} = \max_{H}\{p(H)\}$, where the maximum is taken over all intersection hypotheses $H$ such that $H_{ij} \subseteq H$. The rejection rules are to reject $H_{ij}$ if $\tilde{p}_{ij} \leq \alpha$ and to retain $H_{ij}$ otherwise.

The testing procedure above for the adjusted $p$-value is based on the closure principle, which requires us to construct the weight $w_{ij}(H)$ appropriately. For convenience, we define two indicator variables: let $\delta_{ij}(H) = 0$ if $H_{ij} \in H$ and 1 otherwise, and let $\xi_{ij}(H) = 0$ if $H$ contains any hypothesis from $R_{ij}^S$ or all hypotheses from $R_{ij}^P$ and 1 otherwise. The following three conditions together for the weights will constitute a sufficient condition for using the closure principle and, thus, for the TGP, also.

**Condition 1:**   For any intersection hypothesis $H$, $w_{ij}(H) \geq 0$, $\sum_{j=1}^{m_i} w_{ij}(H) \leq 1$ and $w_{ij}(H) = 0$ if $\delta_{ij}(H) = 0$ or $\xi_{ij}(H) = 0$.

**Condition 2:**   $w_i(H) = (w_{i1}(H), ..., w_{im_i}(H))$ is a vector function of the weights $w_1(H), ..., w_{i-1}(H)$ $(i = 2, ..., m)$ and does not depend on $w_{i+1}(H), ..., w_m(H)$ $(i = 1, ..., m - 1)$.

**Condition 3:**   The weights for $F_1, ..., F_{m-1}$ meet the monotonicity condition, i.e. $w_{ij}(H) \leq w_{ij}(H^*)$, $i = 1, ..., m - 1$, if $H_{ij} \in H$, $H_{ij} \in H^*$, and $H^* \subseteq H$.

## 14.3 Multiple-Endpoint Adaptive Design

In this section, we will discuss adaptive designs for multiple-endpoint trials. Kieser (1999) proposed a test procedure, in which he considered multiple-endpoint tests at each time-point and multiple-endpoint adjustments are made in the same way as classical design based on $\alpha$ spent on each time point (e.g., $\alpha_1$ for the first interim analysis). In contrast, Tang and Geller (1999) proposed a different approach for classical group sequential design, in which, they view different endpoints hierarchically, and fixed sequence tests are constructed based on the importance of the endpoints. The Tang–Geller method is more powerful than Kieser's method. We will extend Tang-Geller's method in our example.

### 14.3.1 *Tang–Geller Method*

Tang and Geller (1999) proposed the following test procedures to group sequential design with multiple endpoints.

Let $M = \{1, 2, ..., m\}$ be the set of indices for the $m$ endpoints. Let $F$ denote a nonempty subset of $M$ and $H_{0,F}$ the null hypothesis $u_i = 0$ for $i \in F$. Let $T_F$ be a test statistic for $H_{0,F}$. Consider a group sequential trial with $K$ analyses. We use $T_{F,t}$ to indicate the dependence of $T_F$ on the analysis time $t$. Let $\{\alpha_{F,t}, t = 1, 2, ..., K\}$ be a one-sided stopping boundary for testing $H_{0,F}$ such that $P_{H_{0,F}}\{T_{F,t} > \alpha_{F,t}$ for some $t \} \leq \alpha$. For a given vector $u$, let $I_u = \{i, u_i = 0\}$.

Tang and Geller (1999) proposed the following two procedures that preserve strong control of type-I error.

**Procedure 1**

Step 1. Conduct interim analyses to test $H_{0,M}$, based on the group sequential boundary $\{\alpha_{M,t}, \ t = 1, 2, ..., K\}$.

Step 2. When $H_{0,M}$ is rejected, say, at time $t^*$, stop the trial and apply the closed testing procedure to test all the other hypotheses $H_{0,F}$ using $T_{F,t^*}$ with $\alpha_{F,t^*}$ as the critical value.

Step 3. If the trial continues to the last analysis without rejection of $H_{0,M}$, then no hypotheses are rejected.

**Proof:** A type-I error occurs if, for some $F \subseteq I_u$, $H_{0,F}$ is rejected, where $u$ denotes the underlying parameter vector (e.g., difference in mean, response rate, or median survival time). According to the closed testing procedure, $H_{0,F}$ can be rejected only if $H_{0,I_u}$ is rejected. Thus, {type-I error occurs} $= \cup_{t=1}^{K}$ {type-I error occurs at time $t$ } $\subseteq \cup_{t=1}^{K}$ {reject $H_{0,I_u}$ at time $t$} $\subseteq \cup_{t=1}^{K}\{T_{I_u,t} > \alpha_{I_u,t}\} = \{T_{I_u,t} > \alpha_{I_u,t}$, for some $t, 1 \leq t \leq K\}$. Hence, the probability of making at least one type-I error is at most $P\{T_{I_u,t} > \alpha_{I_u,t},$ for some $t\} \leq \alpha$.

Procedure 1 does not allow continuation of the trial once the global test crosses its boundary. Tang and Geller (1999) further developed Procedure 2 below, which allows the trial to continue until all hypotheses are rejected or the last analysis is conducted.

**Procedure 2**

Step 1. Conduct interim analyses to test $H_{0,K}$, based on the stopping boundary $\{\alpha_{K,t}, t = 1, 2, ..., K\}$.

Step 2. When $H_{0,M}$ is rejected, say, at time $t^*$, apply the closed testing procedure to test all the other hypotheses $H_{0,F}$ using $T_{F,t^*}$ with $\alpha_{F,t^*}$ as the critical value.

Step 3. If any hypothesis is not rejected, continue the trial to the next stage, in which the closed testing procedure is repeated, with the previously rejected hypotheses automatically rejected without retesting.

Step 4. Reiterate step 3 until all hypotheses are rejected or the last stage is reached.

We can modify Procedure 2 slightly to obtain the following procedure.

**Procedure 3**

Step 1. Conduct interim analyses (IA) to test $H_{0,K}$, based on the group sequential boundary $\{\alpha_{K,t}, t = 1, 2, ..., K\}$.

Step 2. When $H_{0,M}$ is rejected, say, at time $t^*$, apply the closed testing procedure to test all the other hypotheses $H_{0,F}$ using $T_{F,t^{**}}$ with $\alpha_{F,t^{**}}$ as the critical value for any predetermined IA time $t^{**} \leq t^*$.

Step 3. If any hypothesis is not rejected, continue the trial to the next stage, in which the closed testing procedure is repeated, with the previously rejected hypotheses automatically rejected without retesting.

Step 4. Reiterate step 3 until all hypotheses are rejected or the last stage is reached.

### 14.3.2    *Single Primary with Secondary Endpoints*

**Example 14.6    Three-Stage Adaptive Design for NHL Trial**

A phase-III two parallel group non-Hodgkin's lymphoma trial was designed with three analyses. The primary endpoint is progression-free survival (PFS), the secondary endpoints are (1) overall response rate (ORR) including complete and partial response and (2) complete response rate (CRR). The estimated median PFS is 7.8 months and 10 months for the control and test groups, respectively. Assume a uniform enrollment with an accrual period of 9 months and a total study duration of 23 months. The estimated ORR is 16% for the control group and 45% for the test group. The classical design with a fixed sample size of 375 subjects per group will allow for detecting a 3-month difference in median PFS with 82% power at a one-sided significance level of $\alpha = 0.025$. The first IA will be conducted on the first 125 patients/group (or total $N_1 = 250$) based on ORR. The objective of the first IA is to modify the randomization. Specifically, if the difference in ORR (test-control) $\Delta_{ORR} > 0$, the enrollment will continue. If $\Delta_{ORR} \leq 0$, then the enrollment will stop. If the enrollment is terminated prematurely, there will be one final analysis for efficacy based on PFS and possible efficacy claimed on the secondary endpoints. If the enrollment continues, there will be an interim analysis based on PFS and the final analysis of PFS. When the primary endpoint (PFS) is significant, the analyses for the secondary endpoints will be performed for the potential claim on the secondary endpoints. During the interim analyses, the patient enrollment will not stop. The number of patients at each stage is approximately as shown in Figure 14.1.

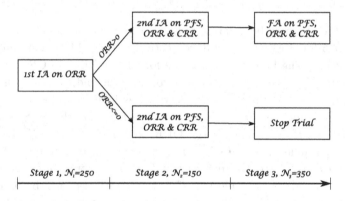

Figure 14.1:   Multiple-Endpoint Adaptive Design

We use Teng–Geller's procedure with MINP and MSP for this trial as illustrated below.

**Inverse-Normal Method**

The test statistic at the $k$th analysis is defined as

$$z_{ik} = \sum_{j=1}^{k} w_{kj} \Phi^{-1}(1 - p_{ij}), \tag{14.32}$$

where the subscript $i$ represents the $i$th endpoint, i.e., 1 for PFS, 2 for

ORR, 3 for CRR. $p_{ij}$ is the stagewise $p$-value for the $i$th endpoint based on the subsample from the $j$th stage.

$$w_{kj} = \sqrt{\frac{N_k}{\sum_{j=1}^{k} N_j}}. \tag{14.33}$$

The first IA is not intended to claim efficacy or futility, but to modify the enrollment (continue or not continue enrollment) based ORR. The stagewise test statistic is given by

$$z_{i1} = (1 - p_{i1}). \tag{14.34}$$

At the second IA, the test statistic is given by

$$Z_{i2} = 0.8\Phi^{-1}(1 - p_{i1}) + 0.6\Phi^{-1}(1 - p_{i2}). \tag{14.35}$$

If the trial continues after the second IA, the test statistic at final analysis will be

$$Z_{i3} = 0.58\Phi^{-1}(1 - p_{i1}) + 0.45\Phi^{-1}(1 - p_{i2}) + 0.68\Phi^{-1}(1 - p_{i3}). \tag{14.36}$$

The OF stopping boundaries on the $z$-scale are $\alpha_1 = 3.490$, $\alpha_2 = 2.468$, $\alpha_3 = 2.015$ for stage 1, 2, and 3, respectively (Table 14.3). For simplicity, the same stopping boundaries are used for PFS, ORR, and CRR.

Denote $H_{0ij}$ the null hypothesis for the $i$th endpoint at $j$th stage. The gatekeeper test procedure is described as follows: Construct the first hypothesis family as $F_1 = H_{011} \cap H_{012} \cap H_{013}$ for the PFS, similarly $F_2 = H_{021} \cap H_{022} \cap H_{023}$ for the ORR, and $F_3 = H_{031} \cap H_{032} \cap H_{033}$. $F_1$ is tested at level $\alpha$; if $F_1$ is not rejected, no further test will be conducted. If $F_1$ is rejected, we further test $F_2$. If $F_2$ is not rejected, no further test will proceed. If $F_2$ is rejected, $F_3$ is tested. All tests will be conducted at the same level $\alpha = 0.025$. The (closed set) gatekeeper procedure ensures the strong control of FWE. Note that due to the correlation between PFS and ORR, we cannot just consider a two-stage weighting test statistic for PFS, even if the hypothesis test for PFS is not performed at the first IA.

Suppose at the first IA, the stagewise $p$-value for the primary endpoint (PFS) is $p_{11} = 0.030$ and the test statistic is $z_{11} = \Phi^{-1}(1 - p_{11}) = 1.881 < \alpha_1$; therefore, the trial continues. At the second IA, the stagewise $p$-value $p_{12} = 0.034$, and the test statistic $z_{12} = 2.6$ is calculated from (14.35). Therefore, the null hypothesis for PFS is rejected and trial stops. Because the PFS is rejected, we can now test ORR. Suppose the stagewise $p$-value for ORR is $p_{21} = 0.002$ and $z_{21} = \Phi^{-1}(1 - p_{21}) = 3.60 > 3.490$;

hence, the null hypothesis for ORR is rejected. Because ORR is rejected, we can proceed with the test for CRR. Suppose that $p_{31} = 0.1$ and $z_{31} = 1.281 < \alpha_1$; $p_{32} = 0.12$ and $z_{32} = 1.73 (< \alpha_2)$ from (14.35). Due to rejection of PFS at the second IA, the trial was stopped. However, the enrollment was not stopped during the interim analyses. At the time when the decision was made to stop the trial, 640 patients (approximately 320 per group) were enrolled. The gatekeeper procedure allows us to proceed to the third analysis of CRR. However, the rejection boundary needs to be recalculated through numerical integration or simulation based on the OB-F spending function. Based on the information time $\sqrt{640/750} = 0.92376$, the new rejection boundary is approximately $\alpha_{33}^* = 2.10$. Suppose that the observed $p_{33} = 0.065$ and the test statistic $z_{33} = 2.3$ is calculated from (14.36). Therefore CRR is also rejected. We can see that PFS, ORR, and CRR were all rejected, but at different times!!! The closed test project allows the rejections of different endpoints at different times (IAs) as illustrated in this example. The calculation is summarized in Table 14.3.

Table 14.3: MINP Based on Hypothetical $p_{ik}$

| IA ($k$) | $\alpha_k$ | PFS | | ORR | | CRR | |
|---|---|---|---|---|---|---|---|
| | | $p_{1k}$ | $z_{1k}$ | $p_{2k}$ | $z_{2k}$ | $p_{3k}$ | $z_{3k}$ |
| 1 | 3.490 | 0.030 | 1.881 | 0.0002 | 3.60 | 0.10 | 1.281 |
| 2 | 2.468 | 0.034 | 2.600 | | | 0.12 | 1.730 |
| 3 | 2.015 | | | | | 0.065 | 2.300 |

### Recursive Two-stage Adaptive Design with MSP

We now use the recursive two-stage adaptive design (Chapter 10) as described in the following steps:

(1) Calculate the sample size based on the classical fixed sample-size design.

For median times of 7.8 months and 10 months for the two groups, an enrollment duration of 9 months, and a trial duration of 23 months, a sample size of 350/group will allow for detecting a 2.2-month difference in PFS with approximately 80% power at one-sided $\alpha = 0.025$.

(2) Design the first two-stage trial.

The IA will be conducted based on a sample size of $n_1 = 150$ subjects per group. Using MSP, we decide the stopping boundaries at IA: $\alpha_1 = 0.01$

and $\beta_1 = \alpha_2 = 0.1832$. From (8.49) or (4.8), we obtain:

$$\alpha_2 = \sqrt{2(\alpha - \alpha_1)} + \alpha_1$$
$$= (2(0.025 - 0.01))^{0.5} + 0.01$$
$$= 0.1832$$

(3) Conduct the first interim analysis.

Assume $p_{11} = 0.030 > \alpha_1$ and the null hypothesis for PFS is not rejected. The trial should proceed to the next stage.

(4) Decide whether to redesign a new two-stage trial.

To determine if we need to redesign a new two-stage trial, the conditional error is calculated as $\pi_2 = \alpha_2 - p_{11} = 0.1832 - 0.03 = 0.1532$. To have 90% conditional power, a total of 241 subjects/group are required based on (11.6) or SAS Macro 11.2 (assumed the standard effect size $= 0.21$). We decided to add a new two-stage design, $n_{21} = 150$ for second IA (the first stage of the second two-stage design), which provides a conditional reject probability of 79%. The stopping boundaries for the second two-stage design are specified as follows: $\alpha_{21} = 0.15$, Let $\beta_{21} = \alpha_{22}$. Thus, we obtain:

$$\alpha_{22} = \sqrt{2(\pi_2 - \alpha_{21})} + \alpha_{21}$$
$$= (2(0.1532 - 0.15))^{0.5} + 0.15$$
$$= 0.23$$

Note that we also need to determine the stopping boundaries for ORR and CRR, but they don't have to be the same, i.e., the stopping boundaries can be different for different endpoints. However, the new stopping boundaries have to be determined for all endpoints at each interim analysis regardless of the endpoint for which the IA was performed. For simplicity, we use the same stopping boundaries for all three endpoints.

(5) Perform the second interim analysis.

Assume $p_{12} = 0.04$. Therefore, the $p$-value for the PFS at the second IA is $p_{11} + p_{12} = 0.03 + 0.04 = 0.07 < \alpha_{21} = 0.15$. Hence, the null hypothesis for the PFS is rejected.

(6) Because the null hypothesis family $F_1$ for PFS is rejected, we proceed to the test for ORR. Assume $p_{21} = 0.007 < \alpha_1 = 0.01$. Hence, the null hypothesis ORR is rejected.

(7) Because ORR is rejected, we proceed to the test for CRR. Assume $p_{31} = 0.05 > \alpha_1 = 0.01$ at the first IA. At the second IA, the test statistic $T_2 = p_{31} + p_{32} = 0.05 + 0.11 = 0.16 > \alpha_{21} = 0.15$. At the last analysis, the

test statistic; for CRR is $T_2 = p_{31} + p_{32} + p_{33} = 0.05 + 0.11 + 0.05 = 0.21 < \alpha_{22} = 0.23$, therefore, the null hypothesis for CRR is rejected (see Table 14.4).

Table 14.4:  RTAD Based on Hypothetical $p_{ik}$

|        |            | PFS      | ORR      | CRR      |
|--------|------------|----------|----------|----------|
| IA $(k)$ | $\alpha_k$ | $p_{1k}$ | $p_{2k}$ | $p_{3k}$ |
| 1      | 0.01       | 0.03     | 0.007    | 0.05     |
| 2      | 0.15       | 0.04     |          | 0.11     |
| 3      | 0.23       |          |          | 0.05     |

## 14.4   Summary and Discussion

In this chapter, we have introduced several important concepts, principles, and test procedures for multiplicity issues. The closure principle is a very useful tool, from which many test procedures are developed including the stepup, stepdown, fixed sequence, and gatekeeper procedures. We introduced Tang and Geller's test procedure for adaptive designs and illustrated its application with trial examples.

## Problems

**14.1** Suppose in Example 14.4, the $p$-values corresponding to the three hypotheses $H_1$, $H_2$, and $H_3$ are $p_1 = 0.007$, $p_2 = 0.008$, and $p_3 = 0.009$. Decide to reject or accept hypotheses $H_1$, $H_2$, and $H_3$ using the multiple testing procedures (1) through (8).

**14.2** In Example 14.6, suppose $p_{11} = 0.032$ but everything else is unchanged. Use Teng–Geller's procedure with MINP to perform the analyses (to reject or accept the hypotheses for the primary and secondary endpoints).

# Chapter 15

# Pick-the-Winners Design

## 15.1 Opportunity

An adaptive seamless phase-II/III design is one of the most attractive adaptive designs. A seamless adaptive design is a combination of traditional phase-II and phase-III trials. In seamless design, there is usually a so-called learning phase that serves the same purpose as a traditional phase-II trial, followed by a confirmatory phase that serves the same objectives as a traditional phase-III trial (Figure 15.1). Compared to traditional designs, a seamless design can reduce sample size and time-to-market for a positive drug candidate. The main feature of a seamless design is the drop-loser mechanism. Sometimes it also allows for adding new treatment arms. A seamless design usually starts with several arms or treatment groups. At the end of the learning phase, inferior arms (losers) are identified and dropped from the confirmatory phase.

Hung, O'Neill, Wang and Lawrence from FDA (2006) articulate that it may be advisable to redistribute the remaining planned sample size of a terminated arm to the remaining treatment arms for comparison so that coupled with use of a proper valid adaptive test, one may enhance the statistical power of the design to detect a dose that is effective (Hung et al., 2006).

In this chapter, we will discuss different methods for seamless designs. Examples are provided to illustrate how to design seamless adaptive trials using an SAS macro.

### 15.1.1 *Impact Overall Alpha Level and Power*

A seamless design can enjoy the following advantages of potential savings by early stopping for futility and efficacy. A seamless design is efficient

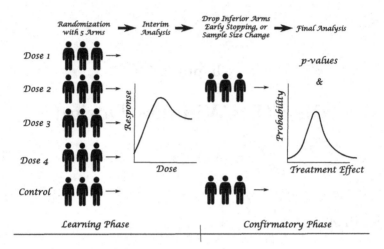

Figure 15.1:   Seamless Design

because there is no lead time between the learning and confirmatory phases, and the data collected at the learning phase are combined for final analysis. A noticeable feature of the seamless phase-II/III design is that there are differences in controlling type-I error rate (alpha) and power between a seamless design and the traditional design with separate phase-II and phase-III trials. In traditional designs, if we view the two phase-II and III trials as a super experiment, the actual $\alpha$ is equal to $\alpha_{II}\alpha_{III}$, where $\alpha_{II}$ and $\alpha_{III}$ are the type-I error rates controlled at phase II and phase III, respectively. If two phase-III trials are required, then $\alpha = \alpha_{II}\alpha_{III}\alpha_{III}$. In seamless phase-II/III design, actual $\alpha = \alpha_{III}$; if two phase-III trials are required, then $\alpha = \alpha_{III}\alpha_{III}$. Thus, the $\alpha$ for a seamless design is actually $1/\alpha_{II}$ times larger than the traditional design. Similarly, in the classical "super experiment," the actual power is equal to $\text{Power}_{II}\,\text{Power}_{III}$, while in a seamless phase-II/III design, actual power is equal to $\text{Power}_{III}$, where $\text{Power}_{II}$ and $\text{Power}_{III}$ are the power for phase-II and III trials, respectively. Therefore, the power for a seamless design is $1/Power_{II}$ times larger than the traditional design.

### 15.1.2   Reduction in Expected Trial Duration

As pointed out by Walton (2006), time between studies has multiple components: (1) analysis of observed data, (2) interpretation of analyzed results, (3) planning next study, (4) resource allocation, (5) selection of, and agreements with, investigators, (6) Institutional Review Board (IRB) submission and approval, and (7) other. In a seamless design, we move the majority of the "planning next study" to up-front, perform analysis at real time, and combined traditional two IRB submissions and approvals into one. Also, in seamless design there is one set of "selection of, agreements with, investigators" instead of two. Adaptive designs require adaptive or dynamic allocation of resources. At the end of traditional phase-IIb design, the analysis and interpretations of results are mainly performed by the sponsor and the "go and no-go" decision making is fully made by the sponsor unless there is a major safety concern. In seamless design, the traditional phase IIb becomes the first phase of the seamless design and IDMC has a big influence on the decision. From that point of view, seamless design is less biased.

There could be competing constraints among "faster," "cheaper," and "better" as noted by Walton (2006; see Figure 15.2). It is challenging to satisfy all goals simultaneously. Decision theory in conjunction with adaptive design is a way to balance the limits to satisfying these goals.

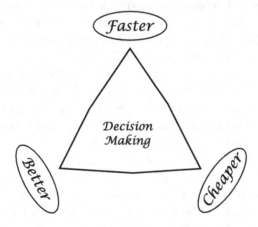

Figure 15.2: Decision Theory for Competing Constraints

### 15.1.3 *Overview of Multiple-Arm Designs*

Multiple-arm dose-response study has been studied since early 1990s. Under the assumption of monotonicity in dose response, Williams (1971, 1972) proposed a test to determine the lowest dose level at which there is evidence for a difference from the control. Cochran (1954), Amitage (1955), and Nam (1987) studied the Cochran–Amitage test for monotonic trend.

For the strong familywise type-I error control, Dunnett's test (1955, 1964) that is based on multivariate normal distribution is most often used. Recently multiple-arm adaptive designs have been studied. A typical multiple-arm confirmatory adaptive design (often called drop-the-loser, drop-arm, or pick-the-winner design or adaptive dose-finding design or phase-II/III seamless design) consists of two stages: a selection stage and a confirmation stage. For the selection stage, a randomized parallel design with several doses and a placebo group is employed for selection of doses. After the best dose is chosen (the winner), the patients of the selected dose group and placebo group continue and enter the confirmation stage. New patients will be recruited and randomized to receive the selected dose or placebo. The final analysis is performed with the cumulative data of patients from both stages (Chang 2011, Maca et al., 2006).

Liu and Hsiao (2011) proposed a seamless design to allow prespecifying probabilities of rejecting the drug at each stage to improve the efficiency of the trial. Posch, Maurer, and Bretz (2011) described two approaches to control the type-I error rate in adaptive designs with sample-size reassessment and/or treatment selection. The first method adjusts the critical value using a simulation-based approach, which incorporates the number of patients at an interim analysis, the true response rates, the treatment selection rule, etc. The second method is an adaptive Bonferroni–Holm test procedure based on conditional error rates of the individual treatment–control comparisons. Posch et al. showed that this procedure controls the type-I error rate, even if a deviation from a preplanned adaptation rule or the time point of such a decision is necessary.

Shun, Lan, and Soo (2008) considered a study starting with two treatment groups and a control group with a planned interim analysis. The inferior treatment group would be dropped after the interim analysis. Such an interim analysis could be based on the clinical endpoint or a biomarker. The unconditional distribution of the final test statistic from the "winner" treatment is skewed and requires numerical integration or simulations for the calculation. To avoid complex computations, they propose a normal approximation approach to calculate the type-I error, the power, the point estimate, and the confidence intervals.

Heritier, Lô and Morgan (2011) studied the type-I error control of seamless unbalanced designs, issues of noninferiority comparison, multiplicity of secondary endpoints, and covariance adjusted analyses. Further extensions of seamless designs also exist, which allow adaptive designs to continue seamlessly either in a subpopulation of patients or in the whole population on the basis of data obtained from the first stage of a phase-II/III design. Jenkins, Stone, and Jennison (2011) proposed a design that adds extra flexibility by also allowing the trial to continue in all patients but with both the subgroup and the full population as coprimary populations when the phase-II and III endpoints are different but correlated time-to-event endpoints.

## 15.2  Pick-the-Winner Design

Suppose in a $K$-group trial, we define the global null hypothesis as $H_G$ : $\mu_0 = \mu_1 = \mu_2 = \ldots = \mu_K$ and the hypothesis test between the selected arm (winner) and the control as

$$H_G : \mu_0 = \mu_s, \ s = \text{selected arm.} \tag{15.1}$$

Chang and Wang (2014) have derived formulations for the two-stage pick-the-winner design with any number of arms. The design starts with all doses under consideration; at the interim analysis, the winner with the best response observed will continue to the second stage with the control group.

Suppose a trial starts with $K$ dose groups (arms) and one control arm (arm 0). The maximum sample size for each group is $N$. The interim analysis will perform on $N_1$ independent observations per group, $x_{ij}$ from $N\left(\mu_i, \sigma^2\right)$ $(i = 0, ..., K; j = 1, ..., N_1)$. The active arm with maximum response at the interim analysis and the control arm will be selected and additional $N_2 = N - N_1$ subjects in each arm will be recruited. Denote by $\bar{x}_i$ the mean of the first $N_1$ observations in the $i$th arm $(i = 0, 1, ..., K)$, and $\bar{y}_i$ the mean of the additional $N_2$ observations $y_{ij}$ from $N\left(\mu_i, \sigma^2\right)$ $(i = 0, S; j = 1, ..., N_2)$. Here, arm $S$ is the active arm selected for the second stage. Let $t_i = \frac{\bar{x}_i}{\sigma}\sqrt{N_1}$ and $\tau_i = \frac{\bar{y}_i}{\sigma}\sqrt{N_2}$, so that, under the $H_G$, $t_i$ and $\tau_i$ are the standard normal distribution with pdf and cdf $\phi$ and $\Phi$, respectively.

Let's define the maximum statistic at the end of stage 1 as

$$T_1 = \max\left(t_1, t_2, ..., t_K\right). \tag{15.2}$$

Based on the theory of order statistics we know that when $t_i$ are drawn independently from an identical cdf $F(t)$, the cdf of $T_1$ is $F_{T_1}(t) = \left[F(t)\right]^K$ and the pdf $f_{T_1}(t) = K\left[F(t)\right]^{K-1} f(t)$. Here $f(t)$ is the pdf associated with the $F(t)$ (Johnson, Kotz, and Balakrishnan, 1994; Zwillinger and

Kokoska, 2000). Therefore, under the $H_G$, the pdf of $T_1$ can be written as

$$f_{T_1}(t) = K \left[\Phi(t)\right]^{K-1} \phi(t).  \tag{15.3}$$

At the final stage, using all data from the winner, we defined the statistic

$$T_2 = T_1\sqrt{\tau} + \tau_i\sqrt{1-\tau} \text{ if } i = S \text{ (arm } i \text{ is selected)}  \tag{15.4}$$

where $\tau = \frac{N_1}{N}$ is the information time at the interim analysis.

Let the indicator $\delta_i = 1$ when $i = S$ (i.e., arm $i$ is selected); otherwise, $\delta_i = 0$. From (15.4), it is convenient to define the cdf of $T_2$ as

$$F_{T_2}(t) = \sum_{i=1}^{K} P\left(\delta_i = 1 \cap T_1\sqrt{\tau} + \tau_i\sqrt{1-\tau} < t\right).  \tag{15.5}$$

Under the $H_G$, the three variables $\delta_i$, $T_1$, and $\tau_i$ are mutually independent, therefore, we have

$$F_{T_2}(t) = \frac{1}{K}\sum_{i=1}^{K} \int_{-\infty}^{\infty} \int_{-\infty}^{\frac{t-\tau_i\sqrt{1-\tau}}{\sqrt{\tau}}} K\left[\Phi(T_1)\right]^{K-1}\phi(T_1)\phi(\tau_i)\,dT_1 d\tau_i$$

$$= \int_{-\infty}^{\infty} \left[\Phi\left(\frac{t-\tau_i\sqrt{1-\tau}}{\sqrt{\tau}}\right)\right]^{K} \phi(\tau_i)\,d\tau_i.  \tag{15.6}$$

Shun, Lan, and Soo (2010) use normal approximation to simplify the distribution of the test statistic under $H_0$ for $K = 2$.

The final test statistic is defined as

$$T_2^* = (T_2 - t_0)/\sqrt{2}.  \tag{15.7}$$

Since $T_2^* \leq z$ is equivalent to $T_2 - t_0 \leq \sqrt{2}z$ and $T_2 - t_0$ and $T_2 + t_0$ have the same distribution under $H_G$, the cdf of $T_2^*$ under $H_G$ is given by the convolution:

$$F_{T_2^*}(z) = \int_{-\infty}^{+\infty} F_{T_2}(t)\phi\left(\sqrt{2}z - t\right)dt$$

$$F_{T_2^*}(z) = \int_{-\infty}^{+\infty} \int_{-\infty}^{\infty} \left[\Phi\left(\frac{t-\tau_i\sqrt{1-\tau}}{\sqrt{\tau}}\right)\right]^{K} \phi(\tau_i)\,d\tau_i\phi\left(\sqrt{2}z - t\right)dt.  \tag{15.8}$$

When the information time $\tau = 1$, (15.8) reduces to a Dunnett test:

$$F_{T_2^*}(z) = \int_{-\infty}^{\infty} \left[\Phi(t)\right]^{K}\phi\left(\sqrt{2}z - t\right)dt.  \tag{15.9}$$

This formulation is much simpler than the mutivariate normal integration.

Theoretically, the drop-arm design can reject $H_0$ at the interim (stage 1) analysis or reject $H_0$ at the final analysis. Here we will focus on the design that only allows us to reject $H_0$ at the final analysis. That is, if the test statistic $\hat{T}_2^* \geq c_\alpha$, the $H_0$ is rejected; otherwise, $H_0$ is not rejected. In such a case, the stopping boundary $c_\alpha$ can be determined using (15.8), that is, $F_{T_2^*}(c_\alpha) = 1 - \alpha$ for a one-sided significance level $\alpha$. Numerical integration or simulation can be used to determine the stopping boundary and power. For $\tau = 0.5$, the numerical integrations (I use *Scientific Workplace*) give $c_\alpha = 2.352, 2.408, 2.451,$ and $2.487$ for $K = 4, 5, 6,$ and 7, respectively, which are consistent with the results provided by the simulations in Table 15.1. The critical value and power of the pick-the-winner design were calculated using SAS Macro 15.1. When the information time $\tau = 1$ (let nStage2=0 in the macro), it reduces to a Dunnett test.

Table 15.1: Critical Value $c_\alpha$ for Classical Pick-the-Winner Design

| Info Time $\tau$ | K | | | | | | |
|---|---|---|---|---|---|---|---|
| | 1 | 2 | 3 | 4 | 5 | 6 | 7 |
| 0.3 | 1.960 | 2.140 | 2.235 | 2.299 | 2.345 | 2.382 | 2.424 |
| 0.5 | 1.960 | 2.168 | 2.278 | 2.352 | 2.407 | 2.452 | 2.487 |
| 0.7 | 1.960 | 2.190 | 2.313 | 2.398 | 2.460 | 2.510 | 2.550 |

Note: 10,000,000 runs per scenario

>>**SAS Macro 15.1:   Pick-the-Winner Design**>>

```
/* The Classical ACTIVE K-arm dropping-Loser Design; */
/* H0: all means are equal. Ha: at least one mean > mean0. */
/* For Dunnett's test, nStage2=0. */
%Macro  WinnerDesign(nSims=1000,  NumOfArms=5,  mu0=0,  sigma=1,
Z_alpha=2.407, nStage1=100, nStage2=100);
data OptnArm;
Set dInput;
Array mu(&NumOfArms); Array xObs(&NumOfArms);
Keep NumOfArms Z_alpha N1 N2 TotalN Power;
nSims=&nSims; NumOfArms=&NumOfArms; Z_alpha=&Z_alpha;
N1=&nStage1; N2=&nStage2;
Power=0;
Do iSim=1 To nSims;
Do i=1 To NumOfArms;
xObs(i) = RAND('NORMAL', mu(i), &sigma/sqrt(N1));
End;
MaxRsp =xObs(1); SelectedArm=1;
Do i=1 To NumOfArms;
```

If xObs(i)> MaxRsp Then Do; SelectedArm=i; MaxRsp=xObs(i); End;
End;
x2 = RAND('NORMAL', mu(SelectedArm), &sigma/Max(1,sqrt(N2)));
FinalxAve = (MaxRsp*N1+x2*N2)/(N1+N2);
x0Ave = RAND('NORMAL', &mu0, &sigma/sqrt(N1+N2));
TestZ=(FinalxAve-x0Ave)*sqrt((N1+N2)/2)/&sigma;
If TestZ >= Z_alpha Then Power=Power+1/nSims;
End;
TotalN=(NumOfArms+1)*N1+2*N2;
output;
Run;
Proc Print data=OptnArm; Run;
%Mend WinnerDesign;
<<**SAS**<<

## Example 15.1    Seamless Design of Asthma Trial

The objective of this trial in asthma patients is to confirm sustained treatment effect, measured as FEV1 change from baseline to 1-year of treatment. Initially, patients are equally randomized to four doses of the new compound and a placebo. Based on early studies, the estimated FEV1 changes at week 4 are 6%, 12%, 13%, 14%, and 15% (with pooled standard deviation 18%) for the placebo (dose level 0) and dose level 1, 2, 3, and 4, respectively. One interim analysis is planned when 60 per group or 50% of patients have the efficacy assessments. The interim analysis will lead to picking the winner (arm with best observed response). The winner and placebo will be used at stage 2. At stage 2, we will enroll 60 patients per group in the winner and control groups. Following are the SAS macro calls.

>>**SAS**>>
Title "Determine Critical Value Z_alpha for 4+1 Arms Winner Design";
Data dInput;
Array mu(4)(0, 0, 0, 0);
%WinnerDesign(nSims=10000000,    NumOfArms=4,    mu0=0,    sigma=1,
Z_alpha=2.352, nStage1=100, nStage2=100);
run;
Title "Determine Power for 4+1 Arms Winner Design";
Data dInput;
Array mu(4)(0.12, 0.13, 0.14, 0.15);
%WinnerDesign(nSims=100000,    NumOfArms=4,    mu0=0.06,    sigma=0.18,
Z_alpha=2.352, nStage1=60, nStage2=60);
run;
<<**SAS**<<

The simulations show that the pick-the-winner design has 95% power with the total sample size of 420.

For the Dunnett test, we let the information time $\tau = 1$ or nStage2 $= 0$ in calling SAS Macro 15.1. As usual, there are two steps: (1) determine or check the critical value Z_alpha, and (2) determine the sample size to achieve the target power. The simulations results indicate the critical value is 2.441 and the total sample size required to achieve 95% power is 510 patients, 80 more than the pick-the-winner design.

**>>SAS>>**
Title "Determine Critical Value Z_alpha for 4+1 Arms Winner Design";
Data dInput;
Array mu(4)(0, 0, 0, 0);
%WinnerDesign(nSims=10000000, NumOfArms=4, mu0=0, sigma=1, Z_alpha=2.441, nStage1=102, nStage2=0);
run;
Title "Determine Power for 4+1 Arms Winner Design";
Data dInput;
Array mu(4)(0.12, 0.13, 0.14, 0.15);
%WinnerDesign(nSims=100000, NumOfArms=4, mu0=0.06, sigma=0.18, Z_alpha=2.441, nStage1=102, nStage2=0);
run;
**<<SAS<<**

If we conduct the interim analysis earlier when 43 per group or 30% patients are enrolled (86 per group in the second stage), we need only 387 patients to achieve 95% power.

## 15.3    Adaptive Dunnett Test

Koenig, Brannath, Bretz, and Posch (2008) proposed the so-called adaptive Dunnett test for pick-the-winners design. While the design allows picking more than one winner, the test procedure that is based on the conditional error principle and the conditional type I error rate of the single-stage Dunnett test.

The conditional error principle says that one can perform any adaptation without inflating the type-I error as long as such adaptations can preserve the conditional error rate. Here the reference test is the classical Dunnett test. In other words, we want to use the same critical value as the Dunnett test but keep the type-I error rate the same when we make the adaptations.

Let the global null hypothesis $H_G : \mu_i = \mu_0, i = 1, ..., K$. The proposed test is a two-stage procedure, in which the conditional type-I error rate for the Dunnett test is calculated at the interim analysis. Assume that the variance $\sigma^2$ is known and treatment means $\bar{x}_0, ..., \bar{x}_K$ from the first stage data with same sizes $N_1$ are calculated. Assume that the information time $\tau = N_1/N$, where $N$ is the preplanned overall sample size $N$ per group. The conditional type-I error rate is then given by

$$A_2 = 1 - \int_{-\infty}^{\infty} \left[ \prod_{i=1}^{K} \Phi \left( c_d \sqrt{\frac{2N}{N - N_1}} - z_{1i} \sqrt{\frac{2N_1}{N - N_1}} + x \right) \right] \phi(x)\, dx,$$

(15.10)

where $Z_i = \frac{\bar{X}_i - \bar{X}_0}{\sigma\sqrt{2/N}}, i = 1, ..., K$, $Z_{1i}$ is similar to $Z_i$ but is based on the data from stage 1, and $c_d$ is the critical value for Dunnett's test at level $\alpha$ with $K$ active treatments; that is, $c_d$ is the $(1 - \alpha)\%$ equicoordinate quantile from a multivariate normal distribution with variance 1 and covariance $1/2$.

Assume a set $S \subset \{1, ..., K\}$ of treatment arms were selected for the second stage. Koenig et al. (2008) proposed the test for $H_G \cap H_0^s$ at the final stage. The $p$-vaue at the final analysis is given by

$$p_2 = 1 - \int_{-\infty}^{\infty} \left[ \prod_{i \in S} \Phi \left( z_{\max} \sqrt{\frac{2N}{N - N_1}} - z_{1i} \sqrt{\frac{2N_1}{N - N_1}} + x \right) \right] \phi(x)\, dx,$$

(15.11)

where $Z_i$ is the overall test statistic for the test arm $i$ against the control at the final stage and $z_{\max}$ is the actually observed maximum of $Z_i$ among all the groups in stage 2. Equation (15.11) is similar to (15.10), with $c_d$ replaced by the observed maximum statistic $\max_{i \in S} z_i$ and the integration performed over the selected arms.

Note that $A_2$ is a function $\mathbf{z}_1$ from the first stage; therefore, they can be calculated only at or after the interim analysis, while $p_2$ appears to be dependent on the data from both stages, but actually it is dependent only on the data from the second stage. This is because if we substitute $Z_i = z_{1i} \sqrt{\frac{N_1}{N}} + Z_{2i} \sqrt{\frac{N - N_1}{N}}$ into (15.10) and $z_{1i}$ is given, we can obtain

$$p_2 = 1 - \int_{-\infty}^{\infty} \left[ \prod_{i \in S} \Phi \left( \sqrt{2} z_{2,\max} + x \right) \right] \phi(x)\, dx,$$

(15.12)

where $Z_{2i}$ is similar to $Z_i$ but based on the data from stage 2 and $z_{2,\max}$ is the actually observed test statistic maximum of $Z_{2i}$ (among all groups in stage 2). The decision rule is when $p_2 \leq A_2$, reject $H_0$; otherwise, accept the null hypothesis. Of course, we assume that for some first stage data $z_1$ the inequality $p_2 \leq A_2$ must be achievable; otherwise, we have to modify the value of $c_d$ to meet the requirement. For other first stage data $z_1$, regardless of what the values are of the data from the second stage, we may never be able to reject the null hypothesis.

As Koenig et al. (2008) pointed out, in the adaptive Dunnett test, we make no assumptions on the selection procedure at interim and allow the interim decision to depend on the interim data as well as on any external information. Thus, it is not required that the treatment group with the largest observed treatment effect at the interim be carried on to the second-stage or that we predetermine how many groups will be selected. However, the method requires the variance to be known and, therefore, the sample sizes to be large in order to obtain valid approximate results. Furthermore, (15.10) is valid when there is no early rejection of $H_0$; that is, the interim analysis is performed solely for arm selection and/or sample-size recalculation.

## 15.4 Summary and Discussion

We have studied the seamless designs that allow for early dropping of losers. Note that the efficiency of a seamless design is sensitive to the sample-size fraction or information time in the end of the learning phase. Therefore, simulations should be done to determine the best information time for the interim analysis.

Practically, the seamless trials require early efficacy readouts. This early efficacy assessment can be the primary endpoint for the trial or surrogate endpoint (biomarker). Because data analysis and interpretation allow exploration of richness of clinical data, the interim analysis should also include some variables other than the primary. Those analyses can be descriptive or the hypothesis-testing kind. Seamless design can also be used for other situations such as a combination of phase-I and phase-II trials. Regarding the logistic issues in a seamless design, please see the papers by the PhRMA adaptive working group (Maca et al., 2006; Quinlan, Gallo, and Krams, 2006).

**Problems**

**15.1** Verify the critical values in Table 15.1 using simulations (SAS Macro 15.1).

**15.2** Suppose in a five-arm phase-II/III combined study, the response rates are 0.3, 0.45, 0.5, 0.47, and 0.55 for the control and four active arms, respectively. Use SAS Macro 15.1 to design the trial with 90% power based on the Dunnett procedure and the pick-the-winner design. Recommend another design and justify your recommendation.

**15.3** Modify SAS Macro 15.1 to allow early stopping for efficacy and futility.

**15.4** Use simulations to study the effect of information time on the sample size and power of the hypothesis test for the pick-the-winner design.

**15.5** Study the pick-the-winner design with a binary endpoint with small sample size.

# Chapter 16

# The Add-Arm Design for Unimodal Response

## 16.1 Introduction

The classical multiple-arm design with the strong familywise type-I error control is a single-stage design with several active arms and a common control arm, in which Dunnett's test (1955, 1964) based on multivariate normal distribution is most used for the multiple comparisons. To improve the design, recently, multiple-arm adaptive designs have been studied. A typical multiple-arm confirmatory adaptive design (often called drop-the-loser, drop-arm, or pick-the-winner design or adaptive dose-finding design, or phase-II/III seamless design) consists of two stages: a selection stage and a confirmation stage. For the selection stage, a randomized parallel design with several doses and a placebo group is employed for selection of doses. After the best dose (the winner) is chosen, the patients of the selected dose group and placebo group will enter the confirmation stage. New patients will be recruited and randomized to receive the selected dose or placebo. The final analysis is performed with the cumulative data of patients from both stages (Chang 2011; Maca, et al., 2006).

Huang, Liu, and Hsiao (2011) proposed a seamless design that allows prespecifying probabilities of rejecting the null hypothesis that the drug is ineffective at each stage to improve the efficiency of the trial. Posch, Maurer, and Bretz (2011) described two approaches to control the type-I error rate in adaptive designs with sample-size reassessment and/or treatment selection. The first method adjusts the critical value using a simulation-based approach, which incorporates the number of patients at an interim analysis, the true response rates, the treatment selection rule, etc. The second method is an adaptive Bonferroni–Holm test procedure based on conditional error rates of the individual treatment–control comparisons. They showed that this procedure controls the type-I error rate, even if a deviation from a pre-planned adaptation rule or the time point of such a decision is necessary.

Shun, Lan, and Soo (2008) considered a study starting with two treatment groups and a control group with a planned interim analysis. The inferior treatment group would be dropped after the interim analysis. Such an interim analysis could be based on the clinical endpoint or a biomarker. The unconditional distribution of the final test statistic from the "winner" treatment is skewed and requires numerical integration or simulations for the calculation. To avoid complex computations, they propose a normal approximation approach to calculate the type-I error, the power, the point estimate, and the confidence intervals. Heritier, Lô and Morgan (2011) studied the type-I error control of the seamless unbalanced designs, the issues of noninferiority comparison, multiplicity of secondary endpoints, and covariance adjusted analyses. Jenkins, Stone, and Jennison (2011) proposed a design that adds extra flexibility by also allowing the trial to continue in the subgroup or the full population with correlated time-to-event endpoints at the selection and the final stages.

The papers mentioned above focus mainly on type-I and type-II error control and mainly for the phase-II/III seamless designs. In contrast, there is another school of research on multiple-arm trials that is mainly for phase-II dose-finding studies, in which selecting a target dose (dose schedule) such as minimum effective dose (MED) is the main purpose with a reasonable control of the type-I error. Early such studies are often based on the assumption of monotonicity in dose response. Williams (1971, 1972) proposed a test to determine the lowest dose level at which there is evidence for a difference from the control. Cochran (1954), Amitage (1955), and Nam (1987) studied the Cochran–Amitage test for monotonic trend. Those methods do not strongly control the type-I error rate.

The MED can be defined as the dose where the mean efficacy outcome is equal to a certain target, with the placebo (or an active control) used as a reference. Mean efficacy is usually assumed to be nondecreasing with dose. Both efficacy and safety endpoints are often taken into consideration when selecting a dose for further studies in phase-III trials, because increasing the dose can result in both higher efficacy and increased adverse event rates. A common approach is to quantify efficacy and adverse event rate trade-off through a utility function that incorporates both efficacy and safety into a measure of overall clinical utility (Berry et al., 2001; Dragalin and Fedorov, 2006; Ivanova et al. 2009, 2012). Such a utility function is typically umbrella-shaped and the goal is to find a dose that maximizes the utility of the drug candidate. The objective in phase II can also be to test efficacy and adverse event rates at the estimated MED or the optimal dose against a control and recommend for further study in phase-III trials (Ivanova et al. 2011). Miller et al. (2007) investigated a two-stage strategy for a dose-ranging study that is optimal across several parametric models. Dragalin et al. (2008) investigated optimal two-stage designs for two correlated binary endpoints that follow a bivariate probit model. Bretz et al. (2005) studied the dose-finding methods under various dose response scenarios including umbrella-shaped response curves. Ivanova et al. (2011) studied a Bayesian two-stage adaptive design for finding MED under the same set of dose response curves and compared the section probability and power against the uniform allocation method.

Besides the type-I and type-II error controls, another critical issue is the estimation of the treatment difference of the multiple-arm adaptive design (Bauer et al., 2010; Bowden and Glimm, 2008; Brannath, Koenig and Bauer, 2006; Carreras and Brannath, 2012; Kathman and Hale, 2007; Stallard and Todd, 2005; Stallard, Todd, Whitehead, 2008). However, this important issue is not the topic of this chapter.

The seamless designs have some similarities to the phase-II dose-finding studies, but there are also differences. For example, the primary objective in a phase-II dose-finding might be to determine MED or ED90; therefore, the probability of selecting the target dose is the most important measure for evaluating a design, while type-I error control is secondary. In contrast, a seamless design focuses on the power of the hypothesis test with the strict control of the type-I error, with the probability of selecting the best arm as secondary. Although the probabilities of selecting the best arm and power are often closely related, they are not one–one mapping. The second difference might be in the endpoint: in phase-II dose-finding study, the endpoint is usually a PD marker, but in the seamless design the endpoint is usually the primary efficacy endpoint for drug approval or its surrogate endpoint. The third different aspect (less obvious) is that phase-II dose-dosing is often about the comparisons of different doses, while seamless design can be about different dose level and dose schedule combinations, drug combinations (this is true for almost all cancer and AIDS drugs), or different drug-delivery methods (e.g., infusion versus infusion).

In this chapter, we will study the 3-stage add-arm adaptive design proposed by Chang and Jing (2014). Its main purpose is for the application of adaptive methods in phase-II/III seamless design with the strict control of the type-I error rate at the target level, and the probability of correct arm selecting is also considered as an important operating characteristic in the design. We will illustrate how to use the proposed method with the seamless designs and phase-II dose-finding studies and compare the add-arm design with three other methods, Dunnett's method with equal sample allocation, the drop-loser design (Chang 2007; Shun, Lan and Soo, 2008), and the Bayesian adaptive design method (Ivanova et al., 2011).

In a classical drop-loser (or drop-arm) design, patients are randomized into all arms (doses) and at the interim analysis, inferior arms are dropped. Therefore, compared to the traditional dose-finding design, this adaptive design can reduce the sample size by not carrying over all doses to the end of the trial, or dropping the losers earlier. However, all the doses have to be explored. For unimodal (including linear or umbrella) response curves, we proposed an effective dose-finding design that allows adding arms at the interim analysis. The trial design starts with two arms; then depending on the response of the two arms and the unimodality assumption, we can decide which new arms to add. This design does not require exploring all arms (doses) to find the best responsive dose; therefore it can further reduce the sample size over the drop-loser design.

The 3-stage add-arm design begins with only two active arms and the placebo (control) group and at the first interim analysis, more arms will be added depending on the observed responses of the two arms and the assumption of a unimodal (including monotonic and umbrella) response curve. The key idea of a drop-arm design is that "some inferior arms don't need to have a large exposure," whereas the central notion of the proposed 3-stage add-arm design is that "some inferior arms don't have to be exposed at all" when the response is unimodal (umbrella-shaped) .

For convenience, we define the global null hypothesis as $H_G : \mu_0 = \mu_1 = \mu_2 = \ldots = \mu_K$ and the hypothesis test between the selected arm (winner) and the control as

$$H_0 : \mu_0 = \mu_s, \ s = \text{selected arm.} \qquad (16.1)$$

In Section 16.2, we will review the commonly used drop-arm designs and derive the exact distribution of the final test statistic. In Section 16.3, we will describe the new 3-stage add-arm design, the rule of picking the winner, and the exact distributions of test statistics. The discussion is based on the design with 4 active arms and the placebo. We call this the $4 + 1$ add-arm design. In Section 16.3, we extend the $4 + 1$ design to $5 + 1$, $6 + 1$, and $7 + 1$ adaptive designs. From that, one can derive any $K + 1$ add-arm designs. Section 16.4 is the comparison of the two adaptive design methods: the drop-arm and the add-arm designs using simulations. The comparisons are carried out under various response curves: monotonic and unimodal response curves. The results show that the new design can gain efficiency in most situations. The new adaptive design is easy to implement. In Section 16.5 we illustrate the new design with a clinical trial, showing a nearly 20% reduction in sample size comparing the drop-arm design. A summary is presented in Section 16.6.

## 16.2 The Add-Arm Design

### 16.2.1 *Design Description*

The add-arm design is a three-stage adaptive design, in which we can use interim analyses and the unimode-response property to determine which doses cannot (are unlikely to) be the arm with best response—thus no exposure to those doses is necessary. Let's take a 4+1 arm design as an example to illustrate the key idea behind the add-arm design.

In the 4+1 arm design, there are $K = 4$ dose levels (active arms) and a placebo arm (dose level 0). Theoretically, if we know dose 2 has a larger response than dose 3, then we know, by the unimode-response assumption, that the best response arm can be either dose 1 or 2, but not dose 4. Therefore, we don't need to test dose 4 at all. Similarly, if we know dose 3 has a larger response than dose 2, then we know, by the unimode-response assumption, that the best response arm can be either dose 4 or 3, but not dose 1. Therefore, we don't need to test dose 1 at all. The problem is that we don't know the true responses for doses 2 and 3. We have to find these out based on the observed responses. Of course, we want the observed rates to reflect the true responses with high probability, which mean the sample size cannot be very small.

We are now ready to fully describe the three-stage 4+1 add-arm design (see Figure 16.1). At the first stage, we randomize subjects into two active and the placebo groups. The second stage is the add-arm stage, at which we determine which arm is to be added based on the observed data from the first stage and the unimodal property of the response curve. At the third or final stage, more subjects will be added to the winner arm and the placebo. The randomization is specified as follows:

- Stage 1: Assign $2.5N_1$ subjects in arms 2, 0, and 3 using randomization ratio $N_1 : N_1/2 : N_1$.
- Stage 2: If $t_2 > t_3$, assign $1.5N_1$ subjects in arms 0 and 1 using an

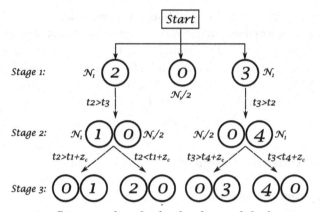

Figure 16.1:   The 4 + 1 Add-Arm Design

$N_1/2 : N_1$ randomization. If $t_2 \leq t_3$, assign $1.5N_1$ subjects in arm 0 and 4 using an $N_1/2 : N_1$ randomization.

• Stage 3: (a) If $t_2 > t_3$ and $t_2 - t_1 > c_R$, select arm 2 as the winner; otherwise select arm 1 as the winner. If $t_2 \leq t_3$ and $t_3 - t_4 > c_R$, select arm 3 as the winner; otherwise select arm 4 as the winner. (b) Assign $2N_2$ subjects in arms 0 and the winner arm using $N_2 : N_2$ randomization.

Therefore, there will be total $4N_1 + 2N_2$ subjects. In the final analysis for the hypothesis test, we will use the data from $N_1 + N_2$ subjects in the winner and $N_1 + N_2$ subjects in arm 0.

You may have noticed that we use an $N_1/2 : N_1 : N_1$ randomization instead of an $N_1 : N_1 : N_1$ randomization. This is because the imbalanced randomization can keep the treatment blinding and balance the confounding factors at both stages. If $N_1$ placebo subjects are all randomized in the first stage, then at the second stage all $N_1$ subjects would be assigned to the active group without randomization, thus unblinding the treatment and potentially imbalancing some (baseline) confounding factors.

A key question is how to determine the constant $c_R$. Before we discuss it, it is convenient to define the term "selection probability," that is, the probability of selecting a dose as the preferred dose for the next stage of the adaptive trial. We noticed that if $c_R = 0$, the design becomes a three-stage pick-the-winner (or the drop–the-loser) design, in which the active arm with the maximum observed response at the current stage is picked as the winner. The problem with this is that the selection probability will be skewed when the response curve is flat. Particularly, the selection probabilities of dose 1, 2, 3, and 4 are $1/6$, $2/6$, $2/6$, and $1/6$, respectively, when in fact all doses have the same response. The real issue with this uneven selection probability is that when, for example, dose 1 has a better response than dose 2, there could still be a large probability of selecting dose 2 or 3 than dose 1 as the winner.

Therefore, we have to force the selection probability equal (or at least approximately equal) for all doses when $H_G$ is true. To this end, we want the selection probability at the second stage to be $1/4$ under $H_G$, i.e.,

$$P(t_2 - t_1 > c_R \cap t_2 > t_3; H_G) = 1/4. \qquad (16.2)$$

For the normal distribution, the selection probability is given by (see Appendix A)

$$P(t_2 - t_1 > c_R \cap t_2 > t_3; H_G) = \int_{-\infty}^{\infty} \Phi(x - c_R)\,\phi(x)\,\Phi(x)\,dx. \qquad (16.3)$$

The numerical integration can be used to determine $c_R$ based on (16.2) and (16.3). It turns out that $c_R = 0.55652$. For the numerical integrations, we find that the replacement of $\infty$ with $10$ and $-\infty$ with $-10$ will not practically impact the precision.

To summarize, the two key ideas in this design are (1) using unimode-response property to determine which arms not to explore, and (2) determining the rule ($c_R$) for picking the winner so that the selection probabilities for all active arms are (at least approximately) equal under a flat response curve.

We are now ready to discuss the test statistics. Theoretically, the add-arm design can reject hypotheses of no treatment effect at the interim and final analyses. Here we will focus on the design that allows rejecting $H_0$ only at the final analysis.

## 16.2.2 *The Interim and Final Test Statistics*

Let $T_1 = \max(t_2, t_3)$, with cdf $F_{T_1}$. It is well known that under $H_G$, the cdf $F_{T_1}(t) = \Phi^2(t)$ and pdf $f_{T_1}(t) = 2\Phi(t)\phi(t)$.

At the second stage, we define the statistic

$$T_2 = \begin{cases} t_1 \text{ if } t_2 \geq t_3 \text{ and } t_2 < t_1 + c_R \text{ (arm 1 is the winner)}, \\ t_2 \text{ if } t_2 \geq t_3 \text{ and } t_2 \geq t_1 + c_R \text{ (arm 2 is the winner)}, \\ t_4 \text{ if } t_2 < t_3 \text{ and } t_3 \geq t_4 + c_R \text{ (arm 3 is the winner)}, \\ t_3 \text{ if } t_2 < t_3 \text{ and } t_3 < t_4 + c_R \text{ (arm 4 is the winner)}. \end{cases} \qquad (16.4)$$

From (16.4), we can write the cdf of $T_2$ as

$$F_{T_2}(t) = P_1(T_2 \leq t) + P_2(T_2 \leq t) + P_3(T_2 \leq t) + P_4(T_2 \leq t),$$

where

$$P_1 = P\left(t_2 \geq t_3 \cap t_2 < t_1 + c_R \cap t_1 \leq t\right)$$
$$P_2 = P\left(t_2 \geq t_3 \cap t_2 \geq t_1 + c_R \cap t_2 \leq t\right)$$
$$P_3 = P\left(t_2 < t_3 \cap t_3 \geq t_4 + c_R \cap t_3 \leq t\right)$$
$$P_4 = P\left(t_2 < t_3 \cap t_3 < t_4 + c_R \cap t_4 \leq t\right)$$

Under the $H_G$, we can prove that the cdf of $T_2$ is

$$F_{T_2}(t) = \int_{-\infty}^{t} \phi(x)\, \Phi^2(x + c_R) + 2\Phi(x - c_R)\, \Phi(x)\, \phi(x)\, dx \qquad (16.5)$$

Thus, the pdf of $T_2$ is given by

$$f_{T_2}(t) = \phi(t)\, \Phi^2(t + c_R) + 2\Phi(t - c_R)\, \Phi(t)\, \phi(t).$$

Numerical integrations or simulations are needed to calculate $F_{T_2}(t)$. $F_{T_2}(t)$ can be used to determine the stopping boundary if the hypothesis test is desirable at the interim analysis.

At the final stage, define a statistic as

$$T_3 = \begin{cases} t_1\sqrt{\tau} + \tau_1\sqrt{1-\tau} & \text{if } t_2 \geq t_3 \text{ and } t_2 < t_1 + c_R \\ t_2\sqrt{\tau} + \tau_2\sqrt{1-\tau} & \text{if } t_2 \geq t_3 \text{ and } t_2 \geq t_1 + c_R \\ t_3\sqrt{\tau} + \tau_3\sqrt{1-\tau} & \text{if } t_2 < t_3 \text{ and } t_3 \geq t_4 + c_R \\ t_4\sqrt{\tau} + \tau_4\sqrt{1-\tau} & \text{if } t_2 < t_3 \text{ and } t_3 < t_4 + c_R \end{cases} \qquad (16.6)$$

Note that $t_i$ is based on $N_1$ subjects in arm $i$, from either stage 1 or stage 2, whereas $\tau_j$ is based on $N_2$ subject in the winner arm $j$ from stage 3. Thus, the cdf of $T_3$ is given by $F_{T_3}(t) = \tilde{P}_1(t) + \tilde{P}_2(t) + \tilde{P}_2(t) + \tilde{P}_4(t)$, where

$$\tilde{P}_1(t) = P\left(t_2 \geq t_3 \cap t_2 < t_1 + c_R \cap t_1\sqrt{\tau} + \tau_1\sqrt{1-\tau} \leq t\right),$$
$$\tilde{P}_2(t) = P\left(t_2 \geq t_3 \cap t_2 \geq t_1 + c_R \cap t_2\sqrt{\tau} + \tau_2\sqrt{1-\tau} \leq t\right),$$
$$\tilde{P}_3(t) = P\left(t_2 < t_3 \cap t_3 \geq t_4 + c_R \cap t_3\sqrt{\tau} + \tau_3\sqrt{1-\tau} \leq t\right),$$
$$\tilde{P}_4(t) = P\left(t_2 < t_3 \cap t_3 < t_4 + c_R \cap t_4\sqrt{\tau} + \tau_4\sqrt{1-\tau} \leq t\right).$$

Under the $H_G$ the cdf of $T_3$ can be written as

$$F_{T_3}(t) = \int_{-\infty}^{\infty} \Phi\left(\frac{t - x\sqrt{\tau}}{\sqrt{1-\tau}}\right) \phi(x)\left[\Phi^2(x + c_R) + 2\Phi(x - c_R)\, \Phi(x)\right] dx.$$
$$(16.7)$$

**Proof.** For the $4+1$ add-arm design ($X_1, X_2, X_3$ are iid from the standard normal distribution), we have

$$P(X_2 - X_1 > c_R \cap X_2 > X_3)$$

$$= \int_{-\infty}^{+\infty} \int_{-\infty}^{x_2} \int_{-\infty}^{x_2-c_R} \phi(x_1) \phi(x_2) \phi(x_3) \, dx_1 dx_3 dx_2$$

$$= \int_{-\infty}^{+\infty} \int_{-\infty}^{x_2} \Phi(x_2 - c_R) \phi(x_2) \phi(x_3) \, dx_3 dx_2$$

$$= \int_{-\infty}^{+\infty} \Phi(x_2 - c_R) \phi(x_2) \Phi(x_2) \, dx_2.$$

Under the $H_G$, due to symmetry, $P_1 = P_4$ and $P_2 = P_3$, but $P_1 \neq P_2$, where

$$P_1 = P(t_2 \geq t_3 \cap t_2 < t_1 + c_R \cap t_1 \leq t)$$

$$P_2 = P(t_2 \geq t_3 \cap t_2 \geq t_1 + c_R \cap t_2 \leq t)$$

$$F_{T_2}(t) = 2P_1(t) + 2P_2(t)$$

$$= 2 \int_{-\infty}^{t} \int_{-\infty}^{t_1+c_R} \int_{-\infty}^{t_2} \phi(t_1) \phi(t_2) \phi(t_3) \, dt_3 dt_2 dt_1$$

$$+ 2 \int_{-\infty}^{t} \int_{-\infty}^{t_2} \int_{-\infty}^{t_2-c_R} \phi(t_1) \phi(t_2) \phi(t_3) \, dt_1 dt_3 dt_2$$

We can further simplify it as

$$F_{T_2}(t) = 2 \int_{-\infty}^{t} \int_{-\infty}^{t_1+c_R} \phi(t_1) \phi(t_2) \Phi(t_2) \, dt_2 dt_1$$

$$+ 2 \int_{-\infty}^{t} \int_{-\infty}^{t_2} \Phi(t_2 - c_R) \phi(t_2) \phi(t_3) \, dt_3 dt_2$$

$$= \int_{-\infty}^{t} \phi(t_1) \Phi^2(t_1 + c_R) \, dt_1 + 2 \int_{-\infty}^{t} \Phi(t_2 - c_R) \Phi(t_2) \phi(t_2) \, dt_2$$

Under the $H_G$, due to symmetry, $\tilde{P}_1 = \tilde{P}_4$ and $\tilde{P}_2 = \tilde{P}_3$, but $\tilde{P}_1 \neq \tilde{P}_2$, where

$$\tilde{P}_1 = P\left(t_2 \geq t_3 \cap t_2 < t_1 + c_R \cap t_1\sqrt{\tau} + \tau_1\sqrt{1-\tau} \leq t\right),$$

$$\tilde{P}_2 = P\left(t_2 \geq t_3 \cap t_2 \geq t_1 + c_R \cap t_2\sqrt{\tau} + \tau_2\sqrt{1-\tau} \leq t\right).$$

$$F_{T_3}(t) = 2\tilde{P}_1 + 2\tilde{P}_2$$

$$= 2\int_{-\infty}^{\infty}\int_{-\infty}^{t_1+c_R}\int_{-\infty}^{t_2}\int_{-\infty}^{\frac{t-t_1\sqrt{\tau}}{\sqrt{1-\tau}}}\phi(\tau_1)\phi(t_1)\phi(t_2)\phi(t_3)\,d\tau_1 dt_3 dt_2 dt_1$$

$$+2\int_{-\infty}^{\infty}\int_{-\infty}^{t_2-c_R}\int_{-\infty}^{t_2}\int_{-\infty}^{\frac{t-t_2\sqrt{\tau}}{\sqrt{1-\tau}}}\phi(\tau_2)\phi(t_1)\phi(t_2)\phi(t_3)\,d\tau_2 dt_3 dt_1 dt_2$$

$$F_{T_3}(t) = 2\int_{-\infty}^{\infty}\int_{-\infty}^{t_1+c_R}\int_{-\infty}^{t_2}\Phi\left(\frac{t-t_1\sqrt{\tau}}{\sqrt{1-\tau}}\right)\phi(t_1)\phi(t_2)\phi(t_3)\,dt_3 dt_2 dt_1$$

$$+2\int_{-\infty}^{\infty}\int_{-\infty}^{t_2-c_R}\int_{-\infty}^{t_2}\Phi\left(\frac{t-t_2\sqrt{\tau}}{\sqrt{1-\tau}}\right)\phi(t_1)\phi(t_2)\phi(t_3)\,dt_3 dt_1 dt_2$$

To further simplify, we have

$$F_{T_3}(t) = 2\int_{-\infty}^{\infty}\int_{-\infty}^{t_1+c_R}\Phi\left(\frac{t-t_1\sqrt{\tau}}{\sqrt{1-\tau}}\right)\phi(t_1)\phi(t_2)\Phi(t_2)\,dt_2 dt_1$$

$$+2\int_{-\infty}^{\infty}\int_{-\infty}^{t_2-c_R}\Phi\left(\frac{t-t_2\sqrt{\tau}}{\sqrt{1-\tau}}\right)\phi(t_1)\phi(t_2)\Phi(t_2)\,dt_1 dt_2$$

$$F_{T_3}(t) = \int_{-\infty}^{\infty}\Phi\left(\frac{t-t_1\sqrt{\tau}}{\sqrt{1-\tau}}\right)\phi(t_1)\Phi^2(t_1+c_R)\,dt_1$$

$$+2\int_{-\infty}^{\infty}\Phi\left(\frac{t-t_2\sqrt{\tau}}{\sqrt{1-\tau}}\right)\Phi(t_2-c_R)\phi(t_2)\Phi(t_2)\,dt_2$$

$$= \int_{-\infty}^{\infty}\Phi\left(\frac{t-t_1\sqrt{\tau}}{\sqrt{1-\tau}}\right)\phi(t_1)\left[\Phi^2(t_1+c_R)+2\Phi(t_1-c_R)\Phi(t_1)\right]dt_1.$$

To test the hypothesis $H_0$, we need to consider the control arm too. Therefore, the final test statistic is defined as

$$T_3^* = (T_3 - t_0)/\sqrt{2}. \qquad (16.8)$$

Without loss of generality, assume $\mu_0 = 0$; thus, $t_0 \sim N(0,1)$. Since $T_3^* \le z$ is equivalent to $\sqrt{2}T_3^* \le \sqrt{2}z$ and $T_3 - t_0$ and $T_3 + t_0$ have the same distribution under $H_G$, the cdf of $T_3^*$ under $H_G$ is given by the convolution:

$$F_{T_3^*}(z) = \int_{-\infty}^{+\infty} F_{T_3}(t)\,\phi\left(\sqrt{2}z - t\right)dt \qquad (16.9)$$

If we allow rejection of $H_0$ only at the final stage; that is, if the test $\hat{T}_3^* \ge c_\alpha$, reject $H_0$, otherwise, retain $H_0$, the stopping boundary $c_\alpha$ can be determined using (16.9); that is, $1 - F_{T_3^*}(c_\alpha) = \alpha$ for a one-sided significance level $\alpha$. Numerical integration or simulation can be used to determine the stopping boundary and power. For $\tau = 0.5$, both the numerical integration (I use *Scientific Workplace*) and the simulation give the rejection boundary $c_\alpha = 2.267$ for a one-sided $\alpha = 0.025$ because for the $4 + 1$ add-arm design with $\tau = 0.5$ and $c_\alpha = 2.352$, we have

$$
1 - \frac{1}{(2\pi)^{\frac{5}{2}}} \int_{-10}^{10} e^{-\frac{(2.267\sqrt{2}-t)^2}{2}} \int_{-10}^{10} \int_{-10}^{\sqrt{2}t-x} e^{-\frac{u^2}{2}} du
$$

$$
\cdot \left( \left( \int_{-10}^{x+0.55652} e^{-\frac{u^2}{2}} du \right)^2 + 2 \int_{-10}^{x-0.55652} e^{-\frac{u^2}{2}} du \int_{-10}^{x} e^{-\frac{u^2}{2}} du \right)
$$

$$
\times e^{-\frac{x^2}{2}} dx dt = 0.0250 = \alpha
$$

□

## >>SAS Macro 16.1:   4+1 Add-Arm Design>>

```
%Macro FourPlus1(nSims=1000000, N1=100, N2=100, c_alpha = 2.267, cR =
0.55652, mu0=0, sigma=1);
data FourPlus1;
Set dInput;
Array mu(4); Array xObs(4); Array SelProb(4);
Keep N1 N2 TotalN Power SelProb1-SelProb4;
N1=&N1; N2=&N2; sigma=&sigma; mu0=&mu0; Power=0;
Do i=1 To 4; SelProb(i)=0; End;
Do iSim=1 To &nSims;
Do i=1 To 4;
xObs(i) = RAND('NORMAL',mu(i), sigma/sqrt(N1));
End;
If xObs(2)>xObs(3) Then
Do;
If      xObs(1)*sqrt(N1)/sigma>      xObs(2)*sqrt(N1)/sigma-&cR      Then
SelectedArm=1;
Else SelectedArm=2;
End;
Else
Do;
If      xObs(4)*sqrt(N1)/sigma>xObs(3)*sqrt(N1)/sigma-&cR      Then
SelectedArm=4;
Else SelectedArm=3;
End;
MaxRsp = xObs(SelectedArm);
x2 = RAND('NORMAL', mu(SelectedArm), sigma/sqrt(N2));
FinalxAve = (MaxRsp*N1+x2*N2)/(N1+N2);
x0Ave = RAND('NORMAL', mu0, sigma/sqrt(N1+N2));
```

```
TestZ=(FinalxAve-x0Ave)*sqrt((N1+N2)/2)/sigma;
If TestZ >= &c_alpha Then Power=Power+1/&nSims;
Do i=1 To 4;
If SelectedArm=i Then SelProb(i)=SelProb(i)+1/&nSims;
End;
End;
TotalN=4*N1+2*N2;
Output;
Run;
Proc Print;
Run;
%Mend FourPlus1;
```
<<**SAS**<<

>>**SAS: Invoking SAS Macro 16.1**>>
```
Title "4+1 Add-Arm Design: Critical value";
Data dInput;
Array mu(4)(0,0,0,0);
%FourPlus1(N1=116,  N2=116,  c_alpha  =  2.267,  cR  =  0.55652,  mu0=0,
sigma=0.9);
Run;
Title "4+1 Add-Arm Design: Power";
Data dInput;
Array mu(4)(0.4,0.58,0.7,0.45);
%FourPlus1(N1=116,  N2=116,  c_alpha  =  2.267,  cR  =  0.55652,  mu0=0.35,
sigma=0.9);
Run;
```
<<**SAS**<<

>>**SAS Macro 16.2:    4+1 Add-Arm Design for Finding MED**>>
```
%Macro FourPlus1AddArmMED(nSims=100000, N1=100, N2=100, c_alpha =
2.267, cR = 0.55652, mu0=0.2, sigma=1, targetResponse=0.715);
* For targeted effective dose or minimum effective dose MED;
* targetResponse = response at MED;
* utility=1/((response-MED)^2+0.0001), MED= the dose with maximum util-
ity;
data FourPlus1;
Set dInput;
Array mu(4); Array xObs(4); ; Array SelProb(4);
Array x1(40000); Array meanX1(4); Array x0(10000); Array xFinal(10000);
Keep N1 N2 TotalN Power SelProb1-SelProb4;
```

```
N1=&N1; N2=&N2; mu0=&mu0; sigma=&sigma; targetResponse= &targetRe-
sponse;
Power=0;
Do i=1 To 4; SelProb(i)=0; End;
Do iSim=1 To &nSims;
Do i=1 To 4;
meanX1(i)=0;
Do j=1 To N1;
x1((i-1)*N1+j)=RAND('NORMAL', mu(i), sigma);
meanX1(i)=meanX1(i)+x1((i-1)*N1+j)/N1;
End;
End;
Do i=1 To 4;
Utility =1/(abs(meanX1(i)-targetResponse)**2+0.00001);
xObs(i) = Utility;
End;
If xObs(2)>xObs(3) Then
Do;
If xObs(1)*sigma/sqrt(N1)>xObs(2)*sigma/sqrt(N1)-&cR Then
SelectedArm=1;
Else SelectedArm=2;
End;
Else
Do;
If xObs(4)*sigma/sqrt(N1)>xObs(3)*sigma/sqrt(N1)-&cR Then
SelectedArm=4;
Else SelectedArm=3;
End;
Do j=1 To N1; xFinal(j)=x1((SelectedArm-1)*N1+j); End;
* Stage 2;
Do j=N1+1 To N1+N2;
xFinal(j) =RAND('NORMAL', mu(SelectedArm), sigma);
End;
* Gnerate response in Placebo;
Do j=1 To N1+N2;
x0(j) =RAND('NORMAL', mu0, sigma);
End;
* Form the final test statistics;
mean0=0; meanSel=0; mean0Sq=0; meanSqSel=0;
```

```
Do j=1 To N1+N2;
mean0=mean0+x0(j)/(N1+N2);
mean0Sq=mean0Sq+x0(j)**2/(N1+N2);
meanSel=meanSel+xFinal(j)/(N1+N2);
meanSqSel=meanSqSel+xFinal(j)**2/(N1+N2);
End;
Variance=abs((mean0Sq-mean0**2)+(meanSqSel-meanSel**2))/(N1+N2);
Testz=(meanSel-mean0)/sqrt(variance);
If TestZ >= &c_alpha Then Power=Power+1/&nSims;
Do i=1 To 4;
If SelectedArm=i Then SelProb(i)=SelProb(i)+1/&nSims;
End;
End;
TotalN=4*N1+2*N2;
Output;
Run;
Proc Print;
Run;
```
<<**SAS**<<

>>**SAS: Invoking SAS Macro 16.2**>>
```
%Mend FourPlus1AddArmMED;
Title "4+1 Add-Arm Design: Critical value";
data dInput;
Array mu(4)(0.2,0.2,0.2,0.2);
%FourPlus1AddArmMED(nSims=100000, N1=45, N2=90, c_alpha = 2.267, cR
= 0.5565, mu0=0.2, sigma=1.65);
Run;
Title "4+1 Add-Arm Design: Power with Emax from Ivanova paper";
data dInput;
Array mu(4)(0.34,0.68,0.76,0.78);
Title "Check Type-I error and Timing of Interim analysis";
%FourPlus1AddArmMED(nSims=100000, N1=45, N2=90, c_alpha = 2.267, cR
= 0.5565, mu0=0, sigma=1.6, targetResponse=0.7); *Normal approximation;
Run;
```
<<**SAS**<<

## 16.3 Extension of Add-Arm Designs

The $4 + 1$ add-arm design can be extended to designs, for example, (1) with more arms, (2) allowing early rejections, and (3) with interim futility stopping (if the nonbinding futility rule is used, the stopping boundary remains unchanged).

### 16.3.1 *The 5+1 Add-Arm Design*

The 5+1 add-arm design consists of 5 active arms and a placebo (control) arm (Figure 16.2). The randomization and dose-selection rules are specified as follows:

- Stage 1: Assign $2.5N_1$ subjects to arms 2, 0, and 4 using randomization ratio $N_1 : N_1/2 : N_1$.
- Stage 2: If $t_2 > t_4$, assign $2.5N_1$ subjects in arms 1, 0, and 3 using an $N_1 : N_1/2 : N_1$ randomization. If $t_2 \leq t_4$, assign $2.5N_1$ subjects in arm 3, 0, and 5 using an $N_1 : N_1/2 : N_1$ randomization.
- Stage 3: (a) If $t_2 > t_4$ and $\max(t_2, t_3) - t_1 < c_R$, select arm 1 as the winner; otherwise select arm 2 or 3 as the winner depending on which has a larger observed response. If $t_2 \leq t_4$ and $\max(t_3, t_4) - t_5 < c_R$, select arm 5 as the winner; otherwise select arm 4 or 3 as the winner depending on which has a larger response. (b) Assign $2N_2$ subjects in arms 0 and the winner arm using $N_2 : N_2$ randomization.

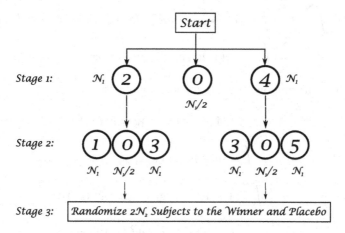

Figure 16.2: The $5 + 1$ Add-Arm Design

Therefore, there will be a total of $5N_1 + 2N_2$ subjects. In the final analysis for the hypothesis test, we will use the data from $N_1 + N_2$ subjects in the winner and $N_1 + N_2$ subjects in arm 0.

For this design, if $c_R = 0$, the selection probabilities are 1/8, 2/8, 2/8, 2/8, and 1/8, for the 5 active doses. To have the equal selection probability under $H_G$, the key is to determine $c_R$. We can prove that the selection probability can be written as

$$P(\max(t_2, t_3) - t_1 < c_R \cap t_2 > t_4; H_G) = \frac{1}{2} - \frac{3}{2} \int_{-\infty}^{\infty} \Phi(x - c_R)\Phi^2(x)\phi(x)dx.$$

(16.10)

The $c_R$ is so determined that the equal selection property under $H_G$ is retained, which is equal to 1/5. Using numerical integration, we obtain $c_R = 0.52153$.

**Proof.** For $5 + 1$ add-arm design, let $P^* = P(\max(X_2, X_3) - X_1 < c_R \cap X_2 > X_4)$. When $H_G$ is true, we have

$$P^* = P(X_2 - X_1 < c_R \cap X_2 > X_4 \cap X_2 > X_3)$$
$$+ P(X_3 - X_1 < c_R \cap X_2 > X_4 \cap X_2 < X_3)$$
$$= \int_{-\infty}^{\infty} \int_{-\infty}^{x_2} \int_{-\infty}^{x_2} \int_{x_2 - c_R}^{\infty} \phi(x_1)\phi(x_2)\phi(x_3)\phi(x_4)\, dx_1 dx_3 dx_4 dx_2$$
$$+ \int_{-\infty}^{\infty} \int_{x_3 - c_R}^{\infty} \int_{-\infty}^{x_3} \int_{-\infty}^{x_2} \phi(x_1)\phi(x_2)\phi(x_3)\phi(x_4)\, dx_4 dx_2 dx_1 dx_3$$

$$P^* = \int_{-\infty}^{\infty} \int_{-\infty}^{x_2} \int_{-\infty}^{x_2} [1 - \Phi(x_2 - c_R)]\,\phi(x_2)\phi(x_3)\phi(x_4)\, dx_3 dx_4 dx_2$$
$$+ \frac{1}{2} \int_{-\infty}^{\infty} \int_{x_3 - c_R}^{\infty} \phi(x_1)\phi(x_3)\Phi^2(x_3)\, dx_1 dx_3.$$

To further carrying out the integration, we obtain

$$P^* = \int_{-\infty}^{\infty} [1 - \Phi(x_2 - c_R)]\,\phi(x_2)\Phi^2(x_2)\, dx_2$$
$$+ \frac{1}{2} \int_{-\infty}^{\infty} [1 - \Phi(x_3 - c_R)]\,\phi(x_3)\Phi^2(x_3)\, dx_3$$
$$= \frac{3}{2} \int_{-\infty}^{\infty} (1 - \Phi(x_2 - c_R))\phi(x_2)\Phi^2(x_2)\, dx_2$$
$$= \frac{1}{2} - \frac{3}{2} \int_{-\infty}^{\infty} \Phi(x_2 - c_R)\Phi^2(x_2)\phi(x_2)\, dx_2$$

$\square$

### 16.3.2 *The 6+1 Add-Arm Design*

The 6+1 add-arm design consists of 6 active arms and a placebo (control) arm (Figure 16.3). The randomization and dose-selection rules are specified as follows:

- Stage 1: Assign $2.5N_1$ subjects in arms 3, 0, and 4 using randomization ratio $N_1 : N_1/2 : N_1$.
- Stage 2: If $t_3 > t_4$, assign $2.5N_1$ subjects in arms 1, 0, and 2 using an $N_1 : N_1/2 : N_1$ randomization. If $t_3 \leq t_4$, assign $2.5N_1$ subjects in arm 5, 0, and 6 using an $N_1 : N_1/2 : N_1$ randomization.
- Stage 3: (a) If $t_3 > t_4$ and $t_3 - \max(t_1, t_2) > c_R$, select arm 3 as the winner; otherwise select arm 1 or 2 as the winner depending on which has a larger observed response. If $t_3 \leq t_4$ and $t_4 - \max(t_5, t_6) > c_R$, select arm 4 as the winner; otherwise select arm 5 or 6 as the winner depending on which has a larger response. (b) Assign $2N_2$ subjects in arms 0 and the winner arm using $N_2 : N_2$ randomization.

Therefore, there will be a total of $5N_1 + 2N_2$ subjects. In the final analysis for the hypothesis test, we will use the data from $N_1 + N_2$ subjects in the winner and $N_1 + N_2$ subjects in arm 0.

For this design, if $c_R = 0$, the selection probabilities are $1/8$, $1/8$, $2/8$, $2/8$, $1/8$, and $1/8$, for the 6 active doses. To have the equal selection probability under $H_G$, the key is to determine $c_R$, which satisfies the following

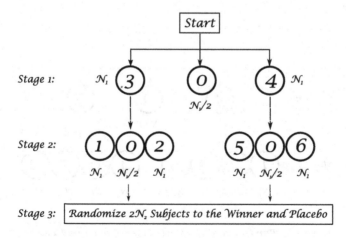

Figure 16.3: The $6 + 1$ Add-Arm Design

condition:

$$P(t_3 - \max(t_1, t_2) > c_R \cap t_3 > t_4; H_G) = \int_{-\infty}^{+\infty} \Phi^2 (x - c_R) \, \Phi (x) \, \phi(x) dx.$$

$$(16.11)$$

From the randomization and the winner selection, we can see that to keep the equal selection property under $H_G$, this probability has to be equal to $1/6$. Using numerical integration methods, we determine $c_R = 0.50094$.

**Proof.** For the $6 + 1$ add-arm design, let $T = \max(X_1, X_2)$. Further, we have

$$P(X_3 - T > c_R \cap X_3 > X_4)$$

$$= \int_{-\infty}^{+\infty} \int_{-\infty}^{x_3} \int_{-\infty}^{x_3 - c_R} 2\Phi (t) \, \phi (t) \, \phi(x_3) \phi (x_4) \, dt dx_4 dx_3$$

$$= \int_{-\infty}^{+\infty} \int_{-\infty}^{x_3} \Phi^2 (x_3 - c_R) \, \phi(x_3) \phi (x_4) \, dx_4 dx_3$$

$$= \int_{-\infty}^{+\infty} \Phi^2 (x_3 - c_R) \, \phi(x_3) \Phi (x_3) \, dx_3 \qquad \square$$

### 16.3.3   The 7+1 Add-Arm Design

The 7+1 add-arm design consists of 7 active arms and a placebo (control) arm (Figure 16.4). The randomization and dose-selection rules are specified as follows:

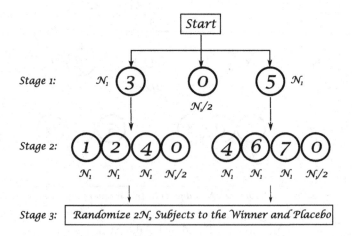

Figure 16.4:   The 7 + 1 Add-Arm Design

- Stage 1: Assign $2.5N_1$ subjects in arms 3, 0, and 5 using randomization ratio $N_1 : N_1/2 : N_1$.
- Stage 2: If $t_3 > t_5$, assign $3.5N_1$ subjects in arms 1, 2, 4, and 0 using an $N_1 : N_1 : N_1 : N_1/2$ randomization. If $t_3 \leq t_5$, assign $3.5N_1$ subjects in arm 4, 6, 7, and 0 using a $N_1 : N_1 : N_1 : N_1/2$ randomization.
- Stage 3: (a) If $t_3 > t_5$ and $\max(t_1, t_2) > \max(t_3, t_4) - c_R$, select arm 1 or 2 as the winner depending on which has a larger response; otherwise select arm 3 or 4 as the winner depending on which has a larger response. If $t_3 \leq t_5$ and $\max(t_7, t_6) > \max(t_5, t_4) - c_R$, select arm 7 or 6 as the winner; otherwise select arm 5 or 4 as the winner depending on which has a larger response. (b) Assign $2N_2$ subjects in arms 0 and the winner arm using a $N_2 : N_2$ randomization.

Therefore, a sample size of $6N_1 + 2N_2$ subjects is required. In the final analysis for the hypothesis test, we will use the data from $N_1 + N_2$ subjects in the winner and $N_1 + N_2$ subjects in arm 0.

For this design, if $c_R = 0$, the selection probabilities are $1/10$, $1/10$, $2/10$, $2/10$, $2/10$, $1/10$, and $1/10$, for the 7 active doses. To have the equal selection probability under $H_G$, the $c_R$ is determined by the following condition:

$$P(t_3 > t_5 \cap t_1 > \max(t_3, t_4) - c_R \cap t_1 > t_2; H_G)$$
$$= \frac{3}{4} \int_{-\infty}^{\infty} \left[1 - \Phi^2(x_3 - c_R)\right] \Phi^2(x_3) \phi(x_3) \, dx_3 = \frac{1}{7} \quad (16.12)$$

From the randomization and the winner selection, we can see that to keep the equal selection property under $H_G$, this probability has to be equal to $1/7$. Using numerical integration methods, we obtain $c_R = 0.48001$.

**Proof.** For the $7 + 1$ add-arm design, we have

$$P^* = P(X_3 > X_5 \cap X_1 > \max(X_3, X_4) - c_R \cap X_1 > X_2)$$
$$= P(X_3 > X_5 \cap X_1 > X_3 - c_R \cap X_3 > X_4 \cap X_1 > X_2) +$$
$$P(X_3 > X_5 \cap X_1 > X_4 - c_R \cap X_3 \leq X_4 \cap X_1 > X_2)$$
$$= \int_{-\infty}^{\infty} \int_{-\infty}^{x_3} \int_{-\infty}^{x_3} \int_{x_3 - c_R}^{\infty} \int_{-\infty}^{x_1} \prod_{i=1}^{5} \phi(x_i) \, dx_2 dx_1 dx_5 dx_4 dx_3 +$$
$$\int_{-\infty}^{\infty} \int_{-\infty}^{x_4} \int_{-\infty}^{x_3} \int_{x_4 - c_R}^{\infty} \int_{-\infty}^{x_1} \prod_{i=1}^{5} \phi(x_i) \, dx_2 dx_1 dx_5 dx_3 dx_4$$

$$P^* = \int_{-\infty}^{\infty} \int_{-\infty}^{x_3} \int_{-\infty}^{x_3} \int_{x_3-c_R}^{\infty} \Phi(x_1)\,\phi(x_1) \prod_{i=3}^{5} \phi(x_i)\, dx_1 dx_5 dx_4 dx_3$$

$$+ \int_{-\infty}^{\infty} \int_{-\infty}^{x_4} \int_{-\infty}^{x_3} \int_{x_4-c_R}^{\infty} \Phi(x_1)\,\phi(x_1) \prod_{i=3}^{5} \phi(x_i)\, dx_1 dx_5 dx_3 dx_4$$

$$P^* = \frac{1}{2} \int_{-\infty}^{\infty} \int_{-\infty}^{x_3} \int_{-\infty}^{x_3} \left[ 1 - \Phi^2 (x_3 - c_R) \right] \prod_{i=3}^{5} \phi(x_i)\, dx_5 dx_4 dx_3$$

$$+ \frac{1}{2} \int_{-\infty}^{\infty} \int_{-\infty}^{x_4} \int_{-\infty}^{x_3} \left[ 1 - \Phi^2 (x_4 - c_R) \right] \prod_{i=3}^{5} \phi(x_i)\, dx_5 dx_3 dx_4$$

$$P^* = \frac{1}{2} \int_{-\infty}^{\infty} \left[ 1 - \Phi^2 (x_3 - c_R) \right] \Phi^2 (x_3)\, \phi(x_3)\, dx_3$$

$$+ \frac{1}{2} \int_{-\infty}^{\infty} \int_{-\infty}^{x_4} \left[ 1 - \Phi^2 (x_4 - c_R) \right] \Phi(x_3)\, \phi(x_3)\, \phi(x_4)\, dx_3 dx_4$$

$$= \frac{3}{4} \int_{-\infty}^{\infty} \left[ 1 - \Phi^2 (x_3 - c_R) \right] \Phi^2 (x_3)\, \phi(x_3)\, dx_3$$

$$P^* = \frac{1}{2} \int_{-\infty}^{\infty} \left[ 1 - \Phi^2 (x_3 - c_R) \right] \Phi^2 (x_3)\, \phi(x_3)\, dx_3$$

$$+ \frac{1}{4} \int_{-\infty}^{\infty} \left[ 1 - \Phi^2 (x_4 - c_R) \right] \Phi^2 (x_4)\, \phi(x_4)\, dx_4$$

$$= \frac{3}{4} \int_{-\infty}^{\infty} \left[ 1 - \Phi^2 (x_3 - c_R) \right] \Phi^2 (x_3)\, \phi(x_3)\, dx_3$$

We provide SAS Macros for $5+1$, $6+1$ and $7+1$ add-arm design in Appendix C.                                                                    □

## 16.4   Comparison of Adaptive Design Methods

### 16.4.1   *Threshold $c_R$ and Stopping Boundary $c_\alpha$*

The first step is to determine the threshold $c_R$ and critical value for rejection of $H_G$, which can be determined using simulations. The results are presented in Table 16.1 for the $4+1$ to $7+1$ add-arm designs with one-sided $\alpha = 0.025$. Each set of results is based on 10,000,000 simulation runs. In Table 16.1, we have also presented the proportion of the $\alpha$ spent on each arm. For instance, for the $4+1$ design, under $H_G$, among all rejections, 20%

Table 16.1: $c_R, c_\alpha$ and Percent of $\alpha$-spent ($\alpha = 0.025, \tau = 0.5$)

| Design | $c_R$ | $c_\alpha$ | (virtual) Dose Level | | | | | | |
|--------|-------|-----------|------|------|------|------|------|------|------|
|        |       |           | 1    | 2    | 3    | 4    | 5    | 6    | 7    |
| 4+1    | 0.5565 | 2.267    | 20.0 | 30.0 | 30.0 | 20.0 | —    | —    | —    |
| 5+1    | 0.5215 | 2.343    | 15.8 | 22.8 | 22.8 | 22.8 | 15.8 | —    | —    |
| 6+1    | 0.5009 | 2.341    | 14.4 | 14.4 | 21.2 | 21.2 | 14.4 | 14.4 | —    |
| 7+1    | 0.4800 | 2.397    | 11.7 | 12.0 | 17.2 | 17.2 | 17.2 | 12.0 | 11.7 |

rejections with the winner being Arm 1, and 30% with the winner being Arm 2, 30% with the winner being Arm 3, and 20% with the winner being Arm 4. We can see that $c_R$ is so determined that it will give equal chance to select any dose when all doses have the same effect, but the $\alpha$ spent on each arm is different. This desirable feature allows one to use the prior knowledge to spend more alpha on the promising doses to achieve more efficient (powerful) design. We further noticed that it is sometimes desirable to have particular $\alpha$-spending among doses by modifying the $c_R$ slightly and the information time $\tau$. When this occurs, the stopping boundaries should be modified accordingly so that the familywise error is controlled. The values $c_R$ and $c_\alpha$ for the add-arm designs with $\alpha = 0.025$ and $\tau = 0.5$ are presented in Table 16.1.

Since these stopping boundaries are determined based on normality or large sample size assumption, we want to know how well they can be applied to the case of small sample size. For sample size $N_1 = N_2 = 30$, the error rate is 0.0278, a small inflation from 0.025. Based on simulations (1,000,000 runs), for sample size $N_1 = N_2 = 100$, the inflation is negligible or within the random fluctuation by the simulation. When the sample size is smaller than 30, the critical value can also be determined by simulations. It is a good practice to check type-I error rate using simulation before running the power simulations. Note that the type-I error will inflated from 0.025 to 0.0274 if using normal distribution approximation for the univariate $t$-test.

## 16.4.2 *Comparison of Seamless Designs*

To compare the power of the add-arm designs against the drop-arm designs, various dose-response curves are considered. The different response curves are obtained by switching the sequence of the doses (Table 16.2). For the drop-arm design, the dose sequence is irrelevant as far as the power is concerned. However, for the add-arm design, a different dose sequence implies a different test order.

For the drop-arm design, there are two stages and the sample size ratio per group at the first stage to the second stage is $N_1/N_2 = 1$ or information time $\tau = 0.5$. From the numerical integrations with $\tau = 0.5$, the rejection boundaries for the $4+1$, $5+1$, $6+1$, and $7+1$ drop-arm designs are 2.352, 2.408, 2.451, and 2.487, respectively.

Table 16.2:    Responses for Difference Response Curves

| Design | Curve Name | Arm 0 | 1 | 2 | 3 | 4 | 5 | 6 | 7 |
|--------|------------|---|-------|-------|-------|-------|-------|-------|-------|
| 4+1 | Linear | 0 | 0.1 | 0.2 | 0.3 | 0.4 | — | — | — |
|      | UM1    | 0 | 0.1 | 0.2 | 0.4 | 0.3 | — | — | — |
|      | UM2    | 0 | 0.1 | 0.4 | 0.3 | 0.2 | — | — | — |
| 5+1 | Linear | 0 | 0.08 | 0.16 | 0.24 | 0.32 | 0.40 | — | — |
|      | UM1    | 0 | 0.08 | 0.16 | 0.24 | 0.40 | 0.32 | — | — |
|      | UM2    | 0 | 0.08 | 0.16 | 0.40 | 0.32 | 0.24 | — | — |
|      | UM3    | 0 | 0.08 | 0.40 | 0.32 | 0.24 | 0.16 | — | — |
| 6+1 | Linear | 0 | 0.067 | 0.133 | 0.200 | 0.267 | 0.333 | 0.400 | — |
|      | UM1    | 0 | 0.067 | 0.133 | 0.200 | 0.267 | 0.400 | 0.333 | — |
|      | UM2    | 0 | 0.067 | 0.133 | 0.200 | 0.400 | 0.333 | 0.267 | — |
|      | UM3    | 0 | 0.067 | 0.133 | 0.400 | 0.333 | 0.267 | 0.200 | — |
|      | UM4    | 0 | 0.067 | 0.400 | 0.333 | 0.267 | 0.200 | 0.133 | — |
| 7+1 | Linear | 0 | 0.057 | 0.114 | 0.171 | 0.229 | 0.286 | 0.343 | 0.400 |
|      | UM1    | 0 | 0.057 | 0.114 | 0.171 | 0.229 | 0.286 | 0.400 | 0.343 |
|      | UM2    | 0 | 0.057 | 0.114 | 0.171 | 0.229 | 0.400 | 0.343 | 0.286 |
|      | UM3    | 0 | 0.057 | 0.114 | 0.171 | 0.400 | 0.343 | 0.286 | 0.229 |
|      | UM4    | 0 | 0.057 | 0.114 | 0.400 | 0.343 | 0.286 | 0.229 | 0.171 |
|      | UM5    | 0 | 0.057 | 0.400 | 0.343 | 0.286 | 0.229 | 0.171 | 0.114 |

Based on 1,000,000 simulation runs for each scenario, the sample size and power are presented in Table 16.3 for the add-arm and drop-arm (DA) designs for different response curves. For the each add-arm design ($\tau = N_1/(N_1 + N_2) = 0.5$), we also present the average power over different response curves. For the drop-arm design, the dose sequence is irrelevant, thus the power is identical for all the response curves.

Note that the total sample size $N_{\max}$ is $(K+1)N_1 + 2N_2$ for the $K+1$ drop-arm design, $4N_1 + 2N_2$ for the $4+1$ add-arm design, $5N_1 + 2N_2$ for the $5+1$ add-arm and the $6+1$ add-arm designs, and $6N_1 + 2N_2$ for the $7+1$ add-arm design.

From the results, we can see that the add-arm designs generally provide a higher average power (2%–5% higher) than drop-arm designs. All add-arm designs (except the $6+1$ design) provide higher power than the corresponding drop-arm designs under all different response curves. The reason for the $6+1$ design not always being higher than the drop-arm design is that it is difficult to identify the better arm in the first stage when

Table 16.3: Power (%) Comparisons

| Design | $N_{\max}$ | Linear | UM1 | UM2 | UM3 | UM4 | UM5 | Average Power | DA Power |
|---|---|---|---|---|---|---|---|---|---|
| 4+1 | 700 | 90.2 | 95.3 | 96.6 | — | — | — | 94.0 | 90.0 |
| 5+1 | 700 | 90.5 | 92.7 | 92.8 | 94.0 | — | — | 92.5 | 89.8 |
| 6+1 | 700 | 81.0 | 81.0 | 91.8 | 94.0 | 89.2 | — | 87.4 | 85.8 |
| 7+1 | 700 | 82.2 | 82.2 | 88.6 | 89.4 | 91.1 | 87.3 | 86.8 | 81.7 |

the responses are similar in the two arms at the first stage. We also want to point out that the linear response arrangement in Table 16.3 is very unlikely to happen since if we are so unsure about response curve (i.e., we thought the response was umbrella-shaped but it was actually linear with a large slope), we should not assume the unimodality at all. On the other hand, if we knew the monotonic response (even when the slope is quite flat), we would have rearranged the dose sequence to more likely make it an umbrella shaped.

In addition, we compare the drop-arm and the add-arm designs under some scenarios that are suspected to be unfavorable to the proposed add-arm design: (1) when the dose responses of the two arms at the first stage are the same and (2) when the response curve is wavelike, but the fluctuation is small. The first dose response curve (named flat in Table 16.4) with an equal response for the two doses at the first stage is $(0.2, 0.2, 0.3, 0.45, 0.3, 0.25)$ for dose sequence $(d_0, d_1, d_2, d_3, d_4, d_5)$ and the second wavelike response curve is $(0.2, 0.2, 0.4, 0.38, 0.42, 0.45)$ for the same dose sequence. We compare the $5 + 1$ add-arm design and $5 + 1$ drop-arm design in terms of power and selection probability. The simulations are based on the standard deviation of 1.5, total sample size of 3500, and one-sided $\alpha$ of 0.025. The simulation results are presented in Table 16.4. From the results we see that the add-arm is superior to the drop-arm design in terms of power and correct selection probabilities.

These kinds of settings may reflect the following practical scenarios. For some disease indications, such as cardiovascular and oncology, the primary efficacy endpoint and the primary safety endpoint are consistent. For

Table 16.4: Comparison of Power and Selection Probability

| Response | Design Method | $N_1/N_2$ | $d_1$ | $d_2$ | $d_3$ | $d_4$ | $d_5$ | Power |
|---|---|---|---|---|---|---|---|---|
| Flat | Add-arm design | 500/500 | 0.00 | 0.05 | 0.89 | 0.05 | 0.01 | 0.88 |
| | Drop-arm design | 438/438 | 0.00 | 0.06 | 0.87 | 0.06 | 0.02 | 0.82 |
| Wave | Add-arm design | 500/500 | 0.00 | 0.32 | 0.14 | 0.21 | 0.32 | 0.91 |
| | Drop-arm design | 438/438 | 0.00 | 0.18 | 0.12 | 0.26 | 0.45 | 0.89 |

example, the composite endpoint of a 30-day death and MI is often the efficacy and safety endpoints for cardiovascular studies. Survival or death is often the efficacy and safety endpoint for cancer trials. In such cases, the dose responses are usually monotonic but we can rearrange the dose sequence so that the responses become a unimodal or umbrella-shaped curve. In this way, the add-arm design will show more powerful than the drop-arm design. At the same time, if several doses have a similar response, the selection probabilities will be similar among doses and lower doses will have a good chance to be selected. This is a desirable feature since higher doses are often associated with a higher cost or lower tolerability, and/or inconvenience.

We want to point out that the doses (arms) can be virtual doses, e.g., different drug combinations or different dose-schedule combinations. To increase power of the add-arm design, we can rearrange the dose (arm) sequence so that the most responsive arms are placed at or near the middle of the response curve. Such an arrangement is based on prior information, but mistakes can happen when the responses among the arms are similar, i.e., the arranged the arm (dose) sequence may not be unimodal. For this reason, comparisons of the designs are conservatively based on the average power over all the response curves for the add-arm design to the power of the drop-loser design (Table 16.3).

The empirical distributions of the test statistics for the drop-arm design and the add-arm design are also investigated. For the drop-arm design, the distributions of the final test statistic appear to be normal under a linear response curve. However, for the add-arm design, the distribution of the final test statistic is skewed under the linear responses.

### 16.4.3    *Comparisons of Phase-II Dose-Finding Designs*

For the phase-II dose-finding trial, we need to define a response-value at the minimum effective dose (MED), $\mu_{MED}$, which will be used to define the utility function:

$$U = \frac{1}{(\mu_i - \mu_{MED})^2}, \qquad (16.13)$$

where $\mu_i$ is the response in arm $i$. Using this utility, we can convert the problem of finding the MED to the problem of finding the dose with the maximum utility $U$ because at or near the MED, the maximum of $U$ is achieved. However, to prevent a numerical overflow in the simulation, we have implemented the utility using

$$U = \frac{1}{\left(\hat{\mu}_i - \mu_{MED}\right)^2 + \varepsilon},\qquad(16.14)$$

where $\varepsilon > 0$ is a very small value (e.g., 0.00000001) introduced to avoid a numerical overflow when the observed $\hat{\mu}_i = \mu_{MED}$.

Ivanova et al. (2012) proposed the Bayesian two-stage adaptive design and compared it with the equal allocation method of Dunnett's test using five different dose-response models, including the $E_{max}$, linear in log-dose, linear, truncated-logistic, and logistic models. The comparisons are based on selection probability (the probability of selecting each arm as the winner) and the power of the hypothesis test against the control. There are five arms including the control arm. Their responses are presented in Table 16.5. The simulations are based on the standard deviation $\sigma$ of 0.65, total sample size of 180 subjects, and one-sided $\alpha$ of .025.

Table 16.5:  Phase II Dose-Finding Models

| Scenario | Model | Mean Response |
|---|---|---|
| 1 | $E_{max}$ | (0.20, 0.34, 0.68, 0.76, 0.78) |
| 2 | Linear in Log-dose | (0.20, 0.27, 0.59, 0.74, 0.80) |
| 3 | Linear | (0.20, 0.23, 0.47, 0.68, 0.80) |
| 4 | Truncated-logistic | (0.20, 0.20, 0.22, 0.54, 0.80) |
| 5 | Logistic | (0.20, 0.21, 0.58, 0.79, 0.80) |

We compare the power and selection probabilities obtained from the two add-arm designs with two different information time, two-drop-arm designs with two different information time, the Bayesian two-stage adaptive design, and the equal allocation design. The simulation results are presented in Table 16.6 through Table 16.10, where the Bayesian design is the Bayesian two-stage adaptive design proposed by Ivanova et al. (2012). From the results we can see that the add-arm designs perform the best in terms of power in all cases and also provide good selection probabilities. However, the Bayesian method provides better selection probabilities in most cases. To improve the selection probability, we can adjust the value $c_R$ based on prior information about dose-response curve in the add-arm design (see a trial example in the next section).

## 16.5  Clinical Trial Examples

### Example 16.1  Phase II Dose-Finding Trial

Anemia is a condition in which the body does not have enough healthy red blood cells. Iron helps make red blood cells. When the body does

Table 16.6:   Power and Selection Probability: $E_{max}$ Model

| Design Method | $N_1/N_2$ | $d_1$ | $d_2$ | $d_3$ | $d_4$ | Power |
|---|---|---|---|---|---|---|
| Add-arm design[1] | 30/30 | 0.01 | 0.56 | 0.31 | 0.12 | 0.98 |
| Add-arm design[2] | 20/50 | 0.02 | 0.52 | 0.32 | 0.13 | 0.98 |
| Drop-arm design[1] | 26/25 | 0.02 | 0.39 | 0.32 | 0.27 | 0.95 |
| Drop-arm design[2] | 20/40 | 0.03 | 0.38 | 0.31 | 0.29 | 0.97 |
| Bayesian design | | 0.19 | 0.67 | 0.10 | 0.04 | 0.89 |
| Equal allocation | | 0.23 | 0.60 | 0.11 | 0.06 | 0.83 |

Table 16.7:   Power and Selection Probability: Linear in Log-Dose

| Design Method | $N_1/N_2$ | $d_1$ | $d_2$ | $d_3$ | $d_4$ | Power |
|---|---|---|---|---|---|---|
| Add-arm design[1] | 30/30 | 0.02 | 0.68 | 0.26 | 0.04 | 0.88 |
| Add-arm design[2] | 20/50 | 0.04 | 0.60 | 0.29 | 0.07 | 0.90 |
| Drop-arm design[1] | 26/25 | 0.03 | 0.55 | 0.26 | 0.15 | 0.81 |
| Drop-arm design[2] | 20/40 | 0.05 | 0.50 | 0.28 | 0.17 | 0.87 |
| Bayesian two-stage | | 0.07 | 0.67 | 0.22 | 0.04 | 0.90 |
| Equal allocation | | 0.11 | 0.62 | 0.22 | 0.05 | 0.84 |

Table 16.8:   Power and Selection Probability: Linear

| Design Method | $N_1/N_2$ | $d_1$ | $d_2$ | $d_3$ | $d_4$ | Power |
|---|---|---|---|---|---|---|
| Add-arm design[1] | 30/30 | 0.00 | 0.19 | 0.56 | 0.25 | 0.93 |
| Add-arm design[2] | 20/50 | 0.00 | 0.25 | 0.50 | 0.24 | 0.91 |
| Drop-arm design[1] | 26/25 | 0.00 | 0.14 | 0.54 | 0.32 | 0.90 |
| Drop-arm Design[2] | 20/40 | 0.00 | 0.17 | 0.49 | 0.33 | 0.92 |
| Bayesian two-stage | | 0.02 | 0.44 | 0.47 | 0.07 | 0.87 |
| Equal allocation | | 0.03 | 0.45 | 0.45 | 0.07 | 0.80 |

Table 16.9:   Power and Selection Probability: Truncated-Logistic

| Design Method | $N_1/N_2$ | $d_1$ | $d_2$ | $d_3$ | $d_4$ | Power |
|---|---|---|---|---|---|---|
| Add-arm design[1] | 30/30 | 0.00 | 0.05 | 0.85 | 0.10 | 0.73 |
| Add-arm design[2] | 20/50 | 0.01 | 0.10 | 0.75 | 0.14 | 0.74 |
| Drop-arm design[1] | 26/25 | 0.04 | 0.05 | 0.78 | 0.12 | 0.60 |
| Dro-arm Design[2] | 20/40 | 0.06 | 0.08 | 0.71 | 0.15 | 0.67 |
| Bayesian two-stage | | 0.00 | 0.04 | 0.79 | 0.17 | 0.86 |
| Equal allocation | | 0.00 | 0.05 | 0.79 | 0.16 | 0.76 |

Table 16.10:   Power and Selection Probability: Logistic

| Design Method | $N_1/N_2$ | $d_1$ | $d_2$ | $d_3$ | $d_4$ | Power |
|---|---|---|---|---|---|---|
| Add-arm design[1] | 30/30 | 0.01 | 0.80 | 0.15 | 0.04 | 0.86 |
| Add-arm design[2] | 20/50 | 0.03 | 0.71 | 0.21 | 0.05 | 0.89 |
| Drop-arm design[1] | 26/25 | 0.02 | 0.65 | 0.17 | 0.16 | 0.80 |
| Dro-arm Design[2] | 20/40 | 0.03 | 0.58 | 0.20 | 0.18 | 0.86 |
| Bayesian two-stage | | 0.04 | 0.76 | 0.18 | 0.02 | 0.90 |
| Equal allocation | | 0.06 | 0.76 | 0.17 | 0.02 | 0.82 |

not have enough iron, it will make fewer red blood cells. This is called iron deficiency anemia (IDA). IDA is the most common form of anemia (Looker, 1997). The majority of IDA is linked to menstrual blood loss, pregnancy, postpartum blood loss, GI bleeding, cancer, or chronic kidney disease (CKD) (Baker, 2000).

The hypothetical drug candidate, FXT, is an IV drug candidate for treating patient with IDA. Serious hypersensitivity reactions and cardiovascular events among other are to be the potential main safety concerns regarding the use of IV iron products. Therefore, the goal is to find the minimum effective dose (MED). It was hypothetically determined that 0.5g/dL is the minimal clinical meaningful change in Hg from baseline.

Suppose 4 active doses (200mg, 300mg, 400mg, 500mg) are to be investigated. The primary endpoint is hemoglobin (Hg) change from baseline to Week 5, which is an objective measure in the lab. Assume an $E_{max}$ model with responses (Hg change from baseline to Week 5) of 0, 0.34, 0.68, 0.76, and 0.78 g/dL for the placebo and 4 active doses with a common standard deviation of 1.6. Because Hg is objectively measured in the lab, the placebo effect, if any, will be minimal.

The target response of MED is determined to be 0.7g/dL, which is somewhat higher than the minimal clinically meaningful difference 0.5g/dL. This is because if we define MED with response 0.5, then there is a 50% probability that the observed response of the MED will be less than 0.5g/dL, regardless of sample size or power. We want the probability of observing response at the target MED>0.5 to be much higher than 50%.

To use the add-arm and drop-arm designs, we first need to define the unimodal utility function using (16.14) so that the MED-finding problem becomes the problem of finding the dose with the maximum utility. The performances of the add-arm and drop-arm designs are evaluated using simulations. The results are presented in Table 16.11.

For the $4+1$ add-arm design with one-sided $\alpha = 0.025$, the critical value $c_\alpha = 2.267$, $c_R = 0.55652$, $N_1 = 45$, $N_2 = 90$, and power = 90%, the total sample size required is 360. For the $4+1$ drop-arm design with $c_\alpha = 2.35$, $N_1 = 48$, $N_2 = 96$, and power = 90%, the total required sample size is

Table 16.11: Selection Probability and Sample Size: AA and DA Designs

| Design method | $d_1$ 200mg | $d_2$ 400mg | $d_3$ 500mg | $d_4$ 300mg | Sample Size |
|---|---|---|---|---|---|
| Add-arm design | 0.074 | 0.430 | 0.362 | 0.164 | 360 |
| Drop-arm design | 0.102 | 0.319 | 0.296 | 0.283 | 432 |

432. The add-arm design can save 72 subjects or 17% sample size from the drop-arm design. In both methods, the type-I error rates are below 2.5% according to 1,000,000 simulation runs.

### Example 16.2    Phase II-III Asthma Trial

Asthma is a chronic disease characterized by airway inflammation. Those affected with the disease experience asthmatic episodes when their airways narrow due to inflammation and they have difficulty breathing. According to the U.S. CDC, about 1 in 12 people (about 25 million) have asthma, and the numbers are increasing every year. About 1 in 2 people (about 12 million) with asthma had an asthma attack in 2008, but many asthma attacks could have been prevented. The number of people diagnosed with asthma grew by 4.3 million from 2001 to 2009. Asthma was linked to 3,447 deaths in 2007. Asthma costs in the U.S. grew from about $53 billion in 2002 to about $56 billion in 2007, about a 6% increase. Greater access to medical care is needed for the growing number of people with asthma.

This hypothetical phase-II/III seamless design is motivated by an actual asthma clinical development program. AXP is a second generation compound in the class of asthma therapies known as 5-LO inhibitors, which block the production of leukotrienes. Leukotrienes are major mediators of the inflammatory response. The company's preclinical and early clinical data suggested that the drug candidate has potential for an improved efficacy and is well tolerated under the total dose of 1600mg.

The objective of the multicenter seamless trial is to evaluate the effectiveness (as measured by FEV1) of oral AXP in adult patients with chronic asthma. Patients were randomized to one of five treatment arms, Arm 0 (placebo), Arm 1 (daily dose of 200mg for 6 weeks), arm 2 (daily dose of 400mg for 4 weeks), arm 3 (daily dose of 500mg 3 weeks), and arm 4 (daily dose of 300mg for 5 weeks). Since the efficacy is usually dependent on both AUC and $C_{max}$ of the active agent, it is difficult to judge at the design stage exactly which dose-schedule combination will be the best. However, based on limited data and clinical judgment, it might be reasonable to assume that the following dose sequence might show a unimodal (umbrella) response curve: Arm 1, Arm 2, Arm 3, and Arm 4. The dose responses are estimated to be: 8%, 13%, 17%, 16%, and 15% for the placebo and the four active arms with a standard deviation of 26%.

We compare the $4 + 1$ add-arm design against the drop-arm design. A total sample size of 600 subjects ($N_1 = N_2 = 100$) for the add-arm design will provide 89% power. We have also tried other different dose sequences, including wavelike sequence; the simulation results show that the power ranges from 88% to 89%, except for the linear response, which provides 86% power. Comparing the drop-arm design, 602 subjects ($N_1 = N_2 = 86$) will provide only 84% power, regardless of dose sequence. Given the good safety profile, the selection probability is much less important than the power. Thus, the slight difference in selection probability is not discussed here.

## Example 16.3    Phase IV Oncology Trial

Multiple myeloma is a cancer of plasma cells (a blood disorder related to lymphoma and leukemia), a type of white blood cell present in bone marrow. Plasma cells normally make antibodies to fight infections. In multiple myeloma, a group of plasma cells (myeloma cells) becomes cancerous and multiplies, raising the number of plasma cells to a higher than normal level. Health problems caused by multiple myeloma can affect one's bones, immune system, kidneys and red blood cell count. Myeloma develops in 1–4 per 100,000 people per year. There is no cure for multiple myeloma, but treatments are available that slow its progression.

The chemical compound $V$ was a newly approved third line (hypothetical) drug for multiple myeloma in addition to several other drugs (labeled $X$, $Y$, $Z$, ...) available for the same disease indication. An investigator wants to know which of the following drug combination will provide the most benefit to the patients: $V + X$, $V + Y$, $V + Z$, or $V + X + Y$. The reasons for such combinations are that the mechanism of action of $V$ is different from $X$, $Y$, and $Z$, while $X$ and $Y$ are similar but with some difference in the mechanism. However, $X$ and $Y$ are very similar to $Z$ in the mechanics of action, thus to combine them ($X + Z$ or $Y + Z$) will not increase the response. To seek the company's sponsorship, the investigator has looked into different designs: the drop-arm design and the add-arm design. For this phase-IV trial, it is determined that the surrogate endpoint of tumor size reduction (partial response + complete response rate) is the primary endpoint. Complete response (CR) is defined as 100% M-protein reduction and partial response (PR) is more than 50% reduction in tumor size.

The standard treatment ($S$) has a response rate of 42%. The estimated rates for $V + X$, $V + Y$, $V + Z$ and $V + X + Y$ are 50%, 54%, 57%, and 60%, respectively. Given such estimates, the $4 + 1$ add-arm design is considered and the arms are arranged as follows: Arm 1: $V + X$, Arm 2: $V + Y$, Arm 3: $V + X + Y$, and Arm 4: $V + Z$ with response sequence: 50%, 54%, 60%, and 57%. With the large sample size assumption, the standard deviation is estimated (somewhat conservatively) $\sigma = \sqrt{p(1-p)} \approx 0.5$ for all the arms, where $p$ is the tumor response rate.

We can see that in this setting, both the correct selection probability and the power are important measures of a trial design. For a total sample size of 300 ($N_1 = N_2 = 100$) and $\alpha = 0.025$, the 4 + 1 add-arm design will provide 88% power and correct selection probability for the best arm is 47%. For the same total sample size ($N_1 = 80$ and $N_2 = 140$), the power of the add-arm design increases to 89% but correct selection probability reduces to 44%. Given that the main objective of the trial is to recommend a best drug combination therapy, the first design with $N_1 = N_2 = 100$ seems a better design.

We know that the constant $c_R$ can also dramatically affect the selection probability and power. For example, if we change $c_R$ from 0.55652 to 0, the correct selection probability will change from 47% to 59% and power will change from 88% to 90%. If the $c_R$ is changed further to $-1$, the correct selection probability will be 74% and power 90%. However, such a deviation (to a more extreme value) from the default value $c_R = 0.5565$ could have a negative effect on the selection probability and power if the response pattern is estimated very inaccurately.

Considering all these factors, the add-arm design with $N_1 = N_2 = 100$ and $c_R = 0$ is recommended. To compare, for the same 90% power, the drop-arm design requires 700 ($N_1 = N_2 = 100$) subjects with the correct selection probability of 58%. Thus, the add-arm design requires 100 fewer subjects or 17% savings in sample size from the drop-arm design in this scenario.

## 16.6   Summary

We studied the effective add-arm adaptive designs. Under unimodal responses (including linear and umbrella responses), the proposed 3-stage add-arm design is usually more powerful that the 2-stage drop-arm design mainly because the former takes advantage of the knowledge of unimodality of responses. If the response is not unimodal, we can use that prior knowledge to rearrange the dose sequence so that it becomes a unimodal response.

In the add-arm design, all arms are usually selected with equal chance when all arms have the same expected response, but the probability of rejection is different even when all arms are equally effective. This feature allows us to effectively use the prior information to place more effective treatments in the middle at the first stage to increase the power.

In an add-arm design, dose levels don't have to be equally placed or based on the dose amount. The arms can be virtual dose levels or combinations of different drugs. Furthermore, the number of arms and the actual dose levels do not have to be prespecified, but instead, they can be decided after the interim analyses.

As mentioned earlier, the constant $c_R$ is usually so chosen to ensure the equal selection probability for a flat response curve. However, this requirement can be relaxed (slightly) if we want to have certain $\alpha$ spending among the arms to boost the correct selection probability and power if there is good information about dose response curve available. We further noticed that the stopping boundary $c_\alpha$ and $\alpha$-spending can be adjusted by modifying the $c_R$ (slightly) and the information time $\tau$.

The distribution of the final test statistic for the drop-arm design appears to be normal under $H_G$ and $H_a$, whereas the distribution of the test statistic of the add-arm design appears to be normal under $H_G$ and skewed under $H_a$.

Sample size can be reestimated at the interim analyses, but the distributions of test statistics and stopping boundaries will be different. The stopping boundary and power can be obtained using computer simulations.

We have assumed that a bigger response in the endpoint is better in previous discussions. For an endpoint for which a smaller value is better, we can change the sign of the variable or use other variable transform methods. When a smaller response rate is better, we can change the proportion of responses to the proportion of nonresponders as the endpoint, but keep the interpretation unchanged.

**Problems**

**16.1** Redesign the trial in Example 16.1 using the target response of MED 0.75g/dL and justify the design you recommend.

**16.2** Redesign the trial in Example 16.2 using the Dunnett, the drop-arm, and the add-arm designs and justify the design you may recommend by comparing the different methods in terms of operating characteristics.

**16.3** Provide examples that the add-arm design might be useful.

# Chapter 17

# Biomarker-Enrichment Design

## 17.1 Introduction

Biomarkers, as compared to a true (primary) endpoint such as survival, can often be measured earlier, more easily, and more frequently; they are less subject to competing risks and less confounded. The utilization of biomarkers will lead to a better target population with a larger effect size, a smaller sample size required, and faster decision making. With the advancement of proteomic, genomic, and genetic technologies, personalized medicine with the right drug for the right patient becomes possible.

Conley and Taube (2004) describe the future of biomarker/genomic markers in cancer therapy: "The elucidation of the human genome and fifty years of biological studies have laid the groundwork for a more informed method for treating cancer with the prospect of realizing improved survival. Advanced in knowledge about the molecular abnormalities, signaling pathways, influence the local tissue milieu and the relevance of genetic polymorphism offer hope of designing effective therapies tailored for a given cancer in particular individual, as well as the possibility of avoiding unnecessary toxicity".

Wang, Hung, and O'Neill (2006) from the FDA have pointed out: "Generally, when the primary clinical efficacy outcome in a phase III trial requires much longer time to observe, a surrogate endpoint thought to be strongly associated with the clinical endpoint may be chosen as the primary efficacy variable in phase II trials. The results of the phase II studies then provide an estimated effect size on the surrogate endpoint, which is supposedly able to help size the phase III trial for the primary clinical efficacy endpoint, where often it is thought to have a smaller effect size".

What exactly is a biomarker? National Institutes of Health Workshop (De Gruttola, 2001) gave the following definitions. *Biomarker* is a characteristic that is objectively measured and evaluated as an indicator of normal biologic processes, pathogenic processes, or pharmacological responses to a therapeutic intervention. *Clinical endpoint* (or outcome) is a characteristic or variable that reflects how a patient feels or functions, or how long a patient survives. *Surrogate endpoint* is a biomarker intended to substitute for a clinical endpoint. Biomarkers can also be classified as classifier, prognostic, and predictive biomarkers, but they are not mutually exclusive.

A **classifier biomarker** is a marker, e.g., a DNA marker, that usually does not change over the course of study. A classifier biomarker can be used to select the most appropriate target population or even for personalized treatment. For example, a study drug is expected to have effects on a population with a biomarker, which is only 20% of the overall patient population. Because the sponsor suspects that the drug may not work for the overall patient population, it may be efficient and ethical to run a trial for only the subpopulations with the biomarker rather than the general patient population. On the other hand, some biomarkers such as RNA markers are expected to change over the course of the study. This type of marker can be either a prognostic or predictive marker.

A **prognostic biomarker** informs the clinical outcomes, independent of treatment. It provides information about the natural course of the disease in an individual with or without treatment under study. A prognostic marker does not inform the effect of the treatment. For example, NSCLC patients receiving either EGFR inhibitors or chemotherapy have better outcomes with a mutation than without a mutation. Prognostic markers can be used to separate good and poor prognosis patients at the time of diagnosis. If the expression of the marker clearly separates patients with an excellent prognosis from those with a poor prognosis, then the marker can be used to aid the decision about how aggressive the therapy needs to be. The poor prognosis patients might be considered for clinical trials of novel therapies that will, hopefully, be more effective (Conley and Taube, 2004). Prognostic markers may also inform the possible mechanisms responsible for the poor prognosis, thus leading to the identification of new targets for treatment and new effective therapeutics.

A **predictive biomarker** informs the treatment effect on the clinical endpoint. A predictive marker can be population-specific: a marker can be predictive for population A but not population B. A predictive biomarker, as compared to true endpoints such as survival, can often be measured earlier, more easily, and more frequently and is less subject to competing risks. For example, in a trial of a cholesterol-lowering drug, the ideal end-point used to evaluate the treatment effect may be death or development of coronary artery disease (CAD). However, such a study usually requires thousands of patients and many years to conduct. Therefore, it is desirable to have a biomarker, such as a reduction in post-treatment cholesterol, if it predicts the reductions in the incidence of CAD. Another example would be an oncology study where the ultimate endpoint is death. However, when a patient has disease progression, the physician will switch the patient's initial treatment to an alternative treatment. Such treatment modalities will jeopardize the assessment of treatment effect on survival because the treatment switching is response-adaptive rather than random (see Chapters 13 and 14). If a marker, such as time-to-progression (TTP) or response rate (RR), is used as the primary endpoint, then we will have much cleaner efficacy assessments because the biomarker assessment is performed before the treatment switching occurs.

In this chapter, we will discuss adaptive designs using classifier, prognostic, and predictive markers. The challenges in marker validations will also be discussed.

## 17.2  Design with Classifier Biomarker

### 17.2.1  *Setting the Scene*

As mentioned earlier, a drug might have different effects in different patient populations. A hypothetical case is presented in Table 17.1, where $RR_+$ and $RR_-$ are the response rates for biomarker-positive and biomarker-negative populations, respectively. In the example, there is a treatment effect of 25% in the 10 million patient population with the biomarker, but only 9% in the 50 million general patient population. The sponsor faces the dilemma of whether to target the general patient population or use biomarkers to select a smaller set of patients that are expected to have a bigger response to the drug.

Table 17.1:  Response Rate and Sample Size Required

|  | Population | $RR_+$ | $RR_-$ | Sample Size |
|---|---|---|---|---|
| Biomarker (+) | 10M | 50% | 25% | 160* |
| Biomarker (−) | 40M | 30% | 25% | |
| Total | 50M | 34% | 25% | 1800 |

Note: *800 subjects screened. Power = 80%.

There are several challenges: (1) the estimated effect size for each subpopulation at the design stage is often very inaccurate; (2) a cost is associated with screening patients for the biomarker; (3) the test for detecting the biomarker often requires a high sensitivity and specificity, and the screening tool may not be available at the time of the clinical trial; and (4) screening patients for the biomarker may cause a burden and impact patient recruitment. These factors must be considered in the design.

Ideally, the utility function should be constructed first in order to decide which population we should target. There are many utility functions from which to choose. For example, the utility can be defined as $U = \Sigma\left(\delta_i N_i - C_i\right)$, where $\delta_i$ is the effect size of the $i$th subpopulation with the size of $N_i$ and $C_i$ is the associated cost or loss.

Suppose we decide to run a trial on population with a biomarker. It is interesting to study how the screening test impacts the expected utility. The target patient size $N$ with biomarker $(+)$ can be expressed as

$$N = N_+ S_e + N_-(1 - S_p),  \tag{17.1}$$

where $N_+$ and $N_-$ are the sizes of patient populations with and without the biomarker, respectively; $S_e$ is the sensitivity of the screening test, i.e., the probability of correctly identifying the biomarker among patients with the biomarker; and $S_p$ is the specificity of the screening test, which is defined as the probability of correctly identifying biomarker-negative among patients without biomarker. The average treatment effect for diagnostic biomarker $(+)$ patients is

$$\Delta = \frac{\Delta_+ N_+ S_e + \Delta_- N_-(1 - S_p)}{N}.  \tag{17.2}$$

If the utility is defined as the overall benefit for the patient population screened as biomarker-positive, i.e., $U = \Delta N$, then the expected utility is given by

$$U_e = \Delta N \ Power.  \tag{17.3}$$

Figure 17.1 shows how the specificity will impact the target population size, the average treatment effect in the target population, and the expected utility under different designs. When the specificity increases, the target population decreases, but the average treatment effect in the target population increases because misdiagnosis of biomarker-negative as positive will reduce the average treatment effect.

Using adaptive design, we can start with the overall patient population. At the interim analysis, a decision can be made whether to go for the

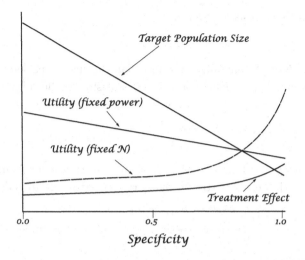

Figure 17.1:  Effect of Biomarker Misclassification

subpopulation or the overall population based on the expected utilities:

(1) If we target for the subpopulation with the biomarker, the expected utility at interim analysis is given by

*(conditional power of subpopulation)* × *(impact of success)*

*−(1 − conditional power of subpopulation)* × *(impact of failure)*

(2) If we target for the full patient population, the expected utility at interim analysis is given by

*(conditional power of full population)* × *(impact of success)*

*−(1 − conditional power of full population)* × *(impact of failure)*

### 17.2.2  *Classical Design with Classifier Biomarker*

Denote treatment difference between the test and control groups by $\delta_+$, $\delta_-$, and $\delta$, for biomarker-positive, biomarker-negative, and overall patient populations, respectively. The null hypothesis for biomarker-positive subpopulation is

$$H_{01} : \delta_+ = 0. \tag{17.4}$$

The null hypothesis for biomarker-negative subpopulation is

$$H_{02} : \delta_- = 0. \tag{17.5}$$

The null hypothesis for overall population is

$$H_0 : \delta = 0. \tag{17.6}$$

Without loss of generality, assume that the first $n$ patients have the biomarker among $N$ patients and the test statistic for the subpopulation is given by

$$Z_+ = \frac{\sum_{i=1}^{n} x_i - \sum_{i=1}^{n} y_i}{n\sigma} \sqrt{\frac{n}{2}} \sim N(0,1) \text{ under } H_0, \tag{17.7}$$

where $x_i$ and $y_i$ $(i = 1, ..., n)$ are the responses in treatment A and B.

Similarly, the test statistic for biomarker-negative group is defined as

$$Z_- = \frac{\left(\sum_{i=n+1}^{N} x_i - \sum_{i=n+1}^{N} y_i\right)}{(N-n)\sigma} \sqrt{\frac{N-n}{2}} \sim N(0,1) \text{ under } H_0. \tag{17.8}$$

The test statistic for overall population is given by

$$Z = \frac{\hat{\delta}}{\sigma}\sqrt{\frac{N}{2}} = T_+\sqrt{\frac{n}{N}} + T_-\sqrt{\frac{N-n}{N}} \sim N(0,1) \text{ under } H_0. \tag{17.9}$$

We choose the test statistic for the trial as

$$T = \max(Z, Z_+). \tag{17.10}$$

It can be shown that the correlation coefficient between $Z$ and $Z_+$ is

$$\rho = \sqrt{\frac{n}{N}}. \tag{17.11}$$

Therefore, the stopping boundary can be determined by

$$\Pr(T \geq z_{2,1-\alpha}|H_0) = \alpha, \tag{17.12}$$

where $z_{2,1-\alpha}$ is the bivariate normal $100(1-\alpha)$-equipercentage point under $H_0$.

The $p$-value corresponding to an observed test statistic $t$ is given by

$$p = \Pr(T \geq t|H_0). \tag{17.13}$$

The power can be calculated using

$$power = \Pr(T \geq z_{2,1-\alpha}|H_a). \tag{17.14}$$

The numerical integration or simulations can be performed to evaluate $z_{2,1-\alpha}$ and the power.

Note that the test statistic for the overall population can be defined as

$$Z = w_1 Z_+ + w_2 Z_-,$$

where $w_1$ and $w_2$ are constants satisfying $w_1^2 + w_2^2 = 1$. In such case, the correlation coefficient between $Z$ and $Z_+$ is $\rho = w_1$.

More generally, if there are $m$ groups under consideration, we can define a statistic for the $g$th group as

$$Z_g = \frac{\hat{\delta}_g}{\sigma} \sqrt{\frac{n_g}{2}} \sim N(0,1) \text{ under } H_0. \tag{17.15}$$

The test statistic for the maximum of these test statistics is given by

$$T = \max \{Z_1, ..., Z_m\}, \tag{17.16}$$

where $\{Z_1, ..., Z_m\}$ is asymptotically $m$-variate standard normal distribution under $H_0$ with expectation $\mathbf{0} = \{0, ..., 0\}$ and correlation matrix $\mathbf{R} = \{\rho_{ij}\}$. It can be easily shown that the correlation between $Z_i$ and $Z_j$ is given by

$$\rho_{ij} = \sqrt{\frac{n_{ij}}{n_i n_j}}, \tag{17.17}$$

where $n_{ij}$ is the number of concordant pairs between the $i$th and $j$th groups.

The asymptotic formulation for power calculation with the multiple tests is similar to that for multiple-contrast tests (Bretz and Hothorn, 2002):

$$\Pr(T \geq z_{m,\,1-\alpha}|H_a)$$
$$= 1 - \Pr(Z_1 < z_{m,\,1-\alpha} \cap ... \cap T_m < z_{m,\,1-\alpha} |H_a)$$
$$= 1 - \Phi_m \left( (\mathbf{z}_{m,\,1-\alpha} - e)\, diag \left( \frac{1}{v_0}, ..., \frac{1}{v_m} \right); \mathbf{0};\ \mathbf{R} \right),$$

where $\mathbf{z}_{m,\,1-\alpha} = (z_{m,\,1-\alpha}, ..., z_{m,\,1-\alpha})$ stands for the $m$-variate normal $100(1 - \alpha)$-equipercentage point under $H_0$, $\mathbf{e} = (E_a(T_0), ..., E_a(T_m))$ and $\mathbf{v} = (v_0, ..., v_m) = \left( \sqrt{V_0(T_0)}, \sqrt{V_1(T_1)}, ..., \sqrt{V_1(T_m)} \right)$ are vectorially summarized expectations and standard errors.

The power is given by

$$p = \Pr(T \geq z_{m,\,1-p}). \tag{17.18}$$

For other types of endpoints, we can use the inverse-normal method, i.e., $Z_g = \Phi(1 - p_g)$ in (17.15), where $p_g$ is the $p$-value for the hypothesis test in the $g$th population group, then (17.17) and (17.18) are still approximately valid.

## Simulation Algorithm

(1) Generate $n_+$ responses for biomarker-positive population (BPP).
(2) Generate $n_-$ responses for biomarker-negative population (BNP).
(3) Compute test statistic $T_+$ for BPP and $T_o$ for overall population.
(4) Compute $T = \max\{T_+, T_o\}$.
(5) Repeat (1)–(4) many times and compute the percentage of the outcomes with $T > Z_c$. This percentage is probability $\Pr(T > Z_c)$.

To determine the critical point $Z_c$ for rejecting the null at $\alpha$ level, run the simulations under the null condition for various $Z_c$ until $\Pr(T > Z_c) \approx \alpha$. To determine the power, run the simulations under the alternative condition; the power is given by $\Pr(T > Z_c)$ or the percentage of the outcomes with $T > Z_c$.

### 17.2.3 *Adaptive Design with Classifier Biomarker*

Let the hypothesis test for biomarker-positive subpopulation at the first stage (size $= n_1$/group) be

$$H_{01} : \delta_+ \leq 0 \qquad (17.19)$$

and the hypothesis test for overall population (size $= N_1$/group) be

$$H_0 : \delta \leq 0 \qquad (17.20)$$

with the corresponding stagewise $p$-values, $p_{1+}$ and $p_1$, respectively. These stagewise $p$-values should be adjusted. A conservative way is used the Bonferroni method or a method similar to Dunnett's method that takes the correlation into consideration. For Bonferroni-adjusted $p$-value and MSP, the test statistic is $T_1 = 2 \min(p_{1+}, p_1)$ for the first stage. The population with a smaller $p$-value will be chosen for the second stage and the test statistic for the second stage is defined as $T_2 = T_1 + p_2$, where $p_2$ is the stagewise $p$-value from the second stage. This method is implemented in SAS Macro 17.1 as described below.

SAS Macro 17.1 is developed for simulating biomarker-adaptive trials with two parallel groups. The key SAS variables are defined as follows: **alpha1** = early efficacy stopping boundary (one-sided), **beta1** = early futility stopping boundary, **alpha2** = final efficacy stopping boundary, **u0p** = response difference in biomarker-positive population, **u0n** = response in biomarker-negative population, **sigma** = asymptotic standard deviation for the response difference, assuming homogeneous variance among groups.

For binary response, sigma $= \sqrt{r_1(1-r_1) + r_2(1-r_2)}$; for normal response, sigma $= \sqrt{2}\sigma$. **np1, np2** = sample sizes per group for the first and second stage for the biomarker-positive population. **nn1, nn2** = sample sizes per group for the first and second stage for the biomarker-negative population. **cntlType** = "strong," for the strong type-I error control and **cntlType** = "weak," for the weak type-I error control, **AveN** = average total sample-size (all arms combined), **pPower** = the probability of significance for biomarker-positive population, **oPower** = the probability of significance for overall population.

### >>SAS Macro 17.1:   Biomarker-Adaptive Design>>

```
%Macro BMAD(nSims=100000, cntlType="strong", nStages=2, u0p=0.2,
u0n=0.1, sigma=1, np1=50, np2=50, nn1=100, nn2=100, alpha1=0.01,
beta1=0.15,alpha2=0.1871);
Data BMAD;
Keep FSP ESP Power AveN pPower oPower;
seedx=1736; seedy=6214; u0p=&u0p; u0n=&u0n; np1=&np1;
np2=&np2; nn1=&nn1; nn2=&nn2; sigma=&sigma;
FSP=0; ESP=0;Power=0; AveN=0; pPower=0; oPower=0;
Do isim=1 to &nSims;
up1=Rannor(seedx)*sigma/Sqrt(np1)+u0p;
un1=Rannor(seedy)*sigma/Sqrt(nn1)+u0n;
uo1=(up1*np1+un1*nn1)/(np1+nn1);
Tp1=up1*np1**0.5/sigma; To1=uo1*(np1+nn1)**0.5/sigma;
T1=Max(Tp1,To1); p1=1-ProbNorm(T1);
If &cntlType="strong" Then p1=2*p1; *Bonferroni;
If p1>&beta1 Then FSP=FSP+1/&nSims;
If p1<=&alpha1 Then Do;
Power=Power+1/&nSims; ESP=ESP+1/&nSims;
If Tp1>To1 Then pPower=pPower+1/&nSims;
If Tp1<=To1 Then oPower=oPower+1/&nSims;
End;
AveN=AveN+2*(np1+nn1)/&nSims;
If &nStages=2 And p1>&alpha1 And p1<=&beta1 Then Do;
up2=Rannor(seedx)*sigma/Sqrt(np2)+u0p;
un2=Rannor(seedy)*sigma/Sqrt(nn2)+u0n;
uo2=(up2*np2+un2*nn2)/(np2+nn2);
Tp2=up2*np2**0.5/sigma; To2=uo2*(np2+nn2)**0.5/sigma;
If Tp1>To1 Then Do;
T2=Tp2; AveN=AveN+2*np2/&nSims;
```

```
End;
If Tp1<=To1 Then Do;
T2=To2; AveN=AveN+2*(np2+nn2)/&nSims;
End;
p2=1-ProbNorm(T2); Ts=p1+p2;
If .<TS<=&alpha2 Then Do;
Power=Power+1/&nSims;
If Tp1>To1 Then pPower=pPower+1/&nSims;
If Tp1<=To1 Then oPower=oPower+1/&nSims;
End;
End;
End;
Run;
Proc Print Data=BMAD (obs=1); Run;
%Mend BMAD;
```
<<**SAS**<<

### Example 17.1    Biomarker-Adaptive Design

Suppose in an active-control two-group trial, the estimated treatment difference is 0.2 for the BPP and 0.1 for the BNP with a common standard deviation of $\sigma = 1$. Using SAS Macro 17.1, we can generate the operating characteristics under the global null hypothesis $H_0 : u_{0p} = 0 \cap u_{0n} = 0$, the alternative hypothesis $H_a : u_{0p} = 0.2 \cap u_{0n} = 0.1$, and the null hypotheses for the subgroups $H_{01}\ u_{0p} = 0 \cap u_{0n} = 0.1$ and $H_{02} : u_{0p} = 0.2 \cap u_{0n} = 0$ (see Table 17.2). Typical SAS macro calls to simulate the global null and the alternative conditions are presented in the following.

Table 17.2:    Simulation Results of Two-Stage Design

| Case | FSP | ESP | Power | AveN | pPower | oPower |
|------|-------|-------|-------|------|--------|--------|
| $H_o$    | 0.876 | 0.009 | 0.022 | 1678 | 0.011 | 0.011 |
| $H_{o1}$ | 0.538 | 0.105 | 0.295 | 2098 | 0.004 | 0.291 |
| $H_{o2}$ | 0.171 | 0.406 | 0.754 | 1852 | 0.674 | 0.080 |
| $H_a$    | 0.064 | 0.615 | 0.908 | 1934 | 0.311 | 0.598 |

$H_{o1}$ and $H_{o2}$ = no effect for BPP and overall population.

>>**SAS: Invoke SAS Macro 17.1**>>
Title "Simulation under global Ho, 2-stage design";
%BMAD(nSims=100000, cntlType="strong", nStages=2, u0p=0, u0n=0, sigma=1.414, np1=260, np2=260, nn1=520, nn2=520, alpha1=0.01, beta1=0.15, alpha2=0.1871);

Title "Simulations under Ha, 2-stage design";
%BMAD(nSims=100000, cntlType="strong", nStages=2, u0p=0.2, u0n=0.1, sigma=1.414, np1=260, np2=260, nn1=520, nn2=520, alpha1=0.01, beta1=0.15, alpha2=0.1871);
**<<SAS<<**

Trial monitoring is particularly important for these types of trials. Assume we have decided the sample sizes $N_2$ per treatment group for overall population at stage 2, of which $n_2$ (can be modified later) subjects per group are biomarker-positive. Ideally, the decision on whether the trial continues for the biomarker-positive patients or overall patients should be dependent on the expected utility at the interim analysis. The utility is the total gain (usually as a function of observed treatment effect) minus the cost due to continuing the trial using BPP or the overall patient population. For simplicity, we define the utility as the conditional power. The population group with larger conditional power will be used for the second stage of the trial. Suppose we design a trial with $n_{1+} = 260$, $n_{1-} = 520$, $p_{1+} = 0.1$, $p_1 = 0.12$, and stopping boundaries: $\alpha_1 = 0.01, \beta_1 = 0.15$, and $\alpha_2 = 0.1871$. For $n_{2+} = 260$, and $n_{2-} = 520$, the conditional power based on MSP is 82.17% for BPP and 99.39% for the overall population. The calculations are presented as follows.

For MSP, the conditional power is given by

$$P_c(p_1, \delta) = 1 - \Phi\left(\Phi^{-1}(1 - \alpha_2 + p_1) - \frac{\delta}{\sigma}\sqrt{\frac{n_2}{2}}\right), \alpha_1 < p_1 \leq \beta_1.$$

For the biomarker-positive population,

$$\Phi^{-1}(1 - 0.1871 + 0.1) = \Phi^{-1}(0.9129) = 1.3588, 0.2\sqrt{260/2} = 2.2804,$$

$$P_c = 1 - \Phi(1.3588 - 2.2804) = 1 - \Phi(-0.9216) = 1 - 0.1783 = 0.8217.$$

For the biomarker-negative population,

$$\Phi^{-1}(1 - 0.1871 + 0.12) = \Phi^{-1}(0.9329) = 1.4977,$$

$$0.2\sqrt{(260 + 520)/2} = 3.9497,$$

$$P_c = 1 - \Phi(1.4977 - 3.9497) = 1 - \Phi(-2.452) = 1 - 0.0071 = 0.9929.$$

Therefore, we are interested in the overall population. Of course, different $n_2$ and $N_2$ can be chosen at the interim analyses, which may lead to different decisions regarding the population for the second stage.

The following aspects should also be considered during design: power versus utility, enrolled patients versus screened patients, screening cost, and the prevalence of biomarker.

## 17.3 Challenges in Biomarker Validation

### 17.3.1 *Classical Design with Biomarker Primary Endpoint*

Given the characteristics of biomarkers, can we use a biomarker as the primary endpoint for late-stage or confirmatory trials? Let's study the outcome in three different scenarios. (1) The treatment has no effect on the true endpoint or the biomarker. (2) The treatment has no effect on the true endpoint but does affect the biomarker. (3) The treatment has a small effect on the true endpoint but has a larger effect on the biomarker. Table 17.3 summarizes the type-I error rates ($\alpha$) and powers for using the true endpoint and biomarker under different scenarios. In the first scenario, we can use either the true endpoint or the biomarker as the primary endpoint because both control the type-I error. In the second scenario, we cannot use the biomarker as the primary endpoint because $\alpha$ will be inflated to 81%. In the third scenario, it is better to use the biomarker as the primary endpoint from a power perspective. However, before the biomarker is fully validated, we don't know which scenario is true; use of the biomarker as the primary endpoint could lead to a dramatic inflation of the type-I error. It must be validated before a biomarker can be used as primary endpoint.

Table 17.3:  Issues with Biomarker Primary Endpoint

| Effect size ratio | Endpoint | Power (alpha) |
|:---:|:---|:---:|
| 0.0/0.0 | True endpoint | (0.025) |
|  | Biomarker | (0.025) |
| 0.0/0.4 | True endpoint | (0.025) |
|  | Biomarker | (0.810) |
| 0.2/0.4 | True endpoint | 0.300 |
|  | Biomarker | 0.810 |

Note: N = 100 per group.  Effect size ratio = effect size of true endpoint to effect size of biomarker.

### 17.3.2 *Treatment-Biomarker-Endpoint Relationship*

Validation of biomarker is not an easy task. Validation here refers to the proof of a biomarker to be a predictive marker, i.e., a marker that can be used as a surrogate marker. Before we discuss biomarker validations, let's take a close look at the 3-way relationships among treatment, biomarker, and the true endpoint. It is important to be aware that the correlations among them are not transitive. In the following example, we will show that it could be the case that there is a correlation ($R_{TB}$) between treatment and the biomarker and a correlation ($R_{BE}$) between the biomarker and the true endpoint, but there is no correlation ($R_{TE}$) between treatment and the true endpoint (Figures 17.2 and 17.3).

The hypothetical example to be discussed is a trial with 14 patients, 7 in the control group and 7 in the test group. The biomarker and true

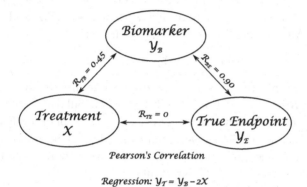

Figure 17.2:   Treatment-Biomarker-Endpoint Three-Way Relationship

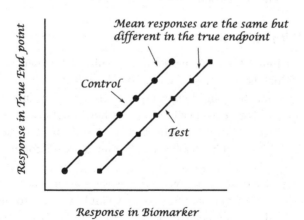

Figure 17.3:   Correlation versus Prediction

endpoint outcomes are displayed in Figure 17.3. The results show that
the Pearson's correlation between the biomarker and the true endpoint is 1
(perfect correlation) in both treatment groups. If the data are pooled from
the two groups, the correlation between the biomarker and the true endpoint is still high, about 0.9. The average response with the true endpoint
is 4 for each group, which indicates that the drug is ineffective compared
with the control. On the other hand, the average biomarker response is
6 for the test group and 4 for the control group, which indicates that the
drug has effects on the biomarker.

Facing the data, what we typically do is to fit a regression model with
the data, in which the dependent variable is the true endpoint $(Y_T)$ and the
independent variables (predictors) are the biomarker $(Y_B)$ and the treatment $(X)$. After model fitting, we can obtain that

$$Y_T = Y_B - 2X. \qquad (17.21)$$

This model fits the data well based on model-fitting $p$-value and $R^2$.
Specifically, $R^2$ is equal to 1, $p$-values for model and all parameters are equal
to 0, where the coefficient 2 in model (17.21) is the separation between the
two lines. Based on (17.21), we would conclude that both biomarker and
treatment affect the true endpoint. However, we know that the treatment
has no effect on the true endpoint at all.

In fact, the biomarker predicts the response in the true endpoint, but
it does not predict the treatment effect on the true endpoint, i.e., it is a
prognostic marker. For more discussions of this topic, see Chang's book on
principles of scientific methods (Chang and Wang, 2014).

### 17.3.3  *Multiplicity and False Positive Rate*

Let's further discuss the challenges from a multiplicity point of view. In
earlier phases or the discovery phase, we often have a large number of
biomarkers to test. Running hypothesis testing on many markers can be
done with either a high false positive rate without multiplicity adjustment
or a low power with multiplicity adjustment. Also, if model selection procedures are used without multiplicity adjustment as we commonly see in
current practice, the false positive rate could be inflated dramatically. Another source of false positive discovery rate is the so-called publication bias.
The last, but not least, source of false positive finding is due to the multiple
testing conducted by different companies or research units. Imagine that
100 companies study the same biomarker, even if familywise type-I error
rate is strictly controlled at a 5% level within each company, there will still

be, on average, 5 companies that have positive findings about the same biomarker just by chance.

### 17.3.4  *Validation of Biomarkers*

We now realized the importance of biomarker validation and would like to review some commonly used statistical methods for biomarker validation.

Prentice (1989) proposed four operational criteria: (1) treatment has a significant impact on the surrogate endpoint; (2) treatment has a significant impact on the true endpoint; (3) the surrogate has a significant impact on the true endpoint; and (4) the full effect of treatment upon the true endpoint is captured by the surrogate endpoint.

Freedman, Graubard, and Schatzkin (1992) argued that the last Prentice criterion is difficult statistically because it requires that the treatment effect is not statistically significant after adjustment of the surrogate marker. They further articulated that the criterion might be useful to reject a poor surrogate marker, but it is inadequate to validate a good surrogate marker. Therefore, they proposed a different approach based on the proportion of treatment effect on the true endpoint explained by biomarkers and a large proportion required for a good marker. However, as noticed by Freedman, this method is practically infeasible due to the low precision of the estimation of the proportion explained by the surrogate.

Buyse and Molenberghs (1998) proposed the internal validation matrices, which include relative effect (RE) and adjusted association (AA). The former is a measure of association between the surrogate and the true endpoint at an individual level, and the latter expresses the relationship between the treatment effects on the surrogate and the true endpoint at a trial level. The practical use of the Buyse–Molenberghs method raises two concerns: (1) a wide confidence interval of RE requires a large sample-size and (2) treatment effects on the surrogate and the true endpoint are multiplicative, which cannot be checked using data from a single trial.

Other methods, such as external validation using meta-analysis and two-stage validation for fast track programs, also face similar challenges in practice. For further readings on biomarker evaluations, Weir and Walley (2006) give an excellent review; Case and Qu (2006) have proposed a method for quantifying the indirect treatment effect via surrogate markers and Alonso et al. (2006) have proposed a unifying approach for surrogate marker validation based on Prentice's criteria.

### 17.3.5   *Biomarkers in Reality*

In reality, there are many possible scenarios: (1) same effective size for the biomarker and true endpoint, but the biomarker response can be measured earlier; (2) bigger effective size for the biomarker and smaller for the true endpoint; (3) no treatment effect on the true endpoint, limited treatment effect on the biomarker; and (4) treatment effect on the true endpoint only occurs after the biomarker response reaches a threshold. Validation of biomarkers is challenging, and the sample size is often insufficient for the full validation. Therefore, validations are often performed to a certain degree and soft validation (e.g., pathway) is scientifically important.

What is the utility of partially validated biomarkers? In the next section, we will discuss how to use prognostic markers in adaptive designs.

## 17.4   Adaptive Design with Prognostic Biomarkers

### 17.4.1   *Optimal Design*

A biomarker before it is proved predictive can only be considered as a prognostic marker. In the following example, we discuss how to use a prognostic biomarker (a marker may also be predictive) in trial design. The adaptive design proposed permits early stopping for futility based on the interim analysis of the biomarker. At the final analysis, the true endpoint will be used to preserve the type-I error. Assume there are three possible scenarios: (1) $H_{01}$: effect size ratio, ESR $= 0/0$; $H_{02}$: effect size ratio; (2) ESR $= 0/0.25$; and (3) $H_a$: effect size ratio, ESR $= 0.5/0.5$, but biomarker response earlier. ESR is the ratio of effect size for true endpoint to the effect size for biomarker. We are going to compare three different designs: classical design and two adaptive designs with different stopping boundaries as shown in Table 17.4.

Based on simulation results (Table 17.4), we can see that the two adaptive designs reduce sample size required under the null hypothesis. However, this comparison is not good enough because it does not consider the prior distribution of each scenario at the design stage.

We have noticed that there are many different scenarios with associated probabilities (prior distribution) and many possible adaptive designs with associated probabilistic outcomes (good and bad). Suppose we have also formed the utility function, the criteria for evaluating different designs. Now let's illustrate how we can use utility theory to select the best design under financial, time, and other constraints.

Table 17.4:  Adaptive Design with Biomarker

| Design | Condition | Power | Expected N/arm | Futility boundary |
|--------|-----------|-------|----------------|-------------------|
| Classical | $H_{01}$ | | 100 | |
| | $H_{02}$ | | 100 | |
| | $H_a$ | 0.94 | 100 | |
| Adaptive | $H_{01}$ | | 75 | |
| | $H_{02}$ | | 95 | $\beta_1 = 0.5$ |
| | $H_a$ | 0.94 | 100 | |
| Adaptive | $H_{01}$ | | 55 | |
| | $H_{02}$ | | 75 | $\beta_1 = 0.1056$ |
| | $H_a$ | 0.85 | 95 | |

Let's assume the prior probability for each of the scenarios mentioned earlier as shown in Table 17.5. For each scenario, we conduct computer simulations to calculate the probability of success and the expected utilities for each design. The results are summarized in Table 17.6.

Based on the expected utility, the adaptive design with the stopping boundary $\beta_1 = 0.5$ is the best. Of course, we can also generate more designs and calculate the expected utility for each design and select the best one.

## 17.4.2  *Prognostic Biomarker in Designing Survival Trial*

An insufficiently validated biomarker such as tumor response rate (RR) can be used in oncology trial for interim decision making as to whether to continue to enroll patients or not to reduce the cost. When the response

Table 17.5:  Prior Knowledge about Effect Size

| Scenario | Effect Size Ratio | Prior Probability |
|----------|-------------------|-------------------|
| $H_{01}$ | 0/0 | 0.2 |
| $H_{02}$ | 0/0.25 | 0.2 |
| $H_a$ | 0.5/0.5 | 0.6 |

Table 17.6:  Expected Utilities of Different Designs

| Design | Classical | Biomarker-adaptive | |
|--------|-----------|--------------------|--------------------|
| | | $\beta_1 = 0.5$ | $\beta_1 = 0.1056$ |
| Expected Utility | 419 | 441 | 411 |

rate in the test group is lower, because of the correlation between RR and survival, it is reasonable to believe the test drug will be unlikely to have a survival benefit. However, even when the trial is stopped earlier due to unfavorable results in response rate, the survival benefit can still be tested. We have discussed this for a non-Hodgkin's lymphoma trial in Chapter 14.

## 17.5    Adaptive Design with Predictive Marker

If a biomarker is proved to be predictive, then we can use it to replace the true endpoint from the hypothesis test point of view. In other words, a proof of treatment effect on predictive marker is a proof of treatment effect on the true endpoint. However, the correlation between the effect sizes of treatment in the predictive (surrogate) marker and the true endpoints is desirable but unknown. This is one of the reasons that follow-up study on the true endpoint is highly desirable in the NDA accelerated approval program.

Changes in biomarker over time can be viewed as stochastic processes (marker processes) and have been used in the so-called threshold regression (Chapter 19). A predictive marker process can be viewed as an external process that covaries with the parent process. It can be used in tracking progress of the parent process if the parent process is latent or only infrequently observed. In this way, the marker process forms a basis for predictive inference about the status of the parent process of a clinical endpoint. The basic analytical framework for a marker process conceives of a bivariate stochastic process $\{X(t), Y(t)\}$ where the parent process $\{X(t)\}$ is one component process and the marker process $\{Y(t)\}$ is the other. Whitmore, Crowder, and Lawless (1998) investigated the failure inference based on a bivariate. The Wiener model has also been used in this aspect, in which failure is governed by the first-hitting time of a latent degradation process. Lee, DeGruttola, and Schoenfeld (2000) apply this bivariate marker model to CD4 cell counts in the context of AIDS survival. Hommel, Lindig, and Faldum (2005) studied a two-stage adaptive design with correlated data.

## 17.6    Summary and Discussion

We have discussed the adaptive designs with classifier, prognostic, and predictive markers. These designs can be used to improve the efficiency by identifying the right population, making decisions earlier to reduce the impact of failure, and delivering the efficacious and safer drugs to market earlier. However, full validation of a biomarker is statistically challenging and sufficient validation tools are not available. Fortunately, adaptive designs with biomarkers can be beneficial even when the biomarkers are not fully validated. The Bayesian approach is an ideal solution for finding an optimal design, while computer simulation is a powerful tool for the utilization of biomarkers in trial design.

## Problems

**17.1** Develop SAS macros or R function for the method described in Section 17.2.2 and conduct a simulation study of the method.

**17.2** Redesign the trial in Example 17.1, assuming the estimated $u_{0p} = 0.2$ and $u_{0n} = 0.05$.

**17.3** Prove that under the global null hypothesis $H_0 : \delta_1 = ... = ...\delta_m = 0$ , the test statistic $T$ in (17.16) has a pdf

$$T \sim m\left[\Phi\left(t\right)\right]^{m-1}\phi\left(t\right),$$

where $\phi$ and $\Phi$ are the standard normal pdf and cdf, respectively.

**17.4** If we arrange the order of the test statistics for different subpopulations from the smallest to the largest, $T_{(1)} \leq T_{(2)} \leq ... \leq T_{(m)}$, we can use the distribution of the order statistics to determine the $p$-values. The cdf of $T_{(i)}$ is given by

$$F_{T_{(i)}}\left(x\right) = \sum_{j=1}^{n} \binom{n}{j} \left[\Phi\left(x\right)\right]^{j}\left[1 - \Phi\left(x\right)\right]^{n-j}.$$

Discuss how to use these $p$-values and the multiple testing procedures you have learned in Chapter 14 to test effectiveness of the drug in each subpopulation. Are there any fundamental challenges with this approach?

# Chapter 18

# Biomarker-Informed Adaptive Design

## 18.1 Introduction

In this chapter, we discuss the biomarker-informed design using the two-level biomarker model proposed by Wang and Chang (2014). We have discussed the pick-the-winner designs where the same endpoint is used for both the interim and final analyses of the study. However, the benefits of such a design or method could be limited if it takes very long to obtain the primary endpoint measurements at the interim. For example, in oncology trials, it usually takes 12–24 months to observe overall survival—the most commonly used and preferred regulatory primary endpoint. The long time needed to reach the interim analyses can present potential operational challenges and may delay bringing a drug to the market.

Considerable interest has been drawn toward the short-term endpoint ("biomarker") informed adaptive seamless phase-II/III designs. These designs incorporate biomarker information at the interim stages of the study. The decision(s) on interim adaptation can be made based upon the biomarker only or on the available joint information of the biomarker and the primary endpoint.

Todd and Stallard (2005) presented a group sequential design for which the interim treatment selection is based upon a biomarker. Stallard (2010) considered a design that uses both the available biomarker and primary endpoint information for treatment selection. He proposed a method for the adjustment of the usual group sequential boundaries to maintain strong control of the familywise type-I error rate. Friede et al. (2011) brought together combination tests for adaptive designs and the closure principle for multiple testing, which allowed them to achieve control of the familywise type-I error rate in the strong sense. Shun et al. (2008) presented a "two-stage winner design" with normal interim and final endpoint, where the unconditional distribution of the final test statistic was derived for the design with two active treatment arms. They also proposed a normal approximation approach for the final distribution. Liu and Pledger (2005), Li, Wang, and Ouyang (2009), and Li, Zhu et al. (2009) considered cases where more than one treatment can be selected at the interim. Scala and Glimm (2011) discussed application of the design when the endpoints are time-to-event data. Jenkins et al. (2010) proposed a design with time-to-event endpoints that allows subgroup selection based upon biomarker at the interim, and methodology was presented which controls the type-I error rate.

Biomarker informed adaptive designs can be helpful for the development of personalized medicine, if the biomarker used at the interim is a good indicator of the primary endpoint.

## 18.2    Motivations and Concepts

To conduct a clinical trial that uses biomarker informed adaptive procedures, statistical simulations are suggested to be performed first in order to understand the operating characteristics, including sample size for a target power, of the design. The conventional approach uses the one-level (individual level only) correlation model, together with historical knowledge, to describe the relationship between the biomarker and the primary endpoint. This approach can easily wrongly estimate the power of a biomarker informed design if there is no well-established knowledge about how the biomarker and the primary endpoint are correlated. When the rank order of mean responses of the biomarker for each treatment group is assumed to be the same as that of the primary endpoint based on historical observations, it is very possible to overestimate the power of the design by the conventional model, as the uncertainty of the historical knowledge has been ignored. In this case, the sample size suggested by simulation may lead to an underpowered trial. The approval rate for NDAs (new drug applications) submitted to the FDA recently is about 40% (2011). This fact indicates that there are trials that are underpowered. It is desirable to propose approaches that lead to a reasonable assessment of the sample size required for biomarker-informed clinical trial designs.

Wang (2013) and Wang and Chang (2014) have proposed a two-level model for biomarker informed adaptive designs. This model considers not only the individual level correlation between the biomarker and the primary endpoint, but also accounts for the variability of the estimated mean level correlation (or "mean level association"). The uncertainty due to a small sample size of historical data about the relationship between the biomarker and primary endpoint is considered in the model. This chapter will describe this two-level model and assess the performance of biomarker informed adaptive designs using this model.

The new model is illustrated in the context of a two-stage winner design with three active treatment arms and a control arm. We assume both biomarker and primary endpoint are normally distributed, the distribution of the final test statistic of the design is proposed, and the type-I error rate control issue is discussed. The new approach is shown to provide a more reasonable and sensible assessment for the biomarker informed adaptive designs.

## 18.3 Issues in Conventional One-Level Correlation Model

The conventional one-level correlation model used for describing the relationship of the two endpoints in a biomarker informed adaptive design considers only the individual level correlation ($\rho$). If the one-level correlation model is used in statistical simulations for biomarker informed designs, the means of the two endpoints have to be specified based on the historical knowledge (as shown in Li, Wang, and Ouyang, 2009). In this way, there would not be much difference in power between different values of correlation coefficient $\rho$ between the biomarker and the primary endpoint.

Friede et al. (2011) point out that the effect of the individual level correlation $\rho$ between the endpoints on power is small if the means of the biomarker in treatment groups are fixed. For example, when the estimated treatment difference in the biomarker is 0.2, the estimated power of their design changes from around 83% to 85% as $\rho$ increases from 0 to 1. Li, Wang, and Ouyang (2009) also mention that the influence of $\rho$ on power is really small when compared to other factors. Their paper showed an increase in simulated power from 70.5% to 73.7% as $\rho$ increased from 0.2 to 0.8.

We ran simulations for a "two-stage winner design" with a survival primary endpoint. The design was assumed to have five active treatment arms and one control arm, with fixed survival means 2.46, 2.71, 3.67, 3.32, 3, and 2.22 for each treatment arm, respectively, and the control fixed biomarker log-means 1.6, 1.7, 2, 1.9, 1.8, and 1.5. The critical value for the final test statistic was obtained by simulation with the type-I error rate at 0.025 level. Our simulation results (Table 18.1) are consistent with

Table 18.1:   Power of Winner Design with One-Level Correlation

| $\rho$ | Cencoring Rate | Sample Size | Power | Power* |
|------|------|------|------|------|
| 0.3 | 0.2 | 216 | 96.5% | 66.7% |
| 0.5 | 0.2 | 216 | 96.1% | 66.3% |
| 0.8 | 0.2 | 216 | 97.4% | 67.7% |

Power* = probability of rejection for the most effective arm

the previous findings, where the interim sample size was 72, and the final sample size was 216.

We can see from Table 18.1 that if the conventional one-level correlation approach is used, when the correlation between the biomarker and the primary endpoint increases from 0.3 to 0.8, the simulated power of two-stage winner design changes from 96.5% to 97.4%. It is only slightly different. This finding violates the presumption that the biomarker informed design should have a better performance when the interim endpoint has a stronger correlation with the final endpoint.

Figure 18.1 illustrates different cases where the individual level correlation $\rho$ between the biomarker and the primary endpoint is the same. Two different biomarkers (A and B) are described in the figure, both of which are correlated with the primary endpoint with correlation coefficient $\rho = 0.9$. Consider two designs, one uses Biomarker A and the other uses biomarker B. Since only $\rho$ is used in the conventional winner design, the two designs with the two different markers will give the same result. In fact, however, the slope of the lines in Figure 18.1 is critical because knowing the slope, we can know how much increase in biomarker in the interim means how much increase in the primary endpoint so that we can make wise decision at the interim analysis. Imagine that if $\rho = 1$, the conventional winner design with biomarker will treat the biomarker as the primary endpoint; thus, the design is equivalent to the pick-the-winner design with the primary endpoint used for both the interim and final analyses. This is obviously inappro-

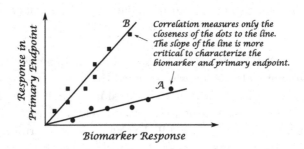

Figure 18.1:   Relationships between Biomarker and Primary Endpoint

priate because two markers can both have linear relationship ($\rho = 1$) but the slopes in the figure can be completely different. Therefore, it is not sufficient to describe the relationship between the biomarker and the primary endpoint by only considering the individual level correlation $\rho$. The slope, which is the rate of change of the primary endpoint with respect to the change in the biomarker, should also be incorporated in the trial design. The conventional one-level correlation model does not incorporate the variability of the slope caused by the uncertainty of historical data, which might easily lead to misestimated power.

## 18.4 Two-Stage Winner Design

A two-stage biomarker-informed winner design is a special multiple-arm design, in which the interim winner is selected based on the responses in the biomarker instead of in the primary endpoint, but the final analysis is based on the primary endpoint. The main difference between this design and the common pick-the-winner design is that in this biomarker-informed winner design the interim endpoint can be different but correlated with the final study primary endpoint. The final comparison of winner treatment with control is performed on the data collected from both stages.

For a two-stage winner design, let $\{X_i^{(j)} | i = 1, ..., n\}$ be the measurements of the biomarker obtained at the interim stage, and $\{Y_i^{(j)} | i = 1, ..., N\}$ be the measurements of the primary endpoint obtained at the final stage. $n$ is the interim sample size per group, and $N$ is the maximum sample size for each group, $n < N$, $j = 0, 1, 2, ..., M$. $M$ is the number of active treatment groups. Let $j = 0$ represent the control group and $j = 1, 2, ..., M$ the active treatment groups. $X_m^{(j)} = \frac{1}{m} \sum X_i^{(j)}$ is the mean of the biomarker measurements for treatment group $j$ and $Y_N^{(j)} = \frac{1}{N} \sum Y_i^{(j)}$ is the mean of the primary endpoint measurements for treatment group $j$.

The decision rule of the winner design is if $\bar{X}_n^{(j)} = \max(\bar{X}_n^{(1)}, \bar{X}_n^{(2)}, ..., \bar{X}_n^{(M)})$ at interim, carry only the best treatment group $j$ and the control group to the end of the study. The option that more than one treatment group will be kept when the interim outcomes are almost the same is not considered, because either treatment group can be selected in this situation. The final assessment will be based on the primary endpoint $Y$ comparing the selected treatment $j$ group and the control group.

## 18.5 Two-Level Relationship Model for Two-Stage Winner Design

To illustrate the proposed two-level relationship model, we consider a two-stage winner design with three active treatment arms ($M = 3$) and a control arm. For simplicity, we further assume both interim and final endpoints are normally distributed. The two-level model can be elaborated as follows.

Assume $u_j^X, j = 0, 1, 2, 3$ are standardized means of biomarker for treatment group $j$, and $\sigma_X^2$ is the common variance. For a fixed $j$, assume $\left\{ X_i^{(j)} | i = 1, ..., n_1 \right\}$ is i.i.d. and $\frac{X_i^{(j)}}{\sigma_X} \sim N\left(u_j^X, 1\right)$. Assume $\left\{ Y_i^{(j)} | i = 1, ..., N \right\}$ is i.i.d. and denote the true mean level correlation between biomarker and primary endpoint by $r_j$ for treatment group $j$; assume $\frac{Y_i^{(j)}}{\sigma_Y} \sim N\left(u_j^Y, 1\right)$ where $u_j^Y = r_j u_j^X$.

In reality, since the true mean level correlation $r_j$ is unknown, an estimate $\hat{r}_j$ is obtained from historical data to describe the estimated mean level correlation. Assume $\hat{r}_j \sim N\left(r_j, \sigma_{r_j}^2\right)$, $\frac{Y_i^{(j)}}{\sigma_Y} | \hat{r}_j \sim N\left(\hat{r}_j u_j^X, 1\right)$. It is easy to show that, under this setting, the unconditional distribution for the primary endpoint is $\frac{Y_i^{(j)}}{\sigma_Y} \sim N\left(u_j^Y, \left(u_j^X\right) \sigma_{r_j}^2 + 1\right)$.

The individual level correlation between the biomarker and the primary endpoint is denoted by $\rho$, where $\rho = Corr(X_i, Y_i)$.

The new variable, $r_j$, incorporated in the model, and the distribution of its estimate $\hat{r}_j$ , accounts for the mean level correlation (or "mean level association") between biomarker and primary endpoint. The uncertainty, due to a small sample size of historical data, about the relationship between the two endpoints should be reflected in the model in this way.

### 18.5.1 *Test Statistic and Its Distribution*

Consider the following hypotheses:

$$H_0 : u_1^Y = u_2^Y = u_3^Y = u_0^Y$$
$$H_a : u_1^Y > u_0^Y \text{ or } u_2^Y > u_0^Y \text{ or } u_3^Y > u_0^Y \quad (18.1)$$

We want to test if there is any treatment that shows significantly better efficacy than the control group.

It is reasonable to assume that when the $H_0$ is true, there is also no treatment effect on biomarker, i.e., $u_1^X = u_2^X = u_3^X = u_0^X$ and $\rho \neq 0$.

Since the variance, $\text{Var}(\bar{Y}_N^{(j)} - \bar{Y}_N^{(0)}) = \left[\left(\hat{u}_j^X\right)^2 \hat{\sigma}_{rj}^2 + \left(\hat{u}_0^X\right)^2 \hat{\sigma}_{r0}^2 + 2\right] \sigma_Y^2 \approx \left[\left(\hat{u}_j^X\right)^2 \hat{\sigma}_{rj}^2 + \left(\hat{u}_0^X\right)^2 \hat{\sigma}_{r0}^2 + 2\right] \hat{\sigma}_Y^2$, we construct the test statistic for comparing the primary endpoint of the $j$th treatment group and the control group as

$$G_j = \sqrt{\frac{N}{\left[\left(\hat{u}_j^X\right)^2 \hat{\sigma}_{rj}^2 + \left(\hat{u}_0^X\right)^2 \hat{\sigma}_{r0}^2 + 2\right] \hat{\sigma}_Y^2}} \left(\bar{Y}_N^{(j)} - \bar{Y}_N^{(0)}\right) \text{ for } j = 1, 2, 3.$$

(18.2)

$G_j$ is expected to approximately follow the standard normal distribution under $H_0$ when the sample size is large. The final test statistic of the study with the given interim selection rule is then:

$$W = G_j, \text{ if } \bar{X}_n^{(j)} = \max\left(\bar{X}_n^{(1)}, \bar{X}_n^{(2)}, \bar{X}_n^{(3)}\right), j = 1, 2, 3.$$

(18.3)

That is, conditional on the interim selection, $W$ takes on the value of the effect from the "winner" treatment group for the final test statistic. It is well understood that the interim treatment selection will skew the distribution of the final test statistic. In the following, the exact distribution of the final test statistic will be derived. As the test statistic is no longer normally distributed, multidimensional numerical integration is needed for its calculation.

The distribution of the final test statistic $W$ could be written as

$$F_W(w) = \sum_{j=1}^{3} \Pr\left(P_{j1} < a_j, P_{j2} > b_j, P_{j3 > c_j}\right),$$

(18.4)

where

$$F_W(w) = \Pr(W < w)$$
$$= \sum_{j=1}^{3} \Pr\left(W < w, \bar{X}_n^{(j)} = \max\left(\bar{X}_n^{(1)}, \bar{X}_n^{(2)}, \bar{X}_n^{(3)}\right)\right)$$
$$= \sum_{j=1}^{3} \Pr\left(G_j < w, \bar{X}_n^{(j)} = \max\left(\bar{X}_n^{(1)}, \bar{X}_n^{(2)}, \bar{X}_n^{(3)}\right)\right)$$
$$= \sum_{j=1}^{3} \Pr\left(G_j < w, \bar{X}_n^{(j)} - \bar{X}_n^{(h)} > 0, \bar{X}_n^{(j)} - \bar{X}_n^{(l)} > 0\right)$$
$$= \Pr\left(P_{j1} < w, P_{j2} > 0, P_{j3} > 0\right),$$

(18.5)

where

$$P_{j1}=G_j, P_{j2}=\frac{\bar{X}_n^{(j)}-\bar{X}_n^{(h)}}{\sqrt{\sigma_X^2/n}}, P_{j2}=\frac{\bar{X}_n^{(j)}-\bar{X}_n^{(l)}}{\sqrt{\sigma_X^2/n}}; \ j=1,2,3, j\neq h, h\neq l, l\neq j.$$

(18.6)

For large sample size $N$, $(P_{j1}, P_{j2}, P_{j3})'$ is approximated from a multivariate normal distribution (using the result from the ratio of two normal distributions to prove),

$$\begin{pmatrix} P_{j1} \\ P_{j2} \\ P_{j3} \end{pmatrix} \sim N \left( \begin{pmatrix} 0 \\ 0 \\ 0 \end{pmatrix}, \sum_j = \begin{pmatrix} 1 & \gamma_j & \gamma_j \\ \gamma_j & 2 & 1 \\ \gamma_j & 1 & 2 \end{pmatrix} \right)$$

(18.7)

and

$$\gamma_j = \sqrt{\frac{n\left[\left(\hat{u}_j^X\right)^2 \hat{\sigma}_{rj}^2 + 1\right]}{N\left[\left(\hat{u}_j^X\right)^2 \hat{\sigma}_{rj}^2 + \left(\hat{u}_0^X\right)^2 \hat{\sigma}_{r0}^2 + 2\right]}} \rho.$$

(18.8)

### 18.5.2    *Type-I Error Rate Control*

As the two-stage winner design is intended for phase-II/III seamless or phase-III trials, it is desirable to preserve the type-I error rate under a target $\alpha$ level. Assuming we have the same amount of historical information on the biomarker and the primary endpoint for each treatment group, from Equation 18.5, the distribution of final test statistic $W$ under $H_0$ is

$$F_0(w) = 3 \int_{-\infty}^{w} \int_0^{\infty} \int_0^{\infty} f(p_1, p_2, p_3)\, dp_3 dp_2 dp_1,$$

(18.9)

where

$$f(p_1, p_2, p_3) = (2\pi)^{-3/2} |\Sigma|^{-1/2} e^{-\frac{1}{2}p'\Sigma^{-1}p} = \frac{(2\pi)^{-3/2}}{(3-2\gamma^2)^{1/2}} e^{-\frac{1}{2}\frac{1}{3-2\gamma^2}v},$$

(18.10)

where $\gamma = \sqrt{\frac{n_1}{2N}}\rho$ and $p = (p_1, p_2, p_3)'$, and

$$v = 2p_1^2 - 2\gamma p_1 p_2 - 2\gamma p_1 p_3 + p_2^2 (2-\gamma^2) + p_2 p_3 (2\gamma^2 - 2) + p_3^2 (2-\gamma^2).$$

(18.11)

Let $w_\alpha$ be the upper $100\alpha$ percent quantile of $F_0$; that is,

$$w_\alpha = F_W^{-1}(1-\alpha|H_0) = F_0^{-1}(1-\alpha).$$

(18.12)

Thus, the type-I error rate is controlled at level $\alpha$ if the one-sided rejection region is $\Omega = \{W : W > w_\alpha\}$.

The stopping boundary $w_\alpha$ could be easily calculated by numerical integration software. See Table 18.2 for numerical values of $w_{0.025}$ for different values of correlation coefficient $\rho$ when interim information time is $1/2$. As expected, the critical value $w_{0.025}$ increases as $\rho$ increases. R code for the calculation of stopping boundaries is presented below:

Table 18.2:   Critical Value of Two-Stage Winner Design

| $\rho$ | 0 | 0.2 | 0.5 | 0.8 | 1 |
|---|---|---|---|---|---|
| $w_{0.025}$ | 1.96 | 2.041 | 2.146 | 2.232 | 2.279 |

Note: Information time $n_1/n = 1/2$.

## >>R Function 18.1:    Stopping Boundary of Biomarker-Informed Design>>

```
##Stopping boundary determined by info time and rho##
##Try stopping boundaries until the "integral" in output achieves 1-alpha.##
library(cubature)
rho = ** #rho takes value between 0 and 1##
mtime = **#interim information between 0 and 1##
r1 = sqrt(0.5*mtime)*rho
w = c(**, . . ., **) ##the numbers to try for the true stopping boundary##
res = c()
for (j in 1:length(w)){
a = w[j]
f = function(p){
3*((2*pi)^(-1.5)*(3-2*r1^2)^(-0.5)*exp(-0.5*(1/(3-2*r1^2))*(3*p[1]^2-2*r1*
p[1]*p[2]-2*r1*p[1]*p[3] + (2 - r1^2)*p[2]^2 + (2-r1^2)*p[2]^2 + (2*r1^2
-2)*p[2]*p[3] + (2-r1^2)*p[3]^2)))
}
intenum=adaptIntegrate(f, lowerLimit=c(-18, 0, 0), upperLimit=c(a, 18, 18))
intenum2=cbind(intenum, a)
res=rbind(res, intenum2) #the stopping boundary is the number that is associated with 1-alpha in column "integral"in "res"##
```
<<R<<

## 18.5.3   *Performance Evaluation of Two-Stage Winner Design*

In this section, we show performance evaluation of the two-stage winner design using the proposed two-level model. As illustrated earlier, when the rank order of mean responses of the biomarker is assumed to be the same as that of the primary endpoint, the power of a two-stage winner design could be easily overestimated if the conventional one-level correlation model is used. It will be shown that the new assessment approach is more reasonable, and can help with determining when a two-stage winner design should be used. As in our earlier study, we consider a two-stage winner design with three active arms and a control arm.

We assume $u_0^X = 1, \sigma_X^2 = 1, u_0^Y = 1, \sigma_Y^2 = 1$—this could always be achieved by scaling—and assume $u_1^Y = 1.1, u_2^Y = 1.5, u_3^Y = 1.3$. We assume that the biomarker and the primary endpoint are positively related; that is, large values of biomarker measurement correspond to large values of the primary endpoint. We consider the following cases when the means of biomarker and primary endpoint are correlated in linear and in nonlinear ways.

If the mean of the biomarker $u^X$ and the mean of primary endpoint $u^Y$ are linearly related, the mean level relationship $r_j$, is the same for all treatment groups. Under our assumption here, $r_1 = r_2 = r_3 = r_0 = 1$. Therefore, $u_1^X = 1.1$, $u_2^X = 1.5$, and $u_3^X = 1.3$ in this case.

Consider the design with interim sample size $n_1 = 52$ and maximum sample size $N = 104$; and $n_1 = 67$ and $N = 134$. The two final size sample sizes will yield 80% and 90% power, respectively, of the corresponding classical design with no interim adaptation.

Table 18.3 (Wang, 2013) lists the simulation results of the two-stage winner design under our setting for the above sample sizes for different values of $\rho$ and $\sigma_r^2$. We can see that, when $\sigma_r^2$ is fixed, the power of the design for different values of $\rho$ is similar. For example, in Table 18.3, when $\sigma_r^2 = 0.2$, the power of the design is around 78–80%. However, when $\rho$ is fixed, the power of the design has a significant change for different values of $\sigma_r^2$. For example, in Table 18.3, for $\rho = 0.5$, the power of the design changes from 87.9% to 78.7% when $\sigma_r^2$ increases from 0 to 0.2. The results indicate that the individual level correlation $\rho$ has only a little influence on the performance of the two-stage winner design, while $\sigma_r^2$, which measures the uncertainty in the mean level correlation estimation has a significant influence on the design performance.

Therefore, it is necessary to consider and incorporate $\sigma_r^2$ when evaluating a two-stage winner design. In the conventional one-level correlation model, since $\sigma_r^2$ is not considered, the power of the design can be easily overestimated. The simulation results also show that the two-stage winner design is not necessarily always better than the corresponding classical design. In our setting here, only when $\sigma_r^2 < 0.2$ does the two-stage winner design show its advantage in terms of power.

Table 18.3: Power of Biomarker-Informed Design

|  |  | $\rho$ |  |  |  |  |
|---|---|---|---|---|---|---|
|  |  | 0 | 0.2 | 0.5 | 0.8 | 1 |
|  | 0 | .881 | .875 | .879 | .883 | .888 |
| $\sigma_r^2$ | 0.1 | .853 | .841 | .840 | .838 | .837 |
|  | 0.2 | .803 | .804 | .787 | .794 | .793 |

Note: Based on 10,000 simulations. $n_1 = 52$, $N = 104$

## 18.5.4 *Parameter Estimation*

In this section, we propose a solution to the question of how to estimate the parameters incorporated in the two-level correlation model using historical data. It is clear that the two-level correlation model incorporates the following parameters: $\sigma_X$, $u_j^X$, $\sigma_Y$, $u_j^Y$, $r_j$, $\sigma_{r_j}^2$, and $\rho$, $j = 0, 1, 2, ..., M$.

Assume there are $n_j$ pairs of historical data for treatment $j$ on biomarker and primary endpoint, $j = 0, 1, 2, ..., M$. Let $s_{x_j}^2$ be the sample variance of biomarker $X_i^{(j)}$ in treatment group $j, i = 1, 2, ..., n_j$, and $\bar{x}^{(j)}$ be the observed sample mean of biomarker in treatment group $j$. Let $s_{y_j}^2$ be the sample variance of primary endpoint $Y_i^{(j)}$ in treatment group $j$, and $\bar{y}^{(j)}$ be the observed sample mean of primary endpoint in treatment group $j$. We suggest that the parameters be estimated in the following natural way:

$$\hat{\sigma}_X^2 = \frac{\sum n_j s_{x_j}^2}{\sum n_j}, \hat{u}_j^X = \frac{\bar{x}^{(j)}}{\hat{\sigma}_X}, \hat{\sigma}_Y^2 = \frac{\sum n_j s_{y.j}^2}{\sum n_j}, \hat{u}_j^Y = \frac{\bar{y}^{(j)}}{\hat{\sigma}_Y}, \hat{r}_j = \frac{\hat{u}_j^Y}{\hat{u}_j^X}, \quad (18.13)$$

$$\hat{\sigma}_{r_j}^2 = Var\left(\frac{\bar{Y}^{(j)}/\sigma_Y}{\bar{X}^{(j)}/\sigma_X}\right). \quad (18.14)$$

Using the approximation to the ratio of two random variables (Stuart and Ord, 1998), we can obtain

$$\hat{\sigma}_{r_j}^2 = \frac{\hat{\sigma}_X^2 \frac{\hat{\sigma}_Y^2}{n} + (\hat{u}_j^Y)^2}{\hat{\sigma}_Y^2 \frac{\hat{\sigma}_X^2}{n} + (\hat{u}_j^X)^2} \left[\frac{\frac{\hat{\sigma}_Y^2}{n}}{\frac{\hat{\sigma}_Y^2}{n} + (\hat{u}_j^Y)^2} - \frac{2}{n} \frac{\rho \hat{\sigma}_X \hat{\sigma}_Y}{\hat{u}_j^X \hat{u}_j^Y} + \frac{\frac{\hat{\sigma}_X^2}{n}}{\frac{\hat{\sigma}_X^2}{n} + (\hat{u}_j^X)^2}\right]. \quad (18.15)$$

$\hat{\rho} = Corr(X, Y)$, which is the observed correlation coefficient of the pooled sample of $X_i^{(j)}$ and $Y_i^{(j)}$, $i = 1, 2, ..., n_j$, $j = 0, 1, 2, ..., M$. Detailed derivation of Equation (18.13) can be find in Wang, Chang, and Menon (2014).

There are times when a common variance is preferred for $r_j$; that is, $\sigma_{r1}^2 = ... = \sigma_{rM}^2 = \sigma_{r0}^2 = \sigma_r^2$ will be assumed. For this case, we suggest

$$\hat{\sigma}_r^2 = \frac{\sum n_j \hat{\sigma}_{r_j}^2}{\sum n_j}. \tag{18.16}$$

The simulation results show that the estimators are practical unbiased.

## 18.6   Hierarchical Model

As an alternative to the model in Section 18.5, we can naturally use the hierarchical (multilevel) model (MEM):

$$\begin{pmatrix} Y_j \\ X_j \end{pmatrix} \sim N\left( \begin{pmatrix} \mu_{yj} \\ \mu_{xj} \end{pmatrix}, \begin{pmatrix} \sigma_y^2 & \rho\sigma_y\sigma_x \\ \rho\sigma_x\sigma_y & \sigma_x^2 \end{pmatrix} \right) \tag{18.17}$$

$$\begin{pmatrix} \mu_{yj} \\ \mu_{xj} \end{pmatrix} \sim N\left( \begin{pmatrix} \mu_{0yj} \\ \mu_{0xj} \end{pmatrix}, \begin{pmatrix} \sigma_{\mu_y}^2 & \rho_\mu\sigma_{\mu_y}\sigma_{\mu_x} \\ \rho_\mu\sigma_{\mu_x}\sigma_{\mu_y} & \sigma_{\mu_x}^2 \end{pmatrix} \right) \tag{18.18}$$

where $j$ = treatment group, $\rho$ and $\rho_\mu$ are the common correlations between individual and mean levels, respectively.

We can rewrite the distribution of $\begin{pmatrix} Y_j \\ X_j \end{pmatrix}$ in terms of the parameters in the parent model (18.18) by multiplying the pdfs (18.17) and (18.18), and integrating $\begin{pmatrix} \mu_{yj} \\ \mu_{xj} \end{pmatrix}$ out, which gives

$$\begin{pmatrix} Y_j \\ X_j \end{pmatrix} \sim N\left( \begin{pmatrix} \mu_{0yj} \\ \mu_{0xj} \end{pmatrix}, \begin{pmatrix} \sigma_{\mu_y}^2 + \sigma_y^2 & \rho_\mu\sigma_{\mu_y}\sigma_{\mu_x} + \rho\sigma_y\sigma_x \\ \rho_\mu\sigma_{\mu_y}\sigma_{\mu_x} + \rho\sigma_y\sigma_x & \sigma_{\mu_x}^2 + \sigma_x^2 \end{pmatrix} \right) \tag{18.19}$$

Note that all model parameters can be reassessed as the clinical trial data accumulated at each interim analysis using MLE or Bayesian posterior distribution.

Let's study this model and discuss how to implement this model into adaptive design. The implementation of biomarker-informed adaptive design with the hierarchical model is straightforward: (1) draw sample $\begin{pmatrix} \mu_{yj} \\ \mu_{xj} \end{pmatrix}$ based on the distribution (18.18); (2) for each sample $\begin{pmatrix} \mu_{yj} \\ \mu_{xj} \end{pmatrix}$, draw $N_1$

samples of ($\frac{Y_j}{X_j}$) from (18.17) for the interim analysis based on biomarker $X$ and determine the winner based on the best response in $X$; (3) draw additional $N_2 = N - N_1$ samples of the primary endpoint $Y$ from the normal distribution $N\left(\mu_{yw}, \sigma_y^2\right)$ in the winner arm $w$ and $N$ samples of $Y$ from $N\left(\mu_0, \sigma_0^2\right)$ for the placebo, and (4) test the hypothesis based on the primary endpoint $Y$ at the final analysis, which will be based on data of the winner arm from the two stages and all the data of $Y$ from the placebo. Here is the R-function for the biomarker-informed design with the hierarchical model.

## >>R Function 18.2: Biomarker-Informed Design with Hierarchical Model>>

```
## u0y[j], u0x[j], rhou, suy sux = parameters of the parent model in group j
## rho, sy, sx = parameters in the lower level model
## Zalpha  = critical point for rejection
## nArms = number of active groups
## N1 and N = sample size per group at interim and final analyses
## probWinners = Probability of selecting the arm as the winner
library(mvtnorm)
powerBInfo=function(uCtl, u0y, u0x, rhou, suy, sux, rho, sy, sx, Zalpha, N1, N,
nArms, nSims)
{
uy=rep(0,nArms); ux=rep(0,nArms); probWinners=rep(0,nArms); power = 0
varcov0=matrix(c(suy^2,rhou*suy*sux,rhou*suy*sux, sux^2),2,2)
varcov=matrix(c(sy^2, rho*sy*sx, rho*sx*sy, sx^2),2,2)
for (i in 1: nSims) {
winnerMarker= -Inf
for (j in 1: nArms) {
u=rmvnorm(1,mean=c(u0y[j],u0x[j]), sigma=varcov0)
uy[j]=u[1]; ux[j]=u[2]
dataStg1=rmvnorm(N1, mean=c(uy[j], ux[j]), sigma=varcov)
meanxMarker=mean(dataStg1[,2])
if (meanxMarker>winnerMarker)
    {winner=j; winnerMarker=meanxMarker; winnerY=dataStg1[,1]}
} ## End of j ##
for (j in 1:nArms) {if (winner==j) {probWinners[j]=probWinners[j]+1/nSims}}
yStg1=winnerY
yStg2=rnorm(N-N1, mean=uy[winner], sd=sy)
yTrt=c(yStg1+yStg2)
yCtl=rnorm(N, mean=uCtl, sd=sy)
```

tValue=t.test(yTrt,yCtl)$statistic
if (tValue>=Zalpha) {power=power+1/nSims}
} ## End of i ##
return (c(power, probWinners))
}
<<**R**<<

To determine the critical value: at the design we run the trial simulation as if $u_{0y} = u_{0x} = 0$ are fixed (i.e., $\sigma_{\mu_x} = \sigma_{\mu_y} = 0$) in the worst-case scenario with $\rho_\mu = \rho = 1$ to control the type-I error rate and critical value. We then use the critical value in our simulations under $H_a$ and check the reality for the power, just as we design a trial with a fixed treatment difference $\varepsilon$ and $\sigma$ and then check what will happen to power if the reality deviates from these two numbers. We use the hierarchical model to see how the power will vary as the parameters vary. Especially, when sample size in the historical trial is small, $\sigma_{\mu_x}$ and $\sigma_{\mu_y}$ will be large, i.e., the precision of $\mu_{0xj}$, $\mu_{0yj}$, and $\rho_\mu$ in the parent model, which are estimated from the historical trial (earlier clinical trials), will be low. When there is a single active arm and a placebo group, the power for this model reduces to

$$\int \text{Power}\,(\varepsilon)\, f\,(\varepsilon)\, d\varepsilon = \int \Phi\left(\frac{\sqrt{n}\varepsilon}{2\sigma} - z_{1-\alpha}\right) f\,(\varepsilon)\, d\varepsilon \le \Phi\left(\frac{\sqrt{n}\bar{\varepsilon}}{2\sigma} - z_{1-\alpha}\right),$$

where $\varepsilon$ is the treatment difference and $f\,(\varepsilon)$ is the pdf of mean treatment difference.

For the purpose of simulation, we consider a placebo and three active arms with responses in the primary endpoint 0, 1, 0.5, and 0.2, respectively. The responses in the biomarker are 2, 1, and 0.5 for the three active arms. We don't need to consider the biomarker response in the placebo arm.

We first try different critical values under the null hypothesis until the simulated power is equal to $\alpha = 0.025$. As a result, we obtain the critical value = 2.772. We then use this critical value to obtained power under the alternative hypothesis using simulations. The results are summarized in Table 18.4 (Wang, 2013). We can see that even $\mu_{0yj}$ does not change, the variability $\sigma_{\mu_y}$ in Equation (18.18) will impact the power significantly. When $\sigma_{\mu_y}$ is larger, the power is less sensitive to the change of $\sigma_y$.

In the two-level relationship model, we study the effect of $\sigma_r^2$ on the power (Table 18.3). Similarly, for the hierarchical model we want to know how the changes of means from $u_{xj}$ to $cu_{xj}$ ($c$ is a constant) in biomarker impact the power. We can see from the simulation results (Table 18.5) that

Table 18.4:  Biomarker-Informed Design with MEM ($\rho$ and $\sigma$ Effects)

| $\sigma_\mu$ | $\rho_\mu$ | $\sigma$ | $\rho$ | Power | Selection Probability |
|---|---|---|---|---|---|
| 0.2 | 0 | 4 | 0.2 | 0.83 | 0.93, 0.06, 0.01 |
| 0.2 | 0.8 | 4 | 0.2 | 0.84 | 0.93, 0.06, 0.01 |
| 0.2 | 0 | 4 | 0.8 | 0.85 | 0.94, 0.06, 0.01 |
| 0.2 | 0.8 | 4 | 0.8 | 0.88 | 0.95, 0.05, 0.01 |
| 2 | 0.8 | 4 | 0.8 | 0.77 | 0.53, 0.28, 0.19 |
| 2 | 0.8 | 3 | 0.8 | 0.80 | 0.52, 0.28, 0.20 |

Note: $\sigma_x = \sigma_y = \sigma$, $n_1 = 100$, $N = 300$.

Table 18.5:  Biomarker-Informed Design with MEM ($\mu$ Effect)

| $u_{x1}$ | $u_{x2}$ | $u_{x3}$ | Power | Selection Probability |
|---|---|---|---|---|
| 0.2 | 0.1 | 0.05 | 0.69 | 0.35, 0.33, 0.32 |
| 2 | 1 | 0.5 | 0.80 | 0.52, 0.28, 0.20 |
| 10 | 5 | 2.5 | 0.97 | 0.95, 0.05, 0.00 |
| 0.5 | 1 | 2 | 0.54 | 0.21, 0.28, 0.52 |
| -2 | -1 | -0.5 | 0.57 | 0.18, 0.36, 0.46 |

$\sigma_x = \sigma_y = \sigma = 3$, $\sigma_{\mu y} = \sigma_{\mu x} = 2$, $\rho_\mu = \rho = 0.8$, $N_1 = 100$, $N = 300$.

the relationship between the primary endpoint means $u_{yj}$ and biomarker mean $u_{xj}$ (see Figure 8.1) has a significance effect on the power.

The typical codes to invoke the R-function 18.2 are presented in the following.

**>>R: Invoke R-Function 18.2>>**
## Determine critical value Zalpha for alpha (power) =0.025 ##
u0y=c(0,0,0); u0x=c(0,0,0)
powerBInfo(uCtl=0, u0y, u0x, rhou=1, suy=0, sux=0, rho=1, sy=4, sx=4, Zalpha=2.772, N1=100, N=300, nArms=3, nSims=100000)
## Power simulation ##
u0y=c(1,0.5,0.2)
u0x=c(2,1,0.5)
powerBInfo(uCtl=0, u0y, u0x, rhou=0.2, suy=0.2, sux=0.2, rho=0.2, sy=4, sx=4, Zalpha=2.772, N1=100, N=300, nArms=3, nSims=5000)
**<<R<<**

## 18.7   Summary

Biomarker-informed adaptive design can shorten the time of drug development and bring the right drug to the right patient earlier, by incorporating a correlated short-term endpoint at the interim stages. Simulations should be performed before conducting such a clinical trial to understand the operating characteristics of the trial design. The conventional one-level correlation model used in simulations for the biomarker-informed adaptive designs might be inappropriate when the relationship between the biomarker and the primary endpoint is not well known. This model considers only the individual level correlation between the interim and final endpoint of the design. Uncertainty of the mean level relationship between the two endpoints is not considered. Hence, the simulation results of a biomarker-informed adaptive design using the conventional one-level model can easily misestimate the power.

The new two-level model incorporates relationships at both the individual and the mean level. It is shown that in a biomarker-informed design, the power is much more sensitive to the relationship between the biomarker and the primary endpoint at the mean level than the correlation at the individual level. Simulations using the two-level relationship model for biomarker informed designs produce more sensible and reasonable results.

The two-level relationship model has been illustrated in the context of a two-stage winner design in this chapter. With the derived distribution of the test statistics and stopping boundary information, the type-I error rate can be controlled. An absolute advantage of the biomarker informed design is not guaranteed. The proposed estimators for the parameters appear to be unbiased by simulations. Hence, based on the prior historical data, we will be able to answer by simulations questions such as which design will provide higher power, the biomarker informed adaptive design or the classical Dunnett design, and, what the sample size should be to achieve a target power. In general, when a good portion of the relationship between the biomarker and the primary endpoint is known, the biomarker informed design is recommended.

The hierarchical model is an alternative way to effectively deal with biomarker utilization in clinical trials. We have discussed how to use simulation to determine the critical value and how different parameters will affect the power and sample size. Such simulation studies should be conducted to decide whether the biomarker-informed design is better than the classical design.

## Problems

**18.1** Explain why correlation ($\rho$) between the primary endpoint and biomarker has only a little effect on power of clinical trial designs.

**18.2** Study the effects of parameters in the hierarchical model in Section 18.6 on the power of the biomarker-informed design.

**18.3** Develop an SAS or R simulation program for the power calculation using the model discussed in Section 8.5.

**18.4** Discuss the pros and cons of the two biomarker-informed adaptive designs in the Chapter.

# Chapter 19

# Survival Modeling and Adaptive Treatment Switching

## 19.1 Introduction to Survival Data Modeling

### 19.1.1 *Basic Terms in Survival Analysis*

Survival analysis, or time-to-event analysis, is a branch of statistics dealing with death (failure) or degradation in biological organisms, mechanical or electronic systems, or other areas. This topic is called reliability theory or reliability analysis in engineering, and duration analysis or duration modeling in economics or sociology.

The lifetime distribution function $F(t)$ is the probability of the event (e.g., death) occurring on or before time $t$, i.e., $F(t) = P(T \le t)$. The survival function $S(t)$ is the probability of an individual surviving longer than $t$, i.e., $S(t) = 1 - F(t)$. Thus, the event density is $f(t) = dF(t)/dt$. The hazard function, or rate $\lambda(t)$, is defined as the event rate at time $t$, conditional on survival until time $t$ or later,

$$\lambda(t)\, dt = P(t < T \le t + dt | T > t) = \frac{f(t)\, dt}{S(t)} = -\frac{S'(t)}{S(t)} dt. \qquad (19.1)$$

Integrating (19.1) with respect to $t$, we obtain $S(t) = \exp(-\Lambda(t))$, where $\Lambda(t) = \int_0^t \lambda(u)\, du$ is called the cumulative hazard function. From (19.1), we can obtain

$$f(t) = \lambda(t) S(t) \qquad (19.2)$$

The expected future (residual) lifetime at a given time $t_0$ is defined as $\frac{1}{S(t_0)} \int_0^\infty t\, f(t + t_0)\, dt = \frac{1}{S(t_0)} \int_{t_0}^\infty S(t)\, dt$.

In survival analysis, we usually have a special type of missing data; i.e., censoring. In practice, survival data involve different types of censoring: (1) left-censoring if a data point (time value) is equal to or below a certain value but it is unknown by how much (e.g., missing adverse event start date), (2) right-censoring if a data point is above a certain value but it is unknown by how much (e.g., lost to follow up), and (3) interval censoring if a data point is somewhere in an interval between two values. Censoring can occur at a fixed time point (e.g., prescheduled clinical trial termination) or at a random time (e.g., early termination). Censoring can be informative or noninformative with respect to time (treatment/medical intervention). If it is noninformative, the censoring time is statistically independent of the failure time. However, the statistical independence of the failure time is a necessary but not a sufficient condition for noninformative censoring; there must be no common parameters between survival and censoring parameters to ensure the censoring is noninformative. Right-censoring is the most common and can be treated as a competing risk (Section 19.3).

### 19.1.2    *Maximum Likelihood Method*

Modeling survival data can be based on a parametric or nonparametric method. Here we will focus on parametric models. A parametric model can be specified for the hazard rate $\lambda(t) \geq 0$, survival time $S(t)$, or degradation process (we will discuss this soon).

The maximum likelihood estimate (MLE) method is commonly used for parameter estimation in survival modeling, which is similar to the MLE for other models, the only difference being the presence of censoring. Specifically, the likelihood can be written as

$$L(\theta) = \prod_{t_i \in \Omega_U} P(T = t_i|\theta) \prod_{t_j \in \Omega_L} P(T \leq t_i|\theta) \prod_{t_i \in \Omega_R} P(T > t_i|\theta)$$

$$\cdot \prod_{t_i \in \Omega_I} P(t_{ia} \leq T < t_{ib}|\theta), \tag{19.3}$$

where $\Omega_U$, $\Omega_L$, $\Omega_R$, $\Omega_I$ are the sets for uncensored, left-, right-, and interval-censored data, respectively; $P(T = t_i|\theta) = f(t_i|\theta)$, $P(T \leq t_i|\theta) = 1 - S(t_i|\theta)$, $P(T > t_i|\theta) = S(t_i|\theta)$, and $P(t_{i,a} < T \leq t_{i,b}|\theta) = S(t_{ia}|\theta) - S(t_{ib}|\theta)$.

The MLE is defined as

$$\hat{\theta}_{mle} = \arg\max L(\theta). \tag{19.4}$$

Under fairly weak conditions (Newey and McFadden, 1994, Theorem 3.3), the maximum likelihood estimator has approximately a normal distribution for a larger sample size $n$,

$$\sqrt{n}\left(\hat{\boldsymbol{\theta}}_{mle} - \boldsymbol{\theta}_0\right) \xrightarrow{d} N\left(\mathbf{0}, I^{-1}\right),$$

where $I$ is the expected Fisher information matrix given by

$$I = E\left[\nabla_{\boldsymbol{\theta}} \ln f\left(x|\boldsymbol{\theta}_0\right) \nabla_{\boldsymbol{\theta}} \ln f\left(x|\boldsymbol{\theta}_0\right)'\right],$$

where the gradient operator is given by $\nabla_{\boldsymbol{\theta}} = \sum_i \frac{\partial}{\partial \theta_i}$.

### 19.1.3 *Overview of Survival Model*

**Proportion Hazard Model**

Proportional hazard models are widely used in practice. Just as the name suggests, a proportional hazard model assumes the hazard is proportional (i.e., independent of time) between any two different groups with covariates $X' = x_1'$ and $X' = x_2'$,

$$h(t) = h_0(t) \exp\left(X'\boldsymbol{\beta}\right), \tag{19.5}$$

where $X'$ is the vector of observed covariates and $\boldsymbol{\beta}$ are the corresponding parameters. If the baseline hazard function is specified (e.g., $h_0(t) = \lambda \rho t^{\rho-1}$), (19.5) represents a parametric proportional hazard model; otherwise, (19.5) is the well-known Cox semiparametric proportional hazard model (Cox, 1972).

**Accelerated Failure Time Model**

When the proportional hazard assumption does not hold, we may use the accelerated failure time model with a hazard function:

$$h(t) = \exp\left(X'\boldsymbol{\beta}\right) h_0\left(\exp\left(X'\boldsymbol{\beta}\right) t\right). \tag{19.6}$$

Different baseline functions $h_0(\cdot)$ will lead to different parametric models. For the exponential model, $h_0(t) = \lambda$ and $S_0(t) = \exp(-\lambda t)$, where $\lambda > 0$; for the Weibull model, $h_0(t) = \lambda \rho t^{\rho-1}$ and $S_0(t) = \exp(-\lambda t^\rho)$, where $\lambda, \rho > 0$; for the Gompertz model, $h_0(t) = \lambda \exp(\gamma t)$ and $S_0(t) = \exp\left(-\lambda\gamma^{-1}\left(\exp(\gamma t) - 1\right)\right)$, where $\gamma, \lambda > 0$; and for the loglogistic model, $h_0(t) = \frac{\exp(\alpha)kt^{k-1}}{1+\exp(\alpha)t^k}$ and $S_0(t) = \frac{1}{1+\exp(\alpha)t^k}$, where $\alpha \in \mathbb{R}, k > 0$.

**Frailty Model**

The notion of frailty provides a convenient way to introduce random effects, association, and unobserved heterogeneity into models for survival data. In its simplest form, a frailty is an unobserved random factor that modifies the hazard function of an individual or related individuals. The term frailty was coined by Vaupel et al. (1979) in univariate survival models, and the model was substantially promoted for its application to multivariate survival data in a seminal paper by Clayton (1978) on chronic disease incidence in families. The simplest form of frailty model with a (unobserved) scale frailty variable $Z$ can be written as

$$h(t, Z, \boldsymbol{X}) = Z h_0(t) \exp\left(\boldsymbol{X}'\boldsymbol{\beta}\right).$$

## Copula Model

Copula modeling is a general approach to formulating different multivariate distributions. The idea is that a simple transformation can be made of each marginal variable in such a way that each transformed marginal variable has a uniform distribution. Once this is done, the dependence structure can be expressed as a multivariate distribution on the obtained uniforms, and a copula is precisely a multivariate distribution on marginally uniform random variables.

In the context of survival analysis, a copula model is often constructed from marginal survival functions instead of marginal distribution functions. If the arguments of the copula function are univariate survival functions $S_1(t_1) = P(X_1 > t_1)$ and $S_2(t_2) = P(X_2 > t_2)$, the copula function $C(S_1, S_2)$ is a legitimate joint (bivariate) survival function $S(t_1, t_2) = P(X_1 > t_1, X_2 > t_2)$ with marginals $S_1$ and $S_2$.

Archimedean copulas are commonly used copulas in survival analysis. Suppose that $\psi : [0, \infty] \to [0, 1]$ is a strictly decreasing convex function such that $\psi(0) = 1$. Then an Archimedean copula can be written as

$$C(S_1, S_2; \theta) = \psi\left(\psi^{-1}(S_1) + \psi^{-1}(S_2)\right), \ S_1, S_1 \in [0, 1], \qquad (19.7)$$

where $\theta$ is the parameter of association. For example, the stable (Gumbel-Hougaard) copula, generated by $\psi^{-1}(s) = (-\ln s)^\theta$, $\theta \geq 1$, can be expressed as

$$S(t_1, t_2; \theta) = \exp\left\{-\left[(-\ln S_1)^\theta + (-\ln S_2)^\theta\right]^{1/\theta}\right\}.$$

Archimedean copulas can be conveniently used for modeling a bivariate survival function with such marginal distributions as Gompertz, Weibull, or even in the semiparametric setup in combination with Kaplan–Meier estimates for the marginal survival functions (Genest and Rivest, 1993). All information concerning dependence between the marginals is contained in the association parameter.

## First-Hitting-Time Model

Many practical problems, such as biomarker or clinical responses, survival time, and random vibrations of a bridge, can be modeled using stochastic processes $X(t)$. When the stochastic process reaches a certain level (i.e., $X(t) = ß$) for the first time, it is called first hitting time (FHT). FHT usually indicates a critical state such as a biological inhibition, death, or bridge collapse. The critical value ß, called the boundary or threshold, can be a constant or function of time $t$. Threshold regression refers to the first-hitting-time models with regression structures that accommodate covariate data (Lee and Whitmore, 2006).

A very commonly used stochastic process is a Wiener process or Brownian motion, which describes, for example, a particle's random motion on the microscope. The macro-behavior (i.e., the average properties for Brownian motion) of the mass is governed by the so-called diffusion equation, which is widely used in science and engineering, the social sciences, and other areas. We will discuss this approach in Section 19.2.

## Multistage Model

A multistage model consists of several stages across a time axis. At each stage, a time-to-event model is applied. In principle, all models mentioned above can be used in multistage models. However, most common multistage models are semi-Markov processes (continuous time, discrete states).

The rationale for using multistage models is that it may not be easy to specify a single model across the entire time course. This is because, for example, the natural course of disease may consist of stages and the time-to-event model is relatively easy to specify for each stage separately. The model within each stage can be the proportional hazard model, frailty model, exponential model, or a combination of them. In principle, a time-dependent hazard model can be approximated by a multistage model with a time-independent hazard rate at each stage, but the number of stages required may have to be large in order to have the desired precision. The time-independent hazard rate $\lambda$ does not have to be a constant; it can include covariates (i.e., $\lambda = \lambda\left(X'\beta\right)$). The examples to illustrate the method in this chapter will focus on Markov or semi-Markov models because their calculations don't require specific software. However, for more complicated multistage models, a software package is required. The transitional probability matrix for a semi-Markov chain is given by

$$P\left(t\right) = e^{At} = I + \sum_{k=1}^{\infty} \frac{A^k t^k}{k!}, \qquad (19.8)$$

where $A = \lim\limits_{h \to 0} (P(h) - I)/h$ with $I$ being the identity matrix. We will discuss the multistage approach in Section 19.3.

## Nonparametric Approach

*Nelson–Aalen Estimator.* Let $Y(t)$ be the number of individuals at risk at (just before) time $t$ and $\tau_i$ the occurrence of the $i$th event. The Nelson–Aalen estimator for the cumulative hazard is given by

$$\hat{\Lambda}(t) = \sum_{\tau_i \leq t} \frac{1}{Y(\tau_i)} \tag{19.9}$$

with variance estimator

$$\hat{\sigma}_\Lambda^2(t) = \sum_{\tau_i \leq t} \frac{1}{Y(\tau_i)^2}.$$

The cumulative hazard $\hat{\Lambda}(t)$ approaches to a normal distribution as the sample size approaches infinity. To improve precision, log-transformation can be used.

*Kaplan–Meier Estimator.* The Kaplan-Meier estimator is given by

$$\hat{S}(t) = \prod_{\tau_k \leq t} S(\tau_k | \tau_{k-1}) = \prod_{\tau_i \leq t} \left\{ 1 - \frac{1}{Y(\tau_i)} \right\} \tag{19.10}$$

with variance

$$\hat{\sigma}_S^2(t) = \hat{S}(t)^2 \sum_{\tau_i \leq t} \frac{1}{Y(\tau_i)^2}.$$

Alternatively, the variance can be estimated using Greenwood's formulation:

$$\hat{\sigma}_S^2(t) = \hat{S}(t)^2 \sum_{\tau_i \leq t} \frac{1}{Y(\tau_i)^2 - Y(\tau_i)}.$$

For a large sample size, $\hat{S}(t)$ has approximately a normal distribution. To improve precision, log-transformation can be used.

Many software packages, such as SAS, R, and STATA, have the built-in capability of performing survival analyses with various models.

## 19.2 First-Hitting-Time Model

### 19.2.1 *Wiener Process and First Hitting Time*

**Definition 19.1** A stochastic process $\{X(t), t \geq 0\}$ is said to be a Brownian motion with a drift $\mu$ if (1) $X(0) = 0$; (2) $\{X(t), t \geq 0\}$ has stationary and independent increments; and (3) for every $t > 0, X(t)$ is normally distributed with mean $\mu t$ and variance $\sigma^2 t$,

$$X(t) \sim \frac{1}{\sqrt{2\pi\sigma^2 t}} \exp\left(-\frac{(x - \mu t)^2}{2\sigma^2 t}\right). \tag{19.11}$$

The covariance of the Brownian motion is $\text{cov}[X(t), X(s)] = \sigma^2 \min\{s, t\}$. The standard Brownian motion $B(t)$ is the Brownian motion with drift $\mu = 0$ and diffusion $\sigma^2 = 1$. The relationship between the standard Brownian motion and Brownian motion with drift $\mu$ and diffusion parameter $\sigma^2$ can be expressed as

$$X(t) = \mu t + \sigma B(t). \tag{19.12}$$

The cdf is given by

$$\Pr\{X(t) \leq y | X(0) = x\} = \Phi\left(\frac{y - x - \mu t}{\sigma\sqrt{t}}\right), \tag{19.13}$$

where $\Phi(\cdot)$ is the cdf of the standard normal distribution.

The first hitting time $T$ is a random variable when $X(t)$ starts from the initial position $X(0) = 0 \in \Omega \backslash ß$ and reaches a given constant boundary $ß = b$ of the domain $\Omega$ (nonnegative values). The FHT for Brownian motion is the inverse-normal distribution:

$$T \sim f(t | \mu, \sigma^2, b) = \frac{b}{\sqrt{2\pi\sigma^2 t^3}} e^{-\frac{(b + \mu t)^2}{2\sigma^2 t}}. \tag{19.14}$$

The cdf corresponding to (19.14) is given by

$$F(t | \mu, \sigma^2, b) = \Phi\left[-\frac{(\mu t + b)}{\sqrt{\sigma^2 t}}\right] + e^{-\frac{2b\mu}{\sigma^2}} \Phi\left[\frac{\mu t - b}{\sqrt{\sigma^2 t}}\right]. \tag{19.15}$$

Note that if $\mu > 0$, then the FHT is not certain to occur and the pdf is improper. Specifically, in this case, $P(t = \infty) = 1 - \exp(-2b\mu/\sigma^2)$.

**Definition 19.2** In general, an FHT model $< X(t), ß >$ has two essential components: (1) a parent stochastic process $\{X(t), t \in T, x \in \mathbb{R}\}$ with initial value $X(0) = 0$, where $T$ is the time space and $\mathbb{R}$ is the state space of the process, and (2) a boundary set or threshold ß, where $ß \subset \mathbb{R}$. Note that ß can be a constant, a function vector of time $t$, or a stochastic process.

### 19.2.2 Covariates and Link Function

In an FHT model, both the parent process $\{X(t)\}$ and boundary ß can have parameters that depend on covariates. As a simple sample, the Wiener process has mean parameter $\mu$ and variance parameter $\sigma^2$. The boundary ß has parameter $x_0$, the initial position. In FHT regression models, these parameters will be connected to linear combinations of covariates using a suitable regression link function,

$$g(\boldsymbol{\theta}) = \boldsymbol{Z}\boldsymbol{\beta}', \qquad (19.16)$$

where $g(\cdot)$ is the link function that has the inverse function $g^{-1}(\cdot)$, $\boldsymbol{\theta}$ is the parameter vector in the FHT model, $\boldsymbol{Z} = (1, Z_1, ..., Z_k)$ is the covariate vector (with a leading unit to include an intercept term), and $\boldsymbol{\beta} = (\beta_0, \beta_1, ..., \beta_k)$ is the associated vector of regression coefficients. The commonly used link functions include the identity and logistic functions.

There are two different covariates: time-independent (e.g., DNA markers) and time-dependent covariates (e.g., RNA markers). The use of time-dependent covariates should be undertaken cautiously since it could be very controversial (see Section 19.3).

We can solve (19.16) for $\boldsymbol{\theta}$:

$$\boldsymbol{\theta} = g^{-1}(\boldsymbol{Z}\boldsymbol{\beta}'). \qquad (19.17)$$

### 19.2.3 Parameter Estimation and Inference

The parameter estimations for FHT models have been dominated by the maximum likelihood method. Consider a latent health status process characterized by a Wiener diffusion process. The FHT for such a process follows an inverse Gaussian distribution. The inverse Gaussian distribution depends on the mean and variance parameters of the underlying Wiener process ($\mu$ and $\sigma^2$) and the initial health status level ($x_0$), i.e., $\boldsymbol{\theta} = (\mu, \sigma, x_0)$. Let $f(t|\boldsymbol{\theta})$ and $F(t|\boldsymbol{\theta})$ be the pdf and cdf of the FHT distribution, respectively. Using (19.17), we can obtain

$$\begin{cases} f(t|\boldsymbol{\theta}) = f(t|g^{-1}(\boldsymbol{Z}\boldsymbol{\beta}')), \\ F(t|\boldsymbol{\theta}) = F(t|g^{-1}(\boldsymbol{Z}\boldsymbol{\beta}')). \end{cases} \qquad (19.18)$$

To form a likelihood function, denote by $Z_i$ ($i = 1, ..., n_e$) the realization of covariate vector $Z$ on the $i$th subject who had an event at time $t_i$, and by $Z_j$ ($j = n_e + 1, ..., n_e + n_s$) the realization of covariate vector $Z$ on the $j$th subject, who is right-censored at time $t_j$. Then the likelihood function is given by

$$L(\beta) = \prod_{i=1}^{n_e} f\left(t_i | g^{-1}\left(Z_i \beta'\right)\right) \prod_{j=n_e+1}^{n_e+n_s} S(t_j | g^{-1}\left(Z_j \beta'\right)). \qquad (19.19)$$

To estimate parameters $\beta$, the likelihood or the log-likelihood function can be used. Numerical gradient methods can be used to find the maximum likelihood estimates for $\beta$. Then the parameter vector $\theta$ can be found using (19.17), and the distribution function $f(t|\theta)$ and $F(t|\theta)$ can be obtained from (19.18).

### 19.2.4 *Applications of First-Hitting-Time Model*

### Example 19.1 The First-Hitting-Time Model for Biological Degradation

A death can be viewed as the final result of the degradation of an individual's health. If we model an individual's health state using a Wiener process, then death can be viewed as the Wiener process reaching a certain threshold ß. The survival analysis becomes the study of the FHT of the process, which has an inverse normal distribution.

Alternatively, if a gamma process is chosen to model the health state, the survival (FHT) will have an inverse gamma distribution. Singpurwalla (1995) and Lawless and Crowder (2001) consider the gamma process as a model for degradation. The Ornstein–Uhlenbeck process can also be used for modeling the biological process. The FHT for the Ornstein–Uhlenbeck process has the Ricciardi–Sato distribution (Ricciardi and Sato, 1988).

### Example 19.2 Treatment Switch in Survival Trial

Survival analysis in a clinical trial with treatment switching is a challenge. In randomized oncology trials, a patient's treatment may be switched in the middle of the study because of a progressive disease (PD), which indicates a failure of the initial treatment regimen. In such cases, the total survival time is the sum of two event times: randomization to switching and switching to death. If the test drug is more effective than the control, then the majority of patients in the control group will switch to the test drug and the survival difference between the two treatment groups will be significantly reduced in comparison with the case without treatment switching. This marker-based treatment switch is not random switching but rather response-adaptive switching. Branson and Whitehead (2002) and Shao et al. (2005) propose different approaches to the problem. Lee et al. (2008) propose a mixture of Wiener processes for clinical trials with adaptive switching and have applied it to an oncology study. It is outlined as follows:

Since the actual or censored survival time can be composed of two intervals, representing the time on the primary therapy and the time on the alternative therapy, the disease may progress at different rates in these two intervals (irrespective of the treatment). We transform survival times from calendar time to the so-called running time, which has the form

$$r = a_1\tau_1 + \tau_2, \tag{19.20}$$

where $\tau_1$ and $\tau_2$ correspond to time to progression and progression to death, respectively, and $a_1$ is a scale parameter to be estimated.

The mixture of Wiener processes with FHT used for the modeling is given by

$$\Pr(S > r) = p\left(1 - F_1\left(r\right)\right) + \left(1 - p\right)\left(1 - F_2\left(r\right)\right). \tag{19.21}$$

The respective lifetime functions $F_j\left(r\right)$ $(j = 1, 2)$ are the same as (19.15) but expressed in terms of running time $r$. The parameter $p$ is to be estimated.

### 19.2.5   *Multivariate Model with Biomarkers*

There are different biomarkers: a pharmacodynamic biomarker informs if a drug has reached its target; a functional response biomarker informs if a drug has affected a target pathway; a pharmacogenomic biomarker (PGx) measures variations in a target; a disease biomarker monitors or predicts disease risk, progression, and improvement; and a surrogate endpoint reflects how a patient feels or physical or mental functions.

Biomarkers, compared with a clinical endpoint such as survival, can often be measured earlier, more easily, and more frequently. They are less subject to competing risks and are less confounded by changes in treatment modalities. Among different biomarkers, some are static, such as DNA markers, while others are time-dependent, such as RNA markers. A time-independent biomarker can be treated as a covariate, whereas a time-dependent marker can be treated in multivariate survival models. There are also models that treat a time-dependent variable as a covariate. However, we will show you that the results from such models can be very misleading. The utility of biomarkers in clinical trial designs, especially in adaptive designs, has been discussed in previous chapters. Here we discuss how to use the biomarker process to assist in tracking the progress of the parent process if the parent process is latent or only infrequently observed. In this way, the marker process forms a basis for a predictive inference about the status of the parent process and its progress toward an FHT. As markers of the parent process, biomarkers offer potential insights into the causal forces that are generating the movements of the parent process (Whitmore, Crowder, and Lawless, 1998).

We now introduce the Whitmore–Crowder–Lawless method (Whitmore et al., 1998). Suppose there are the parent survival process, $X(t)$, and a correlated biomarker process, $Y(t)$. They form a two-dimensional Wiener diffusion process $\{X(r), Y(r)\}$ for $r \geq 0$ and the initial condition $\{X(0), Y(0)\} = \{0, 0\}$. Vector $\{X(r), Y(r)\}$ has a bivariate normal distribution with a mean vector $r\boldsymbol{\mu}$, where $\boldsymbol{\mu} = (\mu_x, \mu_y)'$, $\mu_x \geq 0$, and covariance matrix $r\Sigma$ with $\Sigma = \begin{pmatrix} \sigma_{xx} & \sigma_{xy} \\ \sigma_{yx} & \sigma_{yy} \end{pmatrix}$. The correlation coefficient is $\rho = \sigma_{xy}/\sqrt{\sigma_{xx}\sigma_{yy}}$.

The key is to formulate the probability or pdf for the survival and failing subjects. For a survivor at time $t$, an observed value $Y(t) = y(t)$ for the biomarker constitutes a censored observation of failure time because we know $S > t$. The pdf for survival subjects is given by

$$p_s(y) = \Phi(c_1)\phi(c_2) - e^{\frac{2\mu_x}{\sigma_{xx}}} \Phi\left(c_1 - 2\sqrt{\frac{(1-\rho^2)}{\sigma_{xx}t}}\right) \phi\left(c_2 - \frac{2\sigma_{xy}}{\sigma_{xx}\sqrt{\sigma_{yy}t}}\right),$$

(19.22)

where $\phi$ and $\Phi$ are, respectively, the standard normal pdf and cdf, and

$$\begin{cases} c_1 = \frac{1-\mu_x t - \sigma_{xy}\left(y-\mu_y t\right)}{\sigma_{yy}\sqrt{\sigma_{xx}(1-\rho^2)t}}, \\ c_2 = \frac{y-\mu_y t}{\sqrt{\sigma_{yy}t}}. \end{cases}$$

(19.23)

For a subject who died at time $S = s$ with an observed value $Y(S) = y(s)$ for the biomarker, the joint pdf is

$$p_f(y, s) = \frac{\exp\left(-\frac{1}{2}W^T\Sigma^{-1}W\right)}{2\pi\sqrt{|\Sigma|}s^2},$$

(19.24)

where

$$W^T = \left( \frac{y - \mu_y s}{\sqrt{s}}, \frac{1 - \mu_x s}{\sqrt{s}} \right). \tag{19.25}$$

The probability of surviving longer than time $t$ is

$$P(S > t) = \int_{-\infty}^{\infty} p_s(y)\, dy. \tag{19.26}$$

Numerical methods can be used to calculate $P(S > t)$.

To carry out maximum likelihood estimation of the parameters, we denote the independent sample observations on failing items by $(\hat{y}_i, \hat{s}_i)$, $i = 1, ..., \nu$, and those on surviving items by $\hat{y}_i$, $i = \nu + 1, ..., n$. The log-likelihood can then be written as

$$\ln L(\mu, \Sigma) = \sum_{i=1}^{\nu} \ln p_f(\hat{y}_i, \hat{s}_i) + \sum_{i=\nu+1}^{n} \ln p_s(\hat{y}_i). \tag{19.27}$$

The maximum likelihood estimates of the parameters $\mu$ and $\Sigma$ can be found based on (19.27).

From (19.22) through (19.27), we have assumed the threshold for failure is $x = 1$. If failure is defined as $x = a$, then the estimates $\hat{\mu}_x$, $\hat{\sigma}_{xx}$, and $\hat{\sigma}_{xy}$ from (19.20) should be multiplied by a constant $a$. Other estimates and probabilities are independent of $a$. Thus, no changes are needed.

So far, we have considered a single-marker case. In practice, there is usually more than one relevant marker, while each marker will have a certain degree of correlation with the underlying parent process. We wish to find that the linear combination of the available markers will have the largest possible correlation with the degradation component. Whitmore et al. (1998) extended their method to include a composite marker or a combination of several markers.

Suppose there are $k$ candidate markers available, denoted by $Z(t) = (Z_1(t), ..., Z_k(t))$, with the initial condition $Z(0) = 0$. Assume that vector $Z(t)$, together with the degradation component $X(t)$, forms a $k + 1$ dimensional Wiener process. We define the composite marker denoted by $Y(t)$ as

$$Y(t) = \mathbf{Z}(t)\boldsymbol{\beta}' = \sum_{j=1}^{k} Z_j(t)\beta_j, \tag{19.28}$$

where $\beta = (1, \beta_2, ..., \beta_k)$ is a $k \times 1$ vector of coefficients that we wish to estimate. The linear structure of (19.28) assures that the joint process for $Y(t)$ and $X(t)$ retains its bivariate Wiener form. The parameterization is defined by

$$\mu_y = \mu_Z \beta', \ \sigma_{yy} = \beta \Sigma_{ZZ} \beta', \ \sigma_{yy} = \Sigma_{XZ} \beta', \qquad (19.29)$$

where $\mu_Z$ and $\Sigma_{ZZ}$ denote the $k \times 1$ mean vector and $k \times k$ covariance matrix of markers $Z(t)$ and $\Sigma_{XZ}$ denotes the $1 \times k$ covariate vector of $X(t)$ with $Z(t)$.

The MLEs presented earlier for a single marker can be extended to estimate the optimal composite marker in (19.28). This extension requires rewriting the likelihood function in (19.27) in terms of the new parameterization in (19.29).

## 19.3    Multistage Model

### 19.3.1    *General Framework of Multistage Model*

We consider the time-dependent Markov progressive model in which the probability (density) of transition is usually dependent on the time relative to the previous state but independent of any earlier states. For example, a healthy individual can become a disabled person and then die, as shown in Figure 19.1. The progressive Markov model says that the transition probability from the state "Disabled" to "Death" is a function of time from "Disabled" but is independent of how healthy the person was and how quickly he became a disabled person.

Suppose we have a simple multistage model, as shown in Figure 19.1, that has three states of an individual: health, disabled, and death. Possible transition directions are indicated by arrows, with a corresponding transition probability $F_i(t)$ and density $f_i(t)$ $(i = 1, 2)$, which are the lifetime and event density functions.

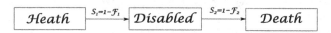

Figure 19.1:    A Simple Multistage Survival Model

After a multistage model is constructed, we need to formulate the likelihood for the MLE of parameters. Similar to the single stage model discussed in Section 19.1, the likelihood formulation $L$ (assume the process starting time $t_0 = 0$) can be classified into the following four different cases:

(1) For subject $i$ disabled at time $t = t_{11i}$ and dead at $t = t_{12i}$, the likelihood is $l_{1i} = f_1(t_{11i}) f_2(t_{12i} - t_{11i})$.

(2) For subject $j$ disabled at time $t = t_{21j}$ and alive (right-censored) at $t = t_{22j}$, the likelihood is $l_{2j} = f_1(t_{21j})(1 - F_2(t_{22j} - t_{21j}))$.

(3) For subject $k$ disabled before or at time $t_{31k}$ (left-censored) and dead at $t = t_{32k}$, the likelihood is $l_{3k} = F_1(t_{31k}) f_2(t_{32k} - t_{31k})$.

(4) For subject $m$ disabled before or at time $t_{41m}$ (left-censored) and alive (right-censored) at $t = t_{42m}$, the likelihood is $l_{4m} = F_1(t_{41m})(1 - F_2(t_{42m} - t_{41m}))$.

Assume there are $n_i$ subjects in category $i$. We label the subjects in such a way that patients 1 to $n_1$ are in category 1, patients $n_1 + 1$ to $n_1 + n_2$ in category 2, patients $n_1 + n_2 + 1$ to $n_1 + n_2 + n_3$ in category 3, and patients $n_1 + n_2 + n_3 + 1$ to $n_1 + n_2 + n_3 + n_4$ in category 4. The likelihood function for the $n$ ($n = n_1 + n_2 + n_3 + n_4$) observations is given by

$$L = \prod_{i=1}^{n_1} l_{1i} \prod_{j=n_1+1}^{n_1+n_2} l_{2j} \prod_{k=n_1+n_2+1}^{n_1+n_2+n_3} l_{3k} \prod_{m=n_1+n_2+n_3+1}^{n_1+n_2+n_3+n_4} l_{4m}. \tag{19.30}$$

By maximizing $L$ in (19.30), we can obtain the MLE of the parameters.

**Example 19.3    Multistage Model for Survival Trial**

In the multistage model in Figure 19.1, we apply an exponential model with constant hazard $\lambda_i$. The transition probability density is $f_i = \lambda_i \exp(-\lambda_i t)$. It follows that $F_i = 1 - \exp(-\lambda_i t)$ and $S_i = 1 - F_i(t) = \exp(-\lambda_i t)$. Suppose there are $n_1$ subjects in category 1 and $n_2$ subjects in category 2, but no left-censored observations, i.e., $n_3 = n_4 = 0$. The likelihood function is given by

$$L = \prod_{i=1}^{n_1} \lambda_1 e^{-\lambda_1 t_{11i}} \lambda_2 e^{-\lambda_2(t_{12i} - t_{11i})} \prod_{j=n_1+1}^{n_2} \lambda_1 e^{-\lambda_1 t_{21j}} e^{-\lambda_2(t_{22j} - t_{21j})}.$$

The log-likelihood is given by

$$\ln L = (n_1 + n_2)\ln\lambda_1 + n_1 \ln\lambda_2 - \lambda_1 \left( \sum_{i=1}^{n_1} t_{11i} + \sum_{j=n_1+1}^{n_1+n_2} t_{21j} \right)$$

$$- \lambda_2 \left( \sum_{i=1}^{n_1} (t_{12i} - t_{11i}) + \sum_{j=n_1+1}^{n_1+n_2} (t_{22j} - t_{21j}) \right).$$

The maximization of $\ln L$ gives

$$\lambda_1 = \frac{n_1 + n_2}{\left( \sum_{i=1}^{n_1} t_{11i} + \sum_{j=n_1+1}^{n_1+n_2} t_{21j} \right)},$$

$$\lambda_2 = \frac{n_1}{\left( \sum_{i=1}^{n_1} (t_{12i} - t_{11i}) + \sum_{j=n_1+1}^{n_1+n_2} (t_{22j} - t_{21j}) \right)}.$$

### 19.3.2 *Covariates and Treatment Switching*

Covariates such as medical treatment, age, race, and disease status may or may not be time-dependent. In Example 19.4, a progressive disease (PD) is an indication of treatment failure and the patient usually has to switch from the initial treatment to an alternative. Thus, treatment for a patient is a time-dependent variable: before PD with one treatment, after PD with another treatment (Figure 19.2).

To consider covariates in a multistage model, we can use a link function as defined in (19.16). Then substitute (19.17) into (19.30) and maximize it to obtain MLEs of the parameters $\beta$.

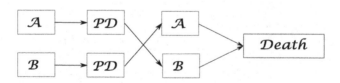

Figure 19.2:   Effect of Treatment Switching

### Example 19.4   Multistage Model for Clinical Trial Treatment Switch

Suppose patients in a two-group oncology clinical trial are randomized to receive either treatment $A$ or $B$. If a progressive disease is observed, meaning the patient has developed a resistance to the drug, then the patient will switch the treatment from $A$ to $B$ or $B$ to $A$ (in practice, there are more options, i.e., different combinations of drugs). The hazard rates are denoted by $\beta_{11}$ for treatment $A$ before PD, $\beta_{21}$ for treatment $A$ after PD, $\beta_{12}$ for treatment $B$ before PD, and $\beta_{22}$ for treatment $B$ after PD.

For simplicity we assume PD is always observed immediately (i.e., no censoring on PD). Thus, a typical patient $i$ initially treated with drug $A$ will have the following two possible likelihood functions:

(1) PD at time $t = t_{11i}$ and death at $t = t_{12i}$, $l_i = \beta_{11}e^{-\beta_{11}t_{11i}}\beta_{21}e^{-\beta_{21}(t_{12i}-t_{11i})}$, where $i = 1, ..., n_1$.

(2) PD at time $t = t_{21i}$ and alive (right-censored) at $t = t_{22i}$, $l_i = \beta_{11}e^{-\beta_{11}t_{21i}}e^{-\beta_{21}(t_{22i}-t_{21i})}$, where $i = n_1 + 1, ..., n_1 + n_2$.

Similarly, a typical patient $i$ initially treated with drug $B$ will have the following two possible likelihood functions:

(1) PD at time $t = t_{31i}$ and death at $t = t_{32i}$, $l_i = \beta_{12}e^{-\beta_{12}t_{31i}}\beta_{22}e^{-\beta_{22}(t_{32i}-t_{31i})}$, where $i = n_1 + n_2 + 1, ..., n_1 + n_2 + n_3$.

(2) PD at time $t = t_{41i}$ and alive (right-censored) at $t = t_{42i}$, $l_i = \beta_{12}e^{-\beta_{12}t_{41i}}e^{-\beta_{22}(t_{42i}-t_{41i})}$, where $i = n_1 + n_2 + n_3 + 1, ..., n_1 + n_2 + n_3 + n_4$.

The likelihood function based on the total $n_1 + n_2 + n_3 + n_4$ observations is the same as (19.30). The log-likelihood function can be given explicitly by

$$\ln L = (n_1 + n_2)\ln\beta_{11} + (n_3 + n_4)\ln\beta_{12} + n_1\ln\beta_{21} + n_3\ln\beta_{22}$$

$$-\beta_{11}\left(\sum_{i=1}^{n_1}t_{11i} + \sum_{i=n_1+1}^{n_1+n_2}t_{21i}\right)$$

$$-\beta_{21}\left(\sum_{i=1}^{n_1}(t_{12i} - t_{11i}) + \sum_{i=n_1+1}^{n_1+n_2}(t_{22i} - t_{21i})\right)$$

$$-\beta_{12}\left(\sum_{i=n_1+n_2+1}^{n_1+n_2+n_3}t_{31i} + \sum_{i=n_1+n_2+n_3+1}^{n_1+n_2+n_3+n_4}t_{41i}\right)$$

$$-\beta_{22}\left(\sum_{i=n_1+n_2+1}^{n_1+n_2+n_3}(t_{32i} - t_{31i}) + \sum_{i=n_1+n_2+n_3+1}^{n_1+n_2+n_3+n_4}(t_{42i} - t_{41i})\right)$$

Letting $\frac{\partial \ln L}{\partial \beta_{jk}} = 0$, we can obtain

$$
\begin{cases}
\beta_{11} = \frac{n_1 + n_2}{\sum_{i=1}^{n_1} t_{11i} + \sum_{i=n_1+1}^{n_1+n_2} t_{21i}}, \\[2mm]
\beta_{12} = \frac{n_3 + n_4}{\sum_{i=1}^{n_1} (t_{12i} - t_{11i}) + \sum_{i=n_1+1}^{n_1+n_2} (t_{22i} - t_{21i})}, \\[2mm]
\beta_{21} = \frac{n_1}{\sum_{i=n_1+n_2+1}^{n_1+n_2+n_3} t_{31i} + \sum_{i=n_1+n_2+n_3+1}^{n_1+n_2+n_3+n_4} t_{41i}}, \\[2mm]
\beta_{22} = \frac{n_3}{\sum_{i=n_1+n_2+1}^{n_1+n_2+n_3} (t_{32i} - t_{31i}) + \sum_{i=n_1+n_2+n_3+1}^{n_1+n_2+n_3+n_4} (t_{42i} - t_{41i})}.
\end{cases}
$$

The relative treatment efficacy between the treatment groups can be measured by the hazard ratio:

$$
\begin{cases}
HR_1 = \frac{\beta_{11}}{\beta_{12}}, \text{ before PD}, \\[2mm]
HR_2 = \frac{\beta_{21}}{\beta_{22}}, \text{ after PD}.
\end{cases}
$$

In practice, cancer drugs are categorized by the number of PDs: newly diagnosed patients usually use first-line drugs, after one PD they use second-line drugs, and so on.

The efficacy should be compared in terms of savings in survival time between the two conditions with and without the new drug $B$. (1) Without drug $B$, the patients would be treated with $A$ initially and then treated with some other available drugs. (2) With drug $B$, the patients will eventually have PD and will be treated with drug $B$ or other drugs. If there are other drugs available (as good as drug $B$) after the PD, then $HR_1 = \frac{\beta_{11}}{\beta_{12}}$ should be used to measure the survival benefit, which implies that PD is a good surrogate marker for survival.

The treatment switching problem has also been studied by Sommer and Zeger (1991), Branson and Whitehead (2002), and Shao, Chang, and Chow (2005) among others.

## 19.4 Summary and Discussion

We have introduced three different methods for modeling survival distribution with response-adaptive treatment switching: the mixed exponential model, the mixture of Wiener process, and the latent event model. The mixture of Wiener processes is very flexible and can model the covariates too, while the mixed exponential method is very simple and can be further developed to include baseline covariates.

From an analysis point of view, the trial should be designed to allow treatment switching, but not crossover. Treatment crossover implies that patients in the control group will be allowed to switch to the test drug. In this case, the treatment difference is difficult to define. If a trial is designed to allow treatment switching but not crossover, then the comparison of the two groups (based on initial randomization) is easy to interpret. Suppose that if progressive disease (PD) is observed for a patient (from either group), the patient will switch to the best alternative treatment available on the market. This way, the control group represents the situation without the test drug, and the test group represents the situation with the test drug. The difference between these two is the patient's net health improvement by adding the test drug to the market. Of course, an oncology trial that does not allow for treatment crossover may be challenging with regard to patient enrollment and may also have some ethical issues.

## Problems

**19.1** Describe the following different survival models and how they differ: (1) proportional Hazard Model, (2) accelerated failure time model, (3) frailty model, (4) Copula model, (5) first-hitting-time model, and (6) multistage model.

**19.2** Explain how the covariates are usually incorporated into a survival model.

**19.3** In Example 19.4, we discussed the multistage model for clinical trial treatment switching. Explain how the benefit of a new drug should be evaluated.

**19.4** We have discussed multistage model with exponential model $f_i = \lambda_i \exp(-\lambda_i t)$ for stage $i$, how do you incorporate the covariates into the model?

# Chapter 20

# Response-Adaptive Allocation Design

## 20.1 Opportunities

Response-adaptive randomization or allocation is a randomization technique in which the allocation of patients to treatment groups is based on the responses (outcomes) of the previous patients. The main purpose is to provide a better chance of randomizing the patients to a superior treatment group based on the knowledge about the treatment effect at the time of randomization. As a result, response-adaptive randomization takes ethical concerns into consideration. The well-known response-adaptive models include the play-the-winner (PW) model and the randomized play-the-winner (RPW) model.

The response-adaptive randomization dose not have to be based on the primary endpoint of the trial; instead, the randomization can be based the response on a biomarker.

In this chapter, we will review traditional randomization methods and discuss the response-adaptive randomization/allocation designs, including the play-the-winner model and the randomized play-the-winner model for two-arm trials, and the generalized urn model for multiple-arm trials with various endpoints. We will explore the properties of these adaptive designs and illustrate the methods with trial examples. Scholars including Zelen (1969); Wei and Durham (1978); Wei, Smythe, and Lin (1990); Stallard and Rosenberger (2002); Hu and Rosenberger (2006); and many others have contributed in this area.

Fiore et al. (2011) use a response-adaptive randomization based on Bayesian posterior distribution of treatment effect given the observed response data and discuss the application as a point-of-care clinical trial with insulin administration. Fava et al. (2003), Walsh et al. (2002), Fava (2010), and Doros et al. (2013) studied two-stage rerandomization adaptive designs and analyses in trials with high placebo effect, which will be discussed in a later section of the chapter.

## 20.2   Traditional Randomization Methods

Let $\boldsymbol{Z}_n$ be the baseline covariate matrix of the first $n$ patients; $\boldsymbol{T}_n$ be the randomization profile (treatment assignment vector) of the first $n$ subjects, in which $T_{nk}$ denotes the possible assignment of treatment $k$ to the $n$th patient; and $\boldsymbol{Y}_n$ be the corresponding response profile of the $n$ subjects. The randomization procedure can generally be designed by the allocation probability $\varphi_n$, which is the conditional probability of assigning the $n$th patient to treatment $k$ $(k = 1, ..., K)$, given the current patient profile and the previous treatment assignments for and responses of the previous $n$ patients.

Randomization methods can be grouped into six different categories: complete, restricted, response-adaptive, covariate-adaptive, covariate-adjusted response-adaptive, and other randomizations.

(1) In the complete randomization, the allocation probability is defined as

$$\varphi_n(k) = E(\boldsymbol{T}_n) = r_k, k = 1, ..., K \qquad (20.1)$$

Here $r_k$ is a constant indexed by treatment $k$. For a balanced design, $r_k = \frac{1}{K}$.

Because of randomness, the complete randomization cannot guarantee the targeted randomization proportion $r_k$ of patients assigned to treatment $k$. Therefore, the restricted randomization is invented.

(2) In restricted randomization, the allocation probability is dependent on the previous treatment assignment:

$$\varphi_n(k) = E(T_{nk}|\boldsymbol{T}_{n-1}) \qquad (20.2)$$

For example, in Efron's biased coin design (1971), the allocation probabilities for the two treatment groups are given by

$$\varphi_n(k) = \begin{cases} r, & \text{if group 1 has more patients} \\ 1 - r, & \text{if group 2 has more patients} \\ 1 - r, & \text{otherwise} \end{cases} \qquad (20.3)$$

where $r$ is a constant between 0 and 1. Block randomization is a restricted randomization.

(3) The allocation probability in the response-adaptive randomization can be written as

$$\varphi_n(k) = E\left(T_{nk}|\boldsymbol{T}_{n-1}, \boldsymbol{Y}_{n-1}\right), \qquad (20.5)$$

which means the allocation probability of the $n$th patient is a function of treatment assignments and responses of the previous $n-1$ patients. We will discuss mainly this randomization scheme in this chapter.

(4) covariate-adaptive randomization

$$\varphi_n(k) = E\left(T_{nk}|\boldsymbol{T}_{n-1}, \boldsymbol{Z}_n\right). \qquad (20.4)$$

In a covariate-adaptive randomization, the treatment of an assignment will not only depend on the previous treatment assignment, but also depend on the baseline covariates of all the patients to date (include the current one). The stratified randomization and stratified block-randomization are two common examples of covariate-adaptive randomizations.

(5) In covariate-adjusted response-adaptive randomization

$$\varphi_n(k) = E\left(T_{nk}|\boldsymbol{T}_{n-1}, \boldsymbol{Y}_{n-1}, \boldsymbol{Z}_n\right). \qquad (20.6)$$

This randomization scheme indicates the probability of treatment assignment will be based on the treatment assignments, baseline covariates, and responses of the previous $n-1$ patients and the covariates of the current patient.

(6) There are other randomizations such as cluster randomization, but we will not discuss them here.

## 20.3 Basic Response-Adaptive Randomizations

### 20.3.1 *Play-the-Winner Model*

The PW model can be easily applied to clinical trials comparing two treatments (e.g., treatment $A$ and treatment $B$) with binary outcomes (i.e., success or failure). For the PW model, it is assumed that the previous subject's outcome will be available before the next patient is randomized. The treatment assignment is based on the treatment response of the previous patient. If a patient responds to treatment $A$, then the next patient will be assigned to treatment $A$. Similarly, if a patient responds to treatment $B$, then the next patient will be assigned to treatment $B$. If the assessment of the previous patients is not available, the treatment assignment can be based on the response assessment of the last available patient. It is obvious that this model lacks randomness.

### 20.3.2  *Randomized Play-the-Winner Model*

The RPW model is a simple probabilistic model used to sequentially randomize subjects in a clinical trial (Coad and Rosenberger, 1999; Wei and Durham, 1978). The RPW model is useful for clinical trials comparing two treatments with binary outcomes. In the RPW model, it is assumed that the previous subject's outcome will be available before the next patient is randomized. At the start of the clinical trial, an urn contains $a_0$ balls representing treatment $A$ and $b_0$ balls representing treatment $B$, where $a_0$ and $b_0$ are positive integers. We denote these balls as either type $A$ or type $B$ balls. When a subject is recruited, a ball is drawn and replaced. If it is a type $A$ ball, the subject receives treatment $A$; if it is a type $B$ ball, the subject receives treatment $B$. When a subject's outcome is available, the urn is updated as follows: A success on treatment $A$ $(B)$ or a failure on treatment $B$ $(A)$ will generate an additional $a_1$ $(b_1)$ type-$B$ balls in the urn. In this way, the urn builds up more balls representing the more successful treatment (Figure 20.1).

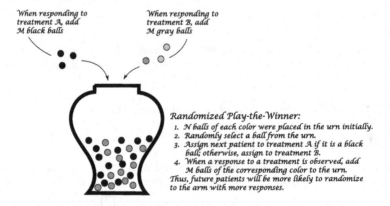

Figure 20.1:  Randomized Play-the-Winner

There are some interesting asymptotic properties with RPW. Let $N_a/N$ be the proportion of subjects assigned to treatment $A$ out of $N$ subjects. Also, let $q_a = 1 - p_a$ and $q_b = 1 - p_b$ be the failure probabilities. Further, let $F$ be the total number of failures. Then, we have (Wei and Durham,

1978):

$$
\begin{cases}
\lim_{N \to \infty} \frac{N_a}{N_b} = \frac{q_b}{q_a}, \\
\lim_{N \to \infty} \frac{N_a}{N} = \frac{q_b}{q_a + q_b}, \\
\lim_{N \to \infty} \frac{F}{N} = \frac{2q_a q_b}{q_a + q_b}.
\end{cases}
\tag{20.7}
$$

Since treatment assignment is based on response of the previous patient in RPW model, it is not optimized with respect to any clinical endpoint. It is desirable to randomize treatment assignment based on some optimal criteria such as minimizing the expected numbers of treatment failures. This leads to the so-called optimal RPW model.

### 20.3.3 *Optimal Randomized Play-the-Winner*

The optimal randomized play-the-winner model (ORPW) is intended to minimize the number of failures in the trial. There are three commonly used efficacy endpoints in clinic trials, namely, simple proportion difference ($p_a - p_b$), the relative risk ($p_a/p_b$), and the odds ratio ($p_a q_b / p_b q_a$), where $q_a = 1 - p_a$ and $q_b = 1 - p_b$ are failure rates. These can be estimated consistently by replacing $p_a$ by $\hat{p}_a$ and $p_b$ by $\hat{p}_b$, where $\hat{p}_a$ and $\hat{p}_b$ are the proportions of observed successes in treatment groups $A$ and $B$, respectively. Suppose that we wish to find the optimal allocation $r = n_a/n_b$ such that it minimizes the expected number of treatment failures $n_a q_a + n_b q_b$, which is mathematically given by (Rosenberger and Lachin, 2002):

$$
r^* = \arg\min_r \{n_a q_a + n_b q_b\}
\tag{20.8}
$$

$$
= \arg\min_r \{\frac{r}{1+r} n\, q_a + \frac{1}{1+r} n\, q_b\}.
$$

For simple proportion difference, the asymptotic variance is given by

$$
\frac{p_a q_a}{n_a} + \frac{p_b q_b}{n_b} = \frac{(1+r)(p_a\, q_a + r\, p_b\, q_b)}{n\, r} = K,
\tag{20.9}
$$

where $K$ is some constant. Solving (20.9) for $n$ yields

$$
n = \frac{(1+r)(p_a\, q_a + r\, p_b\, q_b)}{r K}.
\tag{20.10}
$$

Substituting (20.10) into (20.8), we obtain

$$
r^* = \arg\min_r \left\{ \frac{(r\, p_a + q_b)(p_a q_a + r\, p_b q_b)}{r\, K} \right\}.
\tag{20.11}
$$

Taking the derivative of (20.11) with respect to $r$ and equating to zero, we have

$$r^* = \left(\frac{p_a}{p_b}\right)^{\frac{1}{2}}. \tag{20.12}$$

Note that $r^*$ does not depend on $K$.

Note that the limiting allocation for the RPW rule $\left(\frac{q_b}{q_a}\right)$ is not optimal for any of the three measures and none of the optimal allocation rules yields Neyman allocation given by (Melfi and Page, 1998)

$$r^* = \left(\frac{p_a}{p_b}\frac{q_a}{q_b}\right)^{\frac{1}{2}}, \tag{20.13}$$

which minimizes the variance of the difference in sample proportions (Table 20.1). Note that Neyman allocation would be unethical when $p_a > p_b$ (i.e., more patients receiving the inferior treatment).

Table 20.1:    Asymptotic Variance with RPW

| Measure | $r^*$ | | Asymptotic variance |
|---|---|---|---|
| Proportion difference | $\left(\frac{p_a}{p_b}\right)^{\frac{1}{2}}$ | | $\frac{p_a\,q_a}{n_a} + \frac{p_b\,q_b}{n_b}$ |
| Relative risk | $\left(\frac{p_a}{p_b}\right)^{\frac{1}{2}}$ | $\left(\frac{q_b}{q_a}\right)$ | $\frac{p_a\,q_b^2}{n_a q_a^3} + \frac{p_b\,q_b}{n_b q_a^2}$ |
| Odds ratio | $\left(\frac{p_b}{p_a}\right)^{\frac{1}{2}}$ | $\left(\frac{q_b}{q_a}\right)$ | $\frac{p_a\,q_b^2}{n_a q_a^3 p_b^2} + \frac{p_b q_b}{n_b q_a^2 p_b^2}$ |
| Source: Chow and Chang (2006, p.61). | | | |

Because the optimal allocation depends on the unknown binomial parameters, practically the unknown success probabilities in the optimal allocation rule can be replaced by the current estimate of the proportion of successes (i.e., $\hat{p}_{a,n}$ and $\hat{p}_{b,n}$) observed in each treatment group thus far.

## 20.4    Adaptive Design with Randomized Play-the-Winner

We will use SAS Macro 20.1 below to study the adaptive design using the randomized play-the-winner. There are different ways to design a trial using RPW. We have seen that RPW can reduce the number of failures and increase the number of responses within a trial with fixed sample size. However, it may inflate $\alpha$ using a classical test statistic in conjunction with an unadjusted rejection region. In other words, it may reduce the power, and sample size has to be increased to retain the power. As a result, the increase in sample size may lead to an increase in number of failures. Here are some immediate questions before we design an RPW trial. (1) How many analyses should be used? Should a full or group sequential design be used? (2) How to determine the four parameters in the randomization urn $RPW(a_0, b_0, a_1, b_1)$? (3) What test statistic should be used? (4) How to control $\alpha$ and calculate the power? (5) How to estimate the response rate in each group? We will use the SAS Macro 20.1, RPW, for a two-arm trial with binary endpoint to facilitate the discussion.

In SAS Macro 20.1, the initial numbers of balls in the urn is denoted by **a0** and **b0**. Next **a1** or **b1** balls are added to the urn if a response is observed in arm $A$ or arm $B$. The SAS variables are defined as follows: **RR1**, **RR2** = the response rates in group 1 and 2, respectively, **nSbjs** = total number of subjects (two groups combined), **nMin** ($>0$) = the minimum sample size per group required to avoid an extreme imbalance situation, **nAnlys** = number of analyses (approximately an equal information-time design). All interim analyses are designed for randomization adjustment and only the final analysis is for hypothesis testing. **aveP1** and **aveP2** = the average response rates in group 1 and 2, respectively. **Power** = probability of the test statistic $>$ **Zc**. Note: **Zc** = function of (**nSbjs, nAnlys, a0, b0, a1, b1, nMin**).

**>>SAS Macro 20.1: Randomized Play-the-Winner Design>>**

```
%Macro RPW(nSims=100000, Zc=1.96, nSbjs=200, nAnlys=3, RR1=0.2,
RR2=0.3, a0=1, b0=1, a1=1, b1=1, nMin=1);
Data RPW; Keep nSbjs aveP1 aveP2 Zc Power;
seed1=364; seed2=894; Power=0; aveP1=0; aveP2=0;
Do isim=1 to &nSims;
nResp1=0; nResp2=0; a0=&a0; b0=&b0; Zc=&Zc; N1=0; N2=0;
nSbjs=&nSbjs; nAnlys=&nAnlys; nMax=nSbjs-&nMin;
a=a0; b=b0; r0=a/(a+b);
Do iSbj=1 To nSbjs;
If Mod(iSbj,Round(nSbjs/nAnlys))=0 Then r0=a/(a+b);
rnAss=Ranuni(seed1);
If (rnAss < r0 And N1<nMax) Or N2>=nMax Then
Do;
N1=N1+1; rnRep=Ranuni(seed2);
if rnRep <=&RR1 Then Do;
nResp1=nResp1+1; a=a+&a1;
End;
End;
Else
```

```
Do;
N2=N2+1; rnRep=Ranuni(seed2);
If rnRep <=&RR2 Then Do;
nResp2=nResp2+1; b=b+&b1;
End;
End;
End;
p1=nResp1/N1; p2=nResp2/N2;
aveP1=aveP1+p1/&nSims; aveP2=aveP2+p2/&nSims;
sigma1=sqrt(p1*(1-p1)); sigma2=sqrt(p2*(1-p2));
Sumscf=sigma1**2/(N1/(N1+N2))+sigma2**2/(N2/(N1+N2));
TS = (p2-p1)*Sqrt((N1+N2)/sumscf);
If TS>Zc Then Power=Power+1/&nSims;
End;
Output;
Run;
Proc Print data=RPW; Run;
%Mend RPW;
```
<<**SAS**<<

### Example 20.1    Randomized Play-the-Winner Design

Suppose we are designing an oncology clinical study with tumor response as the primary endpoint. The response rate is estimated to be 0.3 in the control group and 0.5 in the test group. The response rate is 0.4 in both groups under the null condition. We want to design the trial with about 80% power at a one-sided $\alpha$ of 0.025.

We first check the type-I error of a classical two-group design with n = 200 (100/group) using the following SAS macro calls.

>>**SAS**>>
```
%RPW(Zc=1.96, nSbjs=200, nAnlys=200, RR1=0.4, RR2=0.4, a0=1, b0=1,
a1=0, b1=0, nMin=1);
```
<<**SAS**<<

Note that a1 = b1 = 0 represents the classical design. To calculate the power, we run the following code.

>>**SAS**>>
```
%RPW(Zc=1.96, nSbjs=200, nAnlys=200, RR1=0.3, RR2=0.5, a0=1, b0=1,
a1=0, b1=0, nMin=1);
```
<<**SAS**<<

The simulations indicate the power (or type-I error) is 83%. To determine the reject region or the critical point $Z_c$ for a design with RPW(1,1,1,1), we first use $Z_c = 1.96$, the critical point for the classical design in the following SAS macro call:

>>**SAS**>>
%RPW(Zc=1.96, nSbjs=200, nAnlys=200, RR1=0.4, RR2=0.4, a0=1, b0=1, a1=1, b1=1, nMin=1);
<<**SAS**<<

The simulations indicate that the one-sided $\alpha = 0.055$, which is much larger than the target level 0.025. Therefore, using the SAS Macro 20.1 and trial-and-error method, we find that $Z_c = 2.7$ will give the power or $\alpha = 0.025$.

>>**SAS**>>
%RPW(Zc=2.7, nSbjs=200, nAnlys=200, RR1=0.4, RR2=0.4, a0=1, b0=1, a1=1, b1=1, nMin=1);
<<**SAS**<<

Note the previous results are based on full sequential design, i.e., randomization is modified when each response assessment becomes available (assume no delayed response). Practically it is much easier to carry out a group sequential trial. For example, the trial can have five analyses and the randomization is modified at each of the four interim analyses. The final analysis is used for testing the null hypothesis of no treatment effect. We use the following SAS statement to find out that $Z_c$ should be 2.05.

>>**SAS**>>
%RPW(Zc=2.05, nSbjs=200, nAnlys=5, RR1=0.4, RR2=0.4, a0=1, b0=1, a1=1, b1=1, nMin=1);
<<**SAS**<<

Using the following SAS statement, we obtained the power that is 79%, 4% less than the classical design with the same sample size.
>>**SAS**>>
%RPW(Zc=2.05, nSbjs=200, nAnlys=5, RR1=0.3, RR2=0.5, a0=1, b0=1,a1=1, b1=1, nMin=1);
<<**SAS**<<

The results from the above six different scenarios are summarized in Table 20.2.

Table 20.2:  Simulation Results from RPW

| Scenario | nSbjs | aveP1 | aveP2 | Zc | Power |
|---|---|---|---|---|---|
| 1 | 200 | 0.400 | 0.400 | 1.96 | 0.0258 |
| 2 | 200 | 0.300 | 0.500 | 1.96 | 0.8312 |
| 3 | 200 | 0.381 | 0.381 | 1.96 | 0.0553 |
| 4 | 200 | 0.381 | 0.381 | 2.70 | 0.0256 |
| 5 | 200 | 0.395 | 0.396 | 2.05 | 0.0252 |
| 6 | 200 | 0.292 | 0.498 | 2.05 | 0.7908 |

Note: 100,000 Simulation runs.

Similarly we can study the characteristics of different urns by setting the parameters, for example: a0 = 2, b0 = 2, a1 = 1, b1 = 1 for RPW (2,2,1,1). This is left this for readers to practice.

## 20.5   General Response-Adaptive Randomization

For other types of endpoints, we suggest the following allocation probability model:

$$\Pr(trt = i) = f(\hat{\mathbf{u}}),\qquad(20.14)$$

where $\Pr(trt = i)$ is the probability of allocating the patient to the $i$th group and the observed response vector $\hat{\mathbf{u}} = \{u_1, ..., u_M\}$.

We further suggest a specific function for $f$, i.e.,

$$\Pr(trt = i) \propto a_{0i} + b\,\hat{u}_i^m,\qquad(20.15)$$

where $\hat{u}_i$ = the observed proportion, mean, number of events, or categorical score, and $a_{0i}$ and $b$ are constants.

### 20.5.1   *SAS Macro for K-Arm RAR with Binary Endpoint*

The response-adaptive randomization (RAR) algorithm (20.15) has been implemented for the binary response in SAS Macro 20.2 below. The definitions of the SAS variables are defined as follows: **nPts** = the total number of patients, **AveN{i}** = the average number of patients in the $i$th arm, **AveU{i}** = the average response in the $i$th arm, **PowerMax** = the power for testing the response difference between the arm with maximum response and the first arm, **nSims** = number of simulation runs, **nArms** = number of treatment arms, **Zc** = critical point for rejecting the null hypothesis. **a0{i}**, **b** and **m** are the parameters in the model (20.15).

## >>SAS Macro 20.2: Binary Response-Adaptive Randomization>>

```
%Macro RARBin(nSims=1000, nPts=200, nArms=5, b=1, m=1, Zc=1.96);
Data RARBin; Set DataIn;
Keep nPts AveN1-AveN&nArms AveU1-AveU&nArms PowerMax;
Array Ns{&nArms}; Array uObs{&nArms}; Array rP{&nArms};
Array nRsps{&nArms}; Array a0{&nArms}; Array CrP{&nArms};
Array us{&nArms}; Array AveU{&nArms}; Array AveN{&nArms};
PowerMax=0; nArms=&nArms; nPts=&nPts;
Do i=1 To nArms; AveU{i}=0; AveN{i}=0; End;
Do isim=1 to &nSims;
Do i=1 To nArms; nRsps{i}=0; uObs{i}=0; Ns{i}=0; Crp{i}=0; End;
Do iSubject=1 to nPts;
Do i=1 To nArms; rP{i}=a0{i}+&b*uObs{i}**&m; End;
Suma=0; Do i=1 To nArms; Suma=Suma+rP{i}; End;
Do i=1 To nArms; rP{i}=rP{i}/Suma; End;
Do iArm=1 To nArms; CrP{iArm}=0;
Do i=1 To iArm; CrP{iArm}=CrP{iArm}+rP{i}; End;
End;
rn=ranuni(5236); cArm=1;
Do iArm=2 To nArms;
IF CrP{iArm-1}<rn<CrP{iArm} Then cArm=iArm;
End;
Ns(cArm)= Ns(cArm)+1;
* For Binary response;
If ranuni(8364)<us{cArm} Then nRsps{cArm}=nRsps{cArm}+1;
Do i=1 To nArms; uObs{i}=nRsps{i}/max(Ns{i},1); End;
End;
uMax=uObs{1};
Do i=1 to &nArms; If uObs{i}>=uMax Then iMax=i; End;
Se2=0;
Do i=1 to &nArms;
Se2=Se2+uObs{i}*(1-uObs{i})/max(Ns{i},1)*2/nArms;
End;
TSmax=(uObs{iMax}-
uObs{1})*(Ns(1)+Ns{iMax})/2/(nPts/nArms)/Se2**0.5;
If TSmax>&Zc then PowerMax=PowerMax+1/&nSims;
Do i=1 To nArms;
AveU{i}=AveU{i}+uObs{i}/&nSims;
```

```
AveN{i}=AveN{i}+Ns{i}/&nSims;
End;
End;
Output;
Run;
Proc Print Data=RARBin; Run;
%Mend RARBin;
```
<<**SAS**<<

Examples of RAR designs using SAS Macro 20.2 are presented as follows:

>>**SAS**>>
```
Title"Checking Alpha for 2-Group with Classical Design";
Data DataIn;
Array a0{2} (1,1); Array us{2} (0.2,0.2);
%RARBin(nSims=10000, nPts=160, nArms=2, b=0, m=1, Zc=1.96); Run;
Title "Checking Alpha for 2-Group RAR Design";
Data DataIn;
Array a0{2} (1,1); Array us{2} (0.2,0.2);
%RARBin(nSims=100000, nPts=160, nArms=2, b=1, m=1, Zc=2.0); Run;
Title "Power with 2-Group RAR Design";
Data DataIn;
Array a0{2} (1,1); Array us{2} (0.2,0.4);
%RARBin(nSims=100000, nPts=160, nArms=2, b=1, m=1, Zc=2.0); Run;
Title "Checking Alpha for 3-Group RAR Design";
Data DataIn;
Array a0{3} (1,1,1); Array us{3} (0.2,0.2,0.2);
%RARBin(nSims=100000, nPts=160, nArms=3, b=1, m=1, Zc=2.08); Run;
Title "Power with 3-Group RAR Design";
Data DataIn;
Array a0{3} (1,1,1); Array us{3} (0.2,0.3,0.5);
%RARBin(nSims=100000, nPts=160, nArms=3, b=1, m=1, Zc=2.08); Run;
```
<<**SAS**<<

## 20.5.2 *SAS Macro for K-Arm RAR with Normal Endpoint*

Algorithm (20.15) has also been implemented for normal response in SAS Macro 20.3.

## >>SAS Macro 20.3:  Normal Response-Adaptive Randomization>>

```
%Macro   RARNor(nSims=100000,   nPts=100,   nArms=5,   b=1,   m=1,
CrtMax=1.96);
Data RARNor; Set DataIn;
Keep nPts AveN1-AveN&nArms AveU1-AveU&nArms PowerMax;
Array Ns{&nArms}; Array AveN{&nArms}; Array uObs{&nArms};
Array rP{&nArms}; Array AveU{&nArms}; Array cuObs{&nArms};
Array a0{&nArms}; Array CrP{&nArms};
Array us{&nArms}; Array s{&nArms};
PowerMax=0; nArms=&nArms; nPts=&nPts;
Do i=1 To nArms; AveU{i}=0; AveN{i}=0; End;
Do isim=1 to &nSims;
Do i=1 To nArms; cuObs{i}=0; uObs{i}=0; Ns{i}=0; Crp{i}=0; End;
Do iSubject=1 to nPts;
Do i=1 To nArms; rP{i}=a0{i}+&b*uObs{i}**&m; End;
Suma=0; Do i=1 To nArms; Suma=Suma+rP{i}; End;
Do i=1 To nArms; rP{i}=rP{i}/Suma; End;
Do iArm=1 To nArms; CrP{iArm}=0;
Do i=1 To iArm; CrP{iArm}=CrP{iArm}+rP{i}; End;
End;
rn=ranuni(5361); cArm=1;
Do iArm=2 To nArms;
IF CrP{iArm-1}<rn<CrP{iArm} Then cArm=iArm;
End;
Ns(cArm)= Ns(cArm)+1;
* For normal response;
u=Rannor(361)*s{cArm}+us{cArm};
cuObs{cArm}=cuObs{cArm}+u;
Do i=1 To nArms; uObs{i}=cuObs{i}/max(Ns{i},1); End;
End;
se2=0;
 * Assume sigma unknown for simplicity;
Do i=1 To nArms; se2=se2+s{i}**2/max(Ns{i},1)*2/nArms; End;
uMax=uObs{1};
Do i=1 To &nArms; If uObs{i}>=uMax Then iMax=i; End;
TSmax=(uObs{iMax}-
uObs{1})*(Ns(1)+Ns{iMax})/2/(nPts/nArms)/se2**0.5;
If TSmax>&CrtMax then PowerMax=PowerMax+1/&nSims;
```

```
Do i=1 To nArms;
AveU{i}=AveU{i}+uObs{i}/&nSims;
AveN{i}=AveN{i}+Ns{i}/&nSims;
End;
End;
Output;
Run;
Proc Print data=RARNor; Run;
%Mend RARNor;
```
<<**SAS**<<

## Example 20.2    Adaptive Randomization with Normal Endpoint

The objective of this trial in asthma patients is to confirm sustained treatment effect, measured as FEV1 change from baseline to 1-year of treatment. Initially, patients are equally randomized to four doses of the new compound and a placebo. Based on early studies, the estimated FEV1 changes at week 4 are 6%, 12%, 13%, 14%, and 15% (with pooled standard deviation 18%) for the placebo, dose level 1, 2, 3, and 4, respectively.

Using the following SAS macro calls, we can determine that the rejection region is $(2.01, +\infty)$ for 375 subjects and $(1.995, +\infty)$ for 285 subjects. The power is 84% with a total of 375 subjects and 73% with 285 subjects, while the pick-the-winner design in Chapter 15 provides 85% with total sample size 289.

>>**SAS**>>
```
Data DataIn;
Array a0{5} (1, 1, 1, 1, 1); Array us{5} (0.06, 0.06, 0.06, 0.06, 0.06);
Array s{5} (.18, .18, .18, .18, .18);
%RARNor(nPts=375, nArms=5, b=1, m=1, CrtMax=2.01);

Data DataIn;
Array a0{5} (1, 1, 1, 1, 1); Array us{5} (0.06, 0.12, 0.13, 0.14, 0.15);
Array s{5} (.18, .18, .18, .18, .18);
%RARNor(nPts=375, nArms=5, b=1, m=1, CrtMax=2.01);
```
<<**SAS**<<

>>**SAS**>>
```
Data DataIn;
Array a0{5} (1, 1, 1, 1, 1); Array us{5} (0.06, 0.06, 0.06, 0.06, 0.06);
Array s{5} (.18, .18, .18, .18, .18);
%RARNor(nPts=285, nArms=5, b=1, m=1, CrtMax=1.995);
```

Data DataIn;
Array a0{5} (1, 1, 1, 1, 1); Array us{5} (0.06, 0.12, 0.13, 0.14, 0.15);
Array s{5} (.18, .18, .18, .18, .18);
%RARNor(nPts=285, nArms=5, b=1, m=1, CrtMax=1.995);
<<**SAS**<<


### 20.5.3 *RAR for General Adaptive Designs*

Many adaptive designs can be viewed as response-adaptive randomization designs. We are going to illustrate this with the classical group sequential design and the drop-arm design.

For a two-arm group sequential design, the treatment allocation probability to the $i$th arm at the $k$th stage is given by

$$\Pr(trt = i; k) = \frac{H(p_k - \alpha_k) + H(\beta_k - p_k)}{2} - \frac{1}{2}, \tag{20.16}$$

where $i = 1, 2$, and $\alpha_k$ and $\beta_k$ are the stopping boundaries at the $k$th stage, and the step-function is defined as

$$H(x) = \begin{cases} 1, & \text{if } x > 0 \\ 0 & \text{if } x \leq 0 \end{cases}. \tag{20.17}$$

From (20.16), we can see that if $p_k \leq \alpha_k$ (or $p_k \geq \beta_k$), the allocation probability $\Pr(trt = i; k)$ is zero, meaning the trial will stop for efficacy (or futility). If $\alpha_k < p_k < \beta_k$, the allocation probability $\Pr(trt = i; k)$ is 1/2, meaning the patients will be assigned to the two treatment groups with an equal probability. For drop-loser designs, if the dropping-criterion is based on the maximum difference among the observed treatment $\hat{u}_{\max} - \hat{u}_{\min}$ at the interim analysis, then the treatment allocation probability to the $i$th arm at interim analysis is given by

$$\Pr(trt = i) = \frac{H(\hat{u}_i - \hat{u}_{\max} + \delta_{NI})}{\sum_{i=1}^{M} H(\hat{u}_i - \hat{u}_{\max} + \delta_{NI})}, \tag{20.18}$$

where $\hat{u}_i$ is the observed response in the $i$th arm, and $\delta_{NI}$ is the noninferiority margin. $M =$ the total number of arms in the study.


## 20.6 Sequential Parallel Comparison Design

The problem of high placebo responses such as in psychiatry trials leads to difficulties in estimation of the true effect size and ultimately may prevent effective compounds from entering the market or existing drugs from new applications (Doros et al., 2013; Fava et al., 2003). A commonly used classical approach to reduce the placebo effect is the so-called *placebo lead-in* trial design. In this setting, the actual trial is preceded by a phase where all recruited subjects are given the placebo, typically in a single-blinded fashion. After the lead-in periord (phase I), only placebo nonresponders are then randomized and followed up in the second phase of the trial. However, studies have shown that proportions of placebo responders do not differ between studies that do and do not include a placebo lead-in phase (Fava et al., 2003, Walsh et al., 2002). As pointed out by Doros et al., this can be attributed to several aspects of the placebo lead-in design. One of them includes the bias among clinicians who usually have to be unblinded to the fact that patients are on placebo in the initial phase and set low expectations for improvement in this stage. Another drawback of this design relates to the efficiency of the trial that suffers with respect to resources and time of the investigators and subjects. To address this issue, Fava et al. (2003) proposed so-called sequential parallel comparison design (SPCD), in which subjects would be randomized to one of three groups: active drug in both phase I and phase II (DD), placebo in phase I and active drug in phase II (PD), and placebo in both phase I and phase II (PP). Subject allocation to the three groups would be set before the trial, and their sizes would depend on the expected placebo response. The higher the expected placebo response rate, the more subjects would be allocated to the PP and PD arms. A more often used form of SPCD trials has two-phase randomization (Doros et al., 2013, Fava et al., 2003, Walsh et al., 2002), in which, at the beginning of the trial, subjects are randomized to two groups (active drug and placebo, typically with more subjects allocated to placebo than drug). Then, upon the completion of phase I and assessment of actual response to placebo, a second randomization is conducted of placebo nonresponders. This format of SPCD is also called SPD-ReR (rerandomization; Figure 20.2).

The original use of SPCD focused on binary outcomes and the treatment effect is defined as a weighted average of the treatment effects in the two phases, that is, the weighted average of the differences between the rates of responders at the end of phase I and phase II among those on treatment versus those on placebo. Only placebo nonresponders from phase I are taken into account for the estimation of phase-II treatment effect. Chen et al. (2010) and Doros et al. (2013) proposed two different methods of analyzing continuous outcomes in SPCD trials based on ordinary least squares.

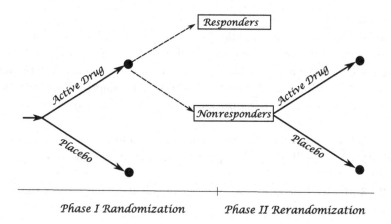

Figure 20.2:   Sequential Parallel Design with Rerandomization

## 20.7   Summary and Discussion

Response-adaptive randomization (RAR) was initially proposed to reduce the number of failures in a trial; however, the overall gain is sometimes limited in two-group design because (1) power is lost as compared to the uniformly most powerful design, and (2) the reduction in number of failures can diminish due to significantly delayed responses. RAR may (although it is unlikely) delay patient enrollment because of the fact that patients enrolled later will have a better chance of being assigned to a better treatment group. If there is heterogeneity in patient enrollment over time (e.g., sicker patients tend to enroll earlier because they cannot wait for long), a bias will be introduced.

RAR may be useful in phase-II/III combination studies, where at the early stages, RAR is used to seamlessly select superior arms. In practice, group (rather than full) sequential response-randomization may be used, where the response data will be unblinded at several prescheduled times. SPCD is a special response-adaptive design, which has practical applications, such as in psychiatry trials.

## Problems

**20.1** Explain the main difference between traditional randomization methods and adaptive randomization. Describe the following randomization methods and when each method should be used: (1) complete randomization, (2) restricted randomization, (3) response-adaptive randomization, (4) covariate-adaptive randomization, and (5) covariate-adjusted response-adaptive randomization.

**20.2** Use simulation to study how the parameters $a_0$, $b_0$, $a_1$, and $b_1$ (Section 20.3.2) will affect the operating characteristics of RPW randomization.

**20.3** Modify Macro 20.3 so that it can calculate and output the mean response per person per trial.

# Chapter 21

# Introductory Bayesian Approach in Clinical Trial

## 21.1 Introduction

The use of adaptive trial designs could greatly improve the efficiency of drug development; the incorporation of the Bayesian approach is one more step further to this direction. Bayesian approaches provide a powerful tool for streamlining sequential learning processes, predicting future results, and synthesizing evidences across different resources. The resulting outcomes using Bayesian approaches are easier to interpret and more informative for decision making.

The Bayesian approach has been widely studied recently in drug development in areas such as clinical trial design (Spiegelhalter, Abrams, and Myles, 2004), pharmacovigilance. (Hauben et al., 2005; Hauben and Reich, 2004), and pharmacoeconomics (Ades, Sculpher, and Sutton, 2006; Iglesias and Claxton, 2006). Goodman (2005), Louis (2005) and Berry (2005) give excellent introductions to using Bayesian methods in clinical trials and discuss relevant issues.

The Bayesian approach can be used to determine the best strategy available at the time. It can be used to monitor trials, predict outcomes, anticipate problems, and suggest early remedies.

In this chapter, a comparative study of frequentist and Bayesian approaches is pursued to objectively evaluate the two different approaches. The differences are identified in various aspects such as learning mechanism, trial design, monitoring, data analysis, and result interpretation. The regulatory aspects of Bayesian approaches are reviewed, challenges in using Bayesian designs are addressed, and steps for planning a Bayesian trial are outlined.

## 21.2    Bayesian Learning Mechanism

We acquire knowledge through a sequence of learning processes. We form a perception about a certain thing based on prior experiences, i.e., prior knowledge. This knowledge is updated when new facts are observed. This learning mechanism is the central idea of the Bayesian approach. Bayes' theorem, the foundation of the Bayesian approach, can be expressed as: Posterior distribution = C(Likelihood • Prior distribution), where C is a normalization constant that can be calculated. The posterior distribution that is used to make inferences about the treatment effect is a combination of evidences from both prior (or historical information sources) and current trials. Note that prior refers to the knowledge before the current trial and posterior distribution is the knowledge after the current trial.

Bayes' rule reveals the important relationships among prior knowledge, new evidence, and updated knowledge (posterior probability). It reflects the human learning process. Whether you are a statistician, a physician, or a regulatory agent, you are using the Bayesian approach constantly, formally or informally, consciously or unconsciously.

The differences between the frequentist and Bayesian approaches are reflected in the learning process. Both frequentist and Bayesian approaches use prior probabilities, but in quite different ways. The frequentist approach uses prior information segmentally, while the Bayesian approach uses the prior rigorously and intelligently. The frequentist approach considers a population parameter to be a fixed number; the Bayesian approach views the population parameter as a random variable with a probability distribution, which can be updated as more information is accumulated. The Bayesian approach can be used to gain knowledge about treatment effect over time; this is illustrated in Figure 21.1. We can see that the uncertainty about the treatment effect is reduced over time.

Drug development is a process that switches between statistics and probability. Statistics is the study of (drawing a conclusion about) population characteristics based on the observed sample; probability is the study of the sample properties based on the characteristics of the population. For example, to design a phase-II trial, we estimate the treatment effect from prior information and use that to calculate the sample size and the probability of success (power); at the end of the trial, we estimate the treatment effect again based on the phase-II trial results, then use that to design the next trial (phase III) and predict power. At the end of the phase-III trial, we estimate the treatment effect again. However, the frequentist and Bayesian approaches make the inference and calculate probability

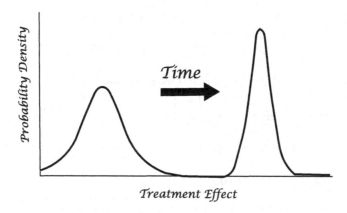

Figure 21.1:   Bayesian Learning Process

differently. The frequentist approach assumes a single known treatment effect at each phase in drug development and calculates sample size based on that single number; the Bayesian approach, on the other hand, realistically uses the posterior distribution of the treatment effect at the end of each phase for sample-size calculation for the next phase. The Bayesian approach also allows for knowledge to be updated when new information becomes available and uses it during the drug development process.

## 21.3   Bayesian Basics

### 21.3.1   *Bayes' Rule*

Denote prior distribution $\pi(\theta)$ and the sample distribution $f(x|\theta)$. The following are four basic Bayesian elements:

(a) The joint distribution of $(\theta, x)$ given by

$$\varphi(\theta, x) = f(x|\theta)\pi(\theta),\qquad(21.1)$$

(b) The marginal distribution of x given by

$$m(x) = \int \varphi(\theta, x)\, d\theta = \int f(x|\theta)\pi(\theta)\, d\theta,\qquad(21.2)$$

(c) The posterior distribution of $\theta$ given by Bayes' formula

$$\pi(\theta|x) = \frac{f(x|\theta)\pi(\theta)}{m(x)},\text{ and}\qquad(21.3)$$

(d) The predictive probability distribution given by

$$P(y|x) = \int P(x|y,\theta)\,\pi(\theta|x)\,d\theta. \tag{21.4}$$

### Example 21.1   Beta Posterior Distribution

Assume that $X \sim Bin(n,p)$ and $p \sim Beta(\alpha,\beta)$.
The sample distribution is given by

$$f(x|p) = \binom{n}{x}p^x(1-p)^{n-x}, \quad x = 0,1,...,n. \tag{21.5}$$

The prior about the parameter $p$ is given by

$$\pi(p) = \frac{1}{B(\alpha,\beta)}p^{\alpha-1}(1-p)^{\beta-1}, \quad 0 \le p \le 1, \tag{21.6}$$

where beta function $B(\alpha,\beta) = \frac{\Gamma(\alpha)\Gamma(\beta)}{\Gamma(\alpha+\beta)}$.
The joint distribution then is given by

$$\varphi(p,x) = \frac{\binom{n}{x}}{B(\alpha,\beta)}p^{\alpha+x-1}(1-p)^{n-x+\beta-1}, \tag{21.7}$$

and the marginal distribution is

$$m(x) = \frac{\binom{n}{x}}{B(\alpha,\beta)}B(\alpha+x,n-x+\beta). \tag{21.8}$$

Therefore, the posterior distribution is given by

$$\pi(p|x) = \frac{p^{\alpha+x-1}(1-p)^{n-x+\beta-1}}{B(\alpha+x,\beta+n-x)} = Beta(\alpha+x,\beta+n-x). \tag{21.9}$$

### Example 21.2   Normal Posterior Distribution

Assume that $X \sim N(\theta,\sigma^2/n)$ and $\theta \sim N(\mu,\sigma^2/n_0)$. The posterior distribution can be written as

$$\pi(\theta|X) \propto f(X|\theta)\,\pi(\theta) \tag{21.10}$$

or

$$\pi(\theta|X) = Ce^{-\frac{(X-\theta)^2 n}{2\sigma^2}}e^{-\frac{(\theta-\mu)^2 n_0}{2\sigma^2}}, \tag{21.11}$$

where $C$ is a constant.

We immediately recognize that (21.11) is the normal distribution of $N\left(\frac{n_0\mu+nX}{n_0+n},\frac{\sigma^2}{n_0+n}\right)$.

We now wish to make predictions concerning future values of $X$, taking into account our uncertainty about its mean $\theta$. We may write $X = (X-\theta)+$

$\theta$, and so can consider $X$ as being the sum of two independent quantities: $(X - \theta) \sim N\left(0, \sigma^2/n\right)$ and $\theta \sim N\left(\mu, \sigma^2/n_0\right)$. The predictive probability distribution is given by (Spiegelhalter et al., 2004),

$$X \sim N\left(\mu, \sigma^2 \left(\frac{1}{n} + \frac{1}{n_0}\right)\right). \tag{21.12}$$

If we have already observed $x_{n_1}$, the mean of the first $n_1$ observations, the predictive distribution is given by

$$X|x_{n_1} \sim N\left(\frac{n_0\mu + n_1 x_{n_1}}{n_0 + n_1}, \sigma^2 \left(\frac{1}{n_0 + n_1} + \frac{1}{n}\right)\right). \tag{21.13}$$

### 21.3.2 *Conjugate Family of Distributions*

A family $F$ of probability distribution on $\Theta$ is said to be conjugate (or closed under sampling) if, for every $\pi \in F$, the posterior distribution $\pi(\theta|x)$ also belongs to $F$.

The main interest of conjugacy becomes more apparent when $F$ is as small as possible and parameterized. When $F$ is parameterized, switching from prior to posterior distribution is reduced to an updating of the corresponding parameters. This is a main reason conjugate priors are so popular, as the posterior distributions are always computable, at least to a certain extent.

The conjugate prior approach, which originated in Raiffa and Schlaifer (1961), can be partially justified through an invariance reasoning. Updating the model should not be radical, e.g., only the values of the parameters not the model or function itself are updated. Commonly used conjugate families are presented in Table 21.1.

For conjugate family distributions, the estimations can easily be obtained and are summarized in Table 21.2.

Table 21.1: Commonly Used Conjugate Families

| Model $f(x|\theta)$ | Prior $\pi(\theta)$ | Posterior $\pi(\theta|x)$ |
|---|---|---|
| Normal $N(\theta, \sigma^2)$ | $N(\mu, \tau^2)$ | $N\left(\frac{\sigma^2\mu + \tau^2 x}{\sigma^2 + \tau^2}, \frac{\sigma^2\tau^2}{\sigma^2 + \tau^2},\right)$ |
| Poisson $P(\theta)$ | $G(\alpha, \beta)$ | $G(\alpha + x, \beta + 1)$ |
| Gamma $G(\nu, \theta)$ | $G(\alpha, \beta)$ | $G(\alpha + \nu, \beta + x)$ |
| Binomial $Bin(n, \theta)$ | $Beta(\alpha, \beta)$ | $Beta(\alpha + x, \beta + n - x)$ |
| Neg. Bin $NB(m, \theta)$ | $Beta(\alpha, \beta)$ | $Beta(\alpha + m, \beta + x)$ |

Table 21.2:   Estimation of Conjugate Families

| Distribution | Conjugate distribution | Posterior expectation |
|---|---|---|
| Normal $N\left(\theta,\sigma^{2}\right)$ | $N\left(\mu,\tau^{2}\right)$ | $\frac{\mu\sigma^{2}+\tau^{2}x}{\sigma^{2}+\tau^{2}}$ |
| Poisson $P\left(\theta\right)$ | $G\left(\alpha,\beta\right)$ | $\frac{\alpha+x}{\beta+1}$ |
| Gamma $G\left(\nu,\theta\right)$ | $G\left(\alpha,\beta\right)$ | $\frac{\alpha+\nu}{\beta+x}$ |
| Binomial $Bin\left(n,\theta\right)$ | $Beta\left(\alpha,\beta\right)$ | $\frac{\alpha+x}{\alpha+\beta+n}$ |
| Neg. Bin $NB\left(m,\theta\right)$ | $Beta\left(\alpha,\beta\right)$ | $\frac{\alpha+n}{\alpha+\beta+x+n}$ |

## 21.4   Trial Design

### 21.4.1   *Bayesian for Classical Design*

We are going to use an example to illustrate some differences between Bayesian and frequentist approaches in trial design.

**Example 21.3   Prior Effect on Power**

Consider a two-arm parallel design comparing a test treatment with a control. Suppose that, based on published data from 3 clinical trials of similar size, the prior probabilities for effect size are 0.1, 0.25, and 0.4 with 1/3 probability for each.

For the 2-arm trial, the power is a function of effect size of $\varepsilon$, i.e,

$$\text{power}\left(\varepsilon\right)=\Phi\left(\frac{\sqrt{n}\varepsilon}{2}-z_{1-\alpha}\right),\qquad(21.14)$$

where $\Phi$ is cdf of the standard normal distribution.

Considering the uncertainty of $\varepsilon$, i.e., prior $\pi\left(\varepsilon\right)$, the expected power

$$\text{P}_{\exp}=\int\Phi\left(\frac{\sqrt{n}\varepsilon}{2}-z_{1-\alpha}\right)\pi\left(\varepsilon\right)d\varepsilon.\qquad(21.15)$$

A numerical integration is usually required for evaluation (21.15).

To illustrate the implication of (21.15), let's assume one-sided $\alpha=0.025$, $z_{1-\alpha}=1.96$, the prior

$$\pi\left(\varepsilon\right)=\left\{\begin{array}{ll}1/3, & \varepsilon=0.1,0.25,0.4\\0, & \text{otherwise.}\end{array}\right.$$

Conventionally we use the mean (median) of the effect size $\bar{\varepsilon}=0.25$ to design the trial and calculate the sample size. For the two-arm balanced design with $\beta=0.2$ or *power* $=80\%$, using the classical approach, the total sample is given by

$$n = \frac{4(z_{1-a} + z_{1-\beta})^2}{\varepsilon^2} = \frac{4(1.96 + 0.842)^2}{0.25^2} = 502.$$

However, if the Bayesian approach is used, the expected power from (21.15) is

$$
\begin{aligned}
&P_{exp}\\
&= \frac{1}{3}\left[\Phi\left(\frac{0.1\sqrt{n}}{2} - z_{1-\alpha}\right) + \Phi\left(\frac{0.25\sqrt{n}}{2} - z_{1-\alpha}\right) + \Phi\left(\frac{0.4\sqrt{n}}{2} - z_{1-\alpha}\right)\right]\\
&= \frac{1}{3}\left[\Phi\left(-0.83973\right) + \Phi\left(0.84067\right) + \Phi\left(2.5211\right)\right]\\
&= \frac{1}{3}\left(0.2005 + 0.7997 + 0.9942\right) = 0.6648 = 66\%.
\end{aligned}
$$

We can see that the expected power is only 66%; therefore, we should increase sample size.

With the Bayesian approach that considers the uncertainty of the effect size, the expected power with a sample-size of 252 is the average of the three powers calculated using the 3 different effect sizes (0.1, 0.25, and 0.4), which turns out to be 66%, much lower than 80% as the frequentist approach claimed. Therefore, to reach the desired power, it is necessary to increase the sample size.

This is an example of a Bayesian–frequentist hybrid approach, i.e., the Bayesian approach is used for the trial design to increase the probability of success given the final statistical criterion of $p$-value $\leq \alpha = 0.025$.

### Example 21.4  Power with Normal Prior

If the prior $\pi(\varepsilon) = N(\mu, \sigma^2/n_0)$, then the expected power can be obtained using the predictive distribution (21.12) and evaluating the chance of the critical event $(X > \frac{1}{\sqrt{n}}z_{1-\alpha}\sigma)$ occurring, which is given by

$$P_{exp} = \Phi\left(\sqrt{\frac{n_0}{n_0 + n}}\left(\frac{\mu\sqrt{n}}{\sigma} - z_{1-\alpha}\right)\right). \tag{21.16}$$

Now let's look at the expected total example size. The total sample size is a function of the effect size $\varepsilon$, i.e.,

$$n(\varepsilon) = \frac{4(z_{1-a} + z_{1-\beta})^2}{\varepsilon^2}. \tag{21.17}$$

Adaptive Design Theory and Implementation

Therefore, the expected total sample size is given by

$$n_{\exp} = \int \frac{4(z_{1-a} + z_{1-\beta})^2}{\varepsilon^2} \pi(\varepsilon)\, d\varepsilon. \qquad (21.18)$$

For flat prior $\pi(\varepsilon) \sim \frac{1}{b-a}, [a \leq \varepsilon \leq b]$,

$$n_{\exp} = \int_a^b \frac{4(z_{1-a} + z_{1-\beta})^2}{\varepsilon^2} \frac{1}{b-a} d\varepsilon$$

$$= \frac{4}{ab}(z_{1-a} + z_{1-\beta})^2. \qquad (21.19)$$

The sample-size ratio $R_n = \frac{n_{\exp}}{n} = \frac{\varepsilon^2}{ab}$. For example $\varepsilon = 0.25, \alpha = 0.025, \beta = 0.8, n = 502, a = 0.1, b = 0.4$ (note that $(a+b)/2 = \varepsilon$), $R_n = \frac{0.25^2}{(0.1)(0.4)} = 1.56$. It indicates again that the frequentist approach could substantially underestimate the sample size required for achieving the target power.

### 21.4.2  Bayesian Power

We want to test the null hypothesis $\theta \leq 0$ against an alternative hypothesis $\theta > 0$. Bayesian significance is defined as $P^B = P(\theta < 0|data) < \alpha_B$. Using the posterior distribution, the Bayesian significance can be easily found.

**Example 21.5   Bayesian Power**

For normal distribution prior and data, the posterior distribution is given by

$$\pi(\theta|x) = N\left(\frac{n_0\mu_0 + n\bar{x}}{n_0 + n}, \frac{\sigma^2}{n_0 + n}\right). \qquad (21.20)$$

Bayesian significance is claimed if the parameter estimate $\bar{x}$ satisfies

$$\bar{x} > \frac{\sqrt{n_0 + n} z_{1-\alpha_B}\sigma - n_0\mu_0}{n}, \qquad (21.21)$$

$$\frac{\sqrt{n_0 + n} z_{1-\alpha_B}\sigma - n_0\mu_0}{n} \frac{\sqrt{n}}{\sigma} + \mu.$$

Therefore, the Bayesian power is given by

$$P_B(n) = 1 - \Phi\left(z_{1-\alpha_B}\sqrt{\frac{n_0}{n} + 1} - n_0\sqrt{n}\frac{\mu_0}{\sigma} + \mu\right), \qquad (21.22)$$

where $\mu$ is the true mean for the population.

## Example 21.6 Trial Design Using Bayesian Power

Suppose in a phase-II two-arm hypotension study with the SBP reduction as the primary endpoint, the estimated treatment effect is normal distribution, i.e., $\theta \sim N\left(\mu, \frac{2\sigma^2}{n_0}\right)$. The trial is designed with a Bayesian power of $(1 - \beta_B)$ at the Bayesian significance level $\alpha_B = 0.2$. For the sample size, the sample mean difference can be expressed as $\hat{\theta} \sim N\left(\theta, \frac{2\sigma^2}{n}\right)$, where $n$ = sample size per group. For a large sample size, we can assume that $\hat{\sigma}$ is constant. Therefore, the sample size $n$ is the solution for the following

$$1 - \Phi\left(z_{1-\alpha_B}\sqrt{\frac{n_0}{n} + 1} - n_0\sqrt{n}\frac{\mu_0}{\sigma} + \mu\right) = 1 - \beta_B. \tag{21.23}$$

That is,

$$z_{1-\alpha_B}\sqrt{\frac{n_0}{n} + 1} - n_0\sqrt{n}\frac{\mu_0}{\sigma} + \mu = z_{\beta_B}. \tag{21.24}$$

Equation (21.24) can be solved numerically for sample size $n$.

### 21.4.3 Frequentist Optimization

#### Simon's Two-Stage Design

Simon's two-stage optimal design (Simon, 1989) is a commonly used design for single-arm oncology trials. The hypothesis testing can be stated as

$$H_0 : R < R_1 \text{ vs. } H_a : R \geq R_2,$$

where $R$ is response rate.

The trial has one interim analysis (IA). At IA, if the observed $\hat{R} < R_0$ or the number of responses is less than a constant $n_{1c}$, then stop the trial for futility. Otherwise trial continues. At the final analysis, if the total number of responses is larger than or equal to $n_c$, then reject $H_0$. Otherwise, accept $H_0$. For a given $\alpha$ and power, different values of $n_{1c}$ and $n_c$ will lead to different maximum sample size and expected sample sizes under $H_0$ and $H_a$. The optimal design minimizes the expected sample size under $H_0$ and the MinMax design minimizes the maximum sample size.

SAS Macro 21.1 below can be used for a single-arm two-stage design with interim futility stopping. For a given constant $n$, the macro will search the best set of designs with sample size ranging from $0.7n$ to $1.5n$. The SAS variables are defined as follows: **Alpha0** = target one-sided significance level, **Alpha** = actual one-sided alpha, **po** and **pa** = response rates under $H_0$ and $H_a$, respectively, **n** = sample size group, **n1** = sample size at interim analysis for early futility stopping, **n1c** = critical value for futility: If the number of responses at the first stage is less than **n1c**, stop for futility; otherwise, continue to the second stage. If the total number of responses from the two stages >= **nc**, claim efficacy. **PrEFSHo** and **PrEFSHa** are the probabilities of early stopping under $H_0$ and $H_a$, respectively. **ExpNo** and **ExpNa** are the expected sample sizes under $H_0$ and $H_a$, respectively.

>>SAS Macro 21.1:   Simon Two-Stage Futility Design>>

```
%Macro TwoStageDesign(n=50, po=0.15, pa=0.3, n1=20, n1c=2, alpha0=0.1);
Data TwoStageBin;
retain alpha power;
drop i p1o p2o p1a p2a n2;
n1=&n1; n1c=&n1c; po=&po; pa=&pa; * Remove "&".;
do n=round(0.7*&n) to round(1.5*&n);
n2=n-&n1;
do nc=n1c to n;
alpha=0;
power=0;
do i=max(n1c,nc-n2) to n1;
p1o=ProbBnml(po, n1,i)-ProbBnml(po, n1,i-1);
p2o=1;
if nc-i>0 then p2o=1-ProbBnml(po, n2,nc-i-1);
alpha=alpha+p1o*p2o;
p1a=ProbBnml(pa, n1,i)-ProbBnml(pa, n1,i-1);
p2a=1;
if nc-i>0 then p2a=1-ProbBnml(pa, n2,nc-i-1);
power=power+p1a*p2a;
end;
if alpha>0.8*&alpha0 && alpha<1.2*&alpha0 then do;
PrEFSHo=ProbBnml(po, n1,n1c-1);
ExpNo=PrEFSHo*n1+(1-PrEFSHo)*n;
PrEFSHa=ProbBnml(pa, n1,n1c-1);
ExpNa=PrEFSHa*n1+(1-PrEFSHa)*n;
output;
end; end; end;
run;
proc print; run;
run;
```

%Mend TwoStageDesign;
**<<SAS<<**

## Example 21.7   Simon Two-Stage Optimal Design

Suppose we design a single-arm, phase-II oncology trial using Simon's two-stage optimal design. The response rates are assumed 0.05 and 0.25 under the null hypothesis and the alternative hypothesis, respectively. For one-sided $\alpha = 0.05$ and power = 80%, the sample size at stage 1 is $n_1 = 9$. The cumulative sample size at stage 2 is $n = 17$. The actual overall $\alpha = 0.047$, the actual power = 0.812. The stopping rules are specified as follows: At stage 1, stop and accept the null hypothesis if the response rate is less than $1/9$. Otherwise, continue to stage 2. The probability of stopping for futility is 0.63 when $H_0$ is true and 0.075 when $H_a$ is true. At stage 2, accept the null hypothesis if the response rate is less than or equal to $2/17$. Otherwise, reject the null hypothesis.

The results can be generated using ExpDesign Studio®, or the following SAS macro call.

**>>SAS>>**
%TwoStageDesign(n=17, po=0.05, pa=0.25, n1=9, n1c=1, alpha0=0.05);
**<<SAS<<**

### 21.4.4   *Bayesian Optimal Adaptive Designs*

Bayesian decision theory can be used to optimize trial designs. The Bayesian approach is decision oriented. A Bayesian views statistical inference as a problem in belief dynamics, or as use of evidence about a phenomenon to revise our knowledge about it. In distinguishing from a frequentist, for a Bayesian, statistical inference cannot be treated entirely independently of the context of the decisions that will be made on the basis of the inferences.

There are many different scenarios of reality with associated probabilities (prior distribution) and many possible adaptive designs with associated probabilistic outcomes (good and bad). Evaluation criterion can be the utility index that can be the aggregation of overall patients' health outcomes. Bayesian optimal design is to achieve the maximum expected utility under financial, time, and other constraints. We will use two-arm designs to illustrate the approach. The three designs we are going to compare are a classical approach with a two-arm phase-II trial followed by a two-arm phase-III trial, and two different group sequential designs (seamless designs).

For each design, the utility is calculated and weighted by its prior probability to obtain the expected utility for the design. The optimal design is the one with maximum expected utility.

**Example 21.8  Bayesian Optimal Design**

Suppose prior knowledge about treatment effect is determined as shown in Table 21.3. We are going to compare the classical design and Bayesian adaptive designs.

Table 21.3:  Prior Knowledge

| Scenario | Effect size | Prior prob. |
|----------|-------------|-------------|
| 1 | 0 | 0.2 |
| 2 | 0.1 | 0.2 |
| 3 | 0.2 | 0.6 |

**The Classical Design:** Assume there is no dose-selection issue. For classical design, we use a phase-II and a phase-III trial (assume that just one phase-III trial is required for approval). For the phase-II trial, we assume $\delta = 0.2$, one-sided $\alpha = 0.1$ and power = 0.8; the total sample-size required is $n_1 = 450$. For the phase-III trial, we assume $\delta = 0.14$ (calculated by $0.2(0) + 0.2(0.1) + 0.6(0.2)$ from Table 21.3), one-sided $\alpha = 0.025$, power = 0.9, the total sample size required is $n = 2144$. If the phase-II does not show statistical significance, we will not conduct the phase-III trial (in practice, this rule is not always followed). The probability of continuing the trial at phase-II is the weighted continual probability in Table 21.4, i.e.,

$$P_c = \Sigma_{i=1}^3 P_c(i)\,\pi(i) = 0.2\,(0.1) + 0.2\,(0.4) + 0.6\,(0.8) = 0.58.$$

Therefore, the expected sample size for phase-II and III trials together is

$$\bar{N} = n_1 + P_c n = 450 + 0.58\,(2144) = 1694.$$

Table 21.4:  Characteristics of Classical Phase II and III Designs

| Scenario, $i$ | Effect size | Prior prob. $\pi$ | Prob. of continue to Phase III, $P_c$ | Phase III Power, $P_3$ |
|---------------|-------------|-------------------|---------------------------------------|------------------------|
| 1 | 0 | 0.2 | 0.1 | 0.025 |
| 2 | 0.1 | 0.2 | 0.4 | 0.639 |
| 3 | 0.2 | 0.6 | 0.8 | 0.996 |

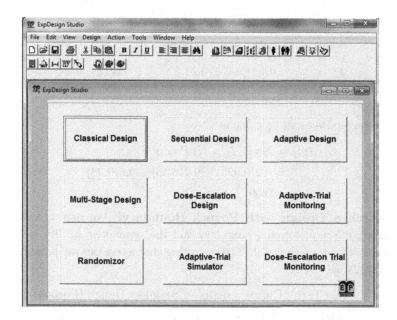

Figure 21.2: ExpDesign Studio for Classical and Adaptive Designs

The expected overall power is given by

$$\bar{P} = \Sigma_{i=1}^{3} P_c(i)\,\pi(i)\,P_3(i)$$
$$= (0.2)(0.1)(0.025) + (0.2)(0.4)(0.639) + (0.6)(0.8)(0.996)$$
$$= 0.53.$$

In conclusion, the classical phase-II trial followed by a phase-III trial has overall power = 53% with expected grand combined sample = 1694.

**Seamless Design with OF Boundary:** Use one-sided $\alpha = 0.025$, power =0.90, with O'Brien–Fleming (OF) efficacy stopping boundary and symmetrical futility stopping boundary. One interim analysis will be conducted when 50% patients are enrolled. We can use the ExpDesign Studio® (Figure 21.2) or SAS Macro 6.1 to simulate the trial. The operating characteristics of the design are summarized in Table 21.5.

Average example size can be calculated as

$$N_{\exp} = \Sigma\pi(i)\,N_{\exp}(i)$$
$$= 0.2(1600) + 0.2(1712) + 0.6(1186)$$
$$= 1374.$$

Table 21.5:   Characteristics of Seamless Design (OF)

| Scenario, $i$ | Effect size | Prior prob. $\pi$ | $N_{exp}$ | Power |
|---|---|---|---|---|
| 1 | 0 | 0.2 | 1600 | 0.025 |
| 2 | 0.1 | 0.2 | 1712 | 0.46 |
| 3 | 0.2 | 0.6 | 1186 | 0.98 |

Average power can be calculated as

$$P_{exp} = \Sigma \pi (i) N_{exp} (i) \, Power (i)$$
$$= 0.2(0.025) + 0.2(0.46) + 0.6(0.98)$$
$$= 0.69$$

**Seamless Design with Pocock Boundary:** We now use Pocock boundary efficacy stopping boundary and the symmetric futility stopping boundary to design the trial. The operating characteristics are summarized in Table 21.6.

Table 21.6:   Characteristics of Seamless Design (Pocock)

| Scenario, $i$ | Effect size | Prior prob. $\pi$ | $N_{exp}$ | Power |
|---|---|---|---|---|
| 1 | 0 | 0.2 | 1492 | 0.025 |
| 2 | 0.1 | 0.2 | 1856 | 0.64 |
| 3 | 0.2 | 0.6 | 1368 | 0.996 |

Average sample-size is given by

$$N_{exp} = \Sigma \pi (i) N_{exp} (i)$$
$$= 0.2(1492) + 0.2(1856) + 0.6(1368)$$
$$= 1490.$$

Average power is given by

$$P_{exp} = \Sigma \pi (i) N_{exp} (i) \, Power (i)$$
$$= 0.2(0.025) + 0.2(0.64) + 0.6(0.996)$$
$$= 0.73.$$

Let's compare the different designs from a financial perspective. Assume per-patient cost in the trial = $50k, dollar value of approval before deducting the trial cost = $1B. Time savings are not included in the calculation. Therefore, the expected utility can be expressed as

Expected utility = (Average power)($80M)–($N_{exp}$)($50K).

The resulting expected utilities for the three designs are summarized in Table 21.7. We can see that the Pocock design is the best among the three designs based on both power and the expected utility.

Table 21.7:   Comparison of Classical and Seamless Designs

| Design | $N_{max}$ | Average $N_{exp}$ | Average power | Expected utility |
|---|---|---|---|---|
| Classical | 1500 | 0.59 | | $0.515B |
| BOF | 1374 | 0.69 | | $0.621B |
| Pocock | 1490 | 0.73 | | $0.656B |

## 21.5   Trial Monitoring

### Conditional and Predictive Powers

The conditional and predictive power can be used to monitor adaptive designs.

Assume $X$ has binomial distribution. Given that $x$ of $n_1$ patients have the response at first stage, what is the probability (conditional power) of having at least $y$ additional responses from $n_2$ additional patients at second stage? The conditional power can be obtained using the frequentist approach:

$$P\left(y|x, n_1, n_2\right) = \sum_{i=y}^{n_2} \binom{n_2}{i} \left(\frac{x}{n_1}\right)^i \left(1 - \frac{x}{n_1}\right)^{n_2-i}. \tag{21.25}$$

Now let's look at Bayesian point of view. For the nonformative prior i.e., $p$ is uniformly distributed in $[0, 1]$, we have

$$P(X = x|p) = \binom{n_1}{x} p^x (1 - p)^{n_1 - x},$$

$$P(a < p < b \cap X = x) = \int_a^b \binom{n_1}{x} p^x (1 - p)^{n_1 - x} dp,$$

$$P(X = x) = \int_0^1 \binom{n_1}{x} p^x (1 - p)^{n_1 - x} dp,$$

and

$$P(a < p < b \mid X = x) = \frac{\int_a^b \binom{n_1}{x} p^x (1-p)^{n_1-x} dp}{\int_0^1 \binom{n_1}{x} p^x (1-p)^{n_1-x} dp}$$

$$= \frac{\int_a^b p^x (1-p)^{n_1-x} dp}{B(x+1, n_1 - x + 1)},$$

where *Beta* function

$$B(x+1, n_1 - x + 1) = \frac{\Gamma(x+1)\Gamma(n_1 - x + 1)}{\Gamma(n_1 + 2)}.$$

Therefore, the posterior distribution of $p$ is a *Beta* distribution

$$\pi(p|x) = \frac{p^x(1-p)^{n_1-x}}{B(x+1, n_1 - x + 1)}. \tag{21.26}$$

The predictive power (to differentiate from frequentist's conditional power) or the predictive probability of having at least $y$ responders out of additional $n_2$ patients is given by

$$P(y|x, n_1, n_2) = \int_0^1 P(X \geq y|p, n_2)\pi(p|x)\, dp$$

$$= \int_0^1 \sum_{i=y}^{n_2} \binom{n_2}{i} p^i (1-p)^{n_2-i} \frac{p^x(1-p)^{n_1-x}}{B(x+1, n_1 - x + 1)} dp.$$

Carrying out the integration, we have

$$P(y|x, n_1, n_2) = \sum_{i=y}^{n_2} \binom{n_2}{i} \frac{B(x+i+1, n_2+n_1-x-i+1)}{B(x+1, n_1 - x + 1)}, \tag{21.27}$$

where we have used the results:

$$\int_0^1 p^a (1-p)^b\, dp = B(a+1, b+1).$$

## 21.6   Analysis of Data

An important feature of the Bayesian approach is that it provides an ideal methodology for synthesizing information. This is often accomplished under the so-called exchangeability assumption. As pointed out by the "Guidance for the Use of Bayesian Statistics in Medical Device Clinical Trials" (FDA, 2006), exchangeability is a key idea in statistical inference in general, but it is particularly important in the Bayesian approach. If the patients in a clinical trial are exchangeable with the target population, then the clinical trial can be used to make inferences about the entire population. Data from different trials are more or less correlated. Exchangeability is a way to characterize the correlation. Suppose we are interested in making inferences on many parameters $\theta_1$, $\theta_2$,..., $\theta_k$ measured on $K$ "units," which may, for example, be true treatment effects in subpopulations, investigative centers, or a sequence of trials. The parameters $\theta_1$, $\theta_2$,..., $\theta_k$ are exchangeable, if the labels (subscripts) are not systematically associated with the values of the parameters. In other words, $\theta_1$, $\theta_2$,..., $\theta_k$ are samples from the same distribution of some "super population." It is important to know that two trials may be exchangeable only after adjustments are made for other confounding factors with the appropriate statistical model (Cornfield, 1976).

In the frequentist approach, the parameter $\theta$ is considered a fixed value; hence, a fixed effect model is used for the analysis. However, in the Bayesian paradigm, the parameter is considered a random variable (hence, $\theta_1$, $\theta_2$,...,$\theta_k$ above can be considered a random sample from a common super population). Therefore, the random-effect model with the exchangeability assumption is used for the analysis. This relationship between subpopulations and super populations can exist on multiple levels—a hierarchical model. Because of the similarity or exchangeability, data can be pooled across patient and disease groups within the same trial, and across trials, using a hierarchical model to obtain more precise estimates.

An example of a hierarchical model is illustrated in the "Guidance for the Use of Bayesian Statistics in Medical Device Clinical Trials" (FDA, 2006). Suppose you want to combine information from a treatment registry of an approved device with results from a new study. A model of two hierarchical levels (the patient level and the study level) is used. In the first (patient) level of the hierarchy, exchangeability is assumed for each of the studies. However, registry patients are not exchangeable with patients in the current study, so patient data from the registry and the current study cannot simply be pooled. The second (study) level of the hierarchy applies a model that assumes that the success probabilities from the registry and the current study are exchangeable after adjustment for covariates. Due to the use of this hierarchical model, the registry provides some information about the success probability for the current study, although not as much information as if the patients in the two groups were pooled directly as in a homogeneous case.

To give a real-life example of the Bayesian approach, in 2003, the FDA approved a drug that combines pravastatin, a cholesterol-lowering agent, with aspirin, based on the use of an exclusively Bayesian analysis of efficacy. The Bayesian approach was used to synthesize information through a meta-analysis of data from five previous pravastatin secondary prevention trials. Hierarchical modeling allowed for diverse sets of patients within the various trials (Berry, 2005).

In contrast, the frequentist approach does not allow for information synergy from different sources (trials) in general, at least in the current regulatory setting.

To illustrate the synergy of evidences, let's consider a very simple example. Suppose we have completed phase-II and phase-III asthma studies that have similar patient populations, similar treatment regimens, etc. The mean difference in efficacy was 7% improvement from baseline FEV1 with a standard deviation of 22% (Standard error = 0.022, n = 200 per group) in the phase-II trial, and 9% improvement with a standard deviation of 20% (Standard error = 0.0126, n = 500 per group) in the phase-III trial. If we use phase II as the prior for phase III, we will have the posterior normal distribution for the percent FEV1 improvement with a mean of 7.5% with a standard deviation 1.1%. We have discussed the treatment effect from the phase-III data on top of the phase-II data, rather than from only the phase-III data.

In practice, because of the heterogeneity of the trials, more complicated hierarchical models have to be used to derive the posterior distribution of treatment effect as mentioned earlier for the combined drug approved by FDA in 2003 (Berry, 2005b).

## 21.7 Interpretation of Outcomes

In addition to $p$-value, confidence interval (CI) is commonly reported as a frequentist outcome of clinical trials. Ironically, frequentist CIs are often misinterpreted as Bayesian credible intervals (BCI) because the concept of CI is difficult to understand and somewhat awkward to interpret. Fortunately, the CI is numerically close to the BCI with a noninformative prior distribution. For this reason, this misunderstanding does not lead to any tragedy.

The concept of a CI is quite difficult for nonstatisticians. For example, assume that our population parameter of interest is the population mean. What is the meaning of a 95% CI in this situation? The correct interpretation is based on repeated sampling. If samples of the same size are drawn repeatedly from a population, and a CI is calculated from each sample, then 95% of these intervals should contain the population mean. We can say that the probability of the true mean falling within this set of intervals with various lower and upper bounds is 95% (Figure 21.3). However, we cannot say that the probability of the true mean falling within a particularly observed (i.e., fixed) CI is 95%.

The frequentist approach considers the treatment effect to be a fixed constant and CIs bound as random variables, while the Bayesian considers the treatment effect to be a random variable and BCIs as fixed constants when data are given. BCI is easy to interpret. For example, if the 95% BCI of the treatment mean is $(1, 3)$, we can say that there is 95% probability that the true mean falls within $(1, 3)$. However, for a CI of $(1, 3)$, we cannot say anything about the location of the true mean. Clearly, BCI is much more informative than frequentist CI and can be used to design a better trial, as discussed in the following example. Note that these posterior probabilities are completely different from power for the hypothesis testing. Power is the probability of showing statistically that the treatment effect is larger than zero, under the assumption of a certain treatment effect, while Bayesian

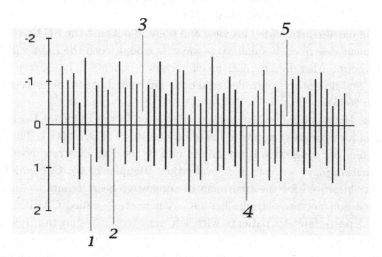

Figure 21.3:   Interpretation of Confidence Interval: Five out of 100 intervals do not cover the population mean (0) with $\alpha = 5\%$

posterior probability is telling us the probabilities associated with different magnitudes of treatment effect. Power is associated with alpha, while the posterior probability is the updated knowledge about the treatment effect and is not associated with alpha.

## 21.8   Regulatory Perspective

Bayesian approaches are accepted by the FDA medical device division, CDRH, which recently issued a FDA draft guidance on the use of Bayesian statistics in medical device clinical trials (FDA, 2006). In CDER FDA, although the frequentist approach, i.e., alpha control, is used in the New Drug Application (NDA) approval criteria, information from other sources has never been ignored. In fact, the FDA uses "prior" information in its decision making on clinical trials, which it refers to as informal use of the Bayesian approach.

Janet Woodcock (FDA acting deputy commissioner for operations) commented at a workshop on Bayesian clinical trials, "Bayesian approaches to clinical trials are of great interest in the medical product development community because they offer a way to gain valid information in a manner that is potentially more parsimonious of time, resources and investigational subjects than our current methods. The need to streamline the product development process without sacrificing important information has become increasingly apparent" (Woodcock, 2004).

Temple also articulated his view and pointed out that the FDA Evidence Document describes, in qualitative ways, how and when the FDA will take into account other data to reach an effectiveness conclusion based on a single study, and how other controlled trial data can contribute to the present case (FDA, 2006).

The Bayesian philosophy is clearly reflected in the Evidence Document criteria for regulatory approval based on one study (FDA, 2006). The drug carvedilol for congestive heart failure can be used to illustrate how prior information plays a role in drug evaluation (Temple, 2005). Carvedilol was already approved for the treatment of congestive heart failure to improve survival and decrease hospitalization. A new study called CAPRICORN studied postinfarction patients with left ventricular dysfunction (ejection fraction less than 40; Dargie, 2001) to study carveldilol use after a heart attack in people with decreased ejection fractions. The primary endpoint was total mortality (TM). However, in the middle of the study, a new endpoint, death plus cardiovascular hospitalization (DPCH), was added by the data monitoring committee (DMC). TM and DPCH became coprimary endpoints. The multiple adjustments were specified, and the familywise alpha was split into two parts: 0.005 for TM and 0.045 for DPCH. This meant that to claim efficacy of the drug, either of the following conditions must have been met: (1) $p$-value for TM less than or equal to 0.005 or (2) $p$-value for DPCH less than or equal to 0.045. The trial results came out as follows: $p$-value for DPCH was much larger than 0.045, but $p$-value for TM was about 0.03. Based on the modified endpoints, efficacy could not be claimed. However, if the DMC had not changed the endpoint, the efficacy of the drug would obviously have been claimed. So, what to do? After extensive discussions, the FDA agreed with the recommendation by the Cardiorenal Advisory Committee to approve the drug. Temple stated that the fairly explicit reasons were that there were very strong priors. Carvedilol was unequivocally effective in congestive heart failure; pooled early heart failure trials showed a survival effect for carvedilol and a large study in moderate to severe heart failure (COPERNICUS) showed a clear survival effect (Packer et al., 2001).

## 21.9 Summary and Discussion

The Bayesian approach can be used in drug development in two different ways: pure Bayesian and hybrid approaches. The pure Bayesian approach can be used for studies before phase III. This is because the Bayesian approach can better incorporate uncertainties at different stages and produce more informative output, such as posterior probability for decision making and streamlining the process of moving from one phase to the next. For phase-III trials, before regulatory agencies accept Bayesian evidence, a Bayesian–frequentist hybrid approach can make better use of the information from earlier phases in the design of phase-III studies, as illustrated in the examples above.

Operational challenges are usually similar for Bayesian trials and frequentist adaptive trials, requiring the ability to rapidly integrate knowledge and experiences from different disciplines into the decision-making process and, hence, require a shift to a more collaborative working environment.

## Problems

**21.1** Based on your understanding, summarize the differences between the frequentist and Bayesian approaches in a clinical trial development program.

**21.2** They are several reasons why the FDA NDA approval rate is much lower (about 40% in recent years) than expected. Use the power difference between the frequentist and Bayesian approaches shown in Example 21.3 to explain why the NDA approval rate is lower than the power since most phase-III clinical trials were designed with 85% to 95% power.

**21.3** Explain the difference between conditional power and predictive power and the difference between confidence interval and Bayesian credible interval.

# Chapter 22

# Adaptive Dose-Escalation Trial

In this chapter, we will introduce two commonly used approaches for oncology dose-escalation trials: (1) the algorithm-based escalation rules and (2) model-based approach. The second approach can be frequentist or Bayesian-based response-adaptive method and can be used in any dose-response trials.

## 22.1  Oncology Dose-Escalation Trial

For nonlife-threatening diseases, since the expected drug toxicity is mild and can be controlled without harm, phase-I trials are usually conducted on healthy or normal volunteers. However, in life-threatening diseases such as cancer and AIDS, phase-I studies are conducted with a limited number of patients due to (1) the aggressiveness and possible harmfulness of cytotoxic treatments, (2) possible systemic treatment effects, and (3) the high interest in the new drug's efficacy in those patients directly.

Drug toxicity is considered as tolerable if the toxicity is manageable and reversible. The standardization of the level of drug toxicity is the Common Toxicity Criteria (CTC) developed by the United States National Cancer Institute (NCI). Any adverse event (AE) related to treatment of CTC category of Grade 3 and higher is often considered a dose-limiting toxicity (DLT). The maximum tolerated dose (MTD) is defined as the maximum dose with a DLT rate that is no more frequent than a predetermined value.

### 22.1.1  *Dose Level Selection*

The initial dose given to the first patients in a phase-I study should be low enough to avoid severe toxicity. The commonly used starting dose is the dose at which 10% mortality ($LD_{10}$) occurs in mice. The subsequent dose levels are usually selected based on the following multiplicative set: $x_i = f_{i-1}x_{i-1}$ $(i = 1, 2, ..., K)$, where $f_i$ is called the dose-escalation factor. The highest dose level should be selected such that it covers the biologically active dose, but remains lower than the toxic dose. A popular dose-escalation factor is called the Fibonacci sequence (2, 1.5, 1.67, 1.60, 1.63, 1.62, 1.62, ...) and modified Fibonacci sequence (2, 1.65, 1.52, 1.40, 1.33, 1.33, ...). Note that the latter is a monotonic sequence and, hence, more appropriate than the former.

### 22.1.2   *Traditional Escalation Rules*

There are usually 5 to 10 predetermined dose levels with modified Fibonacci sequence in a dose escalation study. Patients are treated with the lowest dose first and then gradually escalated to higher doses if there is no major safety concern. The rules for dose escalation are predetermined. The commonly employed set of dose escalation rules is the traditional escalation rules (TER), also known as the "3 + 3" rule. The "3 + 3" rule says to enter three patients at a new dose level and enter another 3 patients when only one DLT is observed. The assessment of the six patients will be performed to determine whether the trial should be stopped at that level or the dose should be increased. Basically, there are two types of the "3 + 3" rules, namely, TER and strict TER (or STER). TER does not allow dose de-escalation, but STER does. The "3+3" TER and STER can be generalized to "$A + B$" TER and STER.

To introduce the $A+B$ escalation rule, let $A, B, C, D$, and $E$ be integers. The notation $A/B$ indicates that there are $A$ toxicity incidences out of $B$ subjects and $>A/B$ means that there are more than A toxicity incidences out of $B$ subjects. We assume that there are $K$ predefined doses and let $p_i$ be the probability of observing a DLT at dose level $i$ for $1 \leq i \leq K$.

### A + B Escalation without Dose Deescalation

The general $A + B$ designs without dose deescalation can be described as follows. Suppose that there are $A$ patients at dose level $i$. If fewer than $C/A$ patients have DLTs, then the dose is escalated to the next dose level $i + 1$. If more than $D/A$ (where $D \geq C$) patients have DLTs, then the previous dose $i - 1$ will be considered the MTD. If no fewer than $C/A$ but no more than $D/A$ patients have DLTs, $B$ more patients are treated at this dose level $i$. If no more than $E$ (where $E \geq D$) of the total of $A+B$ patients experience DLTs, then the dose is escalated. If more than $E$ of the total of $A + B$ patients have DLT, then the previous dose $i - 1$ will be considered the MTD. It can be seen that the traditional "3 + 3" design without dose de-escalation is a special case of the general $A + B$ design with $A = B = 3$ and $C = D = E = 1$. The closed forms of operating characteristics (Lin and Shih, 2001) are given below.

Under the general $A + B$ design without deescalation, the probability of concluding that MTD has been reached at dose $i$ is given by

$$P_i^* = P(MTD = dose\ i) = P\left(\begin{array}{c} \text{escalation at dose } \leq i \text{ and} \\ \text{stop escalation at dose } i+1 \end{array}\right)$$

$$= (1 - P_0^{i+1} - Q_0^{i+1})\left(\prod_{j=1}^{i}(P_0^j + Q_0^j)\right),\ 1 \leq i < K, \qquad (22.1)$$

where

$$P_0^j = \sum_{k=0}^{C-1}\binom{A}{k}p_j^k(1 - p_j)^{A-k},$$

and

$$Q_0^j = \sum_{k=C}^{D}\sum_{m=0}^{E-k}\binom{A}{k}p_j^k(1 - p_j)^{A-k}\binom{B}{m}p_j^m(1 - p_j)^{B-m}.$$

Here $p_j$ is the toxicity (DLT) rate at dose level $j$.

An overshoot is defined as an attempt to escalate to a dose level at the highest level planned, while an undershoot is defined as an attempt to de-escalate to a dose level at a lower dose than the starting dose level. Thus, the probability of undershoot is given by

$$P_1^* = P(MTD < dose\ 1) = (1 - P_0^1 - Q_0^1), \qquad (22.2)$$

and the probability of overshoot is given by

$$P_n^* = P(MTD \geq dose\ K) = \Pi_{j=1}^{K}(P_0^j + Q_0^j). \qquad (22.3)$$

The expected number of patients at dose level $j$ is given by

$$N_j = \sum_{i=0}^{K-1}N_{ji}P_i^*, \qquad (22.4)$$

where

$$N_{ji} = \begin{cases} \frac{AP_0^j + (A+B)Q_0^j}{P_0^j + Q_0^j} & \text{if } j < i+1 \\ \frac{A(1 - P_0^j - P_1^j) + (A+B)(P_1^j - Q_0^j)}{1 - P_0^j - Q_0^j} & \text{if } j = i+1 \\ 0 & \text{if } j > i+1 \end{cases}$$

Note that without consideration of undershoots and overshoots, the expected number of DLTs at dose $i$ can be obtained as $N_i p_i$. As a result, the total expected number of DLTs for the trial is given by $\sum_{i=1}^{K} N_i p_i$.

## A + B Escalation with Dose Deescalation

Basically, the general $A + B$ design with dose deescalation is similar to the design without dose deescalation. However, it permits more patients to be treated at a lower dose (i.e., dose deescalation) when excessive DLT incidences occur at the current dose level. The dose deescalation occurs when more than $D/A$ (where $D \geq C$) or more than $E/(A + B)$ patients have DLTs at dose level $i$. In this case, $B$ more patients will be treated at dose level $i - 1$, provided that only $A$ patients have been previously treated at this prior dose. If more than $A$ patients have already been treated previously, then dose $i - 1$ is the MTD. The deescalation may continue to the next dose level $i - 2$ and so on if necessary. The closed forms of operating characteristics are given by Lin and Shih (2001) as follows.

The probability of concluding that the MTD has been reached at dose $i$ is given by

$$P_i^* = P(MTD = \text{dose } i) = P \left( \begin{array}{c} \text{escalation at dose } \leq i \text{ and} \\ \text{stop escalation at dose } i+1 \end{array} \right)$$

$$= \sum_{k=i+1}^{K} p_{ik}, \tag{22.5}$$

where

$$p_{ik} = (Q_0^i + Q_1^i)(1 - P_0^k - Q_0^k) \left( \prod_{j=1}^{i-1} (P_0^j + Q_0^j) \right) \prod_{j=i+1}^{k-1} Q_2^j, \tag{22.6}$$

$$Q_1^j = \sum_{k=0}^{C-1} \sum_{m=0}^{E-k} \binom{A}{k} p_j^k (1 - p_j)^{A-k} \binom{B}{m} p_j^m (1 - p_j)^{B-m}, \tag{22.7}$$

and

$$Q_2^j = \sum_{k=0}^{C-1} \sum_{m=E+1-k}^{B} \binom{A}{k} p_j^k (1 - p_j)^{A-k} \binom{B}{m} p_j^m (1 - p_j)^{B-m}. \tag{22.8}$$

Also, the probability of undershooting is given by

$$P_1^* = P(MTD < dose\ 1) = \sum_{k=1}^{K} \{ \left( \Pi_{j=1}^{k-1} Q_2^j \right) (1 - P_0^k - Q_0^k) \}, \tag{22.9}$$

and the probability of overshooting is

$$P_K^* = P(MTD \geq dose\ K) = \Pi_{j=1}^K (P_0^j + Q_0^j). \qquad (22.10)$$

The expected number of patients at dose level $j$ is given by

$$N_j = N_{jK}P_K^* + \sum_{i=0}^{K-1} \sum_{k=i+1}^{K} N_{jik}p_{ik}, \qquad (22.11)$$

where

$$N_{jn} = \frac{AP_0^j + (A+B)Q_0^j}{P_0^j + Q_0^j}, \qquad (22.12)$$

$$N_{jik} = \begin{cases} \frac{AP_0^j+(A+B)Q_0^j}{P_0^j+Q_0^j} & \text{if } j < i \\ A+B & \text{if } i \leq j < k \\ \frac{A(1-P_0^j-P_1^j)+(A+B)(P_1^j-Q_0^j)}{1-P_0^j-Q_0^j} & \text{if } j = k \\ 0 & \text{if } j > k \end{cases}, \qquad (22.13)$$

and

$$P_1^j = \sum_{i=C}^{D} \binom{A}{k} p_j^k (1-p_j)^{A-k}. \qquad (22.14)$$

Consequently, the total number of expected DLTs is given by $\sum_{i=1}^K N_i p_i$.

Aiming to increase in-trial patient safety without unnecessary increase in sample size, Lee and Fan (2012) proposed a two-dimesional search algorithm for dose-finding trials of two agents, which uses not only the frequency but also the source of dose-limiting toxicities to direct dose escalations and deescalations. In addition, when the doses of both agents are escalated simultaneously, a more conservative design replaces a default aggressive design to evaluate the resulting dose combination.

### 22.1.3 Simulations Using Traditional Escalation Algorithms

The objective of SAS Macro 22.1 below is to simulate the 3+3 traditional escalation. The SAS variables are defined as follows: **nSims** = number of simulation runs, **nLevels** = number of dose levels, **DeEs** = "true" means that it allows for dose deescalation, otherwise, it does not. **AveMTD** = average observed MTD, **AveNPts** = average number of patient per trial, **AveNRsps** = average number of responses (DLTs) in a trial.

## >>SAS Macro 22.1:    3+3 Dose-Escalation Design>>

```
%Macro TER3p3(nSims=10000, DeEs="true", nLevels=10);
Data TER; Set dInput; Keep AveMTD SdMTD AveNPts AveNRsps;
Array nPts{&nLevels}; Array nRsps{&nLevels}; Array RspRates{&nLevels};
AveMTD=0; VarMTD=0; AveNPts=0; AveNRsps=0; nLevels=&nLevels;
Do iSim=1 to &nSims;
Do i=1 To nLevels; nPts{i}=0; nRsps{i}=0; End;
seedn=Round((Ranuni(281)*100000000));
iLevel=1; TotPts=0; TotRsps=0;
Looper:
If iLevel>&nLevels | iLevel<1 | nPts(iLevel)=6 Then Goto Finisher;
nPts{iLevel}=nPts{iLevel}+3;
rspRate=RspRates{iLevel};
Rsp=RANBIN(seedn,3,rspRate);
nRsps{iLevel}=nRsps{iLevel}+Rsp;
TotPts=TotPts+3; TotRsps=TotRsps+Rsp;
If nPts(iLevel)=3 & nRsps{iLevel}=0 Then Do;
iLevel=iLevel+1;
Goto Looper;
End;
If nPts(iLevel)=3 & nRsps{iLevel}=1 Then Goto Looper;
If nPts(iLevel)=3 & nRsps{iLevel}>1 Then Do;
If &DeEs="false" | iLevel=1 Then Goto Finisher;
iLevel=iLevel-1;
Goto Looper;
End;
If nPts(iLevel)=6 & nRsps{iLevel}<=1 Then Do;
iLevel=iLevel+1;
Goto Looper;
End;
Finisher:
MTD=Min(iLevel-1, nLevels);
AveMTD=AveMTD+MTD/&nSims;
VarMTD=VarMTD+MTD**2/&nSims;
AveNPts=AveNPts+totPts/&nSims;
AveNRsps=AveNRsps+TotRsps/&nSims;
End;
SdMTD=(VarMTD-AveMTD**2)**0.5;
Output;
```

Run;
Proc Print Data=TER; Run;
%Mend TER3p3;
**<<SAS<<**

We will show you later in Example 22.1 how to use this macro.

## 22.2 Continual Reassessment Method

The continual reassessment method (CRM) is a model approach, in which the parameters in the model for the response are continually updated based on the observed response data. The method for updating the parameters can be either frequentist or Bayesian approach.

CRM was initially proposed by O'Quigley (O'Quigley et al., 1990; O'Quigley and Shen, 1996; Babb and Rogatko, 2004) for oncology dose-escalation trial. However, it can be extended to other types of trials (Chang and Chow 2006a). In CRM, the dose-response relationship is continually reassessed based on accumulative data collected from the trial. The next patient who enters the trial is then assigned to the currently estimated MTD level. This approach is more efficient than TER with respect to finding the MTD.

Let's denote prior distribution by $\pi(\theta)$, and the sample distribution by $f(x|\theta)$. In Bayesian approach for CRM, there are four basic elements:

(1) the joint distribution of $(\theta, x)$ given by

$$\varphi(\theta, x) = f(x|\theta)\pi(\theta), \tag{22.15}$$

(2) the marginal distribution of $x$ given by

$$m(x) = \int \varphi(\theta, x)\, d\theta = \int f(x|\theta)\pi(\theta)\, d\theta, \tag{22.16}$$

(3) the posterior distribution of $\theta$ given by Bayes' formula

$$\pi(\theta|x) = \frac{f(x|\theta)\pi(\theta)}{m(x)}, \text{ and} \tag{22.17}$$

(4) the predictive probability distribution given by

$$P(y|x) = \int P(x|y, \theta)\pi(\theta|x)\, d\theta. \tag{22.18}$$

### 22.2.1 Probability Model for Dose-Response

Let $x$ be the dose or dose level, and $p(x)$ be the probability of response or response rate. The commonly used model for dose-response is the logistic model (Figure 22.1).

$$p(x) = [1 + b\exp(-ax)]^{-1}, \qquad (22.19)$$

where $b$ is usually a predetermined constant and $a$ is a parameter to be updated based on observed data.

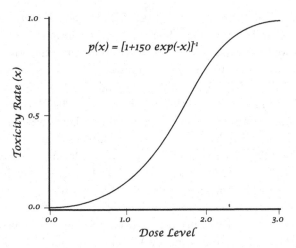

Figure 22.1:   Logistic Toxicity Model

### 22.2.2 Prior Distribution of Parameter

The Bayesian approach requires the specification of prior probability distribution of the unknown parameter $a$.

$$a \sim g_0(a), \qquad (22.20)$$

where $g_0(a)$ is the prior probability.

When very limited knowledge about the prior is available, the non-informative prior can be used.

**Likelihood Function**

The next step is to construct the likelihood function. Given $n$ observations with $y_i$ $(i = 1, ..., n)$ associated with dose $x_{m_i}$, the likelihood function can be written as

$$f_n(\mathbf{r}\,|a) = \prod_{i=1}^{n} [p(x_{m_i})]^{r_i} [1 - p(x_{m_i})]^{1-r_i}, \qquad (22.21)$$

where

$$r_i = \begin{cases} 1, & \text{if response observed for } x_{m_i} \\ 0, & \text{otherwise} \end{cases}. \qquad (22.22)$$

### 22.2.3  *Reassessment of Parameter*

The key is to estimate the parameter $a$ in the response model (22.19). An initial assumption or a prior about the parameter is necessary in order to assign patients to the dose level based on the dose-toxicity relationship. This estimation of $a$ is continually updated based on the cumulative response data observed from the trial thus far. The estimation method can be a Bayesian or frequentist approach. For the Bayesian approach, it leads to the posterior distribution of $a$. For the frequentist approach, maximum likelihood estimate or least square estimate can be used.

**Bayesian approach**

For the Bayesian approach, the posterior probability of parameter $a$ can be obtained as follows:

$$g_n(a|\mathbf{r}) = \frac{f_n(\mathbf{r}|a)g_0(a)}{\int f_n(\mathbf{r}|a)g_0(a)\,da} \qquad (22.23)$$

or

$$g_n(a|\mathbf{r}) = \frac{[p_n(a)]^{r_n} [1 - p_n(a)]^{1-r_n} g_{n-1}(a)}{\int [p_n(a)]^{r_n} [1 - p_n(a)]^{1-r_n} g_{n-1}(a)\,da}, \qquad (22.24)$$

where $p_n(a) = p(x_{m_n})$ is the response rate at the dose level at which the $n$th patient is treated.

After having obtained $g_n(a|\mathbf{r})$, we can update the predictive probability using

$$p(x) = \int [1 + b\exp(-ax)]^{-1} g_n(a|\mathbf{r})\,da. \qquad (22.25)$$

**Maximum likelihood approach**

Note that the Bayesian approach is computationally intensive. Alternatively, we may consider a frequentist approach to simplify the calculation. The maximum likelihood estimate of the parameters is given by

$$\hat{a} = \arg\max_{a}\{f_n(\mathbf{r}\,|\,a)\}. \qquad (22.26)$$

Note that the MLE $\hat{a}$ is only available after both responders and non-responders are observed.

After having obtained $\hat{a}$, we can update the dose-response model or the predictive probability using

$$p(x) = [1 + b\exp(-\hat{a}x)]^{-1}. \tag{22.27}$$

### 22.2.4  *Assignment of Next Patient*

The updated dose-toxicity model is usually used to choose the dose level for the next patient. In other words, the next patient enrolled in the trial is assigned to the currently estimated MTD based on dose-response model (22.25) or (22.27). Practically, this assignment is subject to safety constraints such as limited dose jump. Assignment of patient to the most updated MTD is intuitive. This way, a majority of the patients will be assigned to the dose levels near MTD, which allows for a more precise estimation of MTD with a minimal number of patients.

In practice, it is also not ethical to make a big dose jump. We usually implement a limitation on dose jump, e.g., the dose can only be escalated only one dose level high at one time.

### 22.2.5  *Stopping Rule*

When one of the dose levels reaches a certain number of patients (e.g., 6 patients), the trial will stop. This is because, for example, when there are 6 patients at a dose level, it means that model has predicted the MTD at the same dose level 6 times; thus, it is reasonable to believe this dose level is the MTD. We don't want all dose levels to have 6 patients, it would not be an efficient design.

### 22.3  Alternative Form CRM

The CRM is often presented in an alternative form (e.g.,Yin and Yuan, 2011). In practice, we usually prespecify the doses of interest, instead of any dose. Let $(d_1, ..., d_K)$ be a set of doses and $(p_1, ..., p_K)$ be the corresponding prespecified probability, called the "skeleton," satisfying $p_1 < p_2, ..., < p_K$. The dose-toxicity model of the CRM is assumed, instead of (22.19), to be

$$\Pr(\text{toxicity at } d_i) = \pi_i(a) = p_i^{\exp(a)}, i = 1, 2, ..., K, \tag{22.28}$$

where $a$ is an unknown parameter. Parabolic tangent or logistic structures can also be used to model the dose-toxicity curve.

Let $D$ be the observed data: $y_i$ out of $n_i$ patients treated at dose level $i$ have experienced the dose-limiting toxicity (DLT). Based on the bionamial distribution, the likelihood function is

$$L\left(D|a\right) \propto \prod_{i=1}^{K} \left\{p_i^{\exp(a)}\right\}^{y_i} \left(1 - p_i^{\exp(a)}\right)^{n_i - y_i}. \qquad (22.29)$$

Using Bayes' theorem, the posterior means of the toxicity probabilities at dose $j$ can be computed by

$$\hat{\pi}_i = \frac{1}{\int L\left(D|a\right) g_0\left(a\right) da} \int p_i^{\exp(a)} L\left(D|a\right) g_0\left(a\right) da, \qquad (22.30)$$

where $g_0\left(a\right)$ is a prior distribution for $a$, for example, $a \sim N\left(0, \sigma^2\right)$.

## 22.4 Simulations of CRM

SAS Macro 22.2 CRM below is developed for simulating the trial using CRM, where the logistic response model (22.19) is used. The input SAS variables are defined as follows: **nSims** = number of simulations, **MaxnPts** = maximum total number of patients, **nLevels** = number of dose levels, **b** = model parameter in (22.19), **aMin** and **aMax** = the upper and lower limits for prior on the parameter $a$, **MTRate** = the rate defined for MTD, and **nIntPts** = number of intervals for numerical integration in calculating the posterior. **g0{i}** = prior distribution of the model parameter $a$, **RRo{i}** = true response rates, and **doses{i}** = dose amount. These three arrays should be in the dataset naming **DInput**. The toxicity model can be **ToxModel**="Skeleton" or **ToxModel**="Logist." nPtsForStop = the number of patients required for a dose level to stop the trial. The key output variables are **AveTotalN** = average total number of patients needed, **AveMTD** = average MTD (simulated), **SdMTD** = standard deviation of MTDs.

The logistic toxicity model can be constructed based on the actual dose or on the dose level (1, 2, 3,...). When logistic toxicity model is used, the actual dose (doses{$i$Level}) at each dose level has to be specified in the input dataset. For the skeleton toxicity model, actual dose is not required, but the skeleton, i.e., skeletonP{$i$} has to be given for each dose level.

**>>SAS Macro 22.2:    Continual Reassessment Method>>**

```
%Macro  CRM(nSims=100,  MaxnPts=30,  nLevels=10,  b=100,  aMin=0.1,
aMax=0.3, MTRate=0.3, nIntPts=100, ToxModel="Skeleton", nPtsForStop=6);
Data CRM; Set DInput; Keep MaxnPts AveTotalN nLevels AveMTD SdMTD
DLTS PercentMTD1-PercentMTD&nLevels;
Array nPtsAt{&nLevels}; Array nRsps{&nLevels}; Array g{&nIntPts};
Array Doses{&nLevels}; Array RRo{&nLevels}; Array RR{&nLevels};
Array  g0{&nIntPts};    Array  skeletonP{&nLevels};    Array  PercentMTD
{&nLevels};
seed=2736; nLevels=&nLevels; MaxnPts=&MaxnPts; DLTs=0;
AveMTD=0;VarMTD=0; dx=(&aMax-&aMin)/&nIntPts;
ToxModel=&ToxModel; nPtsForStop=&nPtsForStop;
AveTotalN=0;
Do iLevel=1 to nLevels; PercentMTD(iLevel)=0; End;
Do iSim=1 to &nSims;
Do k=1 To &nIntPts; g{k}=g0{k}; End;
Do i=1 To nLevels; nPtsAt{i}=0; nRsps{i}=0; End;
iLevel=1;  PreLevel=iLevel;
Do iPatient=1 To MaxnPts;
TotalN=iPatient;
iLevel=Min(ilevel, PreLevel+1); * Avoid dose-jump;
iLevel=Min(iLevel, nLevels); PreLevel=iLevel; Rate=RRo{iLevel};
nPtsAt{iLevel}=nPtsAt{iLevel}+1;
r=Ranbin(seed,1,Rate); nRsps{iLevel}=nRsps{iLevel}+r;
** Posterior distribution of a;
c=0;
Do k=1 To &nIntPts;
ak=&aMin+k*dx;
If ToxModel="Logist" Then Rate=1/(1+&b*Exp(-ak*doses{iLevel}));
If ToxModel="Skeleton" Then Rate=skeletonP{iLevel}**Exp(ak);
If r>0 Then L=Rate; Else L=(1-Rate);
g{k}=L*g{k}; c=c+g{k}*dx;
End;
Do k=1 to &nIntPts; g{k}=g{k}/c; End;
** Predict response rate and current MTD;
MTD=iLevel; MinDR=1;
Do i=1 To nLevels;
RR{i}=0;
Do k=1 To &nIntPts;
```

```
ak=&aMin+k*dx;
If  ToxModel="Logist"  Then  RR{i}=  RR{i}+1/(1+&b*Exp(-ak*doses{i}))
*g{k}*dx;
If ToxModel="Skeleton" Then RR{i}= RR{i}+skeletonP{i}**Exp(ak)*g{k}*dx;
End;
DR=Abs(&MTRate-RR{i});
If .<DR <MinDR Then Do; MinDR = DR; iLevel=i; MTD=i; End;
End;
If nPtsAt{iLevel} >= nPtsForStop OR iPatient>= MaxnPts Then Do;
PercentMTD(iLevel) =PercentMTD(iLevel)+1/&nSims; Goto EndTrial;
End;
End;
EndTrial:
Do i=1 To nLevels;
DLTs=DLTs+nRsps{i}/&nSims;
End;
AveMTD=AveMTD+MTD/&nSims;
VarMTD=VarMTD+MTD**2/&nSims; ·
AveTotalN=AveTotalN+TotalN/&nSims;
End;
SdMTD=Max(0,(VarMTD-AveMTD**2))**0.5; Output; Run;
Proc Print Data=CRM; run;
%Mend CRM;
<<SAS<<
```

There are advantages and disadvantages with different dose escalation schemes. For example, the traditional 3+3 escalation is easy to apply but the MTD estimation is usually biased, especially when there are many dose levels. The criteria for evaluation of escalation schemes are listed as follows: number of DLTs, number of patients, number of patients dosed above MTD, accuracy, and precision.

Before a phase-I trial is initiated, the following design characteristics should be checked and defined in the study protocol: (1) starting dose, (2) dose levels, (3) prior information on the MTD, (4) toxicity model, (5) escalation rule, (6) stopping rule, and (7) rules for completion of the sample size when stopping.

**Example 22.1     Adaptive Dose-Finding for Prostate Cancer Trial**

A trial is designed to establish the dose-toxicity relationship and identify MTD for a compound in patients with metastatic androgen independent prostate cancer. Based on preclinical data, the estimated MTD is 230 mg/m$^2$. The modified Fibonacci sequence is chosen for the dose levels (in Table 22.1). There are 8 dose levels anticipated, but more dose levels can be added if necessary. The initial dose level is 30 mg/m$^2$, which is 1/10 of the minimal effective dose level (mg/m$^2$) for 10% deaths (MELD10) of the mouse after verification that no lethal and no life-threatening effects were seen in another species. The toxicity rate (DLT rate) at MTD is defined for this indication as 17%.

Table 22.1:   Dose Levels and DLT Rates

| Dose level $i$ | 1 | 2 | 3 | 4 | 5 | 6 | 7 | 8 |
|---|---|---|---|---|---|---|---|---|
| Dose x | 30 | 45 | 68 | 101 | 152 | 228 | 342 | 513 |
| DLT rate | 0.01 | 0.02 | 0.03 | 0.05 | 0.12 | 0.17 | 0.22 | 0.4 |

The SAS macro calls for TER and STER designs are presented as follows.

**>>SAS>>**
Title "3 + 3 TER and SER Designs";
Data dInput;
Array RspRates{8}(0.01, 0.02, 0.03, 0.05, 0.12, 0.17, 0.22, 0.4);
%TER3p3(nSims=100000, DeEs= "true", nLevels=8);
%TER3p3(nSims=100000, DeEs= "false", nLevels=8);
Run;
**<<SAS<<**

For logistic toxicity model, $p = \frac{1}{1+150\exp(-a\,i)}$ is used, where $i =$ dose level (we can also use actual dose) and the prior distribution for parameter $a$ is flat over $[0, 0.8]$. For the skeleton toxicity model $p_i^{\exp(a)}$, the following skeleton is used: $p_i = (01, .02, .04, .08, .16, .32, .4, .5)$ and a flat prior over $[-0.1, 2]$. The SAS macro calls for CRM designs are presented as follows.

**>>SAS>>**
Title "Bayesian CRM Design—Logistic Model";
Data DInput;
Array g0{100}; Array RRo{8}(.01, .02, .03, .05, .12, .17, .22, .4);
Array Doses{8} (1, 2, 3, 4, 5, 6, 7, 8);

```
Do k=1 To 100; g0{k}=1; End; * Flat prior;
%CRM(nSims=10000, MaxnPts=50, nLevels=8, b=150, aMin=0, aMax=0.8,
MTRate=0.17, ToxModel= "Logist");
Run;
Title "Bayesian CRM Design—Skeleton Model";
Data DInput;
Array g0{100}; Array RRo{8}(.01, .02, .03, .05, .12, .17, .22, .4);
Array skeletonP{8} (.01, .02, .04, .08, .16, .32, .4, .5);
Do k=1 To 100; g0{k}=1; End; * Flat prior;
%CRM(nSims=10000, MaxnPts=50, nLevels=8, aMin=-0.1, aMax=2,
MTRate=0.17, ToxModel= "Skeleton");
```
<<**SAS**<<

The simulation results are presented in Table 22.2. In addition, the percent or the probabilities of selecting different dose levels as the MTD are also obtained from the simulations: for the CRM logistic model they are 0, 0, 0, .0001, 0.4, 0.3446, 0.1159, and 0.1394 for dose 1 to dose 8, respectively. For the CRM skeleton model, the selecting probabilities are 0, 0, 0, 0, 0.1379, 0.5305, 0.1776, and 0.154 for the 8 doses.

Table 22.2: Adaptive Dose-Response Simulation Results

| Method | Mean N | Mean DLTs | Mean MTD | SdMTD |
|---|---|---|---|---|
| TER | 24.5 | 2.71 | 5.97 | 1.43 |
| STER | 26.0 | 3.03 | 5.87 | 1.44 |
| CRM (Logistic) | 12.0 | 2.40 | 5.99 | 1.04 |
| CRM (Skeleton) | 11.5 | 2.53 | 6.35 | 0.90 |

Note the true MTD is dose level 6 (228 mg/m$^2$). The simulation results are summarized in Table 22.2. The average predicted MTD (dose level) is 5.97 with TER and 5.87 with STER, which are underestimated. In contrast, the average MTD for the two CRM with sample-size 12 accurately predict the true MTD. From precision point of view, even with a smaller sample size, the standard deviation of MTD (SdMTD) is much smaller for CRM than for both TER and STER. However, we should be aware that the performance of CRM is dependent on the goodness of the model specification.

## 22.5   Bayesian Model Averaging CRM

There is an important issue in the previous CRM model: the set of prespecified toxicity probabilities (skeleton) in the CRM is somewhat arbitrary or
subjective. Different skeletons can lead to various different conclusions. To
overcome the difficulty, Yin and Yuan (2009) proposed BMA-CRM by using
multiple skeletons in the CRM combined with the Bayesian model average
(BMA) approach.

Let $(M_1, ..., M_K)$ denote a set of prespecified models for the drug under investigation, and let $(p_{k1}, ..., p_{kJ})$ be the corresponding prespecified
probabilities for model $k$. Model $M_k$ in BMA-CRM is

$$\pi_{kj}(a) = p_{kj}^{\exp(a_k)}, j = 1, 2, ..., J, k = 1, 2, ..., K \tag{22.31}$$

Let $\Pr(M_k)$ be the prior model probability, then the likelihood function
under model $M_k$ is

$$L(D|a_k, M_k) \propto \prod_{j=1}^{J} \left\{ p_j^{\exp(a_k)} \right\}^{y_j} \left( 1 - p_j^{\exp(a_k)} \right)^{n_j - y_j}. \tag{22.32}$$

The posterior model probability for model $M_k$ is

$$\Pr(M_k|D) = \frac{L(D|M_k)\Pr(M_k)}{\sum_{i=1}^{K} L(D|M_i)\Pr(M_i)}, \tag{22.33}$$

where $L(D|M_k)$ is the marginal likelihood of model $M_k$ given by

$$L(D|M_k) = \int L(D|a_k, M_k) g_0(a_k|M_k) da_k, \tag{22.34}$$

where $g_0(a_k|M_k)$ is the prior distribution of $a_k$ under model $M_k$.

The BMA estimate for the toxicity probability at each dose level is

$$\bar{\pi}_j = \sum_{k=1}^{K} \hat{\pi}_{kj} \Pr(M_k|D), j = 1, ..., J, k = 1, ..., K, \tag{22.35}$$

where $\hat{\pi}_{kj}$ is the posterior mean of the toxicity probability at dose level $j$
under model $M_k$,

$$\hat{\pi}_{kj} = \int p_{kj}^{\exp(a_k)} \frac{L(D|a_k, M_k) g_0(a_k|M_k)}{\int L(D|a_k, M_k) g_0(a_k|M_k) da_k} da_k. \tag{22.36}$$

By assigning a weight $\hat{\pi}_{kj}$ to $\Pr(M_k|D)$, the BMA automatically favors
the best fitting model and provides a coherent mechanism to account for
the model uncertainty associated with each skeleton.

## 22.6   Summary and Discussion

We have studied the traditional algorithm-based and model-based approaches for dose-response trials. The efficiencies of the approaches are dependent on several aspects, such as the situation in which the next patient is enrolled before we have the response data from the previous patient. In this case, the efficacy of the TER and CRM may be reduced. There may also be a limit for dose escape, which may also reduce the efficiency of the CRM.

In addition to $A + B$ escalation algorithms, many other algorithms have been proposed (Chevret, 2006; Ting, 2006). For example, Shih and Lin (2006) modified $A + B$ and derived closed form solutions for the modified algorithms. They were motivated by the following: (1) in a traditional $A + B$ design, the previous dose level is always declared the maximum tolerated dose and the current dose has no chance at all of being declared the MTD, (2) the starting dose cannot necessarily be the lowest dose, and (3) the design may be a two-stage escalation design used to accelerate the escalation in the early part of the trial with one or two patients per dose level. However, the values from (1) and (2) are questionable because any dose can be the current or previous dose level, and just as with dose jump, dosing the first patient at a higher dose level may put certain individuals at risk, even though the overall toxicity (e.g., number of DLTs) may be reduced.

CRM can be used with other monotonic or nonmonotonic models and can be combined with response-adaptive randomization or a drop-loser design (Chang, 2008).

**Problems**

**22.1** Modify Macro SAS 22.1 using $m+n$ dose-escalation rules.

**22.2** Redesign the trial in Example 22.1 for the following response profile.

Table 22.3:   Dose Levels and DLT Rates

| Dose level $i$ | 1 | 2 | 3 | 4 | 5 | 6 | 7 | 8 |
|---|---|---|---|---|---|---|---|---|
| Dose x | 30 | 45 | 68 | 101 | 152 | 228 | 342 | 513 |
| DLT rate | 0.02 | 0.02 | 0.03 | 0.1 | 0.15 | 0.19 | 0.25 | 0.45 |

**22.3** Develop an SAS or R program for BMA-CRM with Model $M_1$ and $M_2$ specified as

$$\pi_{kj}(a) = p_{kj}^{\exp(a_k)}, j = 1, 2, ..., J, k = 1, 2.$$

# Chapter 23

# Bayesian Design for Efficacy–Toxicity Trade-Off and Drug Combination

## 23.1 Introduction

In this chapter, we will study the more complex Bayesian dose-finding models in two dimensions. Either the outcome has two dimensions (efficacy and toxicity) or the treatment has two dimensions (drug combinations). Going from phase-I to phase-II trials, the objectives gradually switch shift from a single toxicity issue to the combination of toxicity and efficacy, while a combination of drugs is a common way of treating progressive disease such as cancer and AIDs in phase-II and phase-III trials.

Thall et al. (2003) proposed an efficacy–toxicity trade-off model to improve their naive efficacy–toxicity independent model. Ivanova and Wang (2004) propose a nonparametric approach to the design and analysis of two-dimensional dose-finding trials. Wang and Ivanova (2005) proposed a logistic-type regression for dose combinations that used the doses of the two agents as the covariates. Huang et al. (2007) modified the "3 + 3" design for use in the dose-escalation phase of an agent combination trial, where Bayesian adaptive randomization is used. Yin and Yuan (2008) proposed a copula-type model for phase-I drug-combination trial designs. Yin and Yuan (2009) proposed a latent contingency table approach to dose finding for combinations of two agents. Liu and Ning (2013) proposed a Bayesian dose-finding design for drug combination trials with delayed toxicities. In all these approaches, each individual agent in the combination should be carefully studied before the initiation of an agent-combination trial.

## 23.2 Thall–Russell Independent Model

Thall and Cook gave a motivating example in 2004: "Ischemic stroke is the third leading cause of death in the U.S. and the leading cause of disability among the elderly. In Rapid Treatment of Acute Ischemic Stroke I with the trinary outcome case, each patient receives a fixed dose of abciximab (0.25 mg/kg as a bolus followed by 0.125 mg/kg/minute for 12 hours) followed by one of the five doses {0.0, 2.5, 5.0, 7.5, 10.0} units (U) of reteplase. The rationale for this combination arises from the fact that the two major components of a blood clot, the cause of ischemic stroke, are platelets and fibrin. To dissolve the patient's clot, abciximab acts against platelet aggregation, while reteplase, a tissue plasminogen activator, increases the ability of vascular tissues to reestablish blood flow (reperfusion) by degrading fibrin. Patient outcome is evaluated by both physical examination and magnetic resonance imaging. Toxicity is defined as symptomatic intracranial hemorrhage, other severe regimen-related adverse event, or death within 48 hours. Response (efficacy) is defined as reperfusion at 24 hours".

Thall and Russell (1998) propose a Bayesian design that adapts to trial outcomes, both efficacy $(E)$ and toxicity $(T)$. The method accommodates settings with trinary outcomes where $E$ and $T$ are disjoint and it is possible that neither event may occur, and also trials with bivariate binary outcomes, where the patient may experience both events. Denote the probabilities of $E$ and $T$ by

$$\pi(x, \boldsymbol{\theta}) = \{\pi_E(x, \boldsymbol{\theta}), \pi_T(x, \boldsymbol{\theta})\}, \tag{23.1}$$

where $x$ denotes dose and $\boldsymbol{\theta}$ is the model parameter vector, which is continuously reassessed based on the current interim data, $D$. At the same time the desirability of each dose $x$ is determined by using a family of contours characterizing the trade-off between $E$ and $T$ to define a non-Euclidean distance from $E\{\pi_T(x, \boldsymbol{\theta}) | D\}$ to the ideal point $\pi(x^*, \boldsymbol{\theta}) = \pi^*$ (e.g., $\pi^* = (1, 0)$).

Thall-Russell Model (1998) requires $E$ and $T$ to be disjoint, with trinary outcome $Y \in \{E, T, (E \cup T)^c\}$. They propose a three-parameter logistic model (proportional odds model) with

$$logit(\pi_T(x, \boldsymbol{\theta})) = \eta_T(x, \boldsymbol{\theta}) = \mu + x\beta, \tag{23.2}$$

and

$$logit(\pi_E(x, \boldsymbol{\theta}) + \pi_T(x, \boldsymbol{\theta})) = \eta_{E \cup T}(x, \boldsymbol{\theta}) = \mu + \alpha + x\beta. \tag{23.3}$$

The rectangular priors are used, subject to $\alpha > 0$ and $\beta > 0$. Given the interim data $D$, the decision rules are that the dose $x$ is acceptable if

$$\Pr\{\pi_E(x, \boldsymbol{\theta}) > \underline{\pi}_E | D\} > c_E \tag{23.4}$$

and

$$\Pr\left\{\pi_T\left(x,\boldsymbol{\theta}\right)<\bar{\pi}_T|D\right\}>c_T, \tag{23.5}$$

where $\underline{\pi}_E$ and $\bar{\pi}_T$ are fixed lower and upper limits specified by the physician, and $c_E$ and $c_T$ are fixed probability cutoffs.

As pointed out by Thall and Cook (2004): a major limitation of the method is that, in cases where all doses have acceptable toxicity but higher dose levels have substantially higher efficacy, the escalation algorithm does not escalate to the more desirable doses with high probability. Consequently, in such settings it is likely to fail to select a higher dose level that is safe and provides greater efficacy. More generally, the method may fail to reliably determine the best among several acceptable doses. For trinary outcomes, they also found that the three-parameter model, while parsimonious, may be overly restrictive in certain cases. Finally, because it is limited to the case of trinary outcomes, the independent model cannot accommodate settings where the physician wishes to allow the possibility that both $E$ and $T$ may occur.

## 23.3   Efficacy–Toxicity Trade-Off Model

To overcome the limitations of the independent model, Thall and Cook (2004) propose a dose outcome model with correlation between toxicity and efficacy as discussed below.

Given the $J$ doses $d_1, d_2, ..., d_J$ to be considered in the trial, we code dose as $x_j = log(d_j) - J^{-1}\sum_{i=1}^{J}\log\left(d_i\right)$ for use in the regression models underlying the dose-finding method. The toxicity is modeled by

$$logit\left(\pi_T\left(x,\boldsymbol{\theta}\right)\right)=\eta_T\left(x,\boldsymbol{\theta}\right)=\mu_T+x\beta_T. \tag{23.6}$$

The efficacy is modeled by

$$\begin{aligned}\eta_{E|T^c}\left(x,\boldsymbol{\theta}\right)&=logit\left(\pi_{E|T^c}\left(x,\boldsymbol{\theta}\right)\right)\\&=logit\left(\Pr\left(Y=E|Y\neq T\right),x,\boldsymbol{\theta}\right)\\&=\mu_E+x\beta_E.\end{aligned} \tag{23.7}$$

Here $E$, $T$, and $T^C$ represent efficacy, tocixity, and no tocixity. Thus, there are four parameters in the model, i.e., $\theta=(\mu_T,\beta_T,\mu_E,\beta_E)$, where $\beta_T>0$ and $\beta_E>0$.

Given the $i$th patient taking dose $d_{m_i}$ $(1\leq m_i\leq J)$, and having response $y_i$, which is either $E$ (efficacious), $T$ (toxic), or $E\cup T^c$ (neither $E$

nor $T$), the likelihood for the first $n$ patients is given by

$$L\left(D|\theta\right) = \prod_{i=1}^{n} \prod_{y_i = E,T,(E \cup T)^c} \left\{\pi_{y_i}\left(x_{d_{m_i}}\right)\right\}^{I(Y=y_i,)}, \qquad (23.8)$$

where $I\left(Y = y_i\right)$ is an indicator function, taking value either 1 or 0.

After choosing a prior, the posterior probability can be calculated. The next step is to construct the efficacy–toxicity trade-off contours based on experts' opinion (see Figure 23.1 for an example). Along the contours, the preference for any pair of efficacy and toxicity is a constant.

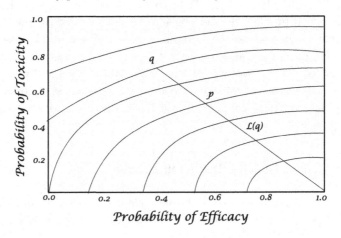

Figure 23.1:    Efficacy–Toxicity Trade-Off Contours for Pentostatin Trail

The authors also provide the dose-finding algorithm (Thall and Cook, 2004).

## 23.4    Odds Ratio Trade-off Model

Yin, Li, and Ji (2006) propose an odds ratio trade-off model. Let $p_j$ and $q_j$ be the pair of toxicity and efficacy probabilities of the dose $d_j$. We define a set of admissible doses, $d_j \in A$, if dose $d_j$ satisfies

$$\Pr\left(p_j < \bar{\pi}_T\right) > c_T \text{ and } \Pr\left(q_j > \underline{\pi}_E\right) > c_E, \qquad (23.9)$$

where $\bar{\pi}_T$ and $\underline{\pi}_E$ are prespecified upper toxicity and lower efficacy boundaries, and $c_T$ and $c_E$ are the fixed probability cutpoints.

The toxicity–efficacy odds ratio for the $j$th dose is given by

$$\omega_j = \frac{p_j/\left(1-p_j\right)}{q_j/\left(1-q_j\right)} = \frac{p_j\left(1-q_j\right)}{q_j\left(1-p_j\right)}, \tag{23.10}$$

which is the ratio of the areas between the lower-right and upper-left rectangles (Figure 23.2). Thus, a dose with a smaller value of $\omega_j$ is more desirable. Figure 23.2 shows the equivalent odds-ratio contours, along which all of the points have the same toxicity–efficacy odds ratio.

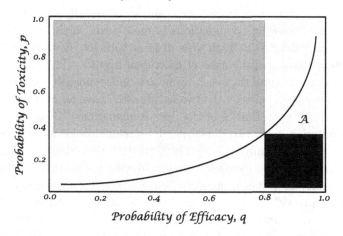

Figure 23.2:   Toxicity–Efficacy Odds Ratio Trade-off Contours

Here are the dose-escalation algorithms described by Lin and Yuan (2011):

(1) Let $j^*$ be the highest tried dose level. If $\Pr\left(p_{j^*} < \bar{\pi}_T\right) > p^\#$ for some chosen cutoff probability of escalation, $p^\# \geq p^*$, we escalate to dose level $j^* + 1$.
(2) Otherwise, the next patient cohort is treated at the dose with the smallest odds ratio in $A$. If $A$ is an empty set, then the trial is terminated and no dose is selected.
(3) Once the maximum sample size is reached, the dose with the minimum toxicity–efficacy odds ratio in $A$ is recommended.

Note that to protect the patient's safety, no dose-jumping is allowed.

## 23.5   Drug Combination

As pointed out by Yin and Yuan (2009), the motivations for combining two agents in medical research are (1) to induce a synergistic treatment effect, to increase the joint dose intensity with nonoverlapping toxicities, and (2) to target various tumor cell susceptibilities and disease pathways. Although there is monotonicity between the toxicity and the drug combinations, it is very difficult to determine the order of such combinations based on the knowledge of single-drug trials. For example, we usually cannot determine which of the following combinations is more toxic, high dose of drug $A$ with low dose drug $B$ or high dose drug $B$ with low dose drug $A$, based on the two dose-toxicity curves of individual agents. This is because we usually cannot assume that each agent acts independently on the patient. "Interactive effects between the two agents often have an enormous impact on the toxicity probabilities of the dose combinations. Consequently, the toxicity ordering in the two-dimensional dose combination space is typically unknown. Without fully understanding the toxicity order, it is difficult to escalate or deescalate the dose correctly during the trial. This difficulty severely limits the application of single agent dose finding designs for agent combination trials" (Yin and Yuan, 2009). Thall and Nguyen (2012) studied the adaptive randomization to improve utility-based dose finding with bivariate ordinal outcomes. In what follows, we will discuss the Yin–Yuan model.

Consider drug combinations of two agents, $J$ different doses of drug $A$ and $K$ different doses of drug $B$. Let $p_j$ be the prespecified toxicity probability (rate) corresponding to $A_j$, the $j$th dose of drug $A$, and let $q_k$ be the prespecified toxicity probability corresponding to $B_k$, the $k$th dose of drug $B$. There are usually the monotonic relationships: $p_1 \leq p_2 \leq \ldots \leq p_J$ and $q_1 \leq q_2 \leq \ldots \leq q_K$. We assume that the dose-toxicity relationships for the two individual agents are reasonably established. We also assume that the toxicity of a combination, $\pi_{jk}$, is no less than those of individual agents, i.e., $\pi_{jk} \geq \max(p_j, q_k)$. For this reason, the dose escalation starts with doses lower than the individual MTDs, say, 40% MTDs.

As in the CRM, we can take $p_j^\alpha$ and $q_k^\beta$ as the true toxicity probability for drug $A$ and drug $B$, respectively, where $\alpha$ and $\beta$ are unknown parameters with prior means centered at one. We link $\pi_{jk}$ with $(p_j^\alpha, q_k^\beta)$ through a copula-type regression model (Nelsen, 1999; Yin, Li, and Ji, 2006):

$$\pi_{jk} = 1 - \left\{ \left(1 - p_j^\alpha\right)^{-\gamma} + \left(1 - q_k^\beta\right)^{-\gamma} - 1 \right\}^{-1/\gamma}, \qquad (23.11)$$

where the association parameter $\gamma > 0$ characterizes the drug–drug interactive effect.

It is obvious that copula model (23.11) has several desirable attributes: $\pi_{jk} \geq \max(p_j, q_k)$, and $\pi_{jk}$ is a monotonic increasing functions of $p_j$ and $q_k$. We can see that the copula model has the following boundary properties: (1) if $p_j^\alpha = q_k^\beta = 0$, then $\pi_{jk} = 0$; (2) if $p_j^\alpha = 0$, then $\pi_{jk} = q_k^\beta$, and if $q_k^\beta = 0$, then $\pi_{jk} = p_j^\alpha$; and (3) if $\max(p_j^\alpha, q_k^\beta) = 1$, then $\pi_{jk} = 1$.

To derive the posterior distribution of the parameters $\alpha$, $\beta$, and $\gamma$, we first construct the likelihood function based on the binomial distribution with probabilities $\pi_{jk}$. Giving data $D$ that $m_{jk}$ out of $n_{jk}$ patients treated with $(A_j, B_k)$ have experienced toxicity, the likelihood is given by

$$L(\alpha, \beta, \gamma | D) \propto \prod_{j=1}^{J} \prod_{k=1}^{K} \pi_{jk}^{m_{jk}} (1 - \pi_{jk})^{n_{jk} - m_{jk}}, \qquad (23.12)$$

and the corresponding posterior distribution is

$$f(\alpha, \beta, \gamma | D) \propto L(\alpha, \beta, \gamma | D) f(\alpha) f(\beta) f(\gamma), \qquad (23.13)$$

where $f(\alpha)$, $f(\beta)$, and $f(\gamma)$ are gamma prior distribution with mean one.

Let $P_{MTD}$, $c_e$, and $c_d$ be the toxicity probability at MTD, the probability cutpoints for dose escalation, and deescalation, respectively. Yin and Yuan (2011) describe the following dose-finding algorithms:

(1) Patients in the first cohort are treated at the lowest dose combination $(A_1, B_1)$.

(2) At the current dose combination $(A_j, B_k)$, perform the following:

   (a) If $\Pr(\pi_{jk} < P_{MTD}) > c_e$, the dose is escalated to an adjacent dose combination with the toxicity probability higher than the current dose and closest to $P_{MTD}$. If the current dose combination is the highest dose combination $(A_J, B_K)$, the doses stay at the same levels.

   (b) If $\Pr(\pi_{jk} > P_{MTD}) > c_d$, the dose is deescalated to an adjacent dose combination with the toxicity probability lower than the current dose and closest to $P_{MTD}$. If the current dose combination is the lowest dose combination $(A_1, B_1)$, the trial is terminated.

   (c) Otherwise, the next cohort of patients continues to be treated at the same dose combination.

(3) Once the maximum sample size is reached, the dose combination with the toxicity probability closest to $P_{MTD}$ is selected as the MTD combination.

## 23.6   Summary

In this chapter, we have discussed a two-dimensional model for clinical trials. Either the outcome has two dimensions (efficacy and toxicity) or the treatment has two dimensions (drug combinations). The implementation of those models is slightly more complicated than for a one-dimensional model. We would like to leave the implementation of computer simulation program using those models for the readers as an exercise.

## Problems

**23.1** Implement the efficacy–toxicity trade-off model in Section 23.3 using SAS or R.

**23.2** Implement the odds-ratio trade-off model in Section 23.4 using SAS or R.

**23.3** Implement the drug combination model in Section 23.5 in SAS or R.

# Chapter 24

# Bayesian Approach to Biosimilarity Trial

## 24.1 Introduction

Biological drugs, such as protein, are large molecule products that are generally produced using a living system or organism and may be manufactured through biotechnology, derived from natural sources, or produced synthetically. The expanded scope of a biological product includes any alpha amino polymer with a specific defined sequence that is greater than 40 amino acids in size and any alpha amino acid polymer that (1) is made entirely by chemical synthesis and (2) is less than 100 amino acids in size.

Unlike small molecule drug products, for which we can make generic versions that contain the exact same active ingredient as the brand-name drug, due to the complexity of the large molecules, generic forms of biological products (called biosimilars or follow-on biologics) can only be similar to the reference product. To prove biosimilarity, stepwise approaches are required to assess the purity, potency, safety, and efficacy.

For generic version of small molecule drugs, the FDA (1984) was authorized to approve generic drug products under the Drug Price Competition and Patent Term Restoration Act, which is also known as the Hatch–Waxman Act. For approval of generic drug products, the FDA recently (February 2012) released three draft guidances about demonstrations of biosimilarity: (1) Scientific Considerations in Demonstrating Biosimilarity to a Reference Product, (2) Quality Considerations in Demonstrating Biosimilarity to a Reference Protein Product, and (3) Biosimilars: Questions and Answers Regarding Implementation of the Biologics Price Competition and Innovation (BPCI) Act of 2009. The FDA suggests the use of a stepwise approach for assessing biosimilarity. The stepwise approach is to evaluate biosimilarity step by step, which is well understood conceptually. However, little or no information regarding criteria for assessment of biosimilarity to be used at each step was mentioned. Similar requirements exist in the EU and Canada. The European Medicines Agency (EMA) has been successful in devising a system for authorizing the marketing of biosimilar products and has approved 14 biosimilars, 13 of which are currently on the market in major countries of the EU. In the U.S., the BPCI Act (as part of the Affordable Care Act) was written into law on 23 March 2010, and gives FDA the authority to approve SBDP (Chow and Ju, 2013).

Generals requirements for biosimilars (351(k) application) are (Sherman (FDA), 2012): (1) analytical studies demonstrating that the biological product is "highly similar" to the reference product notwithstanding minor differences in clinically inactive components; (2) animal studies, including the assessment of toxicity; and (3) a clinical study or studies, including the assessment of immunogenicity and pharmacokinetics (PK) or pharmacodynamics (PD), which must be sufficient to demonstrate safety, purity, and potency in one or more appropriate conditions of use for which the reference product is licensed.

Interchangeable biosimilars imply the two drug products can be exchanged at anytime without comprising the patient's safety and efficacy. The interchangeable product may be substituted for the reference product without the authorization of the health care provider.

The FDA's Draft Guidance outlines FDA's totality-of-the-evidence approach: (1) describes stepwise approach to evidence development, ensuring that development includes only those elements necessary to address residual uncertainty; (2) introduces the concept that only after a thorough review of data from structural and functional analyses can the FDA provide meaningful advice on the scope and extent of necessary animal and human testing; at least one study will be expected (immunogenicity/PK–PD), and comparative safety and effectiveness data may be necessary if residual uncertainty exists; and (3) makes it possible to exceed a current state-of-the-art analysis by evaluating more attributes and combination of attributes at greater sensitivities with multiple complementary methods.

To my knowledge, Prof. Chow's book (2014) is the first monograph on biosimilars from a statistical perspective, which provides excellent source information for the researcher.

## 24.2   Dilemma of Frequentist Noninferiority Trial

Before we study our new methods for the biosimilar products, let's take a look at a controversy about the frequentist noninferiority test.

Table 24.1: Dilemma of Noninferiority Trial

| Trial | Drug | Effect $\mu_i$ | Std Dev. | Sample Size | $p$-Value |
|-------|------|--------|----------|-------------|-----------|
| 1 | Control | 2 | 3.5 | 100 | 0.0227 |
|   | Placebo | 1 | 3.5 | 100 | |
| 2 | Test | 2.8 | 3.5 | 200 | 0.0286 (NI) |
|   | Control | 2 | 3.5 | 100 | |

Note: One-sided $\alpha = 0.025$, $\Delta_{NI} = 0.015 = 50\%$ of the 95% CI lower limit for the treatment difference in trial one.

Suppose we have data from two trials conducted sequentially: a superiority trial for $P$ (Placebo) versus $C$ (the first drug candidate) was conducted first followed by an NI trial with $T$ versus $C$. The hypothetical efficacy data are presented in Table 24.1. In the $P$ versus $C$ trial, $p$-value = 0.0227 < $\alpha = 0.025$; therefore, we claim $C$ superior to $P$. In the second NI trial, $T$ (the second drug candidate or the test drug in the follow-on study) versus $C$ trial with an NI margin of 0.015, the $p$-value for the NI test is = 0.0286 > $\alpha$; hence, we failed to show $T$ noninferior to $C$. However, if we consider the totality of the evidence under the constancy assumption, i.e., considering the data from the two trials all together, we can find the following:

(1) The standard deviation $\sigma_i$ is the same for all groups in the two trials.

(2) The treatment effect $\mu_i$ of the control group, $C$, is consistent between the two trials.

(3) The total sample size in the two trials is the same (200) for the control and test groups.

(4) The treatment effect is 2 for the control and 2.8 for the test groups.

How can we conclude $C$ is significantly better than $P$, and $T$ is not noninferior to $C$? Don't data show clearly that $T$ is better than, or at least as good as $C$? Is there something fundamentally wrong with NI testing?

Furthermore, when $\Delta_{NI} > \mu_C - \mu_T > 0$ and the sample size is large enough, we can reject both $H_{0s} : \mu_C - \mu_T \leq 0$ and $H_{0NI} : \mu_T - \mu_C < -\Delta_{NI}$. The first rejection leads to the conclusion that the control is superior to the test drug. On the other hand, the second rejection leads to the conclusion that the test drug is noninferior to the control. These two conclusions are contradictory.

## 24.3  Synergic Constancy Approach

### 24.3.1  *Conditional Bias of Historical Trial Data*

Under the constancy assumption across the historical and current clinical trials, we can consider the two trials as a single experiment and combine the data together. Let's call this approach the synergic constancy approach.

We denote the observations for the trial outcomes by $X_i$, where $i = 0, 1$, and 2 for the placebo, the brand drug and the follow-on drug, respectively. For simplicity, we assume $X_i$ is normally distributed with $\sigma = 1$. Thus, the means are normally distributed, i.e., $\bar{X}_{1h} \sim N(\mu_1, 1/n_{1h})$ and $\bar{X}_{0h} \sim N(\mu_0, 1/n_{0h})$ in the historical trial and $\bar{X}_{1c} \sim N(\mu_1, 1/n_{1c})$ and $\bar{X}_{2c} \sim N(\mu_2, 1/n_{2c})$ in the current trial. Here the subscripts $h$ and $c$ represent historical and current trials, respectively.

Because we generally approve the drug only when the efficacy is statistically significant, the estimation of treatment difference is positively biased (similar to the positive publication bias) in the historical trial. Furthermore, the sample mean $\bar{X}_{1h}$, conditional on the rejection from the historical trial, is biased upwards (similar to the positive publication bias), while $\bar{X}_{0h}$ conditional on the rejection is biased downwards.

Let the bias be

$$B_0 = E\left(\bar{X}_{0h}|\text{rejection}\right) - \mu_0 \tag{24.1}$$

$$B_1 = E\left(\bar{X}_{1h}|\text{rejection}\right) - \mu_1. \tag{24.2}$$

To reject $H_{0h}$ implies $(\bar{x}_{1h} - \bar{x}_{0h})\sqrt{n^*} \geq z_{1-\alpha}$ or $\bar{x}_{0h} \leq \bar{x}_{1h} - z_{1-\alpha}/\sqrt{n^*}$. Therefore, the expectation of $\bar{x}_{1h}$ is given by

$$E\left(\bar{x}_{0h}\right) = \frac{1}{1 - \Phi_0\left(c_*\right)} \int_{-\infty}^{\infty} \int_{-\infty}^{\bar{x}_{1h} - z_{1-\alpha}/\sqrt{n^*}} \bar{x}_{0h}\, f\left(\bar{x}_{0h}\right) f\left(\bar{x}_{1h}\right) d\bar{x}_{0h} d\bar{x}_{1h}, \tag{24.3}$$

where $1 - \Phi_0\left(c_*\right)$ is equal to power of the hypothesis test $H_{0h}$ in the historical trial,

$$f_0\left(\bar{x}_{0h}\right) = f\left(\bar{x}_{0h}; \mu_0, \frac{1}{n_{0h}}\right), \text{ and } f_1\left(\bar{x}_{1h}\right) = \left(\bar{x}_{1h}; \mu_1, \frac{1}{n_{1h}}\right).$$

Similarly, to reject $H_{0h}$ implies $(\bar{x}_{1h} - \bar{x}_{0h})\sqrt{n^*} \geq z_{1-\alpha}$ or $\bar{x}_{1h} \geq z_{1-\alpha}/\sqrt{n^*} + \bar{x}_{0h}$. The expectation of $\bar{x}_{1h}$ is given by

$$E\left(\bar{x}_{1h}\right) = \frac{1}{1 - \Phi_0\left(c_*\right)} \int_{-\infty}^{\infty} \int_{z_{1-\alpha}/\sqrt{n^*} + \bar{x}_{0h}}^{\infty} \bar{x}_{1h} f\left(\bar{x}_{0h}\right) f\left(\bar{x}_{1h}\right) d\bar{x}_{1h} d\bar{x}_{0h}. \tag{24.4}$$

It is interesting to know that given power, the bias is proportional to the standardized treatment effect, $(\mu_1 - \mu_0)/\sigma$ and

$$B_1 \approx \frac{n_{h0}B_d}{n_{h1} + n_{h0}} \text{ and } B_0 = B_d - B_1. \tag{24.5}$$

The numerical integrations of (24.3) and (24.4) and simulations using SAS Macro 24.1 below provide the same results for the bias in Table 24.2 for a historical, balanced two-group design. From the table, we can see that bias reduces as the sample size or power increases (the bias in mean difference $B_d = B_1 - B_0$).

Table 24.2: Relationship between Bias ($\times(\mu_1 - \mu_0)/\sigma$) and Power

| Power | 0.2 | 0.5 | 0.8 | 0.85 | 0.9 | 0.95 |
|---|---|---|---|---|---|---|
| Bias $B_0$ | −0.630 | −0.204 | −0.0624 | −0.0454 | −0.030 | −0.015 |
| Bias $B_1$ | 0.630 | 0.204 | 0.06244 | 0.0454 | 0.030 | 0.015 |
| Bias $B_d$ | 1.260 | 0.407 | 0.12484 | 0.0909 | 0.060 | 0.030 |

We know that most phase-III trials don't have 80% or 90% power as estimated at the design stage because the drug candidate selection process in a phase-II trial leads to an upward bias. When the treatment effect is overestimated based on phase-II trial data, the power is also overestimated. We will conservatively assume 5% bias in the standardized treatment effect. That is,

$$\frac{B_1}{(\mu_1 - \mu_0)/\sigma} = 5\%. \tag{24.6}$$

Since $(\mu_1 - \mu_0)/\sigma$ is not known, it can be estimated. Thus bias is estimated using (since we assume $\sigma = 1$)

$$\hat{B}_1 = 0.05(\bar{x}_{1h} - x_{0h}). \tag{24.7}$$

## >>SAS Macro 24.1:   Publication Bias>>

```
%Macro Bias(nSims=100000, N0h=1800, N1h=1800, sigma=1, mu0=0,
mu1=0.1, alpha=0.025);
Data Bias;
Keep ph Power mu0 mu1 x0Mean x1Mean dxMean Bias0 Bias1 Biasd;
N0h=&N0h;   N1h=&N1h;   alpha=&alpha;   mu0=&mu0;   mu1=&mu1;
sigma=&sigma;
z_alpha=Probit(1-alpha);
nStar=N1h*N0h/(N1h+N0h);
power=0; x0Mean=0; x1Mean=0; dxMean=0;
```

```
Do iSim=1 To &nSims;
x0h = Rand('normal', mu0, 1/sqrt(N0h));
x1h = Rand('normal',mu1, 1/sqrt(N1h));
deltax=x1h-x0h;
Zph=(x1h-x0h)*sqrt(nStar);
ph=1-ProbNorm(Zph);
If ph<=alpha Then Do;
power=power+1/&nSims;
dxMean=dxMean+deltax/&nSims;
x0Mean=x0Mean+x0h/&nSims;
x1Mean=x1Mean+x1h/&nSims;
End;
End; * end of iSim;
dxMean=dxMean/power;
x0Mean=x0Mean/power;
x1Mean=x1Mean/power;
Bias0=x0Mean-mu0; Bias1=x1Mean-mu1; Biasd=dxMean-(mu1-mu0);
Output;
Run;
Proc Print data=Bias; Run;
%Mend Bias;
<<SAS<<
```

**>>SAS: Invoke SAS Macro 24.1>>**
```
%Bias(nSims=1000000, N0h=1800, N1h=1800, sigma=1, mu0=0, mu1=0.1, al-
pha=0.025);
%Bias(nSims=1000000, N0h=248, N1h=248, sigma=1, mu0=0, mu1=0.1, al-
pha=0.025);
%Bias(nSims=1000000, N0h=2599, N1h=1300, sigma=1, mu0=0, mu1=0.1, al-
pha=0.025);
<<SAS<<
```

### 24.3.2 *Requirements for Biosimilarity or Noninferiority*

To approve the follow-on drug for marketing, there should be two efficacy requirements: (1) the follow-on drug is better than the placebo and (2) the follow-on drug is not worse than the brand drug by the noninferiority margin. The noninferiority margin is considered a trade-off between the efficacy and the other benefits that the new drug might provide, such as being safer, easier to administrate, less invasive, and/or cheaper. If there are no additional benefits of the new drug or the follow-on biologics, a noninferiority trial is not justified and should not be used. In the following discussion, we assume the constancy assumption should approximately hold.

(1) If the constancy between the two trials holds and the trials were conducted under very similar protocols with the same target populations, then we can test (strictly speaking, we don't have randomization between the groups) the follow-on drug in the current trial against the placebo in the historical trial to ensure the test drug is better than placebo, that is,

$$H_{01} : \mu_2 \leq \mu_0. \tag{24.8}$$

Since $\bar{x}_{0h}$ from the historical trial is biased, we define the test statistic as

$$Z_d = \left( \bar{X}_{2c} - (\bar{x}_{0h} - B_0) \right) \sqrt{n_{2c}} \sim N\left( \theta_d, 1 \right), \tag{24.9}$$

where

$$\theta_d = \left( \mu_2 - \bar{x}_{0h} + B_0 \right) \sqrt{n_{2c}}. \tag{24.10}$$

The parameter $\theta_d$ is expected to be zero or close to zero under $H_{01}$. In other words,

$$E\left( \theta_d \right) = \int \theta_d f\left( \bar{x}_{0h} | H_{01} \right) d\bar{x}_{0h} \approx 0.$$

For the sample size calculation, we assume the test drug and the original drug have the same treatment effect $\mu_2 = \mu_1 = \bar{x}_{1h} - B_1$. Assuming $n_{1h} = n_{0h}$, we have $B_1 = -B_0$ and $\hat{\theta}_d = \bar{x}_{1h} - \bar{x}_{0h}$. The sample size in the follow-on group for the test (24.8) is approximately given by

$$n_{2c} = \left( \frac{z_{1-a} + z_{1-\beta}}{\bar{x}_{1h} - \bar{x}_{0h}} \right)^2. \tag{24.11}$$

We assume the observed test statistic $z_{1-p_h}$ obtained from the historical trial for testing $H_{0h} : \mu_1 \leq \mu_0$ is

$$z_{1-p_h} = \frac{\bar{x}_{1h} - \bar{x}_{0h}}{\sqrt{1/n_{1h} + 1/n_{0h}}}. \tag{24.12}$$

From (24.11) and (24.12), we obtain

$$n_{2c} = \frac{n_{1h} n_{0h}}{n_{1h} + n_{0h}} \left( \frac{z_{1-a} + z_{1-\beta}}{z_{1-p_h}} \right)^2. \tag{24.13}$$

If $n_{1h}/n_{0h} = 1$, $\alpha = 0.025$, and $\beta = 0.15$, (24.13) becomes

$$\frac{n_{2c}}{n_{1h}} = \frac{4.5}{z_{1-p_h}^2}. \tag{24.14}$$

(2) To prove the noninferiority, we use the hypothesis test, $H_{02} : \mu_2 < \mu_1 - \Delta_{NI}$, where the noninferiority margin $\Delta_{NI} > 0$ is a trade-off between the efficacy and other benefits the follow-on might provide. This NI margin $\Delta_{NI}$ is not the conventional NI margin which concerns both the clinical and statistical justifications.

To ensure the noninferiority of the follow-on drug to the brand-name drug, we use the hypothesis test

$$H_{02} : \mu_2 \le \mu_1 - \Delta_{NI}, \tag{24.15}$$

at the level of significance $\alpha_{NI}$. If both hypotheses (24.8) and (24.15) are rejected, the efficacy of the follow-on product should be claimed.

To test hypothesis (24.15), it is required that

$$\Pr\left(Z_c > z_{1-\alpha_{NI}} | \mu_2 = \mu_1 - \Delta_{NI}\right) \le \alpha_{NI}, \tag{24.16}$$

where the test statistic is given by

$$Z_c = \frac{\bar{X}_{2c} - w_1(\bar{x}_{1h} - B_1) - (1 - w_1)\bar{X}_{1c} + \Delta_{NI}}{\sqrt{\frac{1}{n_{2c}} + \frac{(1-w_1)^2}{n_{1c}}}} \sim N(\theta_c, 1), \tag{24.17}$$

where

$$\theta_c = \frac{\mu_2 - \mu_1 - w_1\bar{x}_{1h} + w_1 B_1 + \Delta_{NI}}{\sqrt{\frac{1}{n_{2c}} + \frac{(1-w_1)^2}{n_{1c}}}}. \tag{24.18}$$

The parameter is approximately zero or is expected to be zero under global null $H_0 : \mu_1 = \mu_2 = \mu_0$. That is,

$$E(\theta_c) = \int \theta_c f(\bar{x}_{1h}|H_0) d\bar{x}_{1h} \approx 0 \text{ or } \le 0 \text{ for conservative side.}$$

The joint distribution of $Z_c$ and $Z_d$ is a bivariate normal distribution with means $\boldsymbol{\theta} = \left\{\begin{array}{c}\theta_c\\\theta_d\end{array}\right\}$ and covariate matrix $\Sigma = \left[\begin{array}{cc}1 & \sigma_{cd}\\\sigma_{cd} & 1\end{array}\right]$, where

$$\sigma_{cd} = \frac{n_{1c}}{n_{2c}}\frac{1}{\sqrt{n_{1c} + n_{2c}(1-w_1)^2}}.$$

Here $\alpha_{NI}$ should be larger than 0.5. The reason is that when the two drugs are identical in efficacy ($\Delta_{NI} = 0$ or $\mu_2 = \mu_1$) and $\alpha_{NI} = 0.5$ is chosen, the probability of rejecting (24.15) is approximately 50%. The rejection of $H_{02}$ is an additional efficacy requirement to rejection of $H_{01}$. Therefore, $\alpha_{NI}$ should be larger than 0.5 and we suggest using $\alpha_{NI} = 0.6$.

The power (the probability of getting the follow-on approval) is given by

$$\text{Power} = \Pr\left(Z_d \geq z_{1-\alpha} \cap Z_c \geq 0 | \bar{x}_{1h}, \bar{x}_{0h}, \sigma; \mu_1, \mu_2\right). \tag{24.19}$$

The Macro for biosimilar trials is presented in SAS Macro 24.2 and an example is given by Example 24.1 below.

### >>SAS Macro 24.2:  Biosimilar Clinical Trial>>

```
/* nRatio = Nc1/Nc2; CLh = confidence lower limit for (mul-mu0); */
%Macro BiosCT(nSims=100000, x0h=0, x1h=0.1, N0h=1800, N1h=1800,
sigma=1, mu0=0, mu1=0.1, mu2=0.1, nRatio=0.5, deltaNI=0.005, alpha=0.025,
beta=0.15, alpha_NI=0.6, w1=0);
Data BiosCT;
Keep ph Power w1 nRatio x1h x0h mu1 mu2 alpha_NI deltaNI N0h N1h N1c N2c
CLh zph PowerSup PowerNI Zc zd B1 nStar sigma;
x0h=&x0h; x1h=&x1h; nRatio=&nRatio; alpha_NI=&alpha_NI;
N0h=&N0h;   N1h=&N1h;   alpha=&alpha;   beta=&beta;   sigma=&sigma;
w1=&w1;
*Standardize the treatment effects;
mu1=&mu1; mu2=&mu2; deltaNI=&deltaNI;
z_alpha=Probit(1-alpha);
z_beta=Probit(1-beta);
z_NI=Probit(1-alpha_NI);
nStar=N1h*N0h/(N1h+N0h);
B1=0.05*(x1h-x0h);
Zph=(x1h-x0h)*sqrt(nStar)/sigma;
ph=1-ProbNorm(Zph);
CLh=(x1h-x0h)-z_alpha*sigma/Sqrt(nStar);
N2c=nStar*((z_alpha+z_beta)/Zph)**2;
*N2c=N1h*4.5/zph**2;
N1c=nRatio*N2c;
power=0; PowerSup=0; PowerNI=0;
Do iSim=1 To &nSims;
x1c = Rand('normal', mu1, sigma/sqrt(N1c));
x2c = Rand('normal',mu2, sigma/sqrt(N2c));
Zd=Sqrt(N2c)*(x2c-x0h-B1)/sigma;
se=sigma*Sqrt(1/N2c+(1-w1)**2/N1c);
```

```
Zc=(x2c-w1*(x1h-B1)-(1-w1)*x1c+deltaNI)/se;
If Zd>=z_alpha & Zc>=z_NI Then power=power+1/&nSims;
If Zd>=z_alpha Then PowerSup=PowerSup+1/&nSims;
If Zc>=z_NI Then PowerNI=PowerNI+1/&nSims;
End; * end of iSim;
Output;
Run;
Proc Print data=BiosCT; Run;
%Mend BiosCT;
```
<<**SAS**<<

## Example 24.1    Biosimilar Diabetic Trial Design

Diabetes is a problem within the body which causes blood glucose (sugar) levels to rise higher than normal. This is also called hyperglycemia. Insulin is a naturally occurring hormone secreted by the pancreas. Many people with diabetes are prescribed insulin, because their bodies either do not produce insulin (type 1 diabetes) or do not use insulin properly (type 2 diabetes). Type 2 diabetes is the most common form of diabetes. Hemoglobin A1c (HbA1c) is often used for diagnosis of diabetes. A person who has 6.5% or above in HbA1c is considered diabetic.

People with type 1 diabetes must use insulin. For type 2 diabetes healthy eating and exercise can help, but insulin might be needed to help the target blood glucose levels. There are more than 20 types of insulin sold in the United States. These insulin products differ in how they are made, how they work in the body, and how much they cost. It was forecasted that biosimilar insulins (BIs) and insulin analogs will produce $6.1 billion in brand sales in the United States and Europe (France, Germany, Italy, Spain, and United Kingdom) by 2018, saving health care systems $3.8 billion in the process (Heinemann and Hompesch, 2011). The savings will allow more patients to get the treatment benefit and/or can be used in other disease areas to improve patients' health.

The human insulin (HI) molecule has not only a defined primary structure, but also a well-defined secondary and tertiary structure. The manufactured biosimilar human insulin (BHI) has a primary structure that is different from that of HI. It is well known that changes in the structure of HI can affect the safety and efficacy of this therapeutic protein.

This is a biosimilar clinical trial with a BHI for treating diabetes after the early in-vivo studies showed high similarities between the follow-on and original biologics in terms of pharmacokinetic and pharmacodynamic parameters. The primary endpoint is HbA1c after 24 weeks of the treatment.

Patients will be randomized into either the original or the follow-on BHI (or insulin analogs). In the historical trial of the original product with 300 patients per group, it was shown that the original biologic has an mean HbA1c of 8.0%, 0.4% better than the control group (8.4%) with a standard common deviation of $\sigma = 1.8\%$, the noninferiority margin is determined to be $\Delta_{NI} = 0.12\%$ as a trade-off for cost savings. We use SAS Macro 24.2 to assist our designs for the three scenarios: (1) when the treatment effect of the original insulin product is overestimated ($\mu_1 = 8.1\%$), (2) when it is correctly estimated ($\mu_1 = 8\%$), and (3) when it is underestimated ($\mu_1 = 7.9\%$). Since $B_0 = 0.05\,(4\%) = 0.02\%$ is so small, we use the observed value for $\mu_0$, i.e., $\mu_0 = 8.4\%$. We weight the historical data by 20%, i.e., $w_1 = 0.2$. In SAS Macro 24.2 we assume large responses are better, therefore, we have to change the sign of $\mu_1$ and $\mu_2$ as well as their observed values in the historical trial when we invoke the macro.

With power for test $H_{01}$ equal to 95% (beta=0.05) and sample size ratio 0.5, the sample size required is 264 for the test control and 132 for the control group. The design will provide 65% power to reject both $H_{01}$ and $H_{02}$ for scenario 1, 82% power for scenario 2, and 87% power for scenario 3.

**>>SAS: Invoke SAS Macro 24.2>>**

Title "Treatment effect of the original insulin product is overestimated";
%BiosCT(x0h=-8.4, x1h=-8, N0h=300, N1h=300, sigma=1.8, mu0=-8.4, mu1=-8.1, mu2=-8.1, nRatio=0.5, deltaNI=0.12, alpha=0.025, beta=0.05, alpha_NI=0.6, w1=0.2);
Title "Treatment effect of the original insulin product is correctly estimated";
%BiosCT(x0h=-8.4, x1h=-8, N0h=300, N1h=300, sigma=1.8, mu0=-8.4, mu1=-8, mu2=-8, nRatio=0.5, deltaNI=0.12, alpha=0.025, beta=0.05, alpha_NI=0.6, w1=0.2);
Title "Treatment effect of the original insulin product is underestimated";
%BiosCT(x0h=-8.4, x1h=-8, N0h=300, N1h=300, sigma=1.8, mu0=-8.4, mu1=-7.9, mu2=-7.9, nRatio=0.5, deltaNI=0.12, alpha=0.025, beta=0.05, alpha_NI=0.6, w1=0.2);
**<<SAS<<**

## 24.4 Bayesian Approach Combining Preclinical and Clinical Data

To take the stepwise approach that carries the totality of evidence, we discuss a Bayesian approach that integrates the data from animal study and a clinical trial to reduce the sample size in the required clinical trial for efficacy. The key ideas are (1) larger molecules are complex; they involve the primary, secondary, and tertiary structures. Even the folding structure of a long protein molecule can affect the efficacy of the drug. Even if the follow-on product has identical primary and secondary structures, there can still be "residual difference" in structure. For such a structure-similar product, further testing in animal and in human may be necessary. (2) If a structure-similar drug that has a similar dose response curve (not at single point) in animals to the brand drug, then it is reasonable to believe its effect on human will be similar. Therefore, using the data from the animal studies, the size of the clinical trial can be reduced. We want to clarify that (1) here we compare the similarity in the response curve, not the response to a single fixed dose and (2) while knowing that humans and animals are different, i.e., a biologics can be effective in animals but not effective in humans, the present situation is different: we know the brand drug is effective in humans and the follow-on product is similar in structure and similar in dose-response. Given these preconditions, we believe the sample size in the clinical trial can be a smaller one.

Suppose we are conducting a clinical trial for testing the effectiveness of a biosimilar product. We assume a normal model for the primary endpoint:

$$X \sim N\left(\theta, \sigma^2\right), \tag{24.20}$$

where $\theta$ is the treatment difference between the biosimilar drug and original brand drug and $\sigma^2$ is assumed known from the large historical trial(s).

We assume that the prior for the treatment effect of the biosimilar can be decomposed into two parts: (1) the identical treatment effect as the brand, i.e., $\theta$ centered at 0 and (2) skeptical part that has the treatment effect worse than the brand drug by a noninferior amount $\Delta_{NI}$, Specifically, the prior is

$$\pi(\theta) = w_1 \pi_0(\theta) + (1 - w_1)\pi_0(\theta - \Delta_{NI}), \tag{24.21}$$

where $\pi_0(\theta)$ is the prior of treatment difference $\theta$ derived from the historical brand drug trials with sample size $n_0$ and a common standard deviation $\sigma$, that is, $\pi_0(\theta) = N\left(0, \frac{2\sigma^2}{n_0}\right)$ and $\pi_0(\theta - \Delta_{NI}) = N\left(-\Delta_{NI}, \frac{2\sigma^2}{n_0}\right)$. Here the weight $w_1$ is determined by the data from preclinical dose-response studies on animals.

$$w_1 = \frac{1}{1 + \exp\left(-\frac{\bar{d}}{d}\right)}, \tag{24.22}$$

where $d$ is the average distance between the response curves of the two drug forms (the brand and the follow-on products):

$$d = \sqrt{\frac{1}{K} \sum_{i=1}^{K} (\bar{x}_{1i} - \bar{x}_{0i})^2}, \qquad (24.23)$$

where $K$ should be at least 5 points (dose levels) centered at the dose level of interest; $\bar{x}_{1i}$ and $\bar{x}_{0i}$ are the mean responses with dose $i$ in test group and the reference groups, respectively; and $\bar{d}$ is the expected value of $d$ when the two drug forms are truly identical. If we conduct a randomized three-group animal study with two groups treated with the brand biologics and one group treated with the biosimilar, we can estimate $\bar{d}$ based on (24.23) using the data from the two groups treated with the brand drug.

In the follow-on trial, $y_{1i}$ from $N\left(\mu_1, \sigma^2\right)$ and $y_{0i}$ from $N\left(\mu_0, \sigma^2\right)$, $i = 1, ..., n_1$, are the mean responses in the follow-on and original brand groups, respectively. Since the historical study for approval of the original drug is usually larger, we assume either the estimation of $\sigma^2$ from the historical trial(s) is precise in comparison with the smaller follow-on trial or the impact of the variation of $\hat{\sigma}$ is much smaller than that of the mean treatment difference. Therefore, we treat $\sigma$ as if it is a known in the model. The posterior distribution of the treatment difference is a mixed normal distribution

$$f\left(\theta | \boldsymbol{y}_1, \boldsymbol{y}_0\right) = w_1 N \left( \frac{\bar{y}_1 - \bar{y}_0}{n_0 + n_1}, \frac{2\sigma^2}{n_0 + n_1} \right)$$

$$+ (1 - w_1) N \left( \frac{n_0 \left(-\Delta_{IN}\right) + n_1 (\bar{y}_1 - \bar{y}_0)}{n_0 + n_1}, \frac{2\sigma^2}{n_0 + n_1} \right), \qquad (24.24)$$

where $\boldsymbol{y}_1 = (y_{11}, ..., y_{1n_1})'$, $\boldsymbol{y}_0 = (y_{01}, ..., y_{0n_1})'$, and $\bar{y}_1$ and $\bar{y}_0$ are the average responses in the two groups.

To claim biosimilarity, we want the probability of the follow-on product being worse than the brand drug by the noninferiority margin to be very small. In other words, we require the posterior probability

$$F\left(\theta = -\Delta_{NI} | \boldsymbol{y}_1, \boldsymbol{y}_0\right) \leq \alpha, \qquad (24.25)$$

where the nominal level $\alpha$ can be, for example, 5% or 2.5%.

## 24.5   Bayesian Hierarchical Bias Model

Wu (2014) and Wu et al. (2014) propose a Bayesian hierarchical bias model to establish biosimilarity for a composite endpoint (ACR20). We will discuss the model in this section.

### 24.5.1   *Biosimilarity Using Composite Endpoint*

Although, in the past few years, some statistical methods have been proposed for the case of a single primary efficacy endpoint, some biological products are designed to treat medical conditions with improvement measured by several endpoints. For example, rheumatoid arthritis (RA) is a disease of the immune system that leads to the inflammation in the joints. It causes myriad symptoms such as pain, joint swelling, fatigue, weakness, and stiffness. It also leads to loss of physical function and permanent joint damage.

The exact cause of RA is unknown, but it is believed that patients with RA have an over-abundance of tumor necrosis factor (TNF). An increased level of TNF is responsible for joint inflammation. Treatments of mild cases of RA include disease-modifying antirheumatic drugs (DMARDs). However, for moderate to severe cases of RA that do not respond well to DMARDs, intervention using biological products such as TNF blockers may be helpful in slowing down RA progression.

ACR20 improvement criterion (Felson, Anderson, Boers et al., 1995) is defined as 20% or more reduction (improvement) in (1) tender joint count and (2) swollen joint count, and in at least 3 of the following 5 areas: (3) physician global assessment of disease activity, (4) patient global assessment of disease activity, (5) patient assessment of pain, (6) physical disability or functionality, and (7) inflammatory marker: ESR or CRP. In clinical trials studying RA, the current standard measure of efficacy is the ACR20 criteria recommended by the American College of Rheumatology (ACR) Committee. For each individual patient in a trial, it measures if this patient has experienced a clinical response of overall improvement by evaluating the percentage of improvement in a core set of variables during the trial. Therefore, ACR20 is a composite criterion and has served as a working model for other disorders that currently require multiple primary endpoints (Offen et al., 2007). The percent change in each of these variables is also measured at different time points such as 3, 6, and 12 months and one of the time points is used to establish primary efficacy. Other similar but more stringent measures such as ACR50 or ACR70 (i.e., > 50% or >

70% improvement on the same set of endpoints) and other validated scales such as the Disease Activity Score in 28 joints (DAS28) criteria are also adopted.

## 24.5.2   *Study Design and Noninferiority Hypotheses*

Motivated by the desire to decrease sample size, we want our model to allow the evidence from the current biosimilarity trial to meaningfully connect to any similarly conducted historical trials that have evaluated the effect of the licensed reference biological product. Since a standard treatment is already available for the medical condition, including a placebo arm in the current trial will not be ethical. We can use $k$ to index the biological product with $k = 1$ representing the innovator reference product and $k = 2$ the proposed follow-on biological product. In this case, we are interested in testing if, based on the composite endpoint, the proposed biological product is not inferior to the licensed biological product. This noninferiority design may reduce the number of sample subjects needed.

In this two-arm design, patients are randomized to either the original reference or the follow-on generic biological product. For each patient, outcomes on $J$ multiple endpoints will be measured at prespecified follow-up times. These $J$ endpoints can generally be considered as independent measures. We can use $x_{kji}$ to denote the $j$th endpoint ($j = 1, 2, ..., J$) observed in the $i$th patient receiving the product $k$. In this case, we can assume that it is normally distributed as

$$x_{kji} \sim N\left(\mu_{kj}, \sigma_k^2\right) \qquad (24.26)$$

where $k = 1$ or 2, and $i = 1, 2, ..., n_k$. The fixed randomization ratio is therefore equal to $R = n_2/n_1$. $\mu_{kj}$ is the mean response for the $j$th endpoint and $\sigma_k^2$ is the variance which is assumed to be same for all $J$ endpoints but different between the products. In addition, we want to consider combining these $J$ endpoints into a single composite binary efficacy endpoint $y_{ki}$ which can be generally defined as

$$y_{ki} = \begin{cases} 1 \text{ if } \boldsymbol{x}_{ki} \geq \boldsymbol{\omega} \\ 0 \text{ otherwise} \end{cases}, \qquad (24.27)$$

where $\boldsymbol{x}_{ki} = (x_{k1i}, x_{k2i}, ..., x_{kJi})'$ is the random vector of outcomes for the $i$th patient and $\boldsymbol{\omega} = (\omega_1, \omega_2, ..., \omega_J)'$ is a $J$-dimensional vector of cut points for the endpoints common to both biological products, assuming that higher values of $x_{kji}$ are desirable. If we denote the probability of a response on the composite endpoint for product $k$ as $p_k$, then $p_k = P(y_{ki} = 1) = P(\boldsymbol{x}_{ki} > \omega)$, and our noninferiority hypotheses of interest can be constructed as

$$H_0 : p_2 - p_1 \le -\delta \text{ versus } H_a : p_2 - p_1 > -\delta, \qquad (24.28)$$

where $(\delta > 0)$ is the prespecified noninferiority margin for the difference between the two probabilities.

### 24.5.3 *Bayesian Approach*

There are several advantages of approaching this biosimilarity hypothesis testing problem from a Bayesian perspective. First, if the efficacy profile of the licensed reference biological product being compared to a placebo control has been established in a historical trial, and if there are additional historical trials evaluating the effect of this product, then we can incorporate these sources of information into the current trial of biosimilarity. These historical trials can be further assumed to be exchangeable. Also, since multiple endpoints are considered in developing the composite endpoint, the Bayesian approach allows for borrowing between the $J$ multiple endpoints on the precision parameters in addition to the borrowing between historical trials.

The use of the previous data in the model can also means that fewer subjects may be needed for the reference product and more subjects can be randomized to the biosimilar candidate. According to (24.27), $p_k$ is a function of the parameters such that $p_k = f(\mu_{k1}, \mu_{k2}, ..., \mu_{kJ}, \sigma_k^2)$ for $k = 1$ or 2.

### 24.5.4 *Hierarchical Bias Model*

Wu's hierarchical bias model can include any number of historical trials for the licensed reference product, but for simplicity, here we discuss the case with only one historical trial. Let $x_{1hji}$ be the value of the $j$th endpoint observed for the $i$th patient receiving the original reference product $k = 1$ in the historical trial and assume normal distribution:

$$x_{1hji} \sim N\left(\mu_{1hj}, \sigma_1^2\right), \qquad (24.29)$$

where $i = 1, 2, ..., n_{1h}$ and $j = 1, 2, ..., J$.

In the above model, we assume that the historical trial and the current biosimilarity trial share the same within-study variance parameter $\sigma_1^2$, and it is also assumed to be constant across all $J$ endpoints. This assumption allows borrowing strength between the historical trials and also between the $J$ endpoints. In addition, we can represent the $j$th sample mean as $\bar{x}_{1hj}$ which is equal to $(\sum_{i=1}^{n_{1h}} x_{1hji} = 1)/n_{1h}$. Other sample means can be similarly defined.

Additionally, under exchangeability, we consider that the mean parameters, $\mu_{1j}$ of the current biosimilarity trial and $\mu_{1hj}$ of the historical trial, for the original reference product, come from the same distribution (constancy assumption):

$$\mu_{1j}, \mu_{1hj} \sim N\left(\mu_{1j}^0, \sigma_{1b}^2\right), \tag{24.30}$$

where $\mu_{1j}^0$ is the overall mean and $\sigma_{1b}^2$ is the between-trial variance parameter, which is assumed to be the same across the $J$ endpoints. Hierarchical modeling is a logical way of combining historical data when exchangeability between parameters is highly plausible as in the current problem. Modeling the mean endpoints hierarchically recognizes that these historical trials, although using the same licensed reference product, may exhibit slightly different mean endpoints due to possible but small differences in the conduct of the trials, population shift, or changes in medical practice. This variation will be captured by the between-trial variance parameter. This ensures that the current biosimilarity trial is validly connected to the historical trials via the assumption of exchangeability.

For the new generic follow-on product in the current biosimilarity trial, we think of its mean response on the $j$ endpoint, $\mu_{2j}$, as having a bias term from that of the mean endpoint of the original product, $\mu_{1j}$. Therefore, we propose this relationship

$$\mu_{1j} = \mu_{2j} + \zeta_j, \tag{24.31}$$

where $\zeta_j$ represents the bias of $\mu_{2j}$ from $\mu_{1j}$. If $\zeta_j$ is equal to 0, then $\mu_{2j} = \mu_{1j}$ meaning that the follow-on product has the same mean as the licensed reference product on the $j$th endpoint. If $\zeta_j < 0$, then it means the follow-on product exhibits a better effect than the reference product on the $j$th endpoint, and the opposite interpretation follows if $\zeta_j < 0$. Since we do not know the true value of $\zeta_j$, we can assume a model for this bias parameter as

$$\zeta_j \sim N(\theta, \sigma_\zeta^2), \tag{24.32}$$

where $j = 1, 2, ..., J$. We center the expectation of $\zeta_j$ skeptically at the null hypothesis, $\theta$, to allow the data to reflect and influence its true direction and magnitude away from the null value. The null value $\theta$ is the margin on the scale of individual endpoints, such that when this margin is uniformly subtracted from all of the mean responses, the probability of the binary composite endpoint will decrease by exactly the amount of $\delta_{\min}$ as in

$$f(\mu_{k1} - \theta, \mu_{k2} - \theta, ..., \mu_{kJ} - \theta, \sigma_k^2) - f(\mu_{k1}, \mu_{k2}, ..., \mu_{kJ}, \sigma_k^2) = -\delta_{\min}.$$

For ACR20, we let $S_i$ = exact $i$ items from items 3 to 7 achieveing at least 20% improvement, then we have

$$f(\mu_{k1}, \mu_{k2}, ..., \mu_{kJ}, \sigma_k^2)$$
$$= \Phi\left(-\frac{20 - \mu_{k1}}{\sigma_k}\right) \Phi\left(-\frac{20 - \mu_{k2}}{\sigma_k}\right) [\Pr(S_3) + \Pr(S_4) + \Pr(S_5)].$$

This relationship between $\delta_{\min}$ and $\theta$ is one-on-one. Therefore, centering the mean of $\zeta_j$ on $\theta$ also suggests that $\mu_{1j}$ and $\mu_{2j}$ are dissimilar to begin with. We also assume the variance parameter $\sigma_\zeta^2$ to be the same across all $J$ endpoints but a large $\sigma_\zeta^2$ will suggest that this distribution is only weakly informative.

Now that we have completely specified the hierarchical bias model, we can consider the following prior distributions for the parameters. For $\mu_{1j}^0$, we can assume a flat noninformative prior as $\Pr\left(\mu_{1j}^0\right) \propto 1$ for $j = 1, 2, ..., J$ since we have no prior information regarding these overall mean parameters. We can elicit Jeffrey's prior distributions for the remaining variance parameters such that $\Pr(\sigma_{21}) \propto 1/\sigma_1$, $\Pr(\sigma_{22}) \propto 1/\sigma_2$, $\Pr(\sigma_{1b}^2) \propto 1/\sigma_{1b}^2$, and $\Pr(\sigma_\zeta^2) \propto 1/\sigma_\zeta^2$. As a result, the joint posterior distribution of all parameters will be given by the product of all likelihoods and specified densities of the parameters as

$$\Pr\left(\boldsymbol{\mu}_1, \boldsymbol{\mu}_{1h}, \boldsymbol{\mu}_1^0, \boldsymbol{\mu}_2, \boldsymbol{\zeta}, \sigma_1^2, \sigma_{1b}^2, \sigma_2^2, \sigma_\zeta^2 | \boldsymbol{x}_{1j}, \boldsymbol{x}_{1hj}, \boldsymbol{x}_{2j}, j = 1, ...J\right)$$

$$\propto \left(\frac{\Pr\left(\mu_{1j}^0\right)}{\sigma_1^2 \sigma_{1b}^2 \sigma_2^2 \sigma_\zeta^2}\right) \prod_{j=1}^{J} [L\left(\mu_{1j}, \sigma_1^2 | \boldsymbol{x}_{1j}\right) L\left(\mu_{1hj}, \sigma_1^2 | \boldsymbol{x}_{1hj}\right) L\left(\mu_{2j}, \sigma_2^2 | \boldsymbol{x}_{2j}\right),$$

$$\Pr\left(\mu_{1j} | \mu_{1j}^0, \sigma_{1b}^2\right) \Pr\left(\mu_{1hj} | \mu_{1j}^0, \sigma_{1b}^2\right) \Pr\left(\zeta_j | \theta, \sigma_\zeta^2\right)] \qquad (24.33)$$

where $\boldsymbol{\mu}_1, \boldsymbol{\mu}_{1h}, \boldsymbol{\mu}_1^0, \boldsymbol{\mu}_2$, and $\boldsymbol{\zeta} \in R^J$, $\boldsymbol{x}_{1j}$ represent the data on all $n_1$ subjects, $x_{1hj}$ represent the data on all $n_{1h}$ subjects, and $\boldsymbol{x}_{2j}$ represent the data on all $n_2$ subjects for the $j$th endpoint with $j = 1, 2, ..., J$. Note that $\mu_{2j} = \mu_{1j} - \zeta_j$.

Based on the joint density in (24.23), we can find the conditional posterior distributions for the parameters. For the historical trial, the conditional posterior distribution for $\mu_{1hj}$ is given by

$$\mu_{1hj}|\boldsymbol{x}_{1hj} \sim N\left(\tilde{\sigma}_{1h}^2\left(\frac{n_{1h}\bar{x}_{1hj}}{\sigma_1^2} + \frac{\mu_{1j}^0}{\sigma_{1b}^2}\right), \tilde{\sigma}_{1h}^2 = \left(\frac{n_{1h}}{\sigma_1^2} + \frac{1}{\sigma_{1b}^2}\right)^{-1}\right),$$

(24.34)

where $j = 1, 2, ..., J$. The mean of the posterior distribution is a weighted average of the sample mean $\bar{x}_{1hj}$ and $\mu_{1j}^0$. As for the original reference product in the current trial, the mean parameters will have conditional posterior distributions as

$$\mu_{1j}|\boldsymbol{x}_{1j}, \boldsymbol{x}_{2j} \qquad (24.35)$$

$$\sim N\left(\tilde{\sigma}_1^2\left(\frac{n_1\bar{x}_{1j}}{\sigma_1^2} + \frac{n_2(\bar{x}_{2j}+\zeta_j)}{\sigma_1^2} + \frac{\mu_{1j}^0}{\sigma_{1b}^2}\right), \tilde{\sigma}_1^2 = \left(\frac{n_1}{\sigma_1^2} + \frac{n_2}{\sigma_2^2} + \frac{1}{\sigma_{1b}^2}\right)^{-1}\right).$$

The mean of the distribution is given by the weighted average of the sample mean $\bar{x}_{1j}$, $\mu_{1j}^0$, and $(\bar{x}_{2j}+\zeta_j)$. The overall mean parameter $\mu_{1j}^0$ will therefore have conditional posterior distribution given by

$$\mu_{1j}^0 \sim N\left(\frac{\mu_{1j} + \mu_{1hj}}{2}, \tilde{\sigma}_0^2 = \frac{\sigma_{1b}^2}{2}\right). \qquad (24.36)$$

The bias parameters will take on the following conditional posterior distributions

$$\zeta_j \sim N\left(\tilde{\sigma}_\zeta^2\left(\frac{n_2(\mu_{1j} - \bar{x}_{2j})}{\sigma_2^2} + \frac{\theta}{\sigma_\zeta^2}\right), \tilde{\sigma}_\zeta^2 = \left(\frac{n_2}{\sigma_2^2} + \frac{1}{\sigma_\zeta^2}\right)^{-1}\right). \qquad (24.37)$$

However, the mean parameter for the generic follow-on product is completely specified by both $\mu_{1j}$ and $\zeta_j$ as in (24.21); therefore, its posterior distribution will be given by its respective posterior distributions

$$\mu_{2j}|\boldsymbol{x}_{1j}, \boldsymbol{x}_{2j} = \mu_{1j}|\boldsymbol{x}_{1j}, \boldsymbol{x}_{2j} - \zeta_j, j = 1, 2, ..., J \qquad (24.38)$$

As for the within-study variance parameter for the licensed reference product, using the Jeffrey's prior, we get the conditional posterior distribution as the inverse-gamma distribution with shape and scale parameters given by

$$\sigma_1^2|\boldsymbol{x}_{1j}, \boldsymbol{x}_{1hj}, j = 1, ..., J$$

$$\sim IG\left(\frac{J(n_1 + n_{1h})}{2}, \frac{1}{2}\sum_{j=1}^{J}\sum_{i=1}^{n_1}(x_{1ji} - \mu_{1j})^2 + \frac{1}{2}\sum_{j=1}^{J}\sum_{i=1}^{n_{1h}}(x_{1hji} - \mu_{1hj})^2\right).$$

(24.39)

The between-study variance parameter for the licensed reference product will also follow a conditional posterior distribution as an inverse-gamma distribution given by

$$\sigma_{1b}^2 \sim IG\left(J, \frac{1}{2}\sum_{j=1}^{J}\left(\mu_{1j} - \mu_{1j}^0\right)^2 + \frac{1}{2}\sum_{j=1}^{J}\left(\mu_{1hj} - \mu_{1j}^0\right)^2\right). \qquad (24.40)$$

Additionally, the variance parameter for the follow-on product has conditional posterior distribution as

$$\sigma_1^2 | \boldsymbol{x}_{2j}, j = 1, ..., J \sim IG\left(\frac{Jn_2}{2}, \frac{1}{2}\sum_{j=1}^{J}\sum_{i=1}^{n_2}\left(x_{2ji} - (\mu_{1j} - \zeta_j)\right)^2\right). \qquad (24.41)$$

Lastly, the variance parameter for the bias term $\sigma_\zeta^2$ can be shown to be an inverse-gamma distribution

$$\sigma_\zeta^2 \sim IG\left(\frac{J}{2}, \frac{1}{2}\sum_{j=1}^{J}(\zeta_j - \theta)^2\right). \qquad (24.42)$$

Using the conditional posterior distributions in (24.34), (24.35), (24.37), (24.38), (24.39), (24.40), (24.41), and (24.42), we can find the marginal posterior distributions of $\mu_{1j}$, $\sigma_1^2$, $\mu_{2j}$, and $\sigma_2^2$ and, hence, those of $p_k = f(\mu_{k1}, ..., \mu_{kJ}, \sigma_k^2)$ for $k = 1$ or $2$ and perform posterior inference based on the distribution of $p_2 - p_1$. There are two ways to find the marginal posterior densities. One way is to integrate out the conditioning parameters using their conditional posterior densities, but this can be highly intractable. A more viable way is to use Markov chain Monte Carlo (MCMC) methods to simulate the marginal posterior densities from the conditional posterior densities. In this case, since we have close forms for the conditional posterior distributions, we can use Gibbs sampling, one of the widely used MCMC techniques. Using the same Gibbs sampling, we can also simulate the marginal posterior distribution of $p_2 - p_1$. We can directly estimate the posterior probability $\Pr(p_2 - p_1 > -\delta_{\min} | \boldsymbol{x}_{1j}, \boldsymbol{x}_{1hj}, \boldsymbol{x}_{2j}, j = 1, ..., J) = E[I(p2 - p1 > -\delta_{\min}) | \boldsymbol{x}_{1j}, \boldsymbol{x}_{1hj}, \boldsymbol{x}_{2j}, j = 1, 2, ..., J]$. The decision rule is to reject the null hypothesis when this posterior probability is greater than a critical probability $c$ which can be prespecified as high as 95% or 97.5% depending on the clinical significance.

The determination of noninferiority margin and the simulation algorithms as well as a rheumatology trial example are discussed by Wu (2014) and Wu et al. (2014).

## 24.6 Summary

We have introduced the concept of biosimilar trials and discussed the challenges. We studied the dilemma of traditional noninferiority design method and three new methods, the synergic constancy approach: a Bayesian approach that combines preclinical and clinical data for the decision-making, and the Bayesian hierarchical bias model. Biosimilar trial study is an emerging field that opens many opportunities, while at the same time, it puts a lot of challenges in front of researchers.

**Problems**

**24.1** Review regulatory guidance on biosimilar trials and explain the stepwise totality evidence approach in the FDA guidance.

**24.2** Reduce the Bayesian hierarchical bias model to the case with a single endpoint.

**24.3** Use SAS Macro 24.2 to conduct a simulation study of the performance of the synergic constancy approach.

# Chapter 25

# Adaptive Multiregional Trial Design

## 25.1 Introduction

A global multiregional clinical trial (MRCT) is an international clinical trial conducted in multiple countries with a uniform study protocol. Its goal is to get the drug approval in multiple countries. Therefore, it is involved with the health authorities in multiple countries/regions. In a Q&A format, the answer to the ICH E5 Q11 states, a multiregional trial for the purpose of bridging could be conducted in the context of a global development program designed for near simultaneous worldwide registration. The objectives of such a study would be (1) to show that the drug is effective in the region and (2) to compare the results of the study among the regions with the intent of establishing that the drug is not sensitive to ethnic factors. The multiregional trials are built on a common belief that the primary effects of the drug are expected to be the same (consistency principle). Otherwise, the trial can be conducted separately in different countries, and bridging studies can be used if the drug is already approved in some other countries. In recent years, the paradigm of conducting clinical trials starts to shift from bridging studies, which are conducted after a medical product has be approved in one or more of the three major ICH regions (U.S., EU, and Japan), to a simultaneous drug development or global multiregional trials.

A multiregional trial has at least two main objectives. First, it is necessary to show a significant benefit in effect of a new drug in the entire population. Second, one needs to demonstrate that the results for a particular region are consistent with those from the entire population (Ikeda and Bretz, 2010; Shih and Quan, 2013).

A principle for specification of the consistency criterion for a global trial design is to treat all regions equally regardless of the market volumes of individual regions and countries. However, health authorities in different

Table 25.1:   An Example of Global Multiregional Clinical Trial

| Region | Number of Patients | Number of events Tic | Clop | HR (95%CI) |
|--------|--------------------|----------------------|------|------------|
| Asia/Australia | 1714 | 95 | 116 | 0.80 (0.61, 1.04) |
| Cent/Sth America | 1237 | 91 | 104 | 0.86 (0.65, 1.13) |
| Euro/Mid E/Afr | 13859 | 576 | 712 | 0.80 (0.72, 0.90) |
| North America | 1814 | 102 | 82 | 1.25 (0.93) |

Source: Naoyuki Yasuda, ICDRA: Workshop H (25 October 2012)

regions may have different efficacy criteria, e.g., they may have different endpoint measures. In such case, the protocol may need to specify which endpoint for which regions. This complicated situation will not be discussed in detail in this chapter. Instead, we will discuss only the case with the same endpoint for all regions.

Consistency in efficacy is the key to getting the drug approval in all regions. But exactly what does consistency mean here (see Table 25.1 and Figure 25.1 for an example of MRCT results)? There are two types of consistency assessment: (1) the hypothesis testing–based methods, and (2) the observed treatment effect–based methods. Suppose we treat every patient in the world with a study drug and look at the average drug effects in each country or region; we can expect the effects will be different between any two countries or regions. Given the complete population data, how do we define the consistency? If we also consider future patients, how should we define the consistency? If we can define it in these scenarios, we can then propose a meaningful hypothesis test for the consistency and

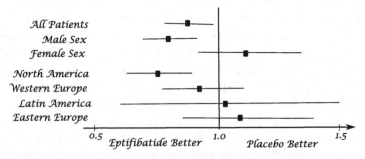

*Odds Ratio of Death or Nonfatal Myocardial Infraction*
*(Horizontal lines are Confidence Intervals)*

Figure 25.1:   Partial Data from a Multiregional Trial
Source: *New England Journal of Medicine*, 1998, 339:436–443.

practically make inference about the consistency with only partial data or a sample of the population in hand. If we define consistency directly based on the observed data, we may still need to understand what the definition means in terms of parameters. Therefore, the definition of consistency based on the parameters is a natural approach and hence why we propose hypothesis-based frequentist and Bayesian approaches.

There are several issues raised by MRCTs in trial design (e.g., sample size distribution across regions), trial conduct and monitoring, and data analysis (e.g., how to use the whole data to assess individual region effect). In assessing global treatment effect, should we propose a "one country/region one vote" or "one person one vote" policy? Or should the regional effect should be weighted inversely by their variance to obtain the most accurate statistical assessment? How should we deal with the Simpson's paradox when it occurs: overall treatment effect exists, but no effect (opposite direction of treatment effect) in regions?

The consistency across regions (CAR) refers to the similarity of treatment effects across regions represented by $\theta_i$, $(i = 1, ..., K)$. The statistical expression of the overall treatment effect $\theta$ is model dependent. For the fixed-effect model, it is a weighted average of the (fixed) individual treatment effects of the participating regions. Weights are proportions of the sample sizes. Hence, the overall treatment effect is trial specific. For a random-effect model, the individual treatment is random, with $\theta$ as its parent mean.

In this chapter, we will discuss the classical and adaptive multiregional clinical trials.

## 25.2 Unified Additional Requirement for Regional Approval in MRCT

### 25.2.1 *Current Consistency Study*

To evaluate the possibility of applying the overall results in an MRCT to the specific region of interest, the Japanese Ministry of Health, Labour and Welfare (MHLW) provides two methods for determining the number of Japanese subjects required for establishing consistency in treatment effect between the Japanese group and the entire group.

For Method 1, the consistency is defined as $D_J > \lambda D$, where $D_J$ and $D$ are the observed treatment effects for the Japanese group and the entire group, respectively. Thus, the sample size for the Japanese group in a

MRCT should satisfy

$$\Pr(D_J > \lambda D) > 1 - \beta',  \tag{25.1}$$

where $\lambda \geq 0.5$ and $\beta' \leq 0.2$.

For Method 2, the consistency is defined globally as $D_1 > 0, D_2 > 0, \dots, D_K > 0$. Thus, the sample size for the Japanese group in an MRCT should satisfy

$$\Pr(D_1 > 0, D_2 > 0, \dots, D_K > 0) > 1 - \beta',  \tag{25.2}$$

where $D_i$ represents the observed treatment effect for region $i$, $i = 1, \dots, K$. and $\beta' \leq 0.2$.

Based on the Japanese MHLW guidance, several statistical methods have been proposed to apply the overall results of the MRCT to the specific region. On the basis of Method 2, Kawai et al. (2008) proposed an approach to partition the total sample size to the individual regions to assure a high probability of observing a consistent trend if the treatment effect is positive and uniform across the regions.

Kawai, Chuang-Stein et al. (2007) discuss the sample size needed for demonstrating the consistency if it exists. Quan, Zhao et al. (2010) derived a formula for sample size from region $i$ based on a general setting with a fixed-effect model without assuming the same treatment effects for all regions. When the true treatment effect of region $i$ is equal to the overall treatment effect, the proportion of patients from region $i$ has the following simple closed-form solution:

$$f_T = \frac{z_{1-\beta'}^2}{\left(z_{1-\alpha} + z_{1-\beta}\right)^2 \left(1 - \lambda\right)^2 + z_{1-\beta'} \left(2\lambda - \lambda^2\right)},$$

where $1 - \beta'$ is the assurance probability.

Luo, Shih, Ouyang, and Delap (2010) and Wang (2009) proposed two-stage MRCT, in which when the observed treatment effect of a specific region from the original global trial fails to meet the prespecified consistency criteria, additional data may be obtained from the region through a follow-up trial. Shao and Chow (2002) proposed the concepts of reproducibility and generalizability for assessing similarity in bridging study.

On the basis of Method 1, Quan, Zhao et al. (2010) discuss the sample size requirement for normal, binary, and survival endpoints. They proposed five definitions of consistency and also calculated the probability of showing consistency for different configuration of sample size allocations and true treatment effects in individual regions. Ko et al. (2010) proposed four criteria to judge whether the treatment is effective in a specific region given the overall result as significant at $\alpha$ level. Tsong et al. (2012) proposed an approach to control the type-I error rate of a specific region adjusted for the regional sample size, then proposed to determine the sample size of a MRCT to accommodate the overall type-I error rate as well as the regional specific type-I error rate. Chen et al. (2012) proposed two conditional decision rules for regional approval, and sample size determination and the relationship between the two rules were also discussed. Quan et al. (2012) proposed the empirical shrinkage estimation approach based on the random effect model to assess the consistency of treatment effect across regions, which presumably could obtain better consistency compared to the fixed effect model. Tsou et al. (2012) proposed consistency criterion to examine whether the overall results can be applied to all participating regions; sample size requirements were also discussed.

Quan, Zhao, Zhang, Roessner, and Aizawa (2009) focused on Method 1 of the multiple regional trials and derived the sample size formula for Japanese population necessary to achieve

$$\Pr\left(\hat{\theta}_t|\hat{\theta} > \pi|\theta_t = u\theta\right) \geq 1 - \gamma,$$

where $\gamma \leq 0.2$.

Kawai, Chuang-Stein, Komiyama, and Li (2007) considered the sample size partitioning such that there is a high probability of observing a consistent trend in treatment effect. Their work is certainly pertinent to Method 2. Assuming variance of the response variable is equal to $\sigma^2$ in all regions, the probability of observing a positive effect in all regions is

$$\Pr\left(\hat{\theta}_n > 0, \forall h = 1, ..., K | \theta_h = \theta, \forall h\right) = \prod_{h=1}^{K} \Phi\left(\frac{\theta}{\sigma}\sqrt{n_n}\right),$$

which is maximized when all regions have equal sample sizes.

Similarly, in a bridging study, Hung, Wang, and O'Neill, (2013) provide the following results: Suppose the drug is approved for marketing in region $m$, the sample size required for a new region $t$ is

$$N_t = N_m \left(\frac{z_{1-\alpha_t} + z_{1-\beta}}{\lambda z_{1-p_t}}\right)$$

$$p_m = \Pr\left(P_m \leq p_m | \theta_m = 0\right) \leq \alpha.$$

$$\Pr\left(P_t \leq p_t | \theta_t^* = \lambda \theta_m^*\right) = \Phi\left(-z_{p_t} + \sqrt{n}\lambda\theta_m^*\right).$$

It should be noted that most of the recent approaches for MRCT utilized the same criteria to assess the consistency no matter how many regions were included in the MRCT. As in Method 1, the rate of retention of the overall result $\lambda$ was considered as a fixed value. Some simulations have shown that the sample size will be double or triple the original sample size even when $\lambda = 0.5$. When more regions are included in an MRCT for consideration, the larger sample size will be required to preserve certain power and probability for the regional approval with this additional requirement. To avoid the need of increasing to too many samples, the value of $\lambda$ should be carefully considered. One approach for determining $\lambda$ is to make it related to the number of regions.

### 25.2.2 *The Unified Regional Requirement*

As mentioned earlier, there are different regional requirement for drug approaches. In this section, we will study the regional requirement that unifies several different approaches. For simplicity, we will focus on the multiregional clinical trial for comparing a test product with a placebo control on a continuous endpoint. Let $\mu_T$ and $\mu_P$ denote the population means for the test drug and placebo control, and $\sigma^2$ the variance which is assumed to be the same for both the test and control group. Let $\mu = \mu_T - \mu_P$ denote the population mean difference. The hypothesis of testing the overall treatment effect is given as

$$H_{10} : \mu \leq 0 \text{ versus } H_{1a} : \mu > 0.$$

Let $N$ denote the total sample size required for all regions combined to detect the expected treatment difference $\mu$ at the desired significance level $\alpha$ and with power $1 - \beta$. Thus,

$$N = 2 \left[ \frac{(z_{1-\alpha} + z_{1-\beta}) \sigma}{\mu} \right]^2$$

where $z_{1-\alpha}$ is the $100(1 - \alpha)$th percentile of the standard normal distribution.

Assume the responses $x_{Ti}$ and $x_{Pi}$ for the test and control groups are normally distributed, $x_{Ti} \sim N\left(\mu_{Ti}, \sigma_i^2\right)$ and $x_{Ti} \sim N\left(\mu_{Pi}, \sigma_i^2\right)$. Let $\mu_i = \mu_{T_i} - \mu_{P_i}$ be the true mean difference for region $i$. We assume that $\sigma_i^2$ is known, which means practically that the sample size is large. Let $D_i$ be the observed mean difference for region $i$ and $D = \sum_{i=1}^{K} N_i D_i / N$ the observed mean difference for the entire group. We have

$$D_i \sim N(\mu_i, \frac{2\sigma_i^2}{N_i}).$$

and

$$D \sim N(\sum_{i=1}^{K} f_i\mu_i, \frac{2\sum_{i=1}^{K} f_i\sigma_i^2}{N}),$$

where $f_i$ is the proportion of patients in the $i$th region, $i = 1, \ldots, K$, $\sum_{i=1}^{K} f_i = 1$.

According to Method 1 and the guidance published by Japanese MHLW, efficacy claim in the $i$th region is

$$D_i > \lambda D. \tag{25.3}$$

Since $D_i$ and $D$ are the observed treatment differences for the region of interest and the entire group, we still have a 50% chance to make a mistake even though $\mu_i = \mu$. Thus, it is better to define the consistency in terms of parameters or true treatment effect and put the consistency requirement in the form of hypothesis test:

$$H_{20} : \mu_i \leq \lambda\mu \text{ versus } H_{2a} : \mu_i > \lambda\mu. \tag{25.4}$$

where $\lambda$ is a constant between 0 and 1.

Given that the overall treatment is effective, i.e., the hypothesis $H_{10} : \mu \leq 0$ (vs. $H_{1a} : \mu > 0$) is rejected, we will claim efficacy of the drug in the region $i$ if $H_{20}$ is rejected.

The test statistics are denoted by $Z$ and $Z_i$ for the overall efficacy ($H_{1a}$) and the additional requirement for region $i$ ($H_{2a}$), respectively.

$$Z = \frac{D}{std\,(D)} = \frac{D}{\sqrt{\frac{2\sigma^2}{N}}}, \tag{25.5}$$

where $\sigma^2 = \sum_{i=1}^{K} f_i\sigma_i^2$. Similarly, we define $\mu = \sum_{i=1}^{K} f_i\mu_i$.

$$Z_i = \frac{D_i - \lambda D}{std(D_i - \lambda D)} = \frac{D_i - \lambda D}{\sqrt{\frac{2(1-2\lambda f_i)\sigma_i^2 + \lambda^2 f_i\sigma^2}{f_i N}}}. \tag{25.6}$$

The unconditional and conditional probabilities of rejection are, respectively,

$$\Pr(Z_i \geq z_{1-\alpha_i}) \tag{25.7}$$

and

$$\Pr(Z_i \geq z_{1-\alpha_i}|Z \geq z_{1-\alpha}). \tag{25.8}$$

We denote the conditional probability by $AP_i$. Thus,

$$AP_i = \frac{\Pr(Z_i \geq z_{1-\alpha_i} \cap Z \geq z_{1-\alpha})}{\Pr(Z \geq z_{1-\alpha})}.$$

The joint distributions of $Z_i$ and $Z$ are bivariate normal distribution. It can be proved (Teng, 2014; Teng and Chang, 2014) that

$$AP_i = \frac{\int_{c^*}^{\infty} \left( \Phi\left(\frac{u-c_2}{c_1}\right) - \Phi\left(\frac{-z_{1-\beta}-c_0 u}{\sqrt{1-c_0^2}}\right) \right) \phi(u)\, du}{\int_{-z_{1-\beta}}^{\infty} \phi(u)\, du}, \tag{25.9}$$

where

$$c_1 = \frac{\lambda f_i}{c_0(1-\lambda f_i)}\sqrt{1-c_0^2},$$

$$c_2 = (\mu - \mu_i)\sqrt{\frac{f_i N}{2\sigma_i^2}} + \frac{z_{1-\alpha_i}}{1-\lambda f_i}\sqrt{1-2\lambda f_i + \frac{\lambda^2 f_i^2}{c_0^2}}, \text{ and}$$

$$c_0 = \sqrt{\frac{f_i \sigma_i^2}{\sigma^2}}, c^* = \frac{c_2\sqrt{1-c_0^2} - z_{1-\beta}c_1}{\sqrt{1-c_0^2} + c_1 c_0}.$$

Quan and Zhang (2010), Uesaka (2009), and Ikeda and Bretz (2010) provide similar results.

When $\alpha_i = 0.5$ or $z_{1-\alpha_i} = 0$, $AP_i$ in formula (25.9) is reduced to $\Pr(D_i > \lambda D|Z > Z_\alpha)$, which is equivalent to the criteria described as "Criteria II" in Ko et al (2010) and "CDR 1" in Chen et al. (2012). We note the assurance probability of this special case as $AP_i^0$. Thus,

$$AP_i^0 = \Pr(D_i > \lambda D|Z > z_{1-\alpha}) \tag{25.10}$$

When $\lambda = 0$, $AP_i$ in formula (25.8) is reduced to Ikeda–Bretz's method (2010), $\Pr(D_i/std(D_i) \geq z_{1-\alpha_i})|Z \geq Z_\alpha) = \Pr(Z_i^* \geq z_{1-\alpha_i}|Z > z_{1-\alpha})$, where $Z_i^* = \frac{\bar{x}_i\sqrt{f_i N}}{\sqrt{2}\sigma_i}$ is the usual test statistic of the following hypothesis test:

$$H_{30} : \mu_i \leq 0 \text{ versus } H_{3a} : \mu_i > 0. \tag{25.11}$$

It is clear that (25.11) is to test whether the treatment is effective in region $i$ at the $\alpha_i$ level. Equation (25.10) is similar to the method proposed in Tsong et al. (2012) and "CDR 2" in Chen et al. (2012). We denote the assurance probability of this special case by $AP_i^*$ and write it as

$$AP_i^* = \Pr(Z_i^* \geq z_{1-\alpha_i} | Z > Z_\alpha). \tag{25.12}$$

Thus, $AP_i^0$ in (25.10) and $AP_i^*$ in (25.12) are the special cases of the unified additional requirement for regional approval in (25.8).

### 25.2.3 Determination of Parameter $\lambda$ and $\alpha_i$

We are going to study what values of $\lambda$ and $\alpha_i$ in (25.3) through (25.8) might be reasonable. We will look at the issue from the sample size and type-I error perspectives, assuming there are true consistencies in efficacy among all regions. In other words, we assume that mean treatment difference and variance are uniform across regions and that the total samples are evenly distributed to each region; namely, $\mu_i = \mu$, $\sigma_i = \sigma$, $f_i = 1/K$, $i = 1, 2, ..., K$. We study the sample size increase for different values of assurance probabilities (AP), different numbers of regions, different values of $\lambda$, and different values of $\alpha_i$.

(1) Sample size required to achieve various assurance probabilities with $\alpha = 0.025$, $\lambda = 0.5$ and $\alpha_i = 0.5$.

Table 25.2: Sample Size Ratio $R$ for Various AP ($AP_i^0$)

| AP | Number of Regions, $K$ | | | | | | |
|---|---|---|---|---|---|---|---|
| | 2 | 3 | 4 | 5 | 6 | 7 | 8 |
| 0.80 | 1.0 | 1.0 | 1.0 | 1.4 | 1.9 | 2.3 | 2.6 |
| 0.85 | 1.0 | 1.0 | 1.5 | 2.0 | 2.6 | 3.0 | 3.5 |
| 0.90 | 1.0 | 1.4 | 2.1 | 2.7 | 3.3 | 4.0 | 4.6 |

Note: $\lambda = 0.5$, $\alpha_i = 0.5$. $R =$ the ratio with vs. without AP

From Table 25.2 we can see that the sample size increases as the number of regions and/or the assurance probability increase. Considering there are usually 4 to 5 regions, the sample size increase for the MRCT is about 50% to 200%.

(2) Determination of the value of $\lambda$ to achieve 80% assurance probability with different number of regions and a fixed $\alpha_i = 0.5$.

From Table 25.3 we can see that for the same sample size, when the number of regions increases, the required $\lambda$ value should decrease for the same assurance probability. Given that 80% AP is considered the minimum AP we need, 4 to 5 regions are common in practice, and 20% to 50% increase

Table 25.3:  $\lambda$ Values for Various Sample Size Ratios

| R | Number of Regions, $K$ | | | | | | |
|------|-------|-------|-------|-------|-------|-------|-------|
|      | 2     | 3     | 4     | 5     | 6     | 7     | 8     |
| 1.0  | 0.727 | 0.614 | 0.527 | 0.454 | 0.389 | 0.331 | 0.278 |
| 1.2  | 0.740 | 0.633 | 0.550 | 0.481 | 0.420 | 0.364 | 0.313 |
| 1.5  | 0.759 | 0.659 | 0.583 | 0.518 | 0.462 | 0.410 | 0.363 |
| 2.0  | 0.786 | 0.697 | 0.629 | 0.572 | 0.522 | 0.476 | 0.434 |

Note: $\alpha_i = 0.5$ and 80% assurance probability

in sample size is practically the upper limit, we suggest $\alpha_i = 0.5$ and for $\lambda = 0.5$, i.e., retaining 50% of the overall efficacy.

(3) Determination of the value of $\alpha_i$ to achieve 80% assurance probability with different number of regions and a fixed $\lambda = 0$.

Table 25.4:  $\alpha_i$ Values for Various Sample Size Ratios

| R | Number of Regions, $K$ | | | | | | |
|------|-------|-------|-------|-------|-------|-------|-------|
|      | 2     | 3     | 4     | 5     | 6     | 7     | 8     |
| 1.0  | 0.071 | 0.151 | 0.219 | 0.274 | 0.318 | 0.355 | 0.385 |
| 1.2  | 0.059 | 0.132 | 0.198 | 0.252 | 0.297 | 0.333 | 0.364 |
| 1.5  | 0.042 | 0.106 | 0.167 | 0.219 | 0.264 | 0.301 | 0.332 |
| 2.0  | 0.022 | 0.069 | 0.120 | 0.168 | 0.211 | 0.248 | 0.280 |

Note: $\lambda = 0$ and 80% assurance probability

From Table 25.4 we can see that for the same sample size, when the number of regions increases, the required $\alpha_i$ value should also increase for the same assurance probability. Given that 80% AP is considered the minimum AP we need, 4 to 5 regions are common in practice, and 20% to 50% increase in sample size is practically the upper limit, we suggest $\alpha_i = 0.25$ for the corresponding value $\lambda = 0$.

(4) Determination of the paired values of $(\lambda, \alpha_i)$ to achieve 80% assurance probability with different number of regions

Table 25.5:  $\alpha_i$ Values for Various $\lambda$ and Sample Size Ratios

| R | $\lambda$ | | | | | | | | |
|------|-------|-------|-------|-------|-------|------|------|------|------|
|      | 0     | 0.1   | 0.2   | 0.3   | 0.4   | 0.45 | 0.48 | 0.52 | 0.57 |
| 1.0  | 0.274 | 0.316 | 0.363 | 0.414 | 0.469 | 0.5  |      |      |      |
| 1.2  | 0.252 | 0.294 | 0.342 | 0.394 | 0.451 |      | 0.5  |      |      |
| 1.5  | 0.219 | 0.261 | 0.309 | 0.364 | 0.424 |      |      | 0.5  |      |
| 2.0  | 0.168 | 0.208 | 0.256 | 0.313 | 0.376 |      |      |      | 0.5  |

Note: five regions ($K=5$) and 80% assurance probability

Based on the results in Table 25.5 and for the same reasons stated in (2) and (3), the following pairs of $(\lambda, \alpha_i)$ seem reasonable: (0, 0.25), (0.1, 0.3), (0.2, 0.35), (0.3, 0.4), (0.4, 0.45), and (0.5, 0.5).

(5) Conditional and unconditional type-I error rates

In the previous two sections we have assumed that the treatment differences and variances are uniform across regions. When the treatment difference in region $i$ is 0, i.e., $\mu_i = 0$, all other treatment differences remain the same: $\mu_j = \mu$, the assurance probability under this setting could be interpreted as the probability of falsely claiming regional approval when there is no treatment effect in region $i$. We define this conditional probability as the conditional type-I error rate for this region:

$$\alpha_i' = \Pr(Z_i \geq z_{1-\alpha_i} | Z \geq z_{1-\alpha}, \mu_i = 0, \underset{j \neq i}{\cap} \mu_j = \mu), \qquad (25.13)$$

where $\mu > 0$ and $Z_i$ and $Z$ are defined in (25.4) and (25.5).

Since the total sample size is determined based on the assumption of $\mu_i = \mu$, it is clear that, when $\mu_i = 0$, the test based on the sample size calculated under the assumption of $\mu_i = \mu$ is underpowered. Thus, we define the unconditional type-I error as follows:

$$\alpha_i'' = \Pr(Z_i \geq z_{1-\alpha_i}, Z \geq z_{1-\alpha} | \mu_i = 0, \underset{j \neq i}{\cap} \mu_j = \mu) \qquad (25.14)$$

The conditional and unconditional errors are summarized in Table 25.6.

Table 25.6: Conditional and Unconditional Error Rates

| | $(K, AP)$ | | | | | | | |
|---|---|---|---|---|---|---|---|---|
| | $(4, 0.8)$ | | $(4, 0.9)$ | | $(5, 0.8)$ | | $(5, 0.9)$ | |
| $(\lambda, \alpha_i)$ | $\alpha_i'$ | $\alpha_i''$ | $\alpha_i'$ | $\alpha_i''$ | $\alpha_i'$ | $\alpha_i''$ | $\alpha_i'$ | $\alpha_i''$ |
| $(0.0, 0.25)$ | 0.201 | 0.362 | 0.239 | 0.295 | 0.220 | 0.316 | 0.247 | 0.265 |
| $(0.1, 0.30)$ | 0.206 | 0.370 | 0.238 | 0.293 | 0.222 | 0.332 | 0.244 | 0.260 |
| $(0.2, 0.35)$ | 0.206 | 0.371 | 0.232 | 0.280 | 0.223 | 0.339 | 0.234 | 0.247 |
| $(0.3, 0.40)$ | 0.204 | 0.366 | 0.219 | 0.256 | 0.223 | 0.335 | 0.216 | 0.225 |
| $(0.4, 0.45)$ | 0.199 | 0.358 | 0.197 | 0.222 | 0.223 | 0.321 | 0.189 | 0.194 |
| $(0.5, 0.50)$ | 0.192 | 0.346 | 0.165 | 0.177 | 0.220 | 0.297 | 0.152 | 0.154 |

Source: Teng and Chang (2014)

We can see given the pair of values $(\lambda, \alpha_i)$ in Table 25.6, the conditional errors mostly range from 0.15 to 0.25 and the unconditional errors range from 0.15 and 0.37, which we think are practically reasonable.

The simulation program of Classical Multiregional Clinical Trial is implemented in SAS Macro 25.1 below, where **nRegs** = number of regions, **Power** = $\Pr(Z > z_{1-\alpha})$, **Powers(i)** = $\Pr(Z > z_{1-\alpha_i})$, **uncondPower** = $\Pr(Z > z_{1-\alpha} \cap Z_i > z_{1-\alpha_i})$, **condPower(i)** = $AP_i$, **mu0** and **mu(i)** are true means of the placebo and the test group in region $i$, **sigma** = common standard deviation, **z_alpha** = $z_{1-\alpha}$ and **z_alphas(i)** = $z_{1-\alpha_i}$, **N(i)** = sample size per treatment (placebo or the test) group in region $i$, and **TotalN** = total sample size per group. The regional consistency requirement is given by (25.4) with $\lambda = 0$.

## >>SAS Macro 25.1:    Classical Multireginal Clinical Trial>>

```
%Macro MRCT(nSims=10000, nRegs=5, mu0=0, sigma=1, z_alpha=1.96);
data MRCT; Set dInput;
Array mu(&nRegs); Array powers(&nRegs); Array z_alphas(&nRegs); Array
t(&nRegs); Array condPowers(&nRegs); Array uncondPowers(&nRegs); Array
N(&nRegs);
Keep TotalN Z_alpha Power powers1-powers&nRegs
condPowers1-condPowers&nRegs uncondPowers1-uncondPowers&nRegs;
Z_alpha=&Z_alpha;
TotalN=0;
Do i=1 To &nRegs;
TotalN=TotalN+N(i); * Total sample size per group;
uncondPowers(i)=0;
powers(i)=0;
End;
Power=0; * Overall power;
Do iSim=1 To &nSims;
MeanEff=0;
Do i=1 To &nRegs;
x0=Rand('normal', &mu0, &sigma/sqrt(N(i)));
xi = Rand('normal',mu(i), &sigma/sqrt(N(i)));
t(i)=(xi-x0)/sqrt(&sigma**2/N(i)+&sigma**2/N(i));
If t(i)>z_alphas(i) Then powers(i)=powers(i)+1/&nSims;
MeanEff=MeanEff+(xi-x0)*N(i)/totalN;
End;
tOverall=MeanEff*sqrt(TotalN/2)/&sigma;
If tOverall>z_alpha Then power=power+1/&nSims;
Do i=1 To &nRegs;
If tOverall>z_alpha & t(i)>z_alphas(i) Then uncondPowers(i) = uncondPowers(i)
+ 1/&nSims;
End;
End;
Do i=1 To &nRegs; condPowers(i)=uncondPowers(i)/power; End;
Output;
Run;
Proc Print data=MRCT; Run;
%Mend MRCT;
```

<<**SAS**<<

## Example 25.1    Multiregional ACS Clinical Trial

Acute coronary syndrome (ACS) refers to any group of symptoms attributed to obstruction of the coronary arteries. The most common symptom prompting diagnosis of ACS is chest pain, often radiating to the left arm or angle of the jaw, pressure-like in character, and associated with nausea and sweating. Acute coronary syndrome usually occurs as a result of one of three problems: ST elevation myocardial infarction (30%), nonST elevation myocardial infarction (25%), or unstable angina (38%; Torres and Moayedi, 2007).

Aggregation of platelets is the pathophysiologic basis of the acute coronary syndromes. EPT, a hypothetical drug candidate, is an inhibitor of the platelet glycoprotein IIb/IIIa receptor, which is involved in platelet aggregation. The sponsor and investigator want to know if inhibition of platelet aggregation with EPT will have an incremental benefit beyond that of heparin and aspirin in reducing the frequency of adverse outcomes in patients with acute coronary syndromes who did not have persistent ST-segment elevation.

A global multiregional clinical trial is considered due to the large sample size required. Patients who had presented with ischemic chest pain within the previous 24 hours and who had either electrocardiographic changes indicative of ischemia (but not persistent ST-segment elevation) or high serum concentrations of creatine kinase MB isoenzymes are to be randomized to receive a bolus and infusion of either EPT or placebo, in addition to standard therapy, for up to 72 hours. The primary endpoint was a composite of death and nonfatal myocardial infarction occurring up to 30 days after the index event. It is estimated that the incidences of the primary endpoint are 165% and 14% for the placebo and the test group, respectively.

We design the trial in the following two options:

(1) The trial is designed for the purpose of market in the United States only and enrolling patients from other regions is for the purpose of meeting the sample size requirement only. This is the same as the classical design with fixed sample size without consideration of regions.

(2) The trial is designed for the international market. We assume the MRCT is to launch in four regions: the USA, Canada, EU, and Japan. We further assume that regional consistency requirement for all countries is defined by (25.4) with $\lambda = 0$ and $\alpha_i = 0.25$ or $z_{1-\alpha_i} = 0.6745$.

Since the SAS macro required that the larger response is better in the hypothesis test, we need to change the event rate to the nonevent rate, that is, $p_1 = 1 - 0.16 = 0.84$ for placebo and $p_2 = 1 - 0.135 = 0.865$ for EPT. With the assumption of a large sample size, the standard deviation is approximately $\sigma = \sqrt{\bar{p}(1-\bar{p})} = \sqrt{0.8525(1-0.8525)} = 0.355$. With these variable transforms, we can invoke SAS Macro 25.1 for our designs.

**>>SAS: Invoke SAS Macro 25.1 for Example 25.1>>**

Title "Checking Critical Value Z_alpha for 4 regions of MRCT";

Data dInput;

Array mu(4)(0.84, 0.84, 0.84, 0.84); Array z_alphas(4)(0.6745, 0.6745, 0.6745, 0.6745); Array N(4)(1400, 1400, 1400, 1400);

%MRCT(nSims=100000, nRegs=4, mu0=0.84, sigma=0.355, Z_alpha=1.96);

Title "Determine Power for the US Market Only";

Data dInput;

Array mu(1)(0.865); Array z_alphas(1)(0.6745); Array N(1)(4200);

%MRCT(nSims=100000, nRegs=1, mu0=0.84, sigma=0.355, Z_alpha=1.96);

Title "Determine Power for the International Market";

Data dInput;

Array mu(4)(0.865, 0.865, 0.865, 0.865); Array z_alphas(4)(0.6745, 0.6745, 0.6745, 0.6745); Array N(4)(1400, 1400, 1400, 1400);

%MRCT(nSims=100000, nRegs=4, mu0=0.84, sigma=0.355, Z_alpha=1.96);

**<<SAS<<**

The sample size required for 90% power is 4200 per treatment group for the classical single region design at the level of $\alpha = 0.025$. For the MRCT, with the power of 90% for the assurance probability $AP_i$ defined in (25.8) for all four regions (not simultaneously met), the required sample size is 5600 subjects per treatment group, or 1400 per group in each region. The overall power increases to 96% with the sample size increase from 4200 for the U.S. market strategy to 5600 per treatment group for the international market strategy.

## 25.3 Optimal Classical MRCT Design

### 25.3.1 *Maximum Power Design*

Given the total example size, the treatment effects for different regions, and the different regional requirements in $\alpha_i$, an optimal design is a design that maximizes the power:

$$Power = \sum_{i \in \Omega} \Pr(Z_i \geq z_{1-\alpha_i}, Z \geq Z_{1-\alpha} | \mu_j, j = 1, ..., K), \qquad (25.15)$$

where $\Omega$ is a subset of regions that are of interest to us and the total sample size $N = N_1 + ... + N_K$ is fixed. If the patient recruitment is not an issue, there is no reason to recruit patients in the regions in which we don't need to get approval. Therefore, we can rewrite the maximum power design as the sample size allocation strategy that maximizes the following probability or power:

$$P_{\max} = \max_{N_1+\cdots+N_K=N} \sum_{i=1}^{K} \Pr(Z_i \geq z_{1-\alpha_i}, Z \geq Z_{1-\alpha} | \mu_j, j = 1, ..., K),$$

(25.16)

### 25.3.2 *Maximum Utility Design*

Getting the drug approval in different regions may have different (commercial) values for different regions to the pharmaceutical company. Therefore, the design that maximizes the utility, however it is defined, might be interesting to the sponsor. Let's denote the value or utility for region $i$ by $u_i$. The maximum utility design

$$P_{\max} = \max_{N_1+\cdots+N_K=N} \sum_{i=1}^{K} u_i \Pr(Z_i \geq z_{1-\alpha_i}, Z \geq Z_{1-\alpha} | \mu_j, j = 1, ..., K),$$

(25.17)

It is obvious that when $u_i \equiv 1$, then the maximum utility design (25.17) reduces to the maximum powerful design (25.16). The utility $u_i$ can be the potential number of patients to be treated in region $i$. Let $Z = (Z, Z_1, ..., Z_K)'$, $\mu = (\mu, \mu_1, ..., \mu_K)'$, and covariate matrix $\Sigma$ has diagonal elements 1, $\sigma_{i1} = \sigma_{1i} = cov\,(Z, Z_i) = cov\left(Z, \sum_{i=1}^{K} \sqrt{\tau_i} Z_i\right) = \frac{N_i}{N}$, and all other elements $cov\,(Z_i, Z_j) = \delta_{ij}$ (Kronecker's delta).

## 25.4 Optimal Adaptive MRCT Design

Since the treatment effects in different regions are unknown, we can design a two-stage trial with one interim analysis. At the interim analysis, the treatment effects in different regions can be estimated, which can be used to reestimate the example size required for each region based on the conditional power or utility:

$$\max_{N_1+\cdots+N_K=K} \sum_{i=1}^{K} u_i \Pr(Z_i \geq z_{1-\alpha_i}, Z \geq Z_{1-\alpha} | D_{1j}, \mu_j = D_{1j}, j = 1, ..., K),$$

(25.18)

where $D_{1j}$ is the treatment difference in the $j$th region, observed at the first stage. Alternatively, for the prefixed total sample size, we can optimize the distribution of the sample size at the second stage in different regions to achieve the maximum power or utility.

SAS Macro 25.2 below is an implementation of the two-stage adaptive multiregional trial that allows sample-size reestimation at the interim based on $\Pr\left(Z_i \geq z_{1-\alpha_i} | z_{1i}\right)$, where $Z_i = w_1 z_{1i} + w_2 z_{2i}$ with fixed weights $w_1$ and $w_2$, $w_1^2 + w_2^2 = 1$. Here, $z_{1i}$ and $z_{2i}$ are the usual $z$-statistics bases on the data from the first and second stages, respectively. In other words, the sample size for the second stage for the region $i$ is adjusted based on

$$\Pr\left(Z_i \geq z_{1-\alpha_i} | z_{1i}\right) = TAP_i, \text{ the targeted value.} \qquad (25.19)$$

At the interim analysis, we can explicitly write the newly estimated sample size required per treatment group for the second stage as

$$n_2 = 2 \left( \frac{z_{1-\alpha_i} - w_1 z_{1i}}{w_2} - z_{1-TAP_i} \right)^2 \left( \frac{\sigma}{\hat{\delta}} \right)^2, \qquad (25.20)$$

Besides, the new sample size for stage 2 should be no more than $r_{\max}$ times the original sample size in that region for stage 2. And we don't allow sample size to be reduced.

The unconditional power is the most important measure of an MRCT, which is defined as the probability of having overall efficacy and meeting the regional consistency requirement, that is,

$$uPower = \Pr(Z_i \geq z_{1-\alpha_i} \cap Z \geq z_{1-\alpha}). \qquad (25.21)$$

Note that the adaptive MRCT allows early futility stopping and sample-size reestimation, but does not allow early efficacy stopping because each region has the consistency requirement which is difficult to meet at the interim analysis with a smaller sample size. Theoretically no type-I error can be made at the interim analysis without rejection. However, the test statistic at the final analysis used is the fixed weight method or MINP to account for the SSR.

In SAS Macro 25.2, the key variables are defined similarly as in SAS Macro 25.1. The key additional variables are **z_beta** is the interim futility stopping boundary and **z_alpha** = the critical value for rejection at the final stage. **TAP** = $TAPi$, **NRmax** = the maximum ratio of the maximum sample size allowed, $N_{max}$, to the original sample size and **NRmin** = the minimum ratio to determine the minimum incremental sample size. This minimum increment can mask the treatment difference or prevent people from calculating the treatment effect on the sample size increment. RegionSig{i} = Significance in region.

**>>SAS Macro 25.2:    Adaptive Multiregional Clinical Trial>>**

```
%Macro MRCTwithSSR(nSims=1000, nRegs=5, mu0=0, sigma=1, z_alpha=
1.96,
z_beta=0, w1=0.707, w2=0.707, TAP=0.8, NRmin=0.25, NRmax=2);
data MRCTwithSSR; Set dInput;
Array mu(&nRegs); Array powers(&nRegs); Array z_alphas(&nRegs); Array
t(&nRegs); Array AveNs(&nRegs);
Array N1(&nRegs); Array N2(&nRegs); Array N2New(&nRegs); Array nFinal
(&nRegs); Array z1(&nRegs); Array z2(&nRegs); Array condPowers(&nRegs);
Array uncondPowers(&nRegs); Array RegionSig(&nRegs);
Keep z_alpha z_beta NRmin NRmax Power powers1-powers&nRegs AveNs1-
AveNs&nRegs AveTotalN condPowers1-condPowers&nRegs uncondPowers1-
uncondPowers&nRegs;
z_alpha=&z_alpha; z_beta=&z_beta; NRmin=&NRmin; NRmax=&NRmax;
w1=&w1/Sqrt(&w1*&w1+&w2*&w2); w2=sqrt(1-w1**2);
Do i=1 To &nRegs;
powers(i)=0; AveNs(i)=0; uncondPowers(i)=0;
End;
AveTotalN=0; IApower=0; Power=0; * Overall power;
Do iSim=1 To &nSims;
Do i=1 To &nRegs;
x0=Rand('normal', &mu0, &sigma/sqrt(N1(i)));
xi = Rand('normal',mu(i), &sigma/sqrt(N1(i)));
z1(i)=(xi-x0)/&sigma*sqrt(N1(i)/2);
End;
* Form IA statistic;
TotalN1=0; Do i=1 To &nRegs; TotalN1=TotalN1+N1(i); End;
Grandz1=0;
Do i=1 To &nRegs;
Grandz1=Grandz1+z1(i)*sqrt(N1(i)/TotalN1);
End;
If z_beta>=Grandz1 Then Do; *Early futile;
AveTotalN=AveTotalN+TotalN1/&nSims;
Do i=1 To &nRegs; AveNs(i)=AveNs(i)+N1(i)/&nSims; End;
End; * End of early stopping;
If z_beta<Grandz1 Then Do; * Trial continues;
* Adjust regional sample size based on conditioal power for the local test.;
Do i=1 To &nRegs;
eSize=z1(i)*sqrt(N(i)/2);
```

```
BFun=(z_alphas(i)- w1*z1(i))/w2;
n2Temp=2*((BFun-Probit(1-&TAP))/eSize)**2; *n per group;
n2Temp=Round(n2Temp, &NRmin*(N1(i)+N2(i))); * Minimum increament;
nFinal(i)=min(max(n2Temp+N1(i), N1(i)+N2(i)), &NRmax*(N1(i)+N2(i)));
End;
Do i=1 To &nRegs; RegionSig(i)=0; End;
Do i=1 To &nRegs;
N2New(i)=nFinal(i)-N1(i);
x0=Rand('normal', &mu0, &sigma/sqrt(N2New(i)));
xi = Rand('normal', mu(i), &sigma/sqrt(N2New(i)));
z2(i)=(xi-x0)/&sigma*sqrt((N2New(i))/2);
T2=w1*z1(i)+w2*z2(i);
If T2>=z_alphas(i) Then RegionSig(i)=1;
End;
TotalN=0;
Do i=1 To &nRegs;
TotalN=TotalN+nFinal(i);
End;
TotalN2new=TotalN-TotalN1;
AveTotalN=AveTotalN+TotalN/&nSims;
Grandz2=0;
Do i=1 To &nRegs;
Grandz2=Grandz2+z2(i)*sqrt(N2New(i)/TotalN2new);
End;
zOverall=w1*Grandz1+w2*Grandz2;
If zOverall>z_alpha Then power=power+1/&nSims;
Do i=1 To &nRegs;
If RegionSig(i)=1 Then Do;
Powers(i)=Powers(i)+1/&nSims;
If zOverall>z_alpha Then uncondPowers(i)=uncondPowers(i)+1/&nSims;
End;
End;
End; * End of stage 2;
End; * End nSims;
Do i=1 To &nRegs; condPowers(i)=uncondPowers(i)/power; End;
Output;
Run;
Proc Print data=MRCTwithSSR; Run;
%Mend MRCTwithSSR;
<<SAS<<
```

**Example 25.2    Adaptive Multiregional ACS Clinical Trial**

For the same ACS trial in Example 25.1, the incidence rates may not be estimated accurately, which may impact the probability of success for the trial. If the treatment effect is smaller than expected but still promising, a larger sample size may be required or we may want to have the ability to adjust the sample size. However, if the treatment effect is very small or the test drug is ineffective, we want to have the ability to stop the trial early due to futility. In summary, we want to design, an adaptive multiregional trial that allows for early futility stopping and sample-size reestimation. We will compare the operating characteristics in two different scenarios: (1) the treatment effect is correctly estimated and (2) the treatment effect is overestimated. We invoke SAS Macro 25.2 using the following SAS code. The results are presented in Table 25.7.

**>>SAS: Invoke SAS Macro 25.2 for Example 25.2 Adaptive ACS MRCT>>**

Title "Checking type-I error rate and sample size under H0";
Data dInput;
Array mu(4)(0.84, 0.84, 0.84, 0.84); Array z_alphas(4)(0.6745, 0.6745, 0.6745, 0.6745); Array N1(4)(1000, 1000, 1000, 1000); Array N2(4)(600, 600, 600, 600);
%MRCTwithSSR(nSims=100000,nRegs=4,      mu0=0.84,      sigma=0.355, z_alpha=1.96, z_beta=0, w1=0.707, w2=0.707, TAP=0.995, NRmin=0.25, NR-max=1.5);
Title "Power for the 4-region Adaptive MRCT with SSR";
Data dInput;
Array mu(4)(0.865, 0.865, 0.865, 0.865); Array z_alphas(4)(0.6745, 0.6745, 0.6745, 0.6745); Array N1(4)(1000, 1000, 1000, 1000); Array N2(4)(600, 600, 600, 600);
%MRCTwithSSR(nSims=100000,nRegs=4,      mu0=0.84,      sigma=0.355, z_alpha=1.96, z_beta=0, w1=0.707, w2=0.707, TAP=0.995, NRmin=0.25, NR-max=1.5);
Title "Example 25.2 scenarion 2—overestimated treatment effect";
Data dInput;
Array mu(4)(0.86, 0.86, 0.86, 0.86); Array z_alphas(4)(0.6745, 0.6745, 0.6745, 0.6745); Array N1(4)(1000, 1000, 1000, 1000); Array N2(4)(600, 600, 600, 600);
%MRCTwithSSR(nSims=100000,nRegs=4,      mu0=0.84,      sigma=0.355, z_alpha=1.96, z_beta=0, w1=0.707, w2=0.707, TAP=0.995, NRmin=0.25, NR-max=1.5);
**<<SAS<<**

Table 25.7:   Comparison of Classical and Adaptive MRCT Designs

| Test Rate $p_2$ | Design | oPower | uPower | cPower $AP_i$ | Average N |
|---|---|---|---|---|---|
| 0.160 | Classical | 0.025 | 0.02 | 0.71 | 5600 |
|       | Adaptive  | 0.025 | 0.02 | 0.72 | 5490 |
| 0.135 | Classical | 0.96  | 0.86 | 0.90 | 5600 |
|       | Adaptive  | 0.98  | 0.90 | 0.92 | 6567 |
| 0.140 | Classical | 0.84  | 0.71 | 0.84 | 5600 |
|       | Adaptive  | 0.90  | 0.78 | 0.86 | 6645 |

Note: $p_1 = 016$, futility boundary z_beta=0, $w_1 = w_2 = 0.707$,
NRmin=0.25, NRmax=1.5, N1=1000, N2=600, TAP=0.995

From the simulation results (Table 25.7), we can see that under $H_0$ ($p_1 = p_2 = 0.16$), the sample for adaptive MRCT is slightly similar than the classical design, while under $H_a$ ($p_1 = 0.16$, $p_2 = 0.135$), the adaptive MRCT has a larger power (uPower) and sample size than those in the classical MRCT. When $p_1 = 0.16$ and the $p_2 = 0.14$, meaning the treatment effect is slightly overestimated, the classical MRCT will reduce the power (uPower) for each regional approval dramatically to 71%, while the adaptive MRCT can retain the probability (uPower) at 78% with an increased average sample size of 6645 per group from the original 5600 per group for the classical MRCT. Although, a sample size of 6645 per group will provide the similar power (77.5% uPower) when the $p_2 = 0.14$, it will not be a cost effective design when the drug is ineffective. Also, when the true treatment effect varies slightly across regions, adaptive MRCT would perform better than the classical MRCT.

The overall power (oPower) based on all regional data combined is less important, which is 84% for the classical MRCT and 90% for adaptive MRCT when $p_1 = 0.16$ and $p_2 = 0.14$. Note that in the Table 15.7, cPower = uPower/oPower.

## 25.5   Bayesian Approach

Drug effects are expected to be different for different regions, but we don't know how much that difference will be or which regions will have larger effects. Therefore, in power calculation it is a good idea to assume different effects for different regions, but we don't have to know which regions are better at the design stage.

The question to be answered is: given the prior that overall treatment effect is significant, what is the posterior that the drug has a positive effect in region $i$?

Let's study a more general case when the variances and sample sizes are difference in the $K$ regions. Let the mixed distribution of random variable $x_i$ be

$$f(x_j) = \sum_{i=1}^{K} w_i f_i \left( x_j; \mu_{ji}, \sigma_i^2 \right), \tag{25.22}$$

where treatment indicator $j = T, C$ and the constant weight $w_i > 0$ satisfying $\sum_{i=1}^{K} w_i = 1$. Assume all $\sigma_i$ are known. The cdf of $x_i$ is given by

$$F(x_j) = \sum_{i=1}^{K} w_i F_i \left( x_j; \mu_{ji}, \sigma_i^2 \right). \tag{25.23}$$

The expected treatment difference

$$\mu = E\left( \bar{x}_T - \bar{x}_C \right) = \mu_T - \mu_C = \sum_{i=1}^{K} w_i \mu_{2i} - \sum_{i=1}^{K} w_i \mu_{1i},$$

where sample size fraction $w_i = \frac{n_i}{n}$. Here $n$ and $n_i$ are the overall sample size per treatment group and sample size per treatment group in region $i$, respectively.

Variance of treatment difference is given by

$$\sigma^2 = var\left( \bar{x}_T - \bar{x}_C \right) = \frac{2}{N^2} \sum_{i=1}^{K} \sum_{m=1}^{n_i} \sigma_i^2 = \frac{1}{n} \sum_{i=1}^{K} w_i \sigma_i^2.$$

For a hypothesis test at a level of significance of $\alpha$, the standard $z$-statistic is given by $T = \left( \bar{x}_T - \bar{x}_C \right) \frac{\sqrt{n/2}}{\sigma}$. Thus, $T|H_0 \sim N(0,1)$ and $T|H_a \sim N(\mu, 1)$.

The Bayesian posterior distribution of the treatment effect $\mu_i$ in region $i$ $(i = 1, ..., K)$ is given by

$$\pi(\mu_i | x) = \int f(x|\mu_i) \pi(\mu_i) d\mu_i,$$

where $f(x|\mu_i)$ is the likelihood function. The prior $\pi(\mu_i)$ for region $i$ is a linear combination of two priors, $\pi_1(\mu_i)$, derived from the data in the other regions, and $\pi_2(\mu_i)$, the skeptic prior based on $H_0$. In other words,

$$\pi(\mu_i) = w \cdot \pi_1(\mu_i) + (1 - w) \pi_2(\mu_i),$$

where

$$\pi_1(\mu_i) = N\left( \mu_{-i}, 1 \right) \text{ and } \pi_2(\mu_i) = N(0, 1).$$

Here the weight $w$ is based on the variability of $\mu_i$ from all regions except region $i$, specifically,

$$w = \frac{1}{1 + \exp\left(-\frac{d}{\bar{d}}\right)},$$

where

$$d = var_{j \neq i}(\bar{x}_j) = \frac{1}{K-1} \sum_{\substack{j=1 \\ j \neq i}}^{K} (\bar{x}_j - \bar{x})^2,$$

and $\bar{d}$ is the expectation of $d$, given that the observed treatment effects in the $K - 1$ regions (excluding region $i$) are the true effects (parameters).

To claim efficacy of the study drug in region $i$, we require that the posterior probability

$$\Pr(\mu_i > \lambda_B \mu | x) > 0.8,$$

where $\lambda_B$ is the overall proportional drug effect retained in region $i$, e.g., $\lambda_B = 0.2$ for 20% of the overall drug effect.

## 25.6   Practical Issues and Challenges

Many of these issues are covered in ICH E5 Q&A addendum. Chuang-Stein, et al. (2013) summarize the issues in MRCT from the clinical, statistical, regulatorical, operational, and commercial perspectives.

From the clinical perspective, There are intrinsic and extrinsic factors, including the choice of control group, choice of endpoints, inclusion and exclusion criteria, and concomitant therapies. Intrinsic factors include genetics, disease etiology, comorbidity, and drug metabolism, which could affect drug–drug interactions. Extrinsic factors include medical practice, disease diagnosis, and how health and comorbidity are managed.

From the statistical perspective, statistical considerations could be discussed in the context of design, interim decision, and analysis. From a design perspective, a sponsor needs to do the following:

(1) Define how to assess the "consistency" of treatment effect across regions.
(2) Articulate how the sample size in each region was determined to support the primary objective on the overall treatment effect and a key secondary objective on treatment effects in prespecified regions.
(3) Decide if randomization will be stratified by regions.

(4) Decide if enrollment to a region will be stopped when enrollment into that region is completed.

From the regulation perspective, sponsors should seek regulatory agreement on the protocol driving multiregional trials. From the commercial perspective, increasingly, pricing and reimbursement considerations are major factors in launching a new medicine in the region/country. From the operational perspective, the issues include (Chuang-Stein, et al. 2013)

(1) Whether the drug will be dispensed centrally or by a regional office
(2) Whether randomization will be done using an interactive voice randomization system
(3) Whether a central laboratory will be used for safety, efficacy, or both
(4) Whether all regions will use the same method (e.g., paper, remote data capture, Internet) to capture the data
(5) Whether enrollment can be initiated in all regions concurrently
(6) How to conduct investigator training (and rater training, if relevant) to ensure consistent study conducted across regions
(7) Whether PRO data will be collected by paper or electronically
(8) What the remediation actions will be if a site does not deliver on enrollment or meet the quality requirement
(9) How to conduct retraining if a site appears not to have understood the assessment procedure or not to have adhered to the protocol

## 25.7 Summary

We have introduced the multiregional clinical trial and discussed the issues and challenges in designing and conducting such trials. We have discussed the concepts of overall significance based on the pooled data and additional requirements for a regional approval of a new drug. The efficacy approval criteria for a region are the combination of these two. The probability of getting a regional approval is the probability $\Pr(Z_i \geq z_{1-\alpha_i}, Z \geq Z_{1-\alpha})$, which is termed uPower in Table 25.7. Practically, each participating region can have different additional approval criteria, we have unified several existing criteria in the form of a hypothesis (25.4). Under such additional requirement for the regional approval (specifically for the condition $\lambda = 0$), we studied the classical and adaptive design with sample size relocation or reestimation using simulations. We have discussed the concepts of optimal classical and adaptive MRCT designs and the potential Bayesian approach for MRCT. In summary, MRCTs present new challenges to us, from all angles: clinical, regulatory, statistical, operational, and commercial aspects. Clinical trial simulation is a powerful tool that can be used to assistant us in dealing with such challenges.

## Problems

**25.1** Develop an SAS or R program for classical MRCT with Japan's consistency criterion (25.3).

**25.2** Develop an SAS or R program for classical MRCT with regional consistency criterion (25.4).

**25.3** For the ACS same trial in Example 25.1, the incidence rates may not be estimated accurately, which may impact the probability of success for the trial. If the treatment effect is larger, a smaller sample size is sufficient or we may want the trial to stop earlier. On the other hand, if the treatment effect is smaller but still promising, a larger sample size may be required or we may want to have the ability to adjust the sample size. However, if the treatment effect is very small or the test drug is ineffective, we want to have the ability to stop the trial early due to futility. In summary, we want to design, an adaptive multiregional trial that allows for early efficacy or futility stopping and sample size reestimation.

Modify SAS Macro 25.2 to allow early efficacy stopping and compare the three methods (classical MRCT, group sequential MRCT, and adaptive MRCT with SSR) with three different scenarios: (1) the treatment effect is correctly estimated, (2) the treatment effect is overestimated, and (3) the treatment effect is underestimated. Use O'Brien–Fleming stopping boundaries (2.7956 and 1.9768 for the interim and final analyses) with the information time 0.5 for the simulation.

**25.4** Use simulation to check the accuracy of the statement: "When the true treatment effect varies across regions, adaptive MRCT would perform better than the classical MRCT."

# Chapter 26

# SAS and R Modules for Group Sequential Design

## 26.1 Introduction

There are two-built-in SAS procedures for group sequential trial designs: SEQDESIGN procedure and SEQTEST procedure. The SEQDESIGN procedure is used to compute the boundary values and required sample sizes for the trial. The SEQTEST procedure is used for monitoring the trial or making decisions at the interim analyses. The SEQTEST procedure is also used for the final analyses to compute parameter estimates, confidence limits, and $p$-values after the trial stops. Our focus will be on SEQDESIGN procedure not SEQTEST procedure.

We start with a three-stage group sequential design for the asthma trial discussed in Example 8.1. In a phase-III asthma study with two dose groups (control and active), the primary efficacy endpoint is the percent change from baseline in FEV1. The estimated FEV1 improvement from baseline is 5% and 12% for the control and active groups, respectively, with a common standard deviation of $\sigma = 22\%$.

The null hypothesis is $H_0$: $\theta \leq 0$ versus the alternative hypothesis $H_a$: $\theta = 7\%$, where $\theta$ is treatment difference. We choose type-I error rate $\alpha = 0.025$ and type-II error rate $\beta = 0.1$ or power $= 0.9$. We choose a balanced two-group three-stage O'Brien–Fleming design. We will only allow early stopping for rejecting the $H_0$. We use equal information time ($\tau_1 = 1/3$, $\tau_2 = 2/3$) for the two interim analyses. The SEQTEST procedure does not provide a flexible futility stopping boundary and will not be used in our examples. The SAS code using SEQDESIGN procedure is presented in the following:

>>**SAS**>>
Proc Seqdesign altref=0.07;
OneSidedOBrienFleming: design nstages=3

525

method=obf

alt=upper

alpha=0.025 beta=0.10;

Samplesize model=twosamplemean(stddev=0.22);

Run;

<<**SAS**<<

The procedure outputs include the following: The maximum sample size is 421.8. The expected sample sizes are 420.8 and 331.6 under $H_0$ and $H_a$, respectively. The stopping boundary on z-scale for the three stages: 3.47109, 2.45443, and 2.00403, with the cumulative sample size $N_1 = 141$, $N_2 = 281$, and $N_3 = 422$, respectively.

## 26.2   SEQDESIGN Procedure

### 26.2.1   *PROC SEQDESIGN Statement*

The syntax of the SEQDESIGN procedure is

   **PROC SEQDESIGN** <options> ;

   <label:> **DESIGN** options ;

   **SAMPLESIZE** <**MODEL**= option> ;

The PROC SEQDESIGN statement and the DESIGN statement are required for the SEQDESIGN procedure. Each DESIGN statement requests a new group sequential design. The label, which must be a valid SAS name, is used to identify the design in the output. The SAMPLESIZE statement computes the required sample sizes for the design specified in each DESIGN statement.

The PROC SEQDESIGN statement invokes the SEQDESIGN procedure. The main options in the PROC SEQDESIGN statement are summarized in Table 26.1.

Table 26.1:   Main Options in Proc SEQDESIGN

| Design Parameter | Description |
| --- | --- |
| ALTREF | Alternative reference |
| BSCALE | Statistic scale for the boundary |
| | |
| **Table Output** | |
| ERRSPEND | Cumulative error spending at each stage |
| PSS | Powers and expected sample sizes |
| STOPPROB | Expected cumulative stopping probabilities |

## 26.2.2 *DESIGN* Statement

The DESIGN statement requests a new group sequential design. You can use multiple DESIGN statements, and each DESIGN statement corresponds to a separate group sequential design. The main options in the DESIGN statement are summarized in Table 26.2.

Table 26.2: Main Options in DESIGN Statement

| Design Parameter | Description |
| --- | --- |
| ALPHA= | Type-I error probability level, $\alpha$ |
| ALT= | Type of alternative hypothesis |
| BETA= | Type-II error probability level |
| INFO= | Information levels |
| NSTAGES= | Number of stages |
| STOP= | Condition for early stopping |
| METHOD= | Methods for boundary values |

ALT=LOWER, UPPER, or TWOSIDED specifies the type of alternative hypothesis in the design. For the hypothesis test $H_0 : \theta = 0$, the keywords LOWER, UPPER, and TWOSIDED correspond to the alternatives of $\theta < 0$, $\theta > 0$, and $\theta \neq 0$, respectively. The default is ALT=TWOSIDED.

INFO=Equal or CUM(*numbers*) specifies relative information levels for all stages in the design, where number is the cumulative relative information levels at different stages. The default is INFO=Equal.

METHOD $=$ *method,* where the option method can be: ERRFUNC-OBF for the O'Brien–Fleming-type cumulative error spending, ERR-FUNCPOC for the Pocock-type cumulative error spending, and ERR-FUNCPOW $<$ ( RHO= ) $>$ for power error-spending function, where the default RHO ($\geq 0.25$) is 2, with 1 mimicking Pocock boundary, and 3 mimicking the O'Brien–Fleming boundary. The option method can also be ERRSPEND (*numbers*), which specifies the relative cumulative error spending at each stage.

If we don't want to use error-spending functions, we can specify the *method* option using OBF for the O'Brien–Fleming method, POC for the Pocock method, or POW $<$ (RHO=$\rho$) $>$ for the power family method (Wang and Tsiatis, 1987; Emerson and Fleming, 1989; Pampallona and Tsiatis, 1994).

## 26.2.3 *SAMPLESIZE* Statement

The SAMPLESIZE statement, SAMPLESIZE <MODEL= option>, computes the required sample sizes or numbers of events (for survival endpoint). The main options in the SAMPLESIZE statement are summarized in Table

26.3.

Table 26.3:  Main Options in SAMPLESIZE Statement

| Design Parameter | Description |
| --- | --- |
| ONESAMPLEMEAN | One-sample Z test for mean |
| ONESAMPLEFREQ | One-sample test for binomial proportion |
| TWOSAMPLEMEAN | Two-sample Z test for mean |
| TWOSAMPLEFREQ | Two-sample test for binomial proportion |
| TWOSAMPLESURVIVAL | Log-rank test for two survival distributions |

We will focus on the two-sample models. The following three options compute the required sample size or number of events for a two-sample group sequential trial.

**MODEL=TWOSAMPLEMEAN** < ( **options** ) > specifies the two-sample Z test for mean difference. The available options are as follows: MEANDIFF=$\theta_1$, STDDEV= $\sigma_a < \sigma_b >$, and WEIGHT= $w_a < w_b >$.

The MEANDIFF= option specifies the alternative reference 1 and is required if the alternative reference is not specified or derived in the procedure. If the MEANDIFF= option is not specified, the specified or derived alternative reference is used. The STDDEV= option specifies the standard deviations $\sigma_a$ and $\sigma_b$. If $\sigma_b$ is not specified, $\sigma_b = \sigma_a$. The default is STDDEV=1. The WEIGHT= option specifies the sample size allocation weights for the two groups. If $w_b$ is not specified, $w_b = 1$ is used. The default is WEIGHT=1, equal sample size for the two groups.

**MODEL=TWOSAMPLEFREQ** < ( **options** ) > specifies the two-sample test for binomial proportions. The available options are as follows: NULLPROP= $p_{0a} < p_{0b} >$; PROP= $p_{1a}$; TEST= PROP, LOGOR, or LOGRR; REF= NULLPROP, PROP, AVGNULLPROP, or AVGPROP; and WEIGHT= $w_a < w_b >$.

The NULLPROP= option specifies proportions $p_a = p_{0a}$ and $p_b = p_{0b}$ in groups $A$ and $B$, respectively, under the null hypothesis. If $p_{0b}$ is not specified, $p_{0b} = p_{0a}$. The default is NULLPROP=0.5. The PROP= option specifies proportion $p_a = p_{1a}$ in group $A$ under the alternative hypothesis. The proportion $p_{1b}$ in group $B$ under the alternative hypothesis is given by $p_{1b} = p_{0b}$. The PROP= option is required if the alternative reference is not specified or derived in the procedure. If the PROP= option is not specified, the specified or derived alternative reference is used to compute $p_{1a}$, the proportion in group $A$ under the alternative hypothesis.

The TEST= option specified the null hypothesis $H_0 : \theta = 0$ in the test. The TEST=PROP option uses the difference in proportions $\theta =$

$(p_a - p_b) - (p_{0a} - p_{0b})$, the TEST=LOGOR (default) option uses the log odds-ratio test $\theta = \delta - \delta_0$, where

$$\delta = \log\left(\frac{p_a (1 - p_b)}{p_b (1 - p_a)}\right), \quad \delta_0 = \log\left(\frac{p_{0a} (1 - p_{0b})}{p_{0b} (1 - p_{0a})}\right)$$

and the TEST=LOGRR option uses the log relative risk test with $\theta = \delta - \delta_0$, where

$$\delta = \log\left(\frac{p_a}{p_b}\right), \quad \delta_0 = \log\left(\frac{p_{0a}}{p_{0b}}\right).$$

The REF= option specifies the hypothesis under which the proportions are used in the sample size computation. The REF=NULLPROP option uses the null proportions $p_{0a}$ and $p_{0b}$, the REF=PROP (default) option uses the alternative proportions $p_{1a}$ and $p_{1b}$, the REF=AVGNULLPROP option uses the average null proportion, and the REF=AVGPROP option uses the average alternative proportion. $w_a$ = sample size ratio for the two groups.

**MODEL=TWOSAMPLESURVIVAL** < **( options )** > specifies the log-rank test for two survival distributions with the null hypothesis $H_0 : \theta = \delta - \delta_0$, where the parameter $\delta = -\log(h_a/h_b)$, $\delta_0$ is the value of $\delta$ under the null hypothesis and the values $h_a$ and $h_b$ are the constant hazard rates for groups $A$ and $B$, respectively.

The available options for the number of events are as follows: NULL-HAZARD= $h_{0a}$ < $h_{0b}$ >, NULLMEDSURVTIME= $t_{0a}$ < $t_{0b}$ >, HAZARD= $h_{1a}$, HAZARDRATIO= $\lambda_1$, and MEDSURVTIME= $t_{1a}$.

The NULLHAZARD= option specifies hazard rates $h_a = h_{0a}$ and $h_b = h_{0b}$ for groups $A$ and $B$, respectively, under the null hypothesis. If $h_{0b}$ is not specified, $h_{0b} = h_{0a}$. The NULLMEDSURVTIME= option specifies the median survival times $t_a = t_{0a}$ and $t_b = t_{0b}$ under the null hypothesis. If $t_{0b}$ is not specified, $t_{0b} = t_{0a}$.

The HAZARD=, MEDSURVTIME=, and HAZARDRATIO= options specify the group $A$ hazard rate $h_{1a}$, the group $A$ median survival time $t_{1a}$, and the hazard ratio $\lambda_1 = h_{1a}/h_{1b}$, respectively, under the alternative hypothesis. The HAZARD=, MEDSURVTIME=, or HAZARDRATIO= option is required if the alternative reference is not specified or derived in the procedure. If these three options are not specified, the specified or derived alternative reference $\theta_1$ is used to compute $h_{1a}$ from the equation:

$$\theta_1 = -\log\frac{h_{1a}}{h_{1b}} - \left(-\log\frac{h_{0a}}{h_{0b}}\right) = -\log\frac{h_{1a}}{h_{0a}}.$$

To derive the sample size, you need to specify additional options: ACC-TIME= $T_a$, FOLTIME= $T_f$, and WEIGHT= $w_a < w_b >$. The ACCTIME= and FOLTIME= options specify the accrual time $T_a$ and follow-up time $T_f$, respectively. The total study time, $T = T_a + T_f$ . The WEIGHT= option specifies the sample size allocation weights for the two groups. The default is WEIGHT=1, equal sample size for the two groups.

## 26.3 Examples with Proc SEQDESIGN

We show how to use Proc SEQDESIGN to design group sequential design with different endpoints. For binary endpoint we use the acute ischemic stroke trial in Example 4.1: A phase-III trial is to be designed for patients with acute ischemic stroke of recent onset. The composite endpoint (death and MI) is the primary endpoint, and the event rate is 14% for the control group and 12% for the test group. This time we choose Pocock stopping boundary and unbalanced design, with sample size ratio 1:2 (more patients in the test group). The trial will have three interim analyses with equal information design and allow early stopping only for rejecting but not for accepting $H_0$.

The SAS code for the design is presented as follows.

>>**SAS**>>
```
Proc Seqdesign altref=0.02;
OneSidedPocock: design nstages=4
method=poc
alt=lower
alpha=0.025 beta=0.10;
Samplesize model=twosamplefreq(nullprop=0.14 test= prop weight=2);
Run;
```
<<**SAS**<<

The SAS output shows the stopping boundary on the z-scale is identical for the four analysis, $z < -2.36130$; the maximum sample size is 16149; and the expected sample size is 15964 and 9520, respectively, under $H_0$ and $H_a$.

Next we study the survival endpoint using the oncology trial in Example 4.3. In a two-arm comparative oncology trial, the primary efficacy endpoint is time-to-progression (TTP). The median TTP is estimated to be 8 months (hazard rate = 0.08664) for the control group, and 10.5 months (hazard rate = 0.06601) for the test group. Assume a uniform enrollment with an accrual period of 9 months and total study duration of 24 months. The log-rank test will be used for the analysis. An exponential survival distribution is assumed for the purpose of sample-size calculation. The classical two-group balanced design requires a sample size of 323 subjects per group.

We design the trial with one interim analysis for rejection $H_0$ when 30% of patients have been enrolled. We choose error spending option with 0.005 on the interim analysis and the rest on the final analysis.

**>>SAS>>**

Proc Seqdesign;
OneSidedErrSpn: design nstages=2 Info = Cum(0.3, 1)
method=ERRSPEND (0.005, 0.025)
alt=upper
alpha=0.025 beta=0.10;
Samplesize model=twoSampleSurvival (
nullMedSurvTime=8, MedSurvTime=10.5
accTime= 9 folTime=24);
Run;

**<<SAS<<**

The SAS output shows the stopping boundary on the z-scale is $z > 2.57583$ for the interim analysis with 176 events ( 650 patients) and $z > 2.02347$ for the final analysis with 586 events (667 patients). The maximum number of events required is 586 and the maximum number of patients required is 677.

## 26.4   SAS SEQTEST and R sgDesign

The purpose of the SEQTEST procedure is to perform the interim and final analyses for clinical trials. At each stage, the data are analyzed with a statistical procedure such as the REG procedure, and a test statistic and its associated information level are computed. The computed test statistic will be compared to the corresponding stopping boundary to make a decision. At the end of a trial, the parameter estimate is computed. The median unbiased estimate, confidence limits, and $p$-value depend on the specified sample space ordering. A sample space ordering specifies the ordering for test statistics that result in the stopping of a trial. That is, for all the statistics in the rejection region and in the acceptance region, the SEQTEST procedure provides three different sample space orderings: the stagewise ordering uses counterclockwise ordering around the continuation region, the LR ordering uses the distance between the observed statistic and its hypothetical value, and the MLE ordering uses the observed maximum likelihood estimate.

An **R** package called gsDesign was developed by Keaven Anderson (2014) for group sequential designs. Compilation is required before using the package. See details in Reference manual at http:// cran.r-project.org/web/packages/gsDesign/index.html.

## Problem

**26.1** Use SAS Proc Seq design to redesign the group sequential trial in Example 5.3 use various stopping boundaries and compare the results obtained from SAS Macro 5.2.

# Chapter 27

# Data Analysis of Adaptive Trial

## 27.1 Introduction

Data analyses of an adaptive trial include point and confidence parameter estimates, and adjusted (conditional and unconditional) $p$-values. The issues surrounding these topics are controversial, even the definitions of bias, confidence interval, and $p$-value are not unique with adaptive trials.

Unlike the bias in a classical trial without adaptation, the concept of bias in adaptive trial is complicated. For example, the first kind of bias concerns the unconditional estimate: Suppose a particular adaptive trial is repeated for infinite times, the unconditional treatment effect is defined as the expected mean treatment differences between the two treatment groups over all the trials regardless of whether the trial is stopped at an interim stage or at the final stage. The difference between the expected mean difference and the truth treatment difference is the bias. We may say that this view of bias is from statisticians' perspective because the statistician can possibly see all these results. The second bias concerns the estimate (called stagewise conditional estimate) conditional on the stage where the trial stopped. Imagine that the trial is repeated infinitely; we estimate the treatment effect by averaging the mean treatment differences over all the trials that stopped at any given stage. The third kind of bias concerns the estimate conditional on the positive results (e.g., mean differences that are statistically significant). Such an estimate of treatment effect can be considered as the regulatory view or patients' views because they usually see only such positive results. The bias of such conditional estimate also directly relates to the publication bias. This bias also exists in classical design with a fixed sample size.

The stagewise conditional estimate is most often studied in the statistical community and is the focus of this chapter. It is interesting to note that we aggregate all type-I errors from different stages and controlled at a $\alpha$ level, but the conditional estimate only concerns the possible results at the stage where the trial actually stopped.

## 27.2  $p$-value Calculation

Denote by $f^o(t) > 0$ and $f^a(t)$ the distributions of the test statistic $T$ under the null hypothesis $H_0$ and the alternative hypothesis $H_a$, respectively. The $p$-value for a one-sided test is defined as $p(t) = \int_t^\infty f^o(\tau)\,d\tau$. To derive the distribution of $p$-value $p(t)$ under $H_a$, we start with the cdf identity: $F_T(t) = F_P(p(t))$. Taking the derivative with respect to $t$ (Kokoska and Zwillinger, 2000, p. 40), we obtain the pdf of the $p$-value:

$$P \sim f_P(p) = f^a(t)\,\frac{1}{|dp(t)/dt|} = \frac{f^a(t)}{f^o(t)},\quad f^o(t) \neq 0. \qquad (27.1)$$

When the null hypothesis $H_0$ is true, $f^a(t) = f^o(t)$, $p$-value $P$ has a uniform distribution in $[0,1]$. However, $p$-value from an adaptive trial does not have this nice property. Not only that, the $p$-value, median, and confidence limits depend on the ordering of the sample space $(k, z)$, where $k$ is the stage number and $z$ is the standardized $Z$ statistic. For instance, at the end of a classical clinical trial, a test statistic $z_1 = 2.3$ is more extreme than $z_2 = 1.8$. In other words, the value of test statistic alone is sufficient to determine the "extremeness" or the sample space orderings. However, in adaptive trial, the definition of extremeness or the ordering is much more complicated, it requires at least a pair of values $(k, z)$. Suppose in a two-stage group sequential trial with $H_0 : \mu \leq 0$ versus $H_a : \mu > 0$, O'Brien–Fleming stopping boundaries with equal information time ($z_{1-\alpha_1} = 2.8$ and $z_{1-\alpha_2} = 1.98$) are used. If we observed the test statistic $z_1 = 2.5$ at the first stage and $z_2 = 2.0$ at the second stage, which value is more extreme? At the first look, we may think $z_1$ is more extreme because $z_1$ is larger than $z_2$, but according to the stopping boundaries, we don't reject $H_0$ at the first stage but reject it at the second stage. Therefore, it is reasonable to consider the pair data $(k, z) = (2, 2.0)$ is more extreme than the pair data $(1, 2.5)$. On the other hand, if the Pocock boundaries ($z_{1-\alpha_1} = 2.18$ and $z_{1-\alpha_2} = 2.18$) are used, we can say $z_1$ is more extreme than $z_2$ because we reject $H_0$ at the first stage. After we define the orderings in the sample space, we can define the $p$-value. That is, with the observed pair of statistics $(k_0, z_0)$ when the trial is stopped, a one-sided upper $p$-value can be computed as

$$\Pr_{\theta=0}\{(k, z) \succeq (k_0, z_0)\}.$$

It is obvious that definition of sample space ordering (denoted by $\succeq$) is somewhat subjective. It can be one of the following.

**Stagewise Ordering**

If the continuation regions of a design are intervals, the stagewise ordering (Fairbanks and Madsen, 1982; Jennison and Turnbull, 2000, pp. 179–180; Tsiatis, Rosner, and Mehta, 1984) uses counterclockwise ordering around the continuation region to compute the $p$-value, unbiased median estimate, and confidence limits. This ordering depends on the stopping region, stopping stage, and standardized statistic at the stopping stage. But it does not depend on information levels beyond the observed stage. For a one-sided design with an upper alternative, $(k', z') \succeq (k_0, z_0)$ if one of the following criteria holds: (1) $k = k'$ and $z' > z$, (2) $k' < k$ and $z' \geq a_{k'}$, the upper efficacy boundary at stage $k'$, or (3) $k' > k$ and $z' < b_k$, the upper futility boundary at stage $k$.

**LR Ordering**

The LR ordering (Chang, 1989) depends on the observed standardized $Z$ statistic $z$, information levels, and a specified hypothetical reference. For the LR ordering under a given hypothesis $H_a : \theta = \theta_g$, we have $(k', z') \succ (k, z)$ if $\left(z' - \theta_g \sqrt{\tau_{k'}}\right) > \left(z - \theta_g \sqrt{\tau_k}\right)$. Under the null hypothesis $H_0 : \theta = 0$, it reduces to $z' > z$ and can be used to derive statistics under $H_0$, such as $p$-values.

The LR ordering is applicable to all designs if all information levels are available. But depending on the boundary shape, some observed statistics $(k, z)$ in the rejection region might be less extreme than the statistics in the acceptance region. That is, the $p$-value for observed statistics in the rejection region might be greater than the significance level.

**MLE Ordering**

The MLE ordering (Emerson and Fleming, 1990) depends only on the observed maximum likelihood estimate. We have $(k', z') \succ (k, z)$ if $\frac{z'}{\sqrt{k'}} > \frac{z}{\sqrt{k}}$. The MLE ordering is applicable to all designs if all information levels are available.

**Score Test Ordering**

The score test ordering (Rosner and Tsiatis, 1988) is to rank the outcomes by values of the score statistic for testing $H_0 : \theta = 0$. That is, $(k', z') \succ (k, z)$ if $z'\sqrt{k'} > z\sqrt{k}$.

## 27.3 Parameter Estimation

Consider the hypothesis test for mean $\mu$:

$$H_0 : \mu \leq 0 \text{ versus } H_a : \mu > 0.$$

Let $x_{ik}$ be the independent observations from the $i$th patient at the $k$th stage ($k = 1, 2$). Assume $x_{ik}$ has the normal distribution $N\left(\mu, \sigma^2\right)$ with known $\sigma$. Denote by $\bar{x}_k$ the stagewise sample mean at the $k$th stage (not based on cumulative data); thus, $\bar{x}_1$ and $\bar{x}_2$ are independent. The test statistic at the first stage of the standard group sequential design can be written as $T_1 = \bar{x}_1\sqrt{n_1}/\sigma$, where $n_1$ is the sample size at the first stage. The stopping rule at the first stage is to stop the trial if $T_1 \geq c_1$ ($p_1 \leq \alpha_1$ on the $p$-scale) and continue otherwise. It is obvious that $T_1 = \bar{x}_1\sqrt{n_1}/\sigma \geq c_1$ implies $x_1 \geq \sigma c_1/\sqrt{n_1}$.

The expectation of the conditional mean at the first stage is

$$\mu_1 = \frac{\int_{\sigma c_1/\sqrt{n_1}}^{\infty} \bar{x}_1 f_{\bar{X}_1}\left(\bar{x}_1\right) d\bar{x}_1}{\int_{\sigma c_1/\sqrt{n_1}}^{\infty} f_{\bar{X}_1}\left(\bar{x}_1\right) d\bar{x}_1}. \qquad (27.2)$$

Because $n_2$ is independent of $x_1$ (i.e., there is no sample size adjustment), the expectation of the conditional mean at the second stage is

$$\mu_2 = \frac{\int_{-\infty}^{\sigma c_1/\sqrt{n_1}} \int_{-\infty}^{\infty} \frac{\bar{x}_1 n_1 + \bar{x}_2 n_2}{n_1 + n_2} f_{\bar{X}_1}\left(\bar{x}_1\right) f_{\bar{X}_2}\left(\bar{x}_2\right) d\bar{x}_2 d\bar{x}_1}{\int_{-\infty}^{\sigma c_1/\sqrt{n_1}} f_{\bar{X}_1}\left(\bar{x}_1\right) d\bar{x}_1}$$

$$= \frac{\int_{-\infty}^{\sigma c_1/\sqrt{n_1}} \frac{n_1\bar{x}_1 + n_2\mu}{n_1 + n_2} f_{\bar{X}_1}\left(\bar{x}_1\right) d\bar{x}_1}{\int_{-\infty}^{\sigma c_1/\sqrt{n_1}} f_{\bar{X}_1}\left(\bar{x}_1\right) d\bar{x}_1}. \qquad (27.3)$$

For normal distribution $f_{\bar{X}_k}\left(\bar{x}_k\right) = N\left(\bar{X}_k; \mu, \sigma^2/n_k\right)$, we have

$$\mu_1 = \frac{1}{1 - \Phi_0\left(c_*\right)} \int_{\sigma c_1/\sqrt{n_1}}^{\infty} \bar{x}_1 \frac{1}{\sqrt{2\pi\sigma^2/n_1}} e^{\frac{-(\bar{x}_1 - \mu)^2 n_1}{2\sigma^2}} d\bar{x}_1$$

$$= \mu + \frac{\sigma \exp\left(-\frac{c_*^2}{2}\right)}{\left[1 - \Phi_0\left(c_*\right)\right]\sqrt{2\pi n_1}}, \qquad (27.4)$$

where $c_* = c_1 - \mu\sqrt{n_1}/\sigma$, and

$$\mu_2 = \frac{1}{\Phi_0\left(c_*\right)} \int_{-\infty}^{\sigma c_1/\sqrt{n_1}} \frac{n_1\bar{x}_1 + n_2\mu}{n_1 + n_2} \frac{1}{\sqrt{2\pi/n_1}} e^{\frac{-(\bar{x}_1 - \mu)^2 n_1}{2\sigma^2}} d\bar{x}_1$$

$$= \frac{n_1}{n_1 + n_2}\left[\mu - \frac{\sigma}{\Phi_0\left(c_*\right)\sqrt{2\pi n_1}} \exp\left(-\frac{c_*^2}{2}\right)\right] + \frac{n_2}{n_1 + n_2}\mu$$

$$= \mu - \frac{n_1\sigma \exp\left(-\frac{c_*^2}{2}\right)}{\left(n_1 + n_2\right)\Phi_0\left(c_*\right)\sqrt{2\pi n_1}}. \qquad (27.5)$$

From (27.4) and (27.5), the expectation of the unconditional mean can be expressed as

$$\mu_{MLE} = [1 - \Phi_0(c_*)]\mu_1 + \Phi_0(c_*)\mu_2 = \mu + \frac{n_2}{n_1 + n_2}\frac{\sigma}{\sqrt{2\pi n_1}}\exp\left(-\frac{c_*^2}{2}\right).$$
(27.6)

The bias of the unconditional estimate can be calculated as

$$\Delta_{bias} = \mu_{MLE} - \mu = \frac{n_2}{n_1 + n_2}\frac{\sigma}{\sqrt{2\pi n_1}}\exp\left(-\frac{c_*^2}{2}\right) < \frac{\sigma}{\sqrt{2\pi n_1}}.$$
(27.7)

For a group sequential design with futility stopping boundary $c_0$, and efficacy stopping boundary $c_1$ on the $z$-scale, the bias is (Emerson, 1988; Jennison and Turnbull, 2000, p.177)

$$\Delta_{bias} = \mu_{MLE} - \mu = \frac{n_2\sigma}{(n_1 + n_2)\sqrt{n_1}}\left\{\phi\left(c_0 - \frac{\mu}{\sigma}\sqrt{n_1}\right) - \phi\left(c_1 - \frac{\mu}{\sigma}\sqrt{n_1}\right)\right\},$$
(27.8)

where $\phi$ is the standard normal pdf.

To calculate $\mu_1$ and $\mu_2$, the standard normal cdf can be approximated by

$$\Phi_0(c) = 1 - \frac{(c^2 + 5.575192695c + 12.77436324)\exp\left(-c^2/2\right)}{\sqrt{2\pi}c^3 + 14.38718147c^2 + 31.53531977c + 2(12.77436324)}.$$
(27.9)

Since the bias is a function true parameter $\mu$, we can use an iterative method to obtain the unbiased estimate of $\mu$. That is, $\hat{\mu} = \mu + Bias(\mu)$; we use $\hat{\mu}^{(k)} = \mu + Bias\left(\hat{\mu}^{(k-1)}\right)$ where $\hat{\mu}^{(k)}$ is the $k$th iterative value and $\mu^{(0)} = \bar{X}$.

To obtain an unbiased estimator is not difficult at all. For example, in a two-stage group sequential design, the sample mean (or MLE) of the treatment effect based on only the data from the second stage is unbiased. However, the estimator will have a large variance. Researchers (Emerson and Fleming, 1990; Emerson and Kittelson, 1997) have studied the biased adjusted estimate by adjusting the estimate from the first stage data using the Rao–Blackwell technique and then combining with the estimate from the second stage data. We will discuss more on this approach in the estimation for adaptive trials with arm selections.

It is interesting, at least to frequentist statisticians, to know if there is a uniformly minimum variance unbiased estimator of $\mu$ in the group sequential setting. Liu and Hall (1999) proved that the sufficient statistics $(T, Z_T)$ is not complete and hence such an estimator generally does not exist, but it only exists in the class of estimators which do not require knowledge of the number of further analyses and their associated information levels that would have occurred had the study continued past termination analysis $T$ (Jennison and Turnbull, 2000, p.178)

In our view, the conditional estimate is more important than the unconditional estimate. The reason is simple: We know from (27.4) and (27.5) that $\bar{x}_1$ is biased upward and $\bar{x}_2$ is biased downward. It doesn't make sense to report $x_k$ with the overall adjustment given by (27.7), especially when the trial stops at stage 2, and adjust $x_2$ downward using (27.5), knowing that $x_2$ is already biased downward. Although both the conditional and overall adjustments can provide unbiased estimates, the conditional adjustment makes much more sense.

Equations (27.3)–(27.8) are valid for two-stage group sequential designs with MINP, MSP, and MPP because the naive mean is determined by the $c_1$ (or $\alpha_1$) and $n_1$ independent of the definition of the test statistic for the two-stage designs. In other words, for two-stage designs, there are always equivalent stopping boundaries for any two adaptive design methods (MSP, MPP, and MINP). However, this conclusion is not applicable to a design with more than two stages because such equivalent boundaries don't exist in general.

In general $K$-stage design, the expectation of the conditional mean at the $n^{th}$ stage is

$$\mu_n = \frac{\int_{\Omega_1} \cdots \int_{\Omega_{n-1}} \int_{-\infty}^{\infty} \frac{\bar{x}_1 n_1 + \cdots + \bar{x}_n n_n}{n_1 + \cdots + n_n} f_{\bar{X}_1 \cdots \bar{X}_n} (\bar{x}_1, ..., \bar{x}_n) \, d\bar{x}_1 ... d\bar{x}_n}{\int_{\Omega_1} \cdots \int_{\Omega_{n-1}} \int_{-\infty}^{\infty} f_{\bar{X}_1 \cdots \bar{X}_n} (\bar{x}_1, ..., \bar{x}_n) \, d\bar{x}_1 ... d\bar{x}_n},$$

$$(27.10)$$

where if $x_i \in \Omega_i$, the trial will continue to the $(i + 1)$th stage.

For an adaptive design with a sample-size adjustment, the calculation of bias is more complicated because sample size at the second stage, $n_2$, is a function of $x_1$. Several sample-size reestimation rules have been proposed such as the conditional power approach. These rules will lead to different functions of $n_2 (x_1)$, and integral (27.4) can only be carried out using numerical methods or simulations.

## 27.4   Confidence Interval

The confidence interval calculation is usually complicated for adaptive designs. There are even several different definitions of confidence intervals dependent on the sample space orderings.

Recall that for the classical design without any adaptations and with the hypothesis $H_0 : \mu \leq \mu_0$, the $100(1 - \alpha)\%$ one-sided confidence interval of $\mu$ can be defined as all the values of $\mu_0$ such that $H_0$ will not be rejected, given observed data $z$. For a group sequential design, we can take the similar approach; we can final a pair $(k_u(\mu_0), z_u(\mu_0))$ such that

$$\Pr_{\mu=\mu_0} \{(T, Z_T) \succeq (k_u(\mu_0), z_u(\mu_0))\} = \alpha. \qquad (27.11)$$

Then the acceptance region

$$A(\mu_0) = \{(k, z) : (k, z) \prec (k_u(\mu_0), z_u(\mu_0))\} \qquad (17.12)$$

defines a one-sided hypothesis test of $H_0 : \mu \leq \mu_0$ with type-I error rate $\alpha$. The $100(1 - \alpha)\%$ one-sided confidence set contains all values $\mu_0$ for which the hypothesis $H_0 : \mu \leq \mu_0$ is accepted. The confidence set is not a continuous region unless the so-called repeated confidence interval at the $k$, $RCI_k$, consists of all possible values for the parameter for which the null hypothesis will not be rejected given the observed value. When $x_{ij}$ is normally distributed and MINP, the $RCI_k$ can be expressed as

$$(\bar{x} - c_k \sigma_{\bar{x}}, \bar{x} + c_k \sigma_{\bar{x}}), \qquad (27.13)$$

where $c_k$ is the stopping boundary at the $k$th stage and $\sigma_{\bar{x}}$ is the standard deviation of $\bar{x}$.

A general approach to obtain $RCI_k$ numerically is through Monte Carlo simulations, but we are not going to discuss the simulation details here.

We now consider a general form of adjusted confidence intervals. Consider the null hypothesis $H_0 : \delta \leq \delta_0$. In general, a $100(1 - \alpha)\%$ confidence interval consists of all $\delta_0$ such that the $H_0$ would not be rejected, given the observed value for the test statistic $T = t$.

For MPP, MSP, and MINP, if the trial is stopped at the first stage, the confidence interval limit $\delta_{01}$ is given by

$$\delta_{01} = \hat{\sigma}\sqrt{\frac{2}{n_1}} \left( \Phi^{-1}(1 - \alpha_1) + z_{1-p_1} \right). \qquad (27.14)$$

When the trial is stopped at the second stage, the confidence bound calculations are different for MPP, MSP, and MINP as discussed below.

(1) For MPP, the test statistic is given by

$$T_2 = \prod_{i=1}^{2} \Phi \left( \frac{\delta}{\hat{\sigma}} \sqrt{\frac{n_i}{2}} - z_{1-p_i} \right).$$

To obtain the confidence limit $\delta_{02}$ for $\delta$, let $T_2 = \alpha_2$ and we obtain

$$\prod_{i=1}^{2} \Phi\left(\frac{\delta_{02}}{\hat{\sigma}}\sqrt{\frac{n_i}{2}} - z_{1-p_i}\right) = \alpha_2. \qquad (27.15)$$

Equation (27.15) can be solved numerically for $\delta_{02}$.

(2) For MSP, the test statistic is given by

$$T_2 = \sum_{i=1}^{2} \Phi\left(\frac{\delta}{\hat{\sigma}}\sqrt{\frac{n_i}{2}} - z_{1-p_i}\right).$$

To obtain the confidence limit $\delta_{02}$ for $\delta$, let $T_2 = \alpha_2$ and we obtain

$$\sum_{i=1}^{2} \Phi\left(\frac{\delta_{02}}{\hat{\sigma}}\sqrt{\frac{n_i}{2}} - z_{1-p_i}\right) = \alpha_2. \qquad (27.16)$$

We can numerically solve (27.16) for $\delta_{02}$.

(3) For MINP, the test statistic test is given by

$$T_2 = \sum_{i=1}^{2} \Phi\left(\frac{\delta}{\hat{\sigma}}\sqrt{\frac{n_i}{2}} - z_{1-p_i}\right).$$

To obtain the confidence limit $\delta_{02}$ for $\delta$, let $T_2 = \alpha_2$ and we obtain

$$1 - \Phi\left(\sum_{i=1}^{2} w_i\left(z_{1-p_i} - \frac{\delta_{02}}{\hat{\sigma}}\sqrt{\frac{n_i}{2}}\right)\right) = \alpha_2. \qquad (27.17)$$

Equation (27.17) can be solved analytically for $\delta_{02}$, i.e.,

$$\delta_{02} = \hat{\sigma}\sqrt{2}\frac{w_1 z_{1-p_1} + w_2 z_{1-p_2} - \Phi^{-1}(1-\alpha_2)}{w_1\sqrt{n_1} + w_2\sqrt{n_2}}. \qquad (27.18)$$

We can now summarize the steps for calculating the confidence intervals as follows:

(1) Using (27.14) through (27.18), calculate $\delta_{0k}$ dependent on MPP, MSP, or MINP, respectively.

(2) The one-sided $(1-\alpha)\%$ overall confidence bound is given by $\delta_c = \max\{\delta_{01}, \delta_{02}\}$.

## 27.5   Parameter Estimation in Trials with Arm Selection

We have discussed drop-the-loser, pick-the-winner, and add-arm designs. There are many other adaptive designs with arm selections, such as Thall,

Simon and Ellenberg (1989), Schaid, Wieand, and Therneau (1990), Stallard and Todd (2005), Stallard and Friede (2008), and Wu and Zhao (2012). The maximum likelihood estimates (MLE) of the selected arm often suffer from two types of bias, as described in Bauer et al. (2010). The first type, selection bias, $B_1(\theta)$, is the positive bias of the selected arm that arises due to the selection method:

$$B_1(\theta) = \sum_{i=1}^{k} E\left[\hat{\theta}_{MLE} - \theta_i | X_i = X_s\right] \Pr\left(X_i = X_s\right). \qquad (27.19)$$

This bias stems from the fact the treatment moving on to stage 2 was the one with the largest observed mean, so the estimate of the treatment effect of the selected arm was likely to be biased upward. Bauer et al. showed that when the true treatment effects of all arms were equal, the bias increased as the timing of the interim analysis became later, and it increased as the number of treatment arms increased. They saw a similar trend in the mean squared error (MSE), with the exception of designs with only 2 arms. In this instance, the MSE remained constant across all possible timings of the interim analysis.

Bauer et al. (2010) then defined the "reporting bias" in this type of design as

$$B_2(\theta) = E\left[\hat{\theta}_{MLE} - \theta_i | X_i = X_s\right] \Pr\left(X_i = X_s\right)$$
$$+ E\left[\hat{\theta}_{MLE} - \theta_i | X_i \neq X_s\right] \Pr\left(X_i \neq X_s\right). \qquad (27.20)$$

While defined as "reporting bias," this examined whether bias still existed when outcome reporting bias was removed. As shown above, the "reporting bias" incorporates the bias of the MLE of the selected arm at the final analysis and the bias of the observed means at the interim analysis for the arms not selected. This bias was typically negative and was most negative with early interim analyses. When the analysis occurs at 100% information (no treatment selection), there was minimal "reporting bias." As the number of arms increased, this type of bias diminished.

The third one, called "positive publication bias," is defined as

$$B_3(\theta) = \sum_{i=1}^{k} E\left[\hat{\theta}_{MLE} - \theta_i | X_i = X_s, \text{ rejecting } H_0\right]$$
$$\times \Pr\left(X_i = X_s, \text{ rejecting } H_0\right). \qquad (27.21)$$

This bias, $B_3(\theta)$, directly relates what patients and doctors will be told or will see in the label.

Over the past several years, there have been several approaches proposed to adjusting the selection bias described by Bauer et al. (20.10). Shen (2001) proposed a "Stepwise Over-Correction" approach for the situation where there were two experimental treatment arms $(k = 2)$. The approach was based upon the first and second moments of the density function for the difference between the observed and true mean of the selected treatment arm, $X_S - \theta_S$. Stallard and Todd (2005) proposed an adjustment inspired by both Whitehead (1986) and Shen (2001).

Cohen and Sackrowitz (1989b) identified a uniformly minimum variance conditional unbiased estimator (UMVCUE) for the mean of the larger of two treatment groups, $\tilde{\theta}_{(1)}$, in a two-stage design when the variances of the two groups were known and equal:

$$\tilde{\theta}_{(1)} = \frac{Z}{2} - \frac{1}{\sqrt{2}} \frac{\phi(W)}{\Phi(W)}, \qquad (27.22)$$

where $Z = X_{(1)} + Y$ and $W = \sqrt{2}\left(Z/2 - X_{(2)}\right)$. This was derived by using the Rao–Blackwell theorem to find an unbiased estimator of $\tilde{\theta}_{(1)}$.

Sampson and Sill (2005) recommended the use of this estimator and developed a confidence interval to be used for hypothesis testing based on the distribution of $\tilde{\theta}_{(1)}$ for a normally distributed endpoint.

### 27.5.1    *Parametric Bootstrap Approach*

Pickard and Chang (2014) proposed the parametric bootstrap approach to the bias and MSE reductions for different endpoints. It is based on using the empirical distribution of the observed responses in each treatment arm, estimating the probability that each arm is the arm with the true maximum response, and comparing these probabilities to those that would be observed if the treatment arms all had equal means.

Let $X_i \sim N\left(\theta_i, \sigma^2/n_i\right), i = 1, ..., k$, be the random variable representing the mean outcome from treatment arm $T_i$. For the purposes described here, $\sigma^2$ is assumed known and equal to 1. At selection time $t$, with $n_1$ patients enrolled to each arm, all treatment arms are ordered based on their observed means, $X_{(1)} < X_{(2)} < ... < X_{(k)}$. The arm with the largest mean $(T_S)$, $X_S = X_{(k)}$, is then selected and carried forward to stage 2. Let $Y \sim N\left(\theta_s, \sigma^2/n_2\right)$ be the random variable representing the mean outcome of the $n_2$ patients enrolled in $T_S$ during the second stage of the study. At the final analysis, the estimated mean of $T_S$, $\hat{\theta}_S$, is calculated using data from all $n_1 + n_2$ patients. When faced with data from such a study, a key question that could be asked is "how likely would it be for the $X_i$ values to be observed in the situation where all $\theta_i$ are equal?" Assume that an estimate for the stage 1 mean of $T_S$ is calculated using a linear combination of all $k$ mean values. One possible choice for the weights used in this linear combination would be the probability of each arm being the one with the largest true mean, that is, $p_{(k)i} = Pr\,(\theta_i = \max(\theta_1, \theta_2, ..., \theta_k)$. The linear combination would then be calculated as

$$\hat{\theta}_S = \sum_{i=1}^{k} p_{(k)i} X_i. \qquad (27.23)$$

If $p_{(k)S}$ approached 1, this would imply that the correct arm was selected and $S$ could be estimated using its MLE, $X_S$. If all $p_{(k)i}$ approached $1/k$, this would suggest that $\theta_1 = \theta_2 = \theta_S$, and a grand mean of all treatment arms should then be used as the stage 1 estimate. These $p_{(k)i}$ values can be calculated as

$$p_{(k)i} = \int_{-\infty}^{\infty} \int_{-\infty}^{X_i} \cdots \int_{-\infty}^{X_i} f\,(x_1, ..., x_k)\,dx_1 \ldots dx_{i-1} dx_{i+1} \ldots dx_k dx_i. \qquad (27.24)$$

Based on Efron's plug-in principle, we have the estimation of $p_{(k)i}$ as

$$\hat{p}_{(k)i} = \int_{-\infty}^{\infty} \int_{-\infty}^{X_i} \cdots \int_{-\infty}^{X_i} \hat{f}\,(x_1, ..., x_k)\,dx_1 \ldots dx_{i-1} dx_{i+1} \ldots dx_k dx_i. \qquad (27.25)$$

Because $\hat{p}_{(k)i}$ is an estimated value, it has some level of variability associated with it. When all $\theta_i$ are equal, $p_{(k)i}$ is equal to $1/k$. In this case, using $1/k$ for $p_{(k)i}$ in (27.24) can reduce the variability of the estimated $\hat{\theta}_S$. However, when $\theta_i$ is very different, using $1/k$ for $p_{(k)i}$ can have a larger bias than using $\hat{p}_{(k)i}$. In general, if we know the parameters $\theta_i$ are approximately equal, we use $1/k$ for $p_{(k)i}$; otherwise, we use $\hat{p}_{(k)i}$ for $p_{(k)i}$ in the estimation. To determine how close the actual situation is to the case of equal $\theta_i$, we can use the vector $(\hat{p}_{(k)1}, ..., \hat{p}_{(k)k})$ to compare to what would be expected when all $\theta_i$ are equal. The Euclidean distance, $d$, is calculated between $(p_{(k)1}, ..., \hat{p}_{(k)k})$ and the vector expected values when there are no differences in the treatment arms are $(1/k, ..., 1/k)$. The value $d$ is then compared to a null distribution of Euclidean distances that arise when $\theta_1 = \theta_2 = ... = \theta_k$. For this null distribution, the means of the treatment arms are all assumed to be $N(0, \sigma^2/n_1)$, and $k$ values are sampled from this distribution to represent observed means for each treatment arm. Null $\hat{p}_{(k)i}^*$ values are calculated for each resampled treatment arm, followed by the calculation of null Euclidean distances, $d^*$. This is repeated for 10,000 simulations to generate a distribution of $d^*$ values. The value $d$ is then compared to this distribution to estimate the probability that similar results could be observed when all treatment arms are equal, $\eta = \Pr(d^* > d)$.

Using the value $\eta$ and $(\hat{p}_{(k)1}, ..., \hat{p}_{(k)k})$, the stage 1 estimate of $T_S$ is calculated as the linear combination of the $k$ stage 1 means:

$$\hat{\theta}^1_{S,boot} = \begin{cases} \sum_{i=1}^{k} \frac{1}{k} X_i, & \text{if } \eta > \eta_c \\ \sum_{i=1}^{k} \left[ (1 - \eta) \hat{p}_{(k)i} + \eta \frac{1}{k} \right] X_i, & \text{if } \eta \le \eta_c. \end{cases} \qquad (27.26)$$

The user-specified variable $\eta_c$ ranges from 0 to 1 and controls the stringency of the bias reduction. Values of $\eta_c$ approaching 0 result in the grand mean more likely to be the stage 1 estimate. The results described here were generated using an $\eta_c$ value of 1. When $\eta$ is large, there is a high probability that all $\theta_i$ are equal, in which case, the grand mean of the treatment arms is used to summarize the treatment effect. Conversely, when $\eta$ is small, then at least one arm has a true mean that largely differs from the rest, and the $\hat{p}_{(k)i}$ values are used as weights. The final point estimate is then calculated as

$$\hat{\theta}_{S,boot} = \frac{n_1}{n_1 + n_2} \hat{\theta}^1_{S,boot} + \frac{n_2}{n_1 + n_2} Y. \qquad (27.27)$$

As an example, assume a study with a normally distributed endpoint was conducted where stage 1 consisted of 40 patients in each of three arms. Let $(X_1, X_2, X_3) = (0.15, 0.05, 0.50)$ with known $\sigma/\sqrt{n_1} = 1/\sqrt{40}$. Using the empirical distributions of the treatment arm means, the probability of being the arm with $\theta_i = \max(\theta_1, \theta_2, ..., \theta_k)$ is calculated to be $(\hat{p}_{(k)1}, ..., \hat{p}_{(k)k}) = (0.056, 0.018, 0.927)$. The Euclidean distance of this vector from $(1/3, 1/3, 1/3)$ is calculated as $d = 0.727$. Comparing this value to the null distribution of $d$ values suggests that there is a probability of 0.0423 that these $\hat{p}_{(k)i}$ values could be observed when all $\theta_i$ are equal, so $\eta = 0.0423$. Thus, the stage 1 estimate is calculated as

$$\hat{\theta}^1_{S,boot} = 0.9577[(0.056)0.15 + (0.018)0.05 + (0.927)0.50] \qquad (27.28)$$
$$+ 0.0423[(0.33)0.15 + (0.33)0.05 + (0.33)0.50]$$
$$= 0.46.$$

The third arm, $T_3$, would then be carried forward to stage 2, where an additional 60 patients would be enrolled to the arm. If it is assumed that the stage 2 mean was 0.39, then the final estimate, $\hat{\theta}_{S,boot}$, is calculated as $0.40(0.46) + 0.60(0.39) = 0.42$.

## 27.5.2 Shrinkage Estimators

Carreras and Brannath (2012) used a shrinkage estimator that was proposed by Lindley (1962) to adjust the estimate based on all observed means when $k = 4$. If the variability among all observed means was relatively small, the adjusted mean of the selected arm based on the shrinkage estimator was closer to the overall grand mean. Conversely, large variability placed more weight on the observed mean of the selected arm. So at the interim analysis, the adjusted estimator,

$$\hat{\theta}_S^{L,1} = CX_S + (1 - C)\,\bar{X}, \tag{27.29}$$

where $C = \max(0, 1 - \frac{(k-3)\sigma^2}{n \sum_{j=1}^{k}(X_j - \bar{X})^2})$ and $\bar{X} = \frac{\sum_{j=1}^{k} X_j}{k}$.

After the interim analysis, $n_2$ patients were then enrolled to the selected arm, and the unbiased mean of the $n_2$ patients, $Y_S$, was calculated. The combined results from the two stages were calculated in the same manner as the MLE, with the exception of the shrinkage estimate we used as the stage 1 estimate:

$$\hat{\theta}_S^{L} = \frac{n_1}{n_1 + n_2}\hat{\theta}_S^{L,1} + \frac{n_2}{n_1 + n_2}Y_S. \tag{27.30}$$

Compared to the MLE, Lindley's shrinkage estimator was shown to have lower Bayes risk with priors that were normal, $\theta_i \sim N(\mu, \tau)$, as defined by Hwang (1993):

$$R_{\mu,\tau}\left(Q_S^L\right) = \int_{-\infty}^{\infty} \cdots \int_{-\infty}^{\infty} E_{\theta}\left\{(Q_S^L - \theta_S)^2 \phi\left(\frac{\theta_1 - \mu}{\tau^2}\right) \cdots \phi\left(\frac{\theta_k - \mu}{\tau^2}\right)\right\}$$
$$\times d\theta_1 \cdots d\theta_k. \tag{27.31}$$

Simulations showed that when there were no differences among the true means of six treatment arms, the shrinkage estimator showed considerably reduced bias and MSE over the MLE. While Bowden and Glimm's (2008) estimator was unbiased, Carreras and Brannath (2012) confirmed it had much higher MSE than the MLE when the interim analysis was conducted later than 50% information time. Earlier interim analyses yielded MSE values similar to the MLE. Stallard and Todd's (2003) estimator tended to overcorrect for the bias in this scenario and also had MSE that was generally higher than the MLE. When the true means of the six treatment arms had a linear relationship, similar trends were observed; however, the differences between the four approaches were smaller. When only one treatment arm was effective, Lindley's (1962) method actually overcorrected for the bias and was the least accurate estimator. In this scenario, all four estimators had very similar MSE (Pickard, 2014). When there were fewer than four treatment arms, Carreras and Brannath recommended using the best linear unbiased predictors (BLUPs) from a random effects model where the treatment arm assignments were random effects:

$$\hat{\theta}_i = \mu + \alpha_i, \tag{27.32}$$

where $\mu$ was the overall grand mean and $\alpha_i$ was the random effect from the $i$th treatment arm. Similar, although diminished, differences among the above-mentioned approaches were observed when only three treatment arms were considered.

Recently, Bowden (2013) proposed several Empirical Bayes estimators that incorporated the information from both stages of a treatment selection design based on methodology used in meta-analyses. These were extensions of the method proposed by Carreras and Brannath (2012), which only incorporated the first stage data in the shrinkage estimator.

### 27.5.3    *Empirical Bayes Estimators*

Pickard (2014) proposed a specific shrinkage estimator, the empirical Bayes estimator. With traditional Bayesian approaches, the hyperparameters of the prior distribution are prespecified based on knowledge (or lack thereof) going into an experiment. An alternative is to let the data determine the hyperparameters. As an example, assuming $k$ arms, each with $n$ observations and means $X_i \sim N(\theta_i, \sigma^2/n)$, $i = 1, \ldots, k$, $\sigma^2$ known and $\theta_i \sim N(\mu, \tau^2)$, use the observed data to identify estimates of $\mu$ and $\tau^2$.

For equal $n$ per arm, to identify estimates of $\mu$ and $\tau^2$, find joint distribution of $\left(X_1, \ldots, X_k, \theta_1, \ldots, \theta_k, \mu, \tau^2\right)$

$$f\left(X_1, \ldots, X_k, \theta_1, \ldots, \theta_k, \mu, \tau^2\right) = \prod_{i=1}^{k} \pi\left(\theta_i\right) f\left(X_i | \theta_i\right) = \left(\frac{1}{2\pi}\right)^{\frac{k+1}{2}} \left(\frac{n}{\tau^2 \sigma^2}\right)^{\frac{k}{2}} \cdot$$

$$\exp\left\{-\frac{1}{2} \sum_{i=1}^{k} \left(\frac{1}{\tau^2} + \frac{n}{\sigma^2}\right) \left(\theta_i - \frac{\frac{nX_i}{\sigma^2} + \frac{\mu}{\tau^2}}{\frac{n}{\sigma^2} + \frac{1}{\tau^2}}\right)^2\right\} \exp\left\{-\sum_{i=1}^{k} \frac{n\left(X_i - \mu\right)^2}{2\left(n\tau^2 + \sigma^2\right)}\right\} \cdot \tag{27.33}$$

Integrating out all $\theta_i$, we obtain

$$\int \cdots \int f\left(X_1, ..., X_k, \theta_1, ..., \theta_k, \mu, \tau^2\right) d\theta_1 \cdots d\theta_k$$

$$= \left(\frac{1}{2\pi}\right)^{\frac{1}{2}} \left(\frac{n}{n\tau^2 + \sigma^2}\right)^{\frac{k}{2}} \exp\left\{-\sum_{i=1}^{k} \frac{n\left(X_i - \mu\right)^2}{2\left(n\tau^2 + \sigma^2\right)}\right\}. \quad (27.34)$$

Solve for the values of $\mu$ and $\tau$ that maximize the likelihood:

$$\hat{\mu} = \frac{\sum_{i=1}^{k} X_i}{k} \text{ and } \hat{\tau} = \max\left(\frac{\sum_{i=1}^{k}(X_i - \hat{\mu})^2}{k} - \frac{\sigma^2}{n}, 0\right). \quad (27.35)$$

The Empirical Bayes estimator of the selected arm is then the expectation of the posterior estimate with a prior distribution:

$$\hat{\theta}_{S,EB} = \frac{\hat{\tau} X_s + \frac{\sigma^2}{n}\hat{\mu}}{\hat{\tau}^2 + \frac{\sigma^2}{n}}. \quad (27.36)$$

Further refinement is needed to address the scenario where only one treatment arm is active, which is a common shortcoming of shrinkage estimators. To perform this adjustment, the circumstance where one arm is largely different from the rest needs to be identified, and the estimate in this circumstance should be close to the MLE.

The $F$-statistic can be used to identify this situation:

$$F = \frac{\sum_{i=1}^{k} n_i\left(X_i - \bar{X}\right)/(k-1)}{\sum_{i=1}^{k}\sum_{j=1}^{n_j}\left(x_{ij} - X_i\right)^2 / \sum_{i=1}^{k}\left(N_i - 1\right)}, \quad (27.37)$$

where $x_{ij}$ is the observed value for the $j$th subject is the $i$th arm and $\bar{X}$ is the grand mean of the arms, weighted by sample size $n_i$.

Pickard (2014) proposed the following estimator:

$$\theta_{S,EB(LT)} = \max\left(\theta_{S,EB}, \theta_{S,MLE}, \frac{\delta_c \sigma}{\sqrt{n_s}}\right), \quad (27.38)$$

$$\log\left(\delta_c\right) = \begin{cases} \log\left(0.01\right) + \frac{\hat{a}+b\log(0.01 F_{0.85})}{\log\frac{F_{0.85}}{F_{0.99}}} \log\frac{0.1}{F_{0.99}}, & \text{if } t_{MLE,k-1} \leq t_{0.90} \\ \log\left(0.01\right) + \frac{\hat{a}+b\log(0.01 F_{0.85})}{\log\frac{F_{0.85}}{F_{0.99}}} \log\frac{F}{F0.99}, & \text{otherwise} \end{cases},$$

$$(27.39)$$

where $\hat{a} = -0.01 - 0.03k + 0.14t + 0.15kt$, $\hat{b} = -1.95 + 0.02k + 0.35log\left(\sum n_i\right) + 0.05t - 0.002\left(N_s\right) - 0.11kt$. $t_{0.90}^*$ is the 90th percentile of $t_{MLE,k-1}$ values that occur when all treatment arms are equal.

## 27.6 Summary

We have discussed the analyses following an adaptive trial, including the $p$-value, parameter estimation, and confidence interval. We see that there are controversies surrounding such analyses, mainly because these quantities are dependent on the sample space (conditional or unconditional) and sample space orderings. As a result, there are different versions of $p$-values and confidence intervals, which make the clinical interpretations very difficult. The estimation bias and variance of the estimation are definitely trade-offs in adaptive design settings. We should balance these two aspects and clinical interpretations as well. In the current practice, the naive, sample mean or MLE is still a common estimation; unadjusted $p$-values and unadjusted confidence intervals are still commonly reported outcomes for an adaptive trial.

**Problems**

**27.1** What are the challenges in data analyses after an adaptive trial?

**27.2** Explain the term "sample-space ordering." Why is it important in the analysis of adaptive trial data?

**27.3** If you are a statistician and a patient, would you use the MLE or bias adjusted estimate in your decision making regarding which drug to take?

# Chapter 28

# Planning, Execution, Analysis, and Reporting

The U.S. FDA released the draft Guidance for Industry, Adaptive Design Clinical Trials for Drugs and Biologics in February 2010. Since then, more than four years has past, no updated or final version has yet been seen. Because it is a draft, it is not recommended for implementation. Adaptive design study has made big progress in the past five years and some of the FDA's views in the draft may be out of date. Nevertheless, there is much valuable information we should be aware of, and everyone who practices adaptive trials should carefully read the draft guidance. The *Journal of Biopharmaceutical Statistics* published a special issue (Liu and Chang, 2010) of discussion papers on the draft adaptive design guidance by the U.S. Food and Drug Administration. In this special discussion issue, technical papers were invited not only to address existing problems with adaptive designs as pointed out by the FDA guidance but also to introduce new designs for clinical trial settings that have not been adequately tackled in the literature.

## 28.1 Validity and Integrity

Both the PhRMA white papers (Gallo et al., 2006a) and the discussion paper (Chang and Chow, 2006b) emphasize the importance of validity and integrity in adaptive trials. Although controlling the overall type-I error rate at the nominal level (alpha) is essential, it does not imply validity and integrity of the trial. The validity of a trial includes internal and external validities. A study that readily allows its findings to be generalized to the population at large has high external validity. Internal validity refers to the degree to which we are successful in eliminating confounding variables and establishing a cause–effect relationship (treatment effect) within the study itself. There are many different ways in which the internal validity of a study could be jeopardized. Threats to internal validity include instrumentation (case report form, coding shift, evaluation criteria), selection bias (failure in randomization at some level, e.g., a less-sick patient may prefer to wait for enrollment in the confirmatory stage instead of the learning stage, but a sicker patient may not be able to wait), and experimental mortality (informed dropouts). The threats to external validity are protocol amendments, including changes in inclusion/exclusion criteria, which could result in a shift in the target patient population (Chow, Chang, and Pong, 2005), and multiple endpoints that do not support a common conclusion.

Ensuring integrity is also critical in a seamless design. Integrity means a solid protocol design, excellent execution, unbiased analyses of trial data, and correct interpretation of the results. Integrity means being ethical and avoiding the out-weighting of the risk–benefit ratio of individual patients, trial patients as a whole, and future patients. Integrity also means that regulatory agencies use appropriate approval criteria that balance risk and benefit. The use of a fixed type-I error rate criterion might, in fact, prevent a low-risk and low-benefit drug from being delivered to patients.

## 28.2 Study Planning

Before the implementation of an adaptive design, it is recommended that the following practical issues be considered. First, determine whether an adaptive design is feasible for the intended trial. For example, will the adaptive design require extraordinary efforts for implementation? Are the level of difficulty and the associated cost justifiable for the gain from the adaptive design? Will the implementation of the adaptive design delay patient recruitment and prolong the duration of the study? Would delayed responses diminish the advantage of the adaptive design? How often will the unblinded analyses be practical, and to whom should the data be unblinded? How should the impact of a Data Monitoring Committee's (DMC's) decisions regarding the trial (e.g., recommending early stopping or other adaptations due to safety concerns) be considered at the design stage? Second, ensure the validity of the adaptive design for the intended trial. For example, will the unblinding cause potential bias in treatment assessment? Will the implementation of the adaptive design destroy the randomness? Third, have an expectation about the degree of flexibility (sensitivity or robustness). For example, will protocol deviations or violations invalidate the adaptive method? How might an unexpected DMC action affect the power and validity of the design? In designing a trial, we should also consider how to prevent premature release of the interim results to the general public using information masks because releasing information could affect the rest of the trial and endanger the integrity of the trial. Regarding study design, we strongly suggest early communication with the regulatory agency and DMC regarding the study protocol and the DMC charter. For broader discussions of planning different adaptive designs, please see the PhRMA full white papers on adaptive design (Chuang et al., 2006; Gallo, 2006; Gaydos et al., 2006; Maca et al., 2006; Quinlan, Gallo, and Krams, 2006).

## 28.3 Working with Regulatory Agency

Dr. Robert Powell from the FDA said that companies should begin a dialogue about adaptive designs with FDA medical officers and statisticians as early as a year before beginning a trial. FDA's Office of Biostatistics Associate Director-Adaptive Design/Pharmacogenomics, Dr. S.J. Wang (2006) addressed some of the expectations for adaptive design submissions. The design: (1) is prospectively planned, (2) has valid statistical approaches on modification of design elements that have alpha control and can be defined in terms of ICH E-9 standard, (3) has valid point estimates and confidence interval estimates, (4) builds on experience from external trials, (5) takes a "learn" and "confirm" approach, (6) has standard operating procedures and infrastructure for adaptive process monitoring to avoid bias, (7) has SOPs on adaptive design decisions, and (8) includes documentation of the actual monitoring process, extent of compliance, and potential effect on study results.

It is important to assure the validity of the adaptive design. Dr. O'Neill said (*The Pink Sheet*, December 18, 2006, p. 24), "We're most concerned about estimating what you think you are estimating ... Is the hypothesis testing appropriate? Do you know what you are rejecting at end of day? Can you say you are controlling the false positive?"

Another reason to communicate with the agency early is that the FDA could be of assistance in sharing the data or at least the disease information or models as Dr. Robert Powell indicated. Building off external data and experience is sometimes a crucial element of adaptive design. Just as Pfizer SVP Dr. Declan Doogan pointed out: Drug development is a knowledge-creating business, we have to increase access to data ... the FDA is sitting on a pile of wonderful data. How can we access that? We could learn much from other people's failures (*The Pink Sheet*, December 18, 2006, p. 24).

The FDA release the draft guidance for Adaptive Design Clinical Trials for Drugs and Biologics in 2010. This guidance gives advice on topics such as (1) what aspects of adaptive design trials (i.e., clinical, statistical, regulatory) call for special consideration, (2) when to interact with FDA while planning and conducting adaptive design studies, (3) what information to include in the adaptive design for FDA review, and (4) issues to consider in the evaluation of a completed adaptive design study. This guidance is intended to assist sponsors in planning and conducting adaptive design clinical studies, and to facilitate an efficient FDA review (FDA, 2010).

FDA's guidance describes the Agency's current thinking on a topic and should be viewed only as recommendations and not requirements. In the guidance, an adaptive design clinical study is defined as a study that includes a prospectively planned opportunity for modification of one or more specified aspects of the study design and hypotheses based on analysis of data (usually interim data) from subjects in the study. Analyses of the accumulating study data are performed at prospectively planned timepoints within the study, can be performed in a fully blinded manner or in an unblinded manner, and can occur with or without formal statistical hypothesis testing.

The adaptations include but not limited to

- study eligibility criteria (either for subsequent study enrollment or for a subset selection of an analytic population)
- randomization procedure
- treatment regimens of the different study groups (e.g., dose level, schedule, duration)
- total sample size of the study (including early termination)
- concomitant treatments used
- planned schedule of patient evaluations for data collection (e.g., number of intermediate timepoints, timing of last patient observation and duration of patient study participation)
- primary endpoint (e.g., which of several types of outcome assessments, which timepoint of assessment, use of a unitary versus composite endpoint or the components included in a composite endpoint)
- election and/or order of secondary endpoints
- analytic methods to evaluate the endpoints (e.g., covariates of final analysis, statistical methodology, type-I error control)

The FDA raises two main concerns with adaptive design: (1) whether the adaptation process has led to design, analysis, or conduct flaws that have introduced bias that increases the chance of a false conclusion that the treatment is effective (a type-I error) and (2) whether the adaptation process has led to positive study results that are difficult to interpret irrespective of having control of type-I error.

The FDA classifies general adaptive designs into two categories: well-understood and less well-understood adaptive designs. The well-understood adaptive designs include

(1) Adaptation of study eligibility criteria based on analyses of pretreatment (baseline) data
(2) Adaptations to maintain study power based on blinded interim analyses of aggregate data
(3) Adaptations based on interim results of an outcome unrelated to efficacy
(4) Adaptations using group sequential methods and the drop-loser designs
(5) Adaptations in the data analysis plan not dependent on within study, between group outcome differences

As suggested in the guidance, a blinded SSR design with a binary, survival, or continuous endpoint requires no alpha adjustment. However, as we have discussed, the unblinded SSR can inflate the alpha to some degree.

For drop-loser designs, the FDA states: Studies with multiple groups (e.g., multiple-dose levels) can be designed to carry only one or two groups to completion out of the several initiated, based on this type of futility analysis done by group. One or more unblinded interim analyses of the apparent treatment effect in each group is examined, and groups that meet the prospective futility criterion are terminated. However, because of the multiplicity arising from the several sequential interim analyses over time with multiple between-group analyses done to select groups to discontinue, statistical adjustments and the usual group sequential alpha spending adjustments need to be made in this case to control type-I error rates.

The guidance stated: "For the group sequential methods to be valid, it is important to adhere to the prospective analytic plan, terminating the group if a futility criterion is met, and not terminating the study for efficacy unless the prospective efficacy criterion is achieved. Failure to follow the prospective plan in either manner risks confounding interpretation of the study results". This seems to be suggesting a futility bonding rule. If it indeed is, a bigger alpha can be used for the group design with a futility boundary.

The less well-understood adaptive designs include

(1) Adaptations for dose selection studies
(2) Adaptive randomization based on relative treatment group responses
(3) Adaptation of sample size based on interim-effect size estimates
(4) Adaptation of patient population based on treatment–effect estimates
(5) Adaptation for endpoint selection based on interim estimate of treatment effect
(6) Adaptations in noninferiority studies

Generally, adaptive designs with well-understood properties can get the FDA's blessing earlier than less well-understood designs. However, the draft guidance was released four years ago. During these four years, research and practice of adaptive designs have made big progress. Some less well-understood designs from yesterday may become well-understood today.

Regarding the interaction with the FDA when planning and conducting an adaptive design, the FDA has stated: The purpose and nature of the interactions between a study sponsor and FDA varies with the study's location (stage) within the drug development program. The increased complexity of some adaptive design studies and uncertainties regarding their performance characteristics may warrant earlier and more extensive interactions than usual. In general, the FDA encorage adaptive designs in early and middle period of drug development, but suggest cautionaly use in late stages of drug development.

FDA will generally not be involved in examining the interim data used for the adaptive decision making and will not provide comments on the adaptive decisions while the study is ongoing. Special protocol assessments (SPA) entail timelines (45-day responses) and commitments that may not be best suited for adaptive design studies. The full review and assessment of a study using less well-understood adaptive design methods can be complex, will involve a multidisciplinary evaluation team, and might involve extended discussions among individuals within different FDA offices before reaching a conclusion. If there has been little or no prior discussion between FDA and the study sponsor regarding the proposed study and its adaptive design features, other information requests following initial FDA evaluation are likely and full completion of study assessment within the SPA 45-day time frame is unlikely. Sponsors are therefore encouraged to have thorough discussions with FDA regarding the study design and the study's place within the development program before considering submitting an SPA request.

## 28.4 Trial Monitoring

In practice, it is recognized that there are often deviations from the study protocol when conducting a clinical trial. It is ethical to monitor the trials to ensure that individual subjects are not exposed, or have limited exposure, to unsafe or ineffective treatment regimens. For this purpose, a Data Monitoring Committee is usually established. The DMC plays a critical role in monitoring clinical trials. There are common issues that affect a DMC's decision, such as short-term versus long-term treatment effects, early termination philosophies, response to early beneficial trends, response to early unfavorable trends, and response where there are no apparent trends (Ellenberg, Fleming, and DeMets, 2002; Pocock, 2005). It is recommended that a DMC be established to monitor the trial when an adaptive design is employed in clinical trials, especially when many adaptations are considered for allowing greater flexibility.

The stopping rule chosen in the design phase serves as a guideline to a DMC (Ellenberg et al., 2002) as it makes a decision to recommend continuing or stopping a clinical trial. If all aspects of the conduct of the clinical trial adhered exactly to the conditions stipulated during the design phase, the stopping rule obtained during the design phase could be used directly. However, there are usually complicating factors that must be dealt with during the conduct of the trial.

Deviation of Analysis Schedule: DMC meetings are typically based on the availability of its members, which may be different from the schedules set at the design phase. The enrollment may be different from the assumption made at the design phase. Deviation in the analysis schedule will affect the stopping boundaries; therefore, the boundaries should be recalculated based on the actual schedules.

Deviation of Efficacy Variable Estimation: The true variability of the response variable is never known, but the actual data collected at interim analysis may show that the initial estimates in the design phase are inaccurate. Deviation in the variability could affect the stopping boundaries. In this case, we may want to know the likelihood of success of the trial based on current data, which is known as conditional and predictive power, and repeated confidence intervals. Similarly, the estimation of treatment difference in response could be different from the initial estimation in the design phase. This could lead to an adaptive design or sample-size reestimation (Jennison and Turnbull, 2000a).

Safety Factors: Efficacy is not the only factor that will affect a DMC's decision. Safety factors are critical for the DMC to make an appropriate recommendation to stop or continue the trial. The term "benefit–risk ratio" is a most commonly used composite criterion to assist in decision making. In this respect, it is desirable to know the likelihood of success of the trial based on current data, i.e., the conditional power or predictive power.

The DMC may also weigh the short-term and long-term treatment effects in its recommendations.

The commonly used tools for monitoring a group sequential design are stopping boundaries, conditional and predictive powers, futility index, and repeated confidence interval. These tools can be used in other adaptive designs. Bayesian monitoring tools are appreciated for different adaptive designs. There are several good books on trial monitoring: *Data Monitoring Committees in Clinical Trials* by Ellenberg, Fleming, and DeMets (2002) and *Statistical Monitoring of Clinical Trials* by Proschan, Lan, and Wittes (2006), among others.

## 28.5  Analysis and Reporting

Data analyses of an adaptive design at interim analysis and at the final stage remain very challenging to statisticians. While they benefit from the flexibility of adaptations, it is a concern that the $p$-value may not be correct and the corresponding confidence interval may not be reliable (EMEA, 2002). It is also a concern that major adaptations could lead to a totally different trial that is unable to address the medical questions or hypotheses that the original trial intended to answer. Although some unbiased estimators of treatment effect for some adaptive designs are available, many issues in data analysis of general adaptive designs are still very debatable from statistical and scientific points of view. It is suggested that both unadjusted and adjusted values be reported, including the adjusted and unadjusted point-estimates, the naive and adjusted confidence intervals, and the adjusted and unadjusted $p$-values. When an unbiased estimate is not available, computer simulations should be performed to assess the magnitude of the bias. It is suggested that in addition to the frequentist results, pharmaceutical companies should make efforts to present Bayesian results because these more-informative results could help the company itself and the FDA to better measure the benefit–risk ratio for a candidate drug.

## 28.6 Clinical Trial Simulation

Traditional drug development is subjective to a large extent, and intuitive decision-making processes are primarily based on individual experiences. Therefore, optimal design is often not achieved. Clinical trial simulation (CTS) is a powerful tool for providing an objective evaluation of development plans and study designs for program optimization and for supporting strategic decision making. CTS is very intuitive and easy to implement with minimal cost and can be done in a short time. The utilities of CTS include, but are not limited to, (1) sensitivity analysis and risk assessment; (2) estimation of probability of success (power); (3) design evaluation and optimization; (4) cost, time, and risk reduction; (5) clinical development program evaluation and prioritization; (6) trial monitoring and interim prediction of future outcomes; (7) prediction of long-term benefit using short-term outcomes; (8) validation of trial design and statistical methods; and (9) streamlining communication among different parties. Within regulatory bodies, CTS has been frequently used for assessing the robustness of results, validating statistical methodology, and predicting long-term benefit in accelerated approvals. CTS plays an important role in adaptive design for the following reasons: First, statistical theory for adaptive designs is often complicated under some relatively strong assumptions, and CTS is useful in modeling very complicated situations with minimum assumptions not only to control type-I error, but also to calculate the power, and to generate many other important operating characteristics such as the expected sample size, conditional power, and unbiased estimates. Second, CTS can be used to evaluate the robustness of the adaptive design against protocol deviations. Moreover, CTS can be used as a tool to monitor trials, predict outcomes, identify potential problems, and provide remedies for resolutions during the conduct of the trials.

In summary, clinical trial simulation is a useful tool for adaptive designs in clinical research. It can help investigators achieve better planning, better designs, better monitoring, and generally better execution of clinical trials. In addition, it can help to (1) streamline the drug development process, (2) increase the probability of success, and (3) reduce the cost and time-to-market in pharmaceutical research and development.

A simplified CTS model is shown in Figure 28.1. The high-level algorithms for the simulations are to simulate the trial under the null hypothesis $m$ times, calculate the test statistic for each simulation, and use the $m$ test statistic values to construct distribution numerically, as well as to simulate the trial under the alternative hypothesis $m$ times, calculate the test

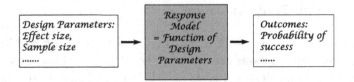

Figure 28.1:   Simplified CTS Model: Gray-Box

statistic, and use the $m$ test statistic values to construct a distribution under $H_a$ numerically. The two distributions can be used to determine the critical region for a given $\alpha$, the $p$-value for given data, and power for a given critical region.

## 28.7   Summary

Adaptive design methods represent new territory in drug development. Using adaptive design, we can increase the chances for the success of a trial with reduced cost. Bayesian approaches provide new tools for optimizing trial design and clinical development program planning by integrating all the relevant knowledge and information available. Clinical trial simulations offer a powerful tool to design and monitor trials. The combination of adaptive design, the Bayesian approach, and trial simulation forms an ultimate statistical instrument for most successful drug development programs.

This innovative approach requires careful upfront planning and the ability to rapidly integrate knowledge and experiences from different disciplines into the decision-making process. It requires integration of new data in real time, where data standardization tools such as CDISC and EDC play critical roles. Last but not least, all of the above require a shift to a more collaborative working environment among disciplines.

## Problems

**28.1** Elaborate how you would use simulation in your adaptive trial design and why it is important.

**28.2** Review and summarize the FDA's and other regulatory agencies' guidance on adaptive design.

**28.3** Plan an adaptive trial including all the necessary steps from beginning to the end.

# Chapter 29

# Debates in Adaptive Designs

In this last chapter, we will discuss most of the controversial issues surrounding adaptive designs. We will review relevant statistical principles and check against adaptive designs. The discussions will be from both statistical and philosophical perspectives. In many ways, this may reflect my personal opinions.

## 29.1  My Standing Point

"We can't solve problems by using the same kind of thinking we used when we created them."—Albert Einstein

"We insist on the fact that statistics should be considered an interpretation of natural phenomena, rather than an explanation."—Christian Robert

"Because we cannot avoid errors, the goal is not to minimize the chance of making errors, but to minimize the impact of the errors."—Mark Chang

There are different paradigms of statistical theory. The different theories represent different philosophies and have provoked much controversy. However, within each paradigm, consistency and completeness are expected with an axiom system. These axioms are often called principles. When a new inference procedure or experiment design violates a principle of an existing theory, there are several possible actions we can take: (1) do not use the new procedure, (2) modify the existing theory or abandon the "principle" so we can explain a new "phenomena" or use a new procedure, or (3) develop a new theory or choose another existing theory.

We cannot completely avoid making errors. Taking clinical trials as an example, we can make a type-I (false positive) or type-II (false negative) error. If one believes that protecting patients from ineffective drugs is of absolute importance, one should use $\alpha = 0$ for the hypothesis test so that no drug (effective or ineffective) will get to the market. On the other hand, if one believes that preventing any effective drug from being delivered to patients is absolutely unacceptable, one should use $\alpha = 1$ so that no drug (effective or ineffective) will be left out. In reality, we should balance the effects of making these two types of errors. In other words, what we really care about is the impact of errors, not the errors themselves.

In statistics, there are many principles; any violation of these principles can be considered an "error" and will have an impact. We all know that in mathematics, statistics, and science, there are many theories that conflict with one another, even though each is internally consistent. In statistics, for example, Bayesian and frequentist approaches have many fundamental differences. An adaptive design may violate principles of one theory, but may be consistent with the principles of other theories. Our action taken, e.g., choosing either classical or adaptive design, is dependent on the impact of that decision.

Statistical analyses and predictions are usually motivated by objectives. The outcome of the analyses and predictions will guide the decision making. When we propose a statistical method (e.g., adaptive design) under a certain condition, we believe the method is preferable to alternative methods based on anticipated consequences or impacts.

The impact is characterized by a loss function in decision theory. This loss function (implicit or explicit) always guides our decision whether we realize it or not. The challenging and also interesting part is that different people have different perspectives on loss, hence the different loss functions. Loss functions are often vague and not explicitly defined, especially when we make decisions in our daily lives. Decision theory makes this loss explicit and deals with it with mathematical rigor.

## 29.2   Decision Theory Basics

In decision theory, statistical models involve three spaces: the observation space $X$, the parameter space $\Theta$, and the action space $A$. Actions are guided by a decision rule $\delta(\mathbf{x})$. An action $\alpha \in A$ always has an associated consequence characterized by the so-called loss function $L(\theta, a)$. In hypothesis testing, the action space is $A = \{\text{accept; reject}\}$.

Because it is usually impossible to uniformly minimize the loss $L(\theta, a)$, in frequentist paradigm, the decision rule $\delta$ is determined such that it will minimize the following average loss:

$$R(\theta, \delta) = E^{X|\theta}(L(\theta, \delta(\mathbf{x})))$$

$$= \int_X L(\theta, \delta(\mathbf{x})) f(\mathbf{x}|\theta) d\mathbf{x}. \qquad (29.1)$$

The rule $a = \delta(\mathbf{x})$ is often called an estimator in estimation problems. Common examples of loss function are *squared error loss* (SEL), $L(\theta, a) = (\theta - a)^2$; *absolute loss*, $L(\theta, a) = |\theta - \alpha|$; the *0-1 loss*, $L(\theta, a) = \mathbf{1}(|\alpha - \theta|)$; etc.

The expected SEL associates variance and bias of an estimator through the following:

$$E^{X|\theta}(\theta - \delta(X))^2 = Var(\delta(X)) + [\text{bias}(\delta(X))]^2,$$

where $\text{bias}(\delta(X)) = E^{X|\theta}(\delta(X))$.

**Definition 29.1** Bayesian expected loss is the expectation of the loss function with respect to posterior measure, i.e,

$$\rho(\delta(\mathbf{x}), \pi) = E^{\theta|X} L(\delta(\mathbf{x}), \theta) = \int_\Theta L(\theta, \delta(\mathbf{x})) \pi(\theta|x) d\theta. \qquad (29.2)$$

An action $a^* = \delta^*(\mathbf{x})$ that minimizes the posterior expected loss is called Bayes action.

By averaging Equation (29.1) over a range of $\theta$ for a given prior $\pi(\theta)$, we can obtain

$$r(\pi, \delta) = E^\pi(R(\theta, \delta))$$

$$= \int_\Theta \int_X L(\theta, \delta(\mathbf{x})) f(\mathbf{x}|\theta) \pi(\theta) d\mathbf{x} d\theta. \qquad (29.3)$$

The two notions by (29.2) and (29.3) are equivalent in the sense that they lead to the same decision.

**Theorem 29.1** An estimator minimizing the integrated risk $r(\pi, \delta)$ can be obtained by selecting, for every $x \in X$, the value $\delta(x)$ which minimizes the posterior expected loss, $\rho(a, \pi)$, because

$$r(\pi, \delta) = \int_X \rho(a, \delta(\mathbf{x})|\mathbf{x}) m(\mathbf{x}) d\mathbf{x}.$$

## 29.3 Evidence Measure

Before we can assess the impact of an error, we have to understand it profoundly. Remember, an error can be viewed as a negation of evidence.

Furthermore, drug development is a sequence of decision-making processes, and decisions are made on the basis of evidence. Therefore, the way in which evidence is measured is critical. The totality of evidence indicating that a drug is beneficial to the patient population is a very complex issue and involves many aspects. However, for simplicity, we will focus on efficacy evidence. We are going to discuss four different measures of evidence: $p$-value, likelihood, Bayes' factor, and the Bayesian $p$-value.

### 29.3.1 *Frequentist p-value*

The $p$-value defined by the conditional probability $\Pr(\text{data}|\text{Ho})$ is the error rate of claiming efficacy, when in fact there is no treatment effect (i.e., the null hypothesis $H_0$ is true). In drug development, the ultimate question is the following: What is the treatment effect given the observed data? That is the exact question that the Bayesian method answers using posterior probability $\Pr(H_a|\text{data})$. However, the frequentist $p$-value for hypothesis testing only tells us the probability of observing at least this treatment difference given that the null hypothesis is true. In other words, $p$-value is a measure of evidence against the null. In this sense, the frequentist approach doesn't answer the question.

There have been extensive discussions on $p$-value (Fisher, 1999). For example, it is believed that there is always a difference between any two treatments (though it might be very small). Therefore, as long as the sample size is large enough, statistical significance will be demonstrated. The $p$-value depends on the power. Furthermore, $p$-value does not provide a consistent measure of evidence because identical $p$-values do not imply identical evidence of treatment effect. Suppose two trials have been conducted. One trial shows a mean treatment difference of 5 with a CI $(0, 10)$ and $p$-value of 0.05, and the other shows a mean treatment difference of 50 with a CI $(0,100)$ and $p$-value of 0.05. Clearly, the second trial has provided stronger evidence supporting the effectiveness of the test drug, even though the $p$-values from the two trials are identical.

### 29.3.2 *Bayes Factor*

As discussed earlier, $p$-value and MLE alone do not provide a good measure for evidence. For a hypothesis test of the null hypothesis $H_0$ (no treatment effect $\theta$) versus the alternative hypothesis $H_a$ (with treatment effect $\theta$), if we consider both the evidence supporting the null hypothesis being true and the evidence supporting the alternative hypothesis being true, an intuitive way to compare them is to take the ratio of the two evidences, the so-called Bayes' factor (BF).

**Definition 29.2** The Bayes factor is the ratio of the posterior probabilities of the null and alternative hypotheses over the ratio of the prior probabilities of the null and the alternative hypotheses, i.e.,

$$BF(x) = \frac{P(\theta \in \Theta_o | x)}{P(\theta \in \Theta_a | x)} \bigg/ \frac{\pi(\theta \in \Theta_0)}{\pi(\theta \in \Theta_a)},\tag{29.4}$$

or

$$BF(x) = \frac{\int_{\Theta_o} f(x | \theta_o) \pi_o(\theta) d\theta}{\int_{\Theta_a} f(x | \theta_a) \pi_a(\theta) d\theta}.\tag{29.5}$$

From (18.4) we know when $\pi(\theta \in \Theta_0) = \pi(\theta \in \Theta_a)$, BF = likelihood ratio.

$$BF = (\text{Likelihood for } \theta \text{ in } Ho)/(\text{Likelihood for } \theta \text{ in } Ha)$$

Reject $H_0$ if $BF \leq k$, where $k$ is a small value, e.g., 0.1. A small value of BF implies strong evidence in favor of $H_a$ or against $H_0$. Note that there are several slightly different definitions of Bayes' factor.

Because of the different methods of measuring the evidence, the same data can lead to different conclusions, which has been stated in Lindley's paradox: When the information ratio (information from current trial versus prior information) is high and $p$-value is just marginally significant against $H_0$, the BF can be greater than 1, and hence support $H_0$ (Lindley, 1957; Spiegelhalter et al., 2004)

### 29.3.3 *Bayesian p-value*

Suppose we want to test the null hypothesis that $H_0 : \theta = 0$ against an alternative hypothesis that $H_a : \theta > 0$.

The frequentist $p$-value is the probability of having the observed treatment difference or larger assuming $\theta = 0$, i.e., $Pr(data$ or more extreme$|\theta = 0)$. The Bayesian $p$-value, calculated from posterior distribution is the probability of $\theta \leq 0$ (no treatment effect) given the observed data, i.e., $Pr(\theta \leq 0 | data)$.

Isn't the Bayesian $p$-value what we are looking for, and not the frequentist $p$-value? Bayesian significance is claimed when the Bayesian $p$-value is less than or equal to the so-called Bayesian significance level $\alpha$, a predetermined constant that does not have to be the same as the frequentist significance level.

### 29.3.4   *Repeated Looks*

One of the difficulties in using the frequentist approach is the issue of multiple testing, or repeated looks. When multiple tests are performed, such as in trials with multiple endpoints and in adaptive trials or pharmacogenomic studies, the false positive rate will be inflated when using naive methods. Therefore, $p$-value adjustment or alpha penalty should be applied in such cases. The problem is that as the number of analyses gets larger, the power for detecting a difference diminishes quickly due to the multiplicity adjustment.

In fact, when the number of looks approaches infinity, the probability of making type-I error is 100%. However, the probability of the BF being less than $\alpha$ is always less than $\alpha$, regardless of the number of looks, i.e., $Pr(BF < \alpha | H_0) \leq \alpha$. This theorem states that when the null hypothesis is true, if we look repeatedly for a BF of less than 10%, strong evidence against the null, this will not occur more than 10% of the time, no matter how many times we look (Royall, 1997). This theorem thus reveals the maximum probability of misleading evidence, but only if we measure the evidence properly.

Because of the controversial issues surrounding multiplicity in classical hypothesis testing based on the Neyman–Pearson theory, the frequentist $p$-value has been strongly criticized from the Bayesian and Fisherian perspectives (Spiegelhalter et al., 2004). Cornfield questioned ironically: "Do we want error control over a single trial, over all the independent trials on the same agent, on the same disease, over the lifetime of an investigator, etc.?" (Cornfield, 1976). Each of these control methods can lead to different adjusted $p$-values and, hence, contradictory statistical conclusions.

### 29.3.5   *Role of Alpha in Drug Development*

As we all know, the frequentist method is fundamentally based on (infinitely) repeated experiments. However, we virtually never repeat (many times) the pivotal clinical trial for the same compound for the same indication. The real replications are the clinical trials of different compounds for the same or different indications. Therefore, we should take a close look at the implications caused by a fixed $\alpha$ enforced by a regulatory body.

From a regulatory point of view, the statistical criterion of a *p*-value $<\alpha$ can be viewed as a simple tool to control the proportion of ineffective drugs on the market. However, that is just one side of the story. We also have to consider the downside, which is the prevention of good drugs from being delivered to patients because of this criterion. To balance the two sides, we can use a benefit–risk ratio or utility. Bayesian decision theory is a powerful tool in this regard. Furthermore, using a fixed $\alpha$ of 5% does not necessarily control the release of ineffective drugs onto the market. For example, if all drug candidates in phase III are efficacious, all drugs on the market will be effective regardless of $\alpha$. Similarly, if all drug candidates in phase III are inefficacious, then all drugs on the market will be ineffective regardless of $\alpha$. The problem is that we don't know the proportion of effective drug candidates in phase-III trials unless the Bayesian approach is adopted.

The frequentist paradigm has played an important historical role in drug development. The frequentist approach, with alpha control at the 5% level, was appropriate because there were many compounds that had major effects. This high standard (error rate $<5\%$) for drug approval has led to the most effective compounds being selected and approved, and at the same time it has prevented a larger number of ineffective drugs from spreading into the market. The frequentist criterion was probably consistent with the benefit–risk measure, had it been developed. However, the situation has changed: given that there are so many drugs already on the market, the margin for improvement is getting smaller, and an active controlled study requires an extremely large sample size that is often not feasible. Even if there are a few remaining drugs with large effects, they will be hard to find using the traditional frequentist method. Given these reasons, the statistical criterion of alpha = 5% could require an unreasonably large benefit–risk ratio. The Bayesian approach is a better alternative, despite its challenges; after all, challenges are the force that drives science forward. Personalized medicine is the future for the patients; however, to be able to effectively develop personalized medicine, advancement in science and technology for drug development is critical.

## 29.4 Statistical Principles

A main purpose of statistical theory is to derive an inference about the probability distribution from observations of a random phenomenon. The distribution model is simple and often an efficient way to describe a past phenomenon and more importantly to predict a future event of a similar nature. David Cox (2006) gives an excellent review of important statistical principles from both frequentist and Bayesian perspectives in his recent book, *Principles of Statistical Inference.*

**Definition 29.3** A parametric statistical model consists of the observation of a random variable $x$, distributed according to $f(x|\theta)$, where only the parameter $\theta$ is unknown and belongs to a vector space $\Theta$ of finite dimension.

Once the statistical model is defined, a main task of the statistical analysis is to lead to an inference (estimation or hypothesis testing) on the parameter $\theta$. In contrast to the probabilistic modeling, the purpose of a statistical analysis is fundamentally an inversion purpose, since it aims at retrieving the "causes," i.e., parameters of the probabilistic generating mechanism, from the "effects" or observations. In early times, statistics was also called "Inverse Probability."

The fiducial approach of Fisher (1956) also relies on this inversion. Let's denote $C$ the cause and $E$ the effect. Consider the relation $E = C + \varepsilon$ where $\varepsilon$ is an error term. It is argued that, if $C$ is known, $E$ is distributed according to the above relation. Conversely, if $E$ is known, $C = E - \varepsilon$ is distributed according to the symmetric distribution. However if $E$ is a random variable and $C$ is a (constant) parameter, to write $C = E - \varepsilon$ does not make $C$ a random variable. The fiducial approach was abandoned after the exposure of fundamental paradoxes (Robert, 1997; Stein, 1959).

**Definition 29.4** A Bayesian statistical model is made of a parametric statistical model, $f(x|\theta)$, and a prior distribution on the parameters, $\pi(\theta)$.

**Theorem 29.2 (Bayes' Theorem)** Bayes theorem can be expressed as

$$\pi(\theta|x) = \frac{f(x|\theta)\,\pi(\theta)}{\int f(x|\theta)\,\pi(\theta)\,d\theta}. \tag{29.6}$$

Bayes's Theorem places causes (observations) and effects (parameters) on the same conceptual level, since both of them have probability distributions. It is considered a major step moving from the notion of an unknown parameter to the notion of a random parameter (Robert, 1997). However, it is important to distinguish $x$ and $\theta$; $x$ is observable, but $\theta$ is latent.

**Definition 29.5** When $x \sim f(x|\theta)$, a function $T$ of $x$ (also called a statistic) is said to be *sufficient* if the distribution of $x$ conditionally on $T(x)$ does not depend on $\theta$.

A sufficient statistic $T(x)$ contains the whole information brought by $x$ about $\theta$.

**Theorem 29.3 (Neymam)** (Hogg, McKean, and Graig, p. 376). Let

$X_1, ..., X_n$ denote a random sample from a distribution that has pdf or pmf. $f(x; \theta)$, $\theta \in \Omega$. The statistic $Y_1 = T_1(X_1, ..., X_n)$ is a sufficient statistic for $\theta$, if and only if there exist two nonnegative functions, $\eta_1$ and $\eta_2$, such that

$$f(x_1; \theta) ... f(x_n; \theta) = \eta_1 [T_1(x_1, ..., x_n); \theta] \eta_2(x_1, ..., x_n), \qquad (29.7)$$

where $\eta_2(x_1, ..., x_n)$ does not depend upon $\theta$.

When the model allows for a minimal sufficient statistic, i.e., for a sufficient statistic which is a function of all the other sufficient statistics, we only have to consider the procedures depending on this statistic.

**Sufficiency Principle** Two observations $x$ and $y$ factorizing through the same value of a sufficient statistic $T$, i.e., such that $T(x) = T(y)$, must lead to the same inference on $\theta$.

Christian Robert (1997) pointed out: "The Sufficiency Principle is only legitimate when the statistical model is actually the one underlying the generation of the observations. Any uncertainty about the distribution of the observations should be incorporated into the model, a modification which almost certainly leads to a change of sufficient statistics. A similar cautionary remark applies to the Likelihood Principle".

**Conditionality Principle** If $m$ experiments $\left( \breve{E}_1, ..., \breve{E}_m, \right)$ on the parameter $\theta$ are available with equal probability to be selected, the resulting inference on $\theta$ should only depend on the selected experiment.

**Stopping Rule Principle** If a sequence of experiments, $\breve{E}_1$, $\breve{E}_2$, ..., $\breve{E}_m$ is directed by a stopping rule, $\tau$, which indicates when the experiments should stop, inference about $\theta$ must depend on $\tau$ only through the resulting sample.

The Bayesian decision is independent of the stopping criterion; therefore, it is not influenced by the subjective motivations which led to the resulting sample size. For example, in a clinical trial, from sponsor perspective, the trial can continue to recruit patients until $p$-value $< \alpha$. The problem is that the regulatory body, physicians and patients, has different loss functions. If the regulatory body has the final say about the loss function, then we unlikely have the stopping rule that allows a trial to continue recruiting patients until $p$-value $< \alpha$. In such case, $p$-value $< \alpha$ can be viewed as a constraint in the minimization using decision theory.

**Likelihood Principle** The information contained by an observation $x$ about $\theta$ is entirely contained in the likelihood function $l(\theta|x)$. Moreover, if $x_1$ and $x_2$ are two observations depending on the same parameter $\theta$, such that there exists a constant $c$ satisfying

$$l_1\left(\theta|x_1\right) = cl_2\left(\theta|x_2\right) \tag{29.8}$$

for every $\theta$, they contain the same information about $\theta$ and must lead to identical inferences.

### Example 29.1    Paradox of Binomial and Negative Binomial Distribution

Suppose, we are interested in the hypothesis testing of a binary endpoint:

$$H_0 : p = 0.5 \text{ vs: } H_a : p > 0.5.$$

The experiment is finished with 3 responses out of 12 patients. However this information is not sufficient for rejecting or accepting the null hypothesis.

Scenario 1: If the total number of patients, N = 12, is predetermined, the number of responses $X$ follows binomial distribution $B(n;p)$, and the frequentist $p$-value of the test is given by

$$\Pr\left(X \geq 9|H_0\right) = \sum_{x=9}^{12} \binom{12}{x} 0.5^x 0.5^{12-x} = 0.073.$$

The null cannot be rejected at a one-sided level $\alpha = 0.05$. The likelihood in this case is given by

$$l_1\left(x|p\right) = \binom{12}{9} p^9 \left(1-p\right)^3 = 220p^9 \left(1-p\right)^3.$$

Scenario 2: If the number of responses, $n = 3$, is predetermined and the experiment continues until 3 responses are observed, then $X$ follows negative binomial $NB(3; 1-p)$ and the frequentist $p$-value of the test is given by

$$\Pr\left(X \geq 9|H_0\right) = \sum_{x=9}^{\infty} \binom{3+x-1}{2} 0.5^x 0.5^3 = 0.0327$$

because $\sum_{x=k}^{\infty} \binom{2+x}{2} \left(\frac{1}{2}\right)^x = \frac{8+5m+m^2}{2^m}$. Therefore the null is rejected at a one-sided level $\alpha = 0.05$. The likelihood in this case is given by

$$l_2\left(x|p\right) = \binom{3+9-1}{2} p^9 \left(1-p\right)^3 = 55p^9 \left(1-p\right)^3.$$

According to the Likelihood Principle, all relevant information is in the likelihood $l(p) = p^9 (1-p)^3$, and therefore, the two scenarios should not lead to different conclusions (rejection or not rejection).

**Maximum Likelihood Estimator (MLE)** When $x \sim f(x|\theta)$ is observed, the maximum likelihood estimator of $\theta$ is defined as

$$\hat{\theta} = Arg \max l(\theta|x), \qquad (29.9)$$

where the notation $Arg \max$ means that the likelihood $l(\theta|x)$ achieves its maximum value at $\hat{\theta}$.

Note that the maximization (29.9) can lead to several maxima. The maximum likelihood estimator is found useful because (1) it is intuitive motivation of maximizing the probability of occurrence; (2) it has strong asymptotic properties (consistency and efficiency); and (3) it is parametrization-invariant.

**Invariance Principle** If $\hat{\theta}$ is the maximum likelihood estimator, then for any function $h\left(\hat{\theta}\right)$, the maximum likelihood estimator of $h(\theta)$ is $h(\hat{\theta})$ (even when $h$ is not one-to-one).

This property is not enjoyed by most other statistical approaches. However, maximum likelihood estimates are often biased. Does it imply that the world is operated biasedly?

**MAP estimator** MAP (maximum a posteriori) estimator is also called the generalized maximum likelihood estimator (GMLE). The GMLE is the largest mode of the $\pi(\theta|x)$. The MLE maximizes $l(\theta)$, while the GLME maximizes $\pi(\theta) l(\theta)$.

## 29.5 Behaviors of Statistical Principles in Adaptive Designs

### 29.5.1 *Sufficiency Principle*

Jennison and Turnbull (2003), Posch, Bauer, and Brannath (2003), and Burman and Sonesson (2006) point out that the adaptive design using a weighted statistic violates the sufficiency principle because it weights the same amount of information from different stages differently. Michael A. Proschan (Burman and Sonesson, 2006, discussion) proved that no test based on the sufficient statistic can maintain level $\alpha$ irrespective of whether the prespecified sample-size rule is followed. Thach and Fisher (2002, p. 436) and Burman and Sonesson highlighted the problem of very different weights. An example (given by Marianne Frisen, in Burman and Sonesson, discussion) of a violation of the sufficiency principle is the use of the median instead of the mean when estimating the expected value of a normal distribution.

The "unweighted test" utilizes the distribution of $N$ to choose a critical level with the desired probability of rejecting the null hypothesis unconditional on $N$ but disregards the observed value of $N$. Because $N$ is part of the minimal sufficient statistic, it is not in accordance with the sufficiency principle and is inefficient (Marianne Frisen, in Burman and Sonesson, 2006, discussion).

Should information (or sufficiency of a statistic) regarding $\theta$ be based on data or data + procedure? We probably can argue that the sufficiency of a statistic should depend not only on the data, but also on the procedure or experiment used to collect the data. The data can contain different amounts of information if they are collected differently. The conclusion that each observation contains the same amount of information is valid in a classical design, but not in an adaptive design, because a later observation contains some information from previous observations due to the dependent sampling procedure. Therefore, an insufficient statistic in classical design can become sufficient under an adaptive design. For example, suppose we want to assess the quantity $\vartheta = \frac{1-R_B}{1-R_A}$, where $R_A$ and $R_B$ are the true response rates in groups $A$ and $B$, respectively. In a classical design with balanced randomization, $\frac{N_A}{N_B}$ is asymptotically approaching 1. However, in the randomized play-the-winner design, $\frac{N_A}{N_B}$ is asymptotically equal to $\vartheta$. Therefore, the same data $\frac{N_A}{N_B}$ could contain different amounts of information in different designs.

It should be apparent that a statistic (e.g., $\bar{X}$) can be a sufficient statistic conditionally but not unconditionally for $\theta$.

### 29.5.2 *Minimum Sufficiency Principle and Efficiency*

Jennison and Turnbull (2006b) raised the question as to when an adaptive design using nonsufficient statistics can be improved upon by a nonadaptive group sequential design. Tsiatis and Mehta (2003) have proved that for any SSR adaptive design, there exists a more powerful group sequential design; however, the group sequential test has to allow analyses at every cumulative information level that might arise in the adaptive design. On the other hand, the weighted method (or MINP) provides great flexibility and when the sample size does not change, it has the same power as the classical group sequential design.

It is really analogous with a two-player game. Player $A$ says if you tell me the sample-size rule, I can find a group sequential design (with as many analyses as I want to have) that is more efficient than the adaptive design. Player $B$ says, if you tell me how many and when you plan the interim analyses, I can produce an adaptive trial with the same number and timing of the analyses that is more flexible, and in case the sample-size does not change, it is identical to the group sequential design.

Interestingly, a group sequential design can also be viewed as a special SSR adaptive design. The adjustment rule at interim analysis is that sample size will not be increased if futility or efficacy is found; otherwise add $n_2$ subjects. Therefore, what Tsiatis and Mehta eventually proved is that there is an SSR design with a discrete sample-size increment that is more efficient than a given SSR with continual sample-size increment.

Uniformly a more powerful design has an important implication: If design $A$ is uniformly more efficient or powerful than design $B$, then $\{\delta; H_0$ is not rejected with design $A\} \subset \{\delta; H_0$ is not rejected with design $B\}$. Because the confidence interval consists of all values of $\delta$ for which $H_0$ is not rejected, $CI_A \subseteq CI_B$.

Jennison and Turnbull (2006) stated, "A design is said to be inadmissible if another design has a lower expected information function and higher power curve. A design that is not inadmissible is said to be admissible. The fundamental theoretical result is a complete class theorem, which states that all admissible designs are solutions of Bayes sequential decision problems. Because Bayes designs are functions of sufficient statistics, any adaptive design defined through nonsufficient statistics is inadmissible and is dominated by a design based on sufficient statistics. This conclusion confirms that violation of the sufficiency principle has a negative impact on the efficiency of an adaptive design." The question is should the information and consequently the sufficiency be procedure dependent?

### 29.5.3 *Conditionality and Exchangeability Principles*

Burman and Sonesson (2006) pointed out that SSR also violates the invariance and conditionality principles because the weighted test depends on the order of exchangeable observations. Marianne Frisen (Burman and Sonesson, discussion) stated similarly: "The 'weighted' test avoids this by forcing a certain error spending. This is done at the cost of violating the conditionality principle. The ordering of the observations is an ancillary statistic for a conclusion about the hypothesis. Thus, by the conditionality principle the test statistic should not depend on the ordering of the realized observations." For a general distribution, not belonging to the exponential family, the weighted test will violate the conditionality principle but not the sufficiency principle (Burman and Sonesson).

If sufficiency and conditionality are important, then the combination of the two is the likelihood principle, which also faces challenges (see examples provided earlier in this chapter). The bottom line is that the world is unpredictable by humans, but it is also deterministic. When it is viewed as random, there will be many paradoxes.

When we talk about exchangeability, we should apply the same data scope to both classical and adaptive designs. The same terminology, "experiment-wise," can imply a different data scope for classical and adaptive designs. For example, in a phase-II and III combined seamless adaptive design, data from phases II (or the learning phase) and III (the confirmatory phase) are combined and viewed as experiment-wise data, while in a classical design, the data from the two phases are analyzed separately simply because we call them two different experiments. Fairly, if we compare the two design approaches at the same data scope, i.e., phase II and III combined, then we will see a very interesting result: the classical design is a special case of an adaptive design using the weighted test, where the weight for the "learning phase" is zero and the weight for the "confirmatory phase" is 1.

Classical design = 0 (learning-phase data) + 1 (confirmatory-phase data)

Adaptives design = $w_1$ ((learning-phase data) + $w_2$ (confirmatory-phase data))

Humans are not memory-less creatures; we should not pretend that we don't have the learning-phase data when we analyze the confirmatory-phase data. Data from different phases of an adaptive trial are often not exchangeable; data from two trials of different phases are not exchangeable in a classical design. Is it just a terminological difference: "phase" or "trial"?

### 29.5.4   *Equal Weight Principle*

Exchangeable observations should be weighted equally in the test statistic. The equal weight principle views exchangeability from the weight perspective. However, the measurement of the information level is not unique. For example, observation $x_i$ can be counted as a unit of information, $1/x_i$ can be counted as a unit of information, or $p_i$ can be counted as unit of information. There are criticisms about the "unequal weights" in sample-size reestimation with the fixed weight approach. However, even in the group sequential design without sample-size reestimation, the "one person/one vote" principle is violated because earlier enrolled patients have more chances to vote in the decision making (rejecting or accepting the null hypothesis) than later enrolled patients. For example, in two-stage group sequential design, the first patient has two chances to "vote," at the interim and final analyses, while the last patient has only one chance to vote, at the final analysis. Moreover, the impact of each individual vote is heavily dependent on the alpha spent on each analysis, i.e., the stopping boundaries.

From an ethical point of view, should there be equal weight for everyone, one vote for one person? Should efficacy be measured by the reduction in number of deaths or by survival time gained? Should it be measured by mean change or percent change from baseline? All these scenarios apply a different "equal weight" system to the sample. Suppose you have a small amount of a magic drug, enough to save only one person in a dying family: the grandfather, the young man, or the little boy. What should you do? If you believe life is equally important for everyone regardless of age, you may randomly (with equal probability) select a person from the family and give him/her the drug. If you believe the amount of survival time saved is important (i.e., one year of prolonged survival is equally important to everyone), then you may give the drug to the little boy because his life expectancy would be the longest among the three family members. If you believe that the impact of a death on society is most important, then you may want to save the young man, because his death would probably have the most negative impact on society. If these different philosophies or beliefs are applied to clinical trials, they will lead to different endpoints and different test statistics with different weights.

It is important to know that even in standard group sequential design, the "one patient/one vote" rule is not honored because patients enrolled earlier at the first stage have at least two votes (two opportunities to vote), one at the interim analysis and the second at the final analysis.

## 29.5.5 *Consistency of Trial Results*

Compared to classical design, adaptive designs naturally allow for an interim look to check the consistency of results from different stages. If $p_1$ and $p_2$ are very different, we may have to look at the reasons, such as baseline difference or gene difference. But should we check this consistency for a classical design too by splitting the data in different ways?

It is also controversial in adaptive designs (including group sequential designs) that we often reject the null hypothesis with less strong evidence, but don't reject the null with stronger evidence. For example, in a two-stage GSD with the O'Brien–Fleming spending function ($\alpha_1 = 0.0025$ and $\alpha_2 = 0.0238$), we will not reject the null when the $p$-value $= 0.003 > \alpha_1$ at the interim look, but we do reject the null when the $p$-value $= 0.022 < \alpha_2$. Why don't we reject the null hypothesis when the evidence against the null is stronger ($p$-value $= 0.003$) and reject $H_0$ when the evidence is much weaker ($p$-value $= 0.022$)?

Unless the test statistic is a monotonic function of the parameter estimator, regardless of how the data were collected, it is always possible to have conflicting results. For example, median and mean have conflicting results, i.e., a rank test statistic conflicts with that from a parametric approach.

### 29.5.6    *Bayesian Aspects*

Two fundamental principles are naturally followed by the Bayesian paradigm with no constraint on the procedures to be considered, namely, the Likelihood Principle and the Sufficiency Principle. On the other hand, the Bayesian approach rejects other principles, such as the notion of un-biasedness. This notion was once a cornerstone of classical statistics and restricted the choice of estimators to those that are, on average, correct (Lehmann, 1983). Our objective is to minimize the impact of errors not the number of errors.

From the frequentist perspective, the most convincing argument in favor of the Bayesian approach is that it intersects widely with the three notions of classical optimality, namely, minimaxity, admissibility, and equivariance. Most estimators that are optimal according to one of these criteria are Bayes estimators or limits of Bayes estimators (the notion of limit depends on the context). Thus, not only is it possible to produce Bayes estimators that satisfy one, two, or three of the optimality criteria, but more importantly, the Bayes estimators are essentially the only ones that achieve this aim (Robert, 1997, Chapters 1 and 10).

The Bayes estimators use uniform representations under loss functions, while the maximum likelihood method does not necessarily lead to an estimator. For example, this is the case for normal mixtures, where the likelihood is not bounded.

An interesting question for a Bayesian approach is, should that which we learn from incremental information many times be the same as that which we learn from the cumulative information all at once? The answer is that it is dependent on the model—the answer is yes for conjugate models, but not for general models.

### 29.5.7 *Type-I Error, p-value, Estimation*

Type-I error control is not very challenging, and most adaptive designs control the familywise error. However, because hypothesis testing is primarily based on the concept of repeated experiments, in what scope the experiment will potentially be repeated is critical. In clinical trials, we virtually never test the same compound for the same indication in a phase-III study repeatedly for many times. For this reason, the implication of control of the experimental error rate $\alpha$ may be totally different from what we initially intended.

The definition, not the calculation, of $p$-value is challenging because there are so many options for an adaptive design. Remember that $p$-value is the probability of the test statistic under the null hypothesis being more extreme than the critical point. The key lies in how the extreme should be defined. Unlike in a classical design, definitions of extremeness of a test statistic can be defined in many different ways in adaptive designs, e.g., stagewise-ordering, sample mean ordering, and likelihood ratio ordering. None of these definitions satisfies simultaneously the concerns raised from statistical, scientific, and ethical angles.

Another relevant question is: should the duality principle between hypothesis testing and the confidence interval be applied to adaptive designs, i.e., the confidence interval consists of all $\delta_0$ that do not lead to rejection of the null hypothesis? If yes, there are many different definitions of confidence intervals, just as with the $p$-values.

Regarding the issues in overall direction of estimation, a very narrow continual band may cause issues. For example, for a group sequential design with stopping boundaries $\alpha_1 = 0$, $\beta_1 = 0.025$, $\alpha_2 = 1$, any data from stage 2 will lead to rejection of $H_0$ regardless of the overall direction of the treatment effect. There are also many other examples of contradictory results between weighted and unweighted methods (one positive and the other negative).

Regarding unbiased estimation, we have proved that the fixed weight method will lead to an unbiased point estimate if the trial does not allow for early stopping. If the trial allows for early stopping, the estimate is biased. What if the trial is designed for no early stopping, but is actually stopped for futility. In such a case, we don't care because the test compound wouldn't be marketed. This implies that we can always design a trial with no stopping and if it continues, we can calculate the naive estimate and claim that it is unbiased.

These controversies encourage us to examine the classical principles more carefully and adapt to the new phenomenon.

### 29.5.8   *The 0-2-4 Paradox*

Let's study further the type-I error, point estimate, confidence interval, and $p$-value through an interesting paradox, called the 0-2-4 paradox.

The 0-2-4 paradox: An experiment is to be conducted to prove that spring water is effective compared to a placebo in certain disease population. To carry out the trial, I need a coin and up to 4 patients. To control type-I error, the coin is used, i.e., **0** patient is needed; to have a unbiased point estimate, a sample-size of **2** patients is required; to obtain the confidence interval and $p$-value, **4** patients are sufficient. The trial is carried out as follows:

(1) To control the type-I error at one-sided $\alpha = 0.05$, I flip the coin 100 times. If the number of heads $n(\text{head}) < 95$, the trial will be stopped without efficacy claim. For this, I don't even need either the water or patients. If the number of heads $n(\text{head}) \geq 95$, the efficacy will be claimed and the trial proceeds to the next step.

(2) To obtain unbiased point estimate, only two patients are needed; one takes the placebo and the other drinks water at random. The unbiased estimate of treatment difference is given by $y - x$, where $x$ and $y$ are the responses from the placebo and water groups, respectively.

(3) To obtain the confidence interval and $p$-value, 4 patients are required: 2 for each group. The confidence interval is given by

$$CI = \delta \pm Z_{1-\alpha}\hat{\sigma},$$

where $\delta = \frac{y_1 + y_2 - x_1 - x_2}{2}$ and $\hat{\sigma}^2 = var\left(\delta\right)$.
The $p$-value is given by

$$p = 1 - \Phi\left(\frac{\delta}{\hat{\sigma}}\right)$$

Here is the problem. The rejection of the null may not be consistent with the confidence interval and $p$-value. To be consistent, I can use 4 patients from Steps 1 to 3.

(4) Spring water is presumably very safe.

(5) It is a cost-effective approach. The water experiment may have a low power, only about 5%, but the cost is very low. Furthermore, when

the water is "proved" to be efficacious statistically, the observed treatment difference is often very big because of small sample size. A big observed treatment difference implies a big market value. Here is the overall picture: The experiment has an extremely low cost and low power, but it has potentially a big market value if the null hypothesis of no treatment effect is rejected.

What if all pharmaceutical companies take spring water as the test drug? If so, then 5% of them will claim efficacy of the water for some indications. What if the water is replaced by some relatively safe, but not efficacious compound? Does this discourage good science—just pick a safe compound and run a small trial? Is doing good science not a cost-effective approach?

To make an analogy, the spring water experiment can be repeated again and again until successful just as different companies can screen the same compounds again and again for the same or different indications until they find something. The water experiment is very easy to conduct and any operational bias can virtually be avoided. In conclusion, don't overemphasize the importance of the type-I error rate, unbiased estimate, adjusted $p$-value, confidence interval, and the operational bias.

## 29.6 Summary

Adaptive designs violate several commonly accepted statistical principles. The violations on one hand remind us to adopt the new approaches with extreme caution. On the other hand, the new approaches may suggest that principles of inference only go so far and that new principles may be desirable. Indeed, adaptive designs present great challenges to frequentist statistics and conventional thinking in development. Group sequential designs have been widely used in clinical trials; however, there are many controversial issues with these designs that are only fully realized when we widen the concept to a more general category of adaptive designs (GSD can be viewed as an adaptive design with discrete values of sample-size adjustment, i.e., 0 increase if futility or efficacy; add $n_2$ subjects otherwise). Those controversial issues include $p$-values and estimations. Should $p$-values and estimations be unconditional or conditional? Should they be conditional on statistical significance or stagewise-conditional? Should a test statistic be ordered by stage, by the mean, or by something else? The concepts of $p$-value and unbiasedness are based on repeated experiments, but what does this mean in clinical trials? The likelihood principle, which is equivalent to the conjunction of the frequentist sufficiency and the conditionality principles, denies the importance of hypothesis testing. All of these considerations seem to suggest that we should use other approaches, such as Bayesian approaches and decision theory. It is obvious that efficiency in clinical trials is not identical to the power of hypothesis testing. In clinical trials, the concept of efficiency often includes the power, the time to market, and the operationally flexibility. Overemphasizing the power can be very misleading when evaluating adaptive designs. This simple fact is often overlooked.

One fundamental difficulty in using decision theory is that different beneficial bodies have different utilities; therefore, if a decision involves multiple decision-making bodies, the decision becomes extremely challenging. For example, if a regulatory body enforces the $\alpha$ criterion, we can use decision theory and incorporate the condition $p < \alpha$ as a constraint. This is not an ideal solution because $p < \alpha$ is not the best criterion, and the interactions between sponsors and the FDA will alter opinions.

We describe the deterministic world as a random phenomenon because of our limited capabilities. Many controversial issues raised by the different statistical theories about this virtual random world can be reduced to a single, most important question: Should information level be dependent on the (experimental) procedure?

# Appendix A

# Random Number Generation

## A.1  Random Number

To perform clinical trial simulations, we need to take random samples. Typically, random sampling is based on the computer-generated, uniformly distributed random numbers over (0,1). The computer-generated "random" number is not a true random because the sequence of the numbers is determined by the so-called seed, an initial number. Other random variates from a nonuniform distribution are usually obtained by applying a transformation to uniform variates. There are usually several algorithms available to generate random numbers with a specific distribution. The algorithms differ in speed, accuracy, and the memory required.

## A.2  Uniformly Distributed Random Number

One of the commonly used methods to generate pseudorandom numbers starts with an initial value $x_0$, called the seed, and then recursively computes successive values $x_n, n \geq 1$, by letting

$$x_n = ax_{n-1} \quad module \ m, \qquad (A.1)$$

where $a$ and $m$ are given positive integers. (A.1) means that $ax_{n-1}$ is divided by $m$ and the remainder is taken as the value of $x_n$. Thus, each $x_n$ is either $0, 1, ...,$ or $m - 1$ and the quantity $x_n/m$ is called a pseudorandom number, which is approximately uniformly distributed on $(0, 1)$. This method is called linear congruential method. The positive integer $a$ directly impacts the quality of the random deviates. $m$ is the period of the sequence of the random numbers. The number $a$ should be carefully chosen such that it will lead to a large $m$. Park and Miller (1988) have suggested

$a = 7^5 = 16807$, or $m = 2^{31} - 1 = 2147483647$. Please be aware that not all built-in random number generators from software products are good.

## A.3    Inverse CDF Method

It is well known that if $X$ is a scalar random variable with a continuous cumulative distribution function (cdf) $F$, then the random variable $U = F(X)$ has a U(0,1) distribution. Hence, we have $X = F^{-1}(U)$. This fact provides the so-called inverse cdf technique for generating random numbers with the distribution $F$ by using the random numbers from the uniform distribution. The inverse cdf relationship exists between any two continuous (nonsingular) random variables. If $X$ is a continuous random variable with cdf $F$ and $Y$ is a continuous random variable with cdf $G$, then $X = F^{-1}(G(Y))$ over the ranges of positive support. Using this kind of relationship is actually trying to match percentile points of one distribution ($F$) with those of another distribution ($G$). The advantages of the inverse method is simple. However, the closed form of $F^{-1}$ is not always available. When $F$ does not exist in closed form, the inverse cdf method can be applied by solving the equation $F(x) - u = 0$ numerically.

The inverse cdf method also applies to discrete distributions. Suppose the discrete random variable $X$ has mass points of $m_1 < m_2 < m_3 < ...$ with probabilities of $p_1, p_2, p_3, ...$ and the distribution function

$$F(x) = \sum_{i \in m_i \leq x} p_i. \tag{A.2}$$

To use the inverse cdf method for this distribution, we first generate a realization $u$ of the uniform random variable $U$. We then deliver the realization of the target distribution as $x$, where $x$ satisfies the relationship

$$F(x_{(-)}) < u \leq F(x). \tag{A.3}$$

## A.4    Acceptance–Rejection Methods

The acceptance–rejection method is another elegant method for random number generation. For generating realizations of a random variable $X$ with a distribution $f$, the acceptance–rejection method makes use of realizations of another random variable $Y$ with a simpler distribution of $g$. Further, the pdf $g$ can be scaled to majorize $f$, using some constant $c$, i.e., $c\,g(x) > f(x)$ for all $x$. To gain efficiency, the difference $\varepsilon = c\,g(x) - f(x) > 0$ should be small for all $x$. The density $g$ is called the majorizing density and $cg$ is called the majorizing function.

**Algorithm A.1:** The Acceptance–Rejection Method to Convert Uniform Random Numbers

1. Generate $y$ from the distribution with density function $g$.
2. Generate $u$ from a uniform (0,1) distribution.
3. If $u < f(y)/cg(y)$, then take $y$ as the desired realization; otherwise, return to step 1.

Unlike the inverse cdf method, the acceptance–rejection can apply immediately to multivariate random variables.

Most software packages have certain capabilities to generate different random variables. We can use them to generate specific random variables. SAS Macro A.1 is an example using SAS random function for the exponential distribution to generate the mixed exponential distribution.

**>>SAS Macro A.1:   Mixed Exponential Distribution>>**
```
%Macro RanVars(nObs=100, Lamda1=1, Lamda2=1.5, w1=0.6, w2=0.4);
Data RVars;
Drop iObs;
Do iObs=1 To &nObs;
xMixEXP=&w1/&Lamda1*Ranexp(782)+&w2/&Lamda2*Ranexp(323);
Output;
End;
Run;
Proc Print Data=RVars; Run;
%Mend RanVars;
```
**<<SAS<<**

An example of using this SAS macro is presented below.

**>>SAS>>**
```
TITLE "Random Variables";
%RanVars(nObs=10, Lamda1=1, Lamda2=1.5, w1=0.6, w2=0.4);
```
**<<SAS<<**

## A.5   Multivariate Distribution

Many statistical software products such as SAS and ExpDesign Studio® provide built-in functions for generating variates of univariate random numbers. However, Some of them may not provide random number generators for multivariate random numbers. Here we provide a method to generate random variables from multivariate normal distribution.

The multivariate normal distribution is given by

$$f\left(\mathbf{x}\right) = \left(\frac{1}{2\pi}\right)^{n/2} |\mathbf{M}|^{-1/2} \exp\left(-\frac{\mathbf{x}^T\mathbf{M}\mathbf{x}}{2}\right), \qquad (A.4)$$

where $\mathbf{M} = \{m_{kl}\}$ is the covariance matrix.

Let $\mathbf{u} = (u_1, ..., u_n)$ be n independent variables from the standard normal distribution and $A$ be the triangle matrix

$$A = \begin{pmatrix} a_{11} & 0 & \cdots & 0 \\ a_{21} & a_{22} & \cdots & 0 \\ \cdots & \cdots & \cdots & \cdots \\ a_{n1} & a_{n2} & \cdots & a_{nn} \end{pmatrix}. \qquad (A.5)$$

Let $\boldsymbol{\xi} = \mathbf{Au}$ or

$$\begin{cases} \xi_1 = a_{11}u_1 \\ \xi_2 = a_{21}u_1 + a_{22}u_2 \\ \cdots\cdots \\ \xi_n = a_{n1}u_1 + a_{n2}u_2 + ... + a_{nn}u_n. \end{cases} \qquad (A.6)$$

It is obvious that the expectation $E(\xi_k) = 0 \ (k = 1, ..., n)$. Furthermore, we have

$$E(u_k u_l) = \delta_{kl} = \begin{cases} 1, & k = l \\ 0, & k \neq l. \end{cases} \qquad (A.7)$$

Therefore, it can be obtained that

$$E\left(\xi_k \xi_l\right) = E\left(\left(\Sigma_{i=1}^k a_{ki}u_i\right)\left(\Sigma_{j=1}^l a_{kj}u_j\right)\right) = \Sigma_{j=1}^k a_{kj}a_{lj} = \left(\mathbf{AA}^T\right)_{kl}. \qquad (A.8)$$

Comparing the corresponding elements in $\mathbf{AA}^T = \mathbf{M}$, we can obtain:

$$a_{kl} = \frac{m_{kl} - \Sigma_{j=1}^{l-1} a_{kj}a_{lj}}{\sqrt{m_{ll} - \Sigma_{j=1}^{l-1} a_{lj}^2}}, \quad (1 \leq l \leq k \leq n). \qquad (A.9)$$

For convenience, we have defined $\Sigma_{j=1}^0 a_{kj}a_{lj} = 0$.

**Algorithm A.2** The Generation of Random Numbers $\xi_i$ from Multivariate Normal Distribution

1. Calculate $a_{kl}$ using (A.9) for $1 \leq l \leq k \leq n$.

2. Generate $n$ independent random numbers $u_i$ $(i = 1, ..., n)$ from the standard normal distribution.

3. Generate $\xi_i$ using (A.6).

Algorithm A.2 is implemented in SAS Macro A.2, which can be used to generate the standard multivariate normal distribution. The SAS variables are defined as follows: **nVars** = number of variables, **sSize** = square of nVars, **nObs** = number of observations to be generated, **ss{i}** = covariate matrix, **x{i}** = the outputs multivariates.

### >>SAS Macro A.2:  Multivariate Normal Distribution>>

```
%Macro RanVarMNor(sSize=4, nVars=2, nObs=10);
Data nVars; SET CorrMatrix; keep x1-x&nVars;
Array a{&sSize}; Array xNor{&nVars}; Array x{&nVars};
Array ss{&sSize}; * Correlation matrix;
* Checovsky decomposition;
Do k=1 To &nVars; Do L=1 To k;
Saa=0; Sa2=0;
Do j=1 to L-1;
Saa=Saa+a{&nVars*(k-1)+j}*a{&nVars*(L-1)+j};
Sa2=Sa2+a{&nVars*(L-1)+j}*a{&nVars*(L-1)+j};
End;
nkL=&nVars*(k-1)+L;
a{nkL}=(ss{nkL}-Saa)/Sqrt(ss{&nVars*(L-1)+L}-Sa2);
End; End;
Do iObs=1 to &nObs;
Do iVar=1 to &nVars; xNOR{iVar}=Rannor(762); End;
Do iVar=1 to &nVars;
x{iVar}=0;
Do i=1 To iVar;
x{iVar}=x{iVar}+a{&nVars*(iVar-1)+i}*xNor{i};
End;
End;
Output;
End;
Run;
Proc Print data=nVars(obs=100); Run;
Proc corr data=nVars; Run;
%Mend RanVarMNor;
```

**<<SAS<<**

An example of an SAS macro call to generate the standard multivariate normal variables is given as follows.

```
>>SAS>>
TITLE "Standard Multivariate Normal Variables";
Data CorrMatrix;
Array ss{9} (1, .1, .5,
             .1, 1, .5,
             .5, .5, 1);
%RanVarMNor(sSize=9, nVars=3, nObs=10000);
Run;
<<SAS<<
```

Using the standard multivariate normal variables, we can transform
them into general multivariate normal variables as shown below.

```
>>SAS>>
Title "General Multivariate Normal Variables";
Data Final; Keep ys1-ys3;
Set nVars;
Array ys{3}; Array x{3};
Array sigma{3} (1, 2, 3);
Array means{3} (0, 1, 3);
Do iVar=1 To 3;
ys{iVar}=x{iVar}*sigma{iVar}+means{iVar};
End;
Title "Check the outputs";
Proc print data=Final; Run;
Proc means data=Final; Run;
Proc corr data=Final; Run;
<<SAS<<
```

# Appendix B

# A Useful Utility

```
>>SAS>>
Title "Create Sample dataset myData with variable id and x";
Data myData;
do i=1 to 100;
id=i; output;
x=id**2-100*id;
End;
Run;
Title "Randomize the order of records in dataset myData";
Data RanOrder;
Set myData;
RowId=ranuni(0); output;
Run;
Proc Sort data=RanOrder;
By RowId;
Run;
Proc Print; Run;
Title "Randomly select n (here n=70) observations";
Data RanPartOfmyData;
Set RanOrder;
newId=_N_;
If newId<=70 Then Output;
Run;
*Sort records in the original order;
Proc Sort Data=RanPartOfmyData;
by id;
Run;
Proc Print; Run;
<<SAS<<
```

# Appendix C

# SAS Macros for Add-Arm Designs

## C.1 The 5+1 Add-Arm Design

**>>SAS Macro C.3:    The 5+1 Add-Arm Design>>**

```
/* Larger mean or response means better */
/* SelProb(i) = the probability of selecting arm i. */
%Macro FivePlus1(nSims=10000, N1=100, N2=100, c_alpha = 2.343, cR =
0.52153, mu0=0, sigma=1);
Data FivePlus1;
Set dInput;
Array mu(5); Array xObs(5); Array SelProb(5);
Keep N1 N2 TotalN Power SelProb1-SelProb5;
N1=&N1; N2=&N2; Power=0;
Do i=1 To 5;
SelProb(i)=0;
End;
Do iSim=1 To &nSims;
Do i=1 To 5;
xObs(i) = RAND('NORMAL', mu(i), &sigma/sqrt(N1));
End;
If xObs(2)>xObs(4) Then Do;
If    xObs(1)*sqrt(N1)/&sigma>max(xObs(2),xObs(3))*sqrt(N1)/&sigma-&cR
Then SelectedArm=1;
Else If xObs(2)> xObs(3) Then SelectedArm=2;
Else SelectedArm=3;
End;
If xObs(2)<=xObs(4) Then Do;
If    xObs(5)*sqrt(N1)/&sigma>max(xObs(4),xObs(3))*sqrt(N1)/&sigma-&cR
Then SelectedArm=5;
```

```
Else If xObs(4)>xObs(3) Then SelectedArm=4;
Else SelectedArm=3;
End;
MaxRsp=xObs(SelectedArm);
x2 = RAND('NORMAL', mu(SelectedArm), &sigma/sqrt(N2));
FinalxAve = (MaxRsp*N1+x2*N2)/(N1+N2);
x0Ave = RAND('NORMAL', 0, &sigma/sqrt(N1+N2));
TestZ=(FinalxAve-x0Ave)*sqrt((N1+N2)/2)/&sigma;
If TestZ >= &c_alpha Then Power=Power+1/&nSims;
Do i=1 To 5;
If SelectedArm=i Then SelProb(i)=SelProb(i)+1/&nSims;
End;
End; * end iSims;
TotalN=5*N1+2*N2;
Output;
Run;
Proc print;
Run;
%Mend;
<<SAS<<
```

## >>SAS: Invoking Macro C.1>>

```
Title "5+1 Add-Arm Design: Critical Value and Type-I Error";
data dInput;
Array mu(5)(0,0,0,0,0);
%FivePlus1(nSims=1000000, N1=100, N2=100, c_alpha = 2.343, cR = 0.52153,
mu0=0);Run;
Title "5+1 Add-Arm Design: Power";
data dInput;
Array mu(5)(0.4,0.38,0.3,0.25,0.15);
%FivePlus1(nSims=1000000, N1=100, N2=100, c_alpha = 2.343, cR = 0.52153,
mu0=0);
Run;
<<SAS<<
```

## C.2   The 6+1 Add-Arm Design

### >>SAS Macro C.4:   The 6+1 Add-Arm Design>>

```
/* Larger mean or response means better */
/* SelProb(i) = the probability of selecting arm i. */
```

```
%Macro SixPlus1(nSims=10000, N1=100, N2=100, c_alpha = 2.341, cR =
0.50094, mu0=0, sigma=1);
Data SixPlus1;
Set dInput;
Array mu(6); Array xObs(6); Array SelProb(6);
Keep N1 N2 TotalN Power SelProb1-SelProb6;
N1=&N1; N2=&N2; Power=0;
Do i=1 To 6;
SelProb(i)=0;
End;
Do iSim=1 To &nSims;
Do i=1 To 6;
xObs(i) = RAND('NORMAL', mu(i), &sigma/sqrt(N1));
End;
If xObs(3)>xObs(4) Then Do;
If xObs(3)*sqrt(N1)/&sigma>max(xObs(1), xObs(2))*sqrt(N1)/&sigma+&cR
Then SelectedArm=3;
Else If xObs(1)>xObs(2) Then SelectedArm=1;
Else SelectedArm=2;
End;
If xObs(3)<=xObs(4) Then Do;
If xObs(4)*sqrt(N1)/&sigma>max(xObs(5), xObs(6))*sqrt(N1)/&sigma+&cR
Then SelectedArm=4;
Else If xObs(5)>xObs(6) Then SelectedArm=5;
Else SelectedArm=6;
End;
MaxRsp=xObs(SelectedArm);
x2 = RAND('NORMAL', mu(SelectedArm), &sigma/sqrt(N2));
FinalxAve = (MaxRsp*N1+x2*N2)/(N1+N2);
x0Ave = RAND('NORMAL', 0, &sigma/sqrt(N1+N2));
TestZ=(FinalxAve-x0Ave)*sqrt((N1+N2)/2)/&sigma;
If TestZ >= &c_alpha Then Power=Power+1/&nSims;
Do i=1 To 6;
If SelectedArm=i Then SelProb(i)=SelProb(i)+1/&nSims;
End;
End; * end iSims;
TotalN=5*N1+2*N2;
Output;
Run;
```

```
Proc print data=SixPlus1;
Run;
%Mend;
<<SAS<<
```

>>SAS: Invoking Macro C.2>>

```
Title "6+1 Add-Arm Design: Critical Value and Type-I Error";
data dInput;
Array mu(6)(0,0,0,0,0,0);
%SixPlus1(nSims=1000000, N1=80, N2=80, c_alpha = 2.343, cR = 0.52153,
mu0=0);Run;
Title "6+1 Add-Arm Design: Power";
data dInput;
Array mu(6)(0.4,0.38,0.3,0.25,0.15, 0.8);
%SixPlus1(nSims=1000000, N1=80, N2=80, c_alpha = 2.343, cR = 0.52153,
mu0=0);
Run;
<<SAS<<
```

## C.3    The 7+1 Add-Arm Design

>>SAS Macro C.5:    The 7+1 Add-Arm Design>>

```
/* Larger mean or response means better */
/* SelProb(i) = the probability of selecting arm i. */
%Macro   SevenPlus1(nSims=10000,   N1=100,   N2=100,   c_alpha  =  2.397,
cR=0.48001, mu0=0, sigma=1);
Data SevenPlus1;
Set dInput;
Array mu(7); Array xObs(7); Array SelProb(7);
Keep N1 N2 TotalN Power SelProb1-SelProb7;
N1=&N1; N2=&N2; Power=0;
Do i=1 To 7;
SelProb(i)=0;
End;
Do iSim=1 To &nSims;
Do i=1 To 7;
xObs(i) = RAND('NORMAL', mu(i), &sigma/sqrt(N1));
End;
If xObs(3)>xObs(5) Then Do;
If max(xObs(1), xObs(2))*sqrt(N1)/&sigma>max(xObs(3), xObs(4))*sqrt(N1)/
```

```
&sigma-&cR Then Do;
If xObs(1)>xObs(2) Then SelectedArm=1; Else SelectedArm=2; End;
Else If xObs(3)>xObs(4) Then SelectedArm=3; Else SelectedArm=4;
End;
If xObs(3)<=xObs(5) Then Do;
If max(xObs(7), xObs(6))*sqrt(N1)/&sigma>max(xObs(5), xObs(4))*sqrt(N1)/
&sigma-&cR Then Do;
If xObs(7)>xObs(6) Then SelectedArm=7; Else SelectedArm=6; End;
Else If xObs(5)>xObs(4) Then SelectedArm=5; Else SelectedArm=4;
End;
MaxRsp=xObs(SelectedArm);
x2 = RAND('NORMAL', mu(SelectedArm), &sigma/sqrt(N2));
FinalxAve = (MaxRsp*N1+x2*N2)/(N1+N2);
x0Ave = RAND('NORMAL', 0, &sigma/sqrt(N1+N2));
TestZ=(FinalxAve-x0Ave)*sqrt((N1+N2)/2)/&sigma;
If TestZ >= &c_alpha Then Power=Power+1/&nSims;
Do i=1 To 7;
If SelectedArm=i Then SelProb(i)=SelProb(i)+1/&nSims;
End;
End; * end iSims;
TotalN=5*N1+2*N2;
Output;
Run;
Proc print data=SevenPlus1;
Run;
%Mend;
```
<<**SAS**<<

## >>SAS: Invoking Macro C.3>>

```
Title "7+1 Add-Arm Design: Critical value and Type-I Error";
data dInput;
Array mu(7)(0,0,0,0,0,0,0);
%SevenPlus1(nSims=10000, N1=100, N2=100, c_alpha = 2.397, cR =0.48001,
mu0=0, sigma=2);
Title "7+1 Add-Arm Design: Power";
data dInput;
Array mu(7)(0.4,0.38,0.3,0.25,0.15, 0.8,0.1);
%SevenPlus1(nSims=10000, N1=100, N2=100, c_alpha = 2.397, cR =0.48001,
mu0=0, sigma=2);
Run;
```
<<**SAS**<<

# Appendix D

# Implementing Adaptive Designs in R

R is a language and environment for statistical computing and graphics. It is a GNU project which is similar to the S language and environment which was developed at Bell Laboratories (formerly AT&T, now Lucent Technologies) by John Chambers and colleagues. R can be considered as a different implementation of S. There are some important differences, but much code written for S runs unaltered under R. The R compiler is available at http://www.r-project.org/.

In this appendix, the R functions that mimic the SAS Macros in each chapter are presented. We purposely made the code very similar to the SAS macros so that those who know SAS but are new to R programming can understand more easily. For those who have some experience in R programming, you are encourage to make modifications or simplifications using the advantages of built-in R functions or the R language. Some such examples are presented in Chapter 13.

### Sample-Size Based on Conditional Power in Chapter 11

The sample-size required at the second stage based on the conditional power (11.5) is implemented in R Function D.1. The R variables are defined as follows: **nAdjModel** = "MIP," "MSP," "MPP," or "MINP;" **alpha0** = overall $\alpha$ level; **alpha1** = efficacy stopping boundary at the first stage; **eSize** = standardized effect size; **cPower** = the conditional power; **p1** = the stagewise $p$-value at the first stage; **w1** and **w2** = weights for Lehmacher–Wassmer method; and **n2New** = new sample size required for the second stage to achieve the desired conditional power.

**>>R Function D.1: Sample-Size Based on Conditional Power>>**

```
nByCPower = function(nAdjModel, a2, eSize, cPower, p1, w1, w2){
if (nAdjModel=="MIP") {BFun = qnorm(1-a2)}
if (nAdjModel=="MSP") {
BFun = qnorm(1-max(0.000001,a2-p1))
```

```
}
if (nAdjModel=="MPP") {BFun =qnorm(1- a2/p1)}
if (nAdjModel=="MINP") {
BFun = (qnorm(1-a2)- w1*qnorm(1-p1))/w2
}
2*((BFun-qnorm(1-cPower))/eSize)^2
}
```
<<R<<

**>>R Example>>**
```
pw1=nByCPower("MSP",.1,.3,.4,.05,.6,.4)
pw1
```
<<R<<

## Sample-Size Reestimation in Chapter 11

R-function D.2 TwoArmNStgAdpDsg is developed to simulate a two-arm n-stage adaptive design with a normal, binary, or survival endpoint using "MIP," "MSP," "MPP," "MINP," or "UWZ." The sample-size adjustment can be "CHW" based on (11.4) or the conditional power method (11.6). The sample-size adjustment is allowed only at the first interim analysis, and the sample-size adjustment affects only the final stagewise sample size, **ux** and **uy** = the means, response rates, or hazard rates for the two groups, **Ns[k]** = sample size per group at the stage k. **nMinIcr** = minimum sample-size increment for the conditional power approach only (this info is blinded to sponsor), **n2new** = the reestimated sample-size per group at the second stage, and **eSize** = the standardized effect size. **nSims** = number of simulation runs, **nStgs** = number of stages, **alpha0** = overall $\alpha$; and **EP** = "normal," "binary," or "survival." **Model** = "MSP," "MSP," "MPP," "MINP," or "UWZ." **Nadj** = "N" for the case without SSR, **Nadj** = "Y" for the case with SSR; and **nAdjModel** = "CHW" for SSR or other values based on the conditional power. **cPower** = conditional power, **DuHa** =1, **Nmax** = the maximum sample size allowed, **N0** = the initial sample size, **sigma** = standard deviation for normal endpoint, **tAcr** = accrual time, **tStd** = study duration, **power** = initial target power for the trial. **Aveux**, **Aveuy**, and **AveN** = average simulated responses (mean, proportion, or hazard rate) and sample size, **FSP[i]** = futility stopping probability at the $i$th stage, **ESP[i]** = efficacy stopping probability at the $i$th stage, **alpha[i]** and **beta[i]** = efficacy and futility stopping boundaries at the $i$th stage.

## >>R Function D.2:    Sample-Size Reestimation>>

```
TwoArmNStgAdpDsg = function (nSims=1000000, nStgs=2, ux=0, uy=1,
NId=0, a2=0.025, EP= "normal", Model= "MSP", Nadj= "Y",
nAdjModel= "MSP", cPower=0.9, DuHa=1, Nmax=300, N0=200,
nMinIcr=1, sigma=3, tAcr=10, tStd=24, Ns, alpha, beta) {
power=0; AveN=0; Aveux=0; Aveuy=0; cumN=0
for (i in 1:nStgs-1) {cumN=cumN+Ns[i]}
for (k in 1:nStgs) {
sumWs[k]=0
for (i in 1:k) {sumWs[k]=sumWs[k]+Ws[i]^2}
sumWs[k]=sqrt(sumWs[k])
}
u=(ux+uy)/2
if (EP== "normal") {sigma=sigma}
if (EP== "binary") {sigma=(u*(1-u))^0.5}
if (EP== "survival") {
expTerm=exp(-u*tStd)*(1-exp(u*tAcr))/(tAcr*u)
sigma=u*(1+expTerm)^(-0.5)
}

for (i in 1:nStgs) { FSP[i]=0; ESP[i]=0 }
for (iSim in 1:nSims) {
ThisN=0; Thisux=0; Thisuy=0
for (i in 1:nStgs) {TSc[i]=0}
TS=0
if (Model== "MPP") {TS=1}
EarlyStop=0
for (i in 1:nStgs) {
uxObs=rnorm(1)*sigma/sqrt(Ns[i])+ux
uyObs=rnorm(1)*sigma/sqrt(Ns[i])+uy
Thisux=Thisux+uxObs*Ns[i]
Thisuy=Thisuy+uyObs*Ns[i]
ThisN=ThisN+Ns[i]
TS0 = (uyObs-uxObs+NId)*sqrt(Ns[i]/2)/sigma
if (Model== "MIP") {TS=1-pnorm(TS0)}
if (Model== "MSP") {TS=TS+(1-pnorm(TS0))}
if (Model== "MPP") {TS=TS*(1-pnorm(TS0))}
if (Model== "MINP") {
for (k in 1:nStgs) {
```

```
TSc[k]=TSc[k]+Ws[i]/sumWs[k]*TS0
}
TS=1-pnorm(TSc[i])
}
if (Model=="UWZ") {
nT=(Thisuy-Thisux)/ThisN+NId
TS0=nT*sqrt(ThisN/2)/sigma
TS=1-pnorm(TS0)
}
if (TS>beta[i]) { FSP[i]=FSP[i]+1/nSims; EarlyStop=1 }
else if (TS<=alpha[i]) {
power=power+1/nSims
ESP[i]=ESP[i]+1/nSims
EarlyStop=1
}
else if (i==1 & Nadj=="Y") {
eSize=DuHa/(abs(uyObs-uxObs)+0.0000001)
nFinal=min(Nmax, max(N0,eSize*N0));
if (nAdjModel != "CHW") {
eSize=(uyObs-uxObs+NId)/sigma;
n2New=nByCPower(nAdjModel, a2, eSize,
cPower, TS, ws[1], ws[2]);
mT=min(Nmax,Ns[1]+n2New+nMinIcr/2)
nFinal=round(mT, nMinIcr)
}
if (nStgs>1) {Ns[nStgs]= max(1,nFinal-cumN)}
}
if (EarlyStop==1) i=nStgs+1
}
Aveux=Aveux+Thisux/ThisN/nSims
Aveuy=Aveuy+Thisuy/ThisN/nSims
AveN=AveN+ThisN/nSims
}
power=round(power,3);  AveN=round(AveN)
Aveux=round(Aveux,4); Aveuy=round(Aveuy,4)
FSP=round(FSP,3); ESP=round(ESP,3)
return (cbind(Model, power, Aveux, Aveuy, AveN, FSP, ESP, alpha, beta,
cPower))}
<<R<<
```

**>>R Example>>**

Ns = c(100,100); alpha = c(0.005, 0.205); beta = c(0.25, 0.205)

Ws = c(1,1); ESP = c(0,0); FSP = c(0,0); sumWs = c(0,0);

TSc = c(0,0)

AD1=TwoArmNStgAdpDsg(nSims=100000, nStgs=2,

ux=0, uy=0, NId=0, a2=0.025, EP="normal",

Model="MSP", Nadj="N", nAdjModel="MSP",

cPower=0.9, DuHa=1, Nmax=300, N0=200,

nMinIcr=1, sigma=3, tAcr=10, tStd=24, Ns, alpha, beta)

AD2=TwoArmNStgAdpDsg(nSims=100000, nStgs=2,

ux=0, uy=1, NId=0, a2=0.025, EP="normal",

Model="MSP", Nadj="Y", nAdjModel="MSP",

cPower=0.9, DuHa=1, Nmax=300, N0=200,

nMinIcr=1, sigma=3, tAcr=10, tStd=24, Ns, alpha, beta)

AD1; AD2

**<<R<<**

## Biomarker-Adaptive Design in Chapter 17

R Function D.3 is developed for simulating biomarker-adaptive trials with two parallel groups. The key R variables are defined as follows: **alpha1** = early efficacy stopping boundary (one-sided), **beta1** = early futility stopping boundary, **alpha2** = final efficacy stopping boundary, **u0p** = response difference in biomarker-positive population, **u0n** = response difference in biomarker-negative population. **sigma** = asymptotic standard deviation for the response difference, assuming homogeneous variance among groups; for binary response, sigma $=\sqrt{r_1(1-r_1)+r_2(1-r_2)}$; for normal response, sigma $= \sqrt{2}\sigma$. **np1, np2** = sample sizes per group for the first and second stage for the biomarker-positive population. **nn1, nn2** = sample sizes per group for the first and second stage for the biomarker-negative population. **cntlType** = "strong," for the strong type-I error control and **cntlType** = "weak," for the weak type-I error control, **AveN** = average total sample-size (all arms combined), **pPower** = the probability of significance for biomarker-positive population, **oPower** = the probability of significance for overall population.

## >>R Function D.3:  Biomarker-Adaptive Design>>

BMAD = function(nSims=10, cntlType="strong", nStages=2, u0p=0.2,

u0n=0.1, sigma=1, np1=50, np2=50, nn1=100, nn2=100, alpha1=0.01,

beta1=0.15, alpha2=0.1871) {

FSP=0; ESP=0; Power=0; AveN=0; pPower=0; oPower=0

for (isim in 1:nSims) {

```
up1=rnorm(1)*sigma/sqrt(np1)+u0p
un1=rnorm(1)*sigma/sqrt(nn1)+u0n
uo1=(up1*np1+un1*nn1)/(np1+nn1)
Tp1=up1*sqrt(np1)/sigma
To1=uo1*sqrt((np1+nn1))/sigma
T1=max(Tp1,To1)
p1=1-pnorm(T1)
if (cntlType=="strong") {p1=2*p1}
if (p1>beta1) {FSP=FSP+1/nSims}
if (p1<=alpha1) {
Power=Power+1/nSims; ESP=ESP+1/nSims
if (Tp1>To1) {pPower=pPower+1/nSims}
if (Tp1<=To1) {oPower=oPower+1/nSims}
}
AveN=AveN+2*(np1+nn1)/nSims
if (nStages==2 & p1>alpha1 & p1<=beta1) {
up2=rnorm(1)*sigma/sqrt(np2)+u0p
un2=rnorm(1)*sigma/sqrt(nn2)+u0n
uo2=(up2*np2+un2*nn2)/(np2+nn2)
Tp2=up2*sqrt(np2)/sigma
To2=uo2*sqrt(np2+nn2)/sigma
if (Tp1>To1) {
T2=Tp2
AveN=AveN+2*np2/nSims
}
if (Tp1<=To1) {
T2=To2
AveN=AveN+2*(np2+nn2)/nSims
}
p2=1-pnorm(T2)
TS=p1+p2
if (TS<=alpha2) {
Power=Power+1/nSims
if (Tp1>To1) {pPower=pPower+1/nSims}
if (Tp1<=To1) {oPower=oPower+1/nSims}
}
}
}
return (cbind(FSP, ESP, Power, AveN, pPower, oPower))
```

```
}
<<R<<
```

**>>R Example>>**

```
# Simulation under global Ho, 2-stage design
bmad1=BMAD(nSims=100000, cntlType="strong", nStages=2, u0p=0,
u0n=0, sigma=1.414, np1=260, np2=260, nn1=520, nn2=520,
alpha1=0.01, beta1=0.15, alpha2=0.1871)

# Simulations under Ha, single-stage design
bmad2=BMAD(nSims=100000, cntlType="strong", nStages=1, u0p=0.2,
u0n=0.1, sigma=1.414, np1=400, np2=0, nn1=800, nn2=0, alpha1=0.025);
# Simulation under global Ho, 2-stage design
bmad3=BMAD(nSims=100000, cntlType="strong", nStages=2, u0p=0,
u0n=0, sigma=1.414, np1=260, np2=260, nn1=520, nn2=520,
alpha1=0.01, beta1=0.15, alpha2=0.1871)
# Simulations under Ha, 2-stage design
bmad4=BMAD(nSims=100000, cntlType="strong", nStages=2, u0p=0.2,
u0n=0.1, sigma=1.414, np1=260, np2=260, nn1=520, nn2=520,
alpha1=0.01, beta1=0.15, alpha2=0.1871)
bmad1; bmad2; bmad3; bmad4
<<R<<
```

## Randomized Play-the-Winner Design in Chapter 15

R Function D.4 is developed to simulate RPW designs. The variables are defined as follows: the initial number of balls in the urn is denoted by **a0** and **b0**. Next **a1** or **b1**-balls added to the urn if a response is observed in arm $A$ or arm $B$. The SAS variables are defined as follows: **RR1, RR2** = the response rates in group 1 and 2, respectively, **nSbjs** = total number of subjects (two groups combined), **nMin** ($>0$) = the minimum sample size per group required to avoid an extreme imbalance situation, **nAnlys** = number of analyses (approximately an equal information-time design). All interim analyses are designed for randomization adjustment and only the final analysis for hypothesis testing. **aveP1** and **aveP2** = the average response rates in group 1 and 2, respectively. **Power** = probability of the test statistic > **Zc**. Note: **Zc** = function of (**nSbjs, nAnlys, a0, b0, a1, b1, nMin**).

**>>R Function D.4: Randomized Play-the-Winner Design>>**

```
RPW = function(nSims=1000, Zc=1.96, nSbjs=200, nAnlys=3,
RR1=0.2, RR2=0.3, a0=1, b0=1, a1=1, b1=1, nMin=1) {
```

```
set.seed(21823)
Power=0; aveP1=0; aveP2=0; aveN1=0; aveN2=0
for (isim in 1:nSims) {
nResp1=0; nResp2=0; N1=0; N2=0
nMax=nSbjs-nMin
a=a0; b=b0; r0=a/(a+b)
for (iSbj in 1:nSbjs) {
nIA=round(nSbjs/nAnlys)
if (iSbj/nIA==round(iSbj/nIA)) {r0=a/(a+b)}
if ((rbinom(1,1,r0)==1 & N1<nMax) | N2>=nMax) {
N1=N1+1
if (rbinom(1,1,RR1)==1) {nResp1=nResp1+1; a=a+a1}
}
else
{
N2=N2+1
if (rbinom(1,1,RR2)==1) { nResp2=nResp2+1; b=b+b1 }
}
}
aveN1=aveN1+N1/nSims; aveN2=aveN2+N2/nSims
p1=nResp1/N1; p2=nResp2/N2
aveP1=aveP1+p1/nSims; aveP2=aveP2+p2/nSims
sigma1=sqrt(p1*(1-p1)); sigma2=sqrt(p2*(1-p2))
sumscf=sigma1^2/(N1/(N1+N2))+sigma2^2/(N2/(N1+N2))
TS = (p2-p1)*sqrt((N1+N2)/sumscf)
if (TS>Zc) {Power=Power+1/nSims}
}
return (cbind(nSbjs, aveN1, aveN2, aveP1, aveP2, Zc, Power))
}
<<R<<
```

## >>R Example>>

```
rpw1=RPW(nSims=1000, Zc=1.96, nSbjs=200, nAnlys=200, RR1=0.4,
RR2=0.4, a0=1, b0=1,a1=0, b1=0, nMin=1)
rpw2=RPW(nSims=1000, Zc=1.96, nSbjs=200, nAnlys=200, RR1=0.3,
RR2=0.5, a0=1, b0=1,a1=0, b1=0, nMin=1)
rpw3=RPW(nSims=10000, Zc=2.035, nSbjs=200, nAnlys=5, RR1=0.4,
RR2=0.4, a0=2, b0=2,a1=1, b1=1, nMin=1)
rpw4=RPW(nSims=1000, Zc=2.035, nSbjs=200, nAnlys=5, RR1=0.3,
RR2=0.5, a0=2, b0=2,a1=1, b1=1, nMin=1)
```

rpw1; rpw2; rpw3; rpw4

<<**R**<<

## Continual Reassessment Method in Chapter 22

R Funcrion D.5 is for trial simulation trial using CRM. The input variables are defined as follows: **b** = model parameter in (22.19), **aMin** and **aMax** = the upper and lower limits for prior on the parameter $a$. The definitions of other variables are the same as SAS Macro 22.2.

>>**R Function D.5:**    **Continual Reassessment Method**>>

```
CRM = function(nSims=100, nPts=30, nLevels=10, b=100, aMin=0.1,
aMax=0.3, MTRate=0.3, nIntPts=100, ToxModel= "Skeleton", nPtsForStop=6)
{
nPtsAt = c(1); nRsps = c(1); RR = c(1); g0 = c(1); PercentMTD= c(1)
DLTs=0; AveMTD=0; VarMTD=0; AveTotalN=0
dx=(aMax-aMin)/nIntPts
for (k in 1:nIntPts) {g0[k]=g[k]}
for (i in 1:nLevels) { PercentMTD[i]=0 }
for (iSim in 1:nSims) {
for (k in 1:nIntPts) {g[k]=g0[k]}
for (i in 1:nLevels) { nPtsAt[i]=0; nRsps[i]=0}
iLevel=1; PreLevel=1
for (iPtient in 1:nPts) {
TotalN=iPtient
TotalN=iPtient
iLevel=min(iLevel, PreLevel+1); #Avoid dose-jump
iLevel=min(iLevel, nLevels)
PreLevel=iLevel
Rate=RRo[iLevel]
nPtsAt[iLevel]=nPtsAt[iLevel]+1
r= rbinom(1, 1, Rate)
nRsps[iLevel]=nRsps[iLevel]+r
# Posterior distribution of a
c=0
for (k in 1:nIntPts) {
ak=aMin+k*dx
f (ToxModel== "Logist") { Rate=1/(1+b*exp(-ak*doses[iLevel]))}
if (ToxModel== "Skeleton") { Rate=skeletonP[iLevel]^exp(ak)}
if (r>0) {L=Rate}
if (r <= 0) {L=1-Rate}
g[k]=L*g[k]; c=c+g[k]*dx
```

```
}
for (k in 1:nIntPts) {g[k]=g[k]/c}
# Predict response rate and current MTD
MTD=iLevel; MinDR=1
for (i in 1:nLevels) {
RR[i]=0
for (k in 1:nIntPts) {
ak=aMin+k*dx
if (ToxModel=="Logist") { RR[i]= RR[i]+1/(1+b*exp(-ak*doses[i]))*g[k]*dx}
if (ToxModel=="Skeleton") { RR[i]= RR[i]+skeletonP[i]^exp(ak)*g[k]*dx}
}
DR=abs(MTRate-RR[i])
if (DR <MinDR) { MinDR = DR; iLevel = i; MTD = i }
}
if (nPtsAt[iLevel] >= nPtsForStop) {
PercentMTD[iLevel] =PercentMTD[iLevel]+1/nSims
break()
}
}
for (i in 1:nLevels) {DLTs=DLTs+nRsps[i]/nSims}
AveMTD=AveMTD+MTD/nSims
VarMTD=VarMTD+MTD^2/nSims
AveTotalN=AveTotalN+TotalN/nSims
}
SdMTD=sqrt(VarMTD-AveMTD^2)
return (cbind(AveTotalN, nLevels, AveMTD, SdMTD, DLTs))
}
<<R<<

>>R Example>>
#Logistic Model
g= c(1); doses = c(1)
RRo = c(0.01,0.02,0.03,0.05,0.12,0.17,0.22,0.4)
for (k in 1:100) {g[k]=1}; # Flat prior
for (i in 1:8) {doses[i]=i}
CRM(nSims=500, nPts=30, nLevels=8, b=150, aMin=0, aMax=3,
MTRate=0.17, ToxModel="Logist", nPtsForStop=6)

#Skeleton Model
g = c(1);
```

```
RRo = c(0.01,0.02,0.03,0.05,0.12,0.17,0.22,0.4)
skeletonP=c(0.01,0.02,0.04,0.08,0.16,0.32,0.4,0.5)
for (k in 1:100) {g[k]=1}; # Flat prior
CRM(nSims=500, nPts=20, nLevels=8, aMin=-0.1, aMax=2,
MTRate=0.17, ToxModel="Skeleton", nPtsForStop=6)
<<R<<
```

# Bibliography

Ades, A.E., Sculpher, M., and Sutton, A. et al. (2006). Bayesian methods for evidence synthesis in cost-effectiveness analysis. *Pharmacoeconomics*, 24(1):1–19.

Alonso, A., Molenberghs, G., Geys, H., Buyse, M., and Vangeneugden, T. (2006). A unifying approach for surrogate marker validation based on Prentice's criteria. *Statististical Medicine* 25:205–221. Published online 11 October 2005 in Wiley InterScience (www.interscience.wiley.com). DOI: 10.1002/sim.2315.

Anderson, K. (2014). gsDesign: Group Sequential Design. R package version 2.8-8. http://cran.r-project.org/web/packages/gsDesign/index.html

Arbuck, S.G. (1996). Workshop on phase I study design. *Annals of Oncology*, 7:567–573.

Armitage, P. (1955). Tests for linear trends in proportions and frequencies. *Biometrics*, 11:375–86.

Armitage, P., McPherson, C., and Rowe, B. (1969). Repeated significance tests on accumulating data. *Journal of the Royal Statistical Society*, Series A, 132:235–244.

Atkinson, A.C. (1982). Optimum biased coin designs for sequential clinical trials with prognostic factors. *Biometrika*, 69:61–67.

Atkinson, A.C. and Donev, A.N. (1992). *Optimum Experimental Designs*. Oxford University Press, New York.

Babb, J., Rogatko, A., and Zacks, S. (1998). Cancer phase I clinical trials. Efficient dose escalation with overdose control. *Statistics in Medicine*, 17: 1103–1120.

Babb, J.S. and Rogatko, A. (2001). Patient specific dosing in a cancer phase I clinical trial. *Statistics in Medicine*, 20:2079–2090.

Babb, J.S. and Rogatko, A. (2004). Bayesian methods for cancer phase I clinical trials. In *Advances in Clinical Trial Biostatistics*. Geller, N.L., editor, New York: Marcel Dekker.

Bandyopadhyay, U. and Biswas A. (1997). Some sequential tests in clinical trials based on randomized play-the-winner rule. *Calcutta Statistical Association Bulletin*, 47:67–89.

Banerjee, A. and Tsiatis, A.A. (2006). Adaptive two-stage designs in phase II clinical trials. *Statistics in Medicine*, In press.

Banik, N., Kohne, K., and Bauer, P. (1996). On the power of Fisher's combination test for two stage sampling in the presence of nuisance parameters. *Biometrical Journal*, 38:25–37.

Bauer, P. (1989). Multistage testing with adaptive designs (with Discussion). *Biometrie und Informatik in Medizin und Biologie*, 20:130–148.

Bauer, P. and Brannath, W. (2004). The advantages and disadvantages of adaptive designs for clinical trials. *Drug Discovery Today*, 9, 351–57.

Bauer, P. and Kieser, M. (1999). Combining different phases in development of medical treatments within a single trial. *Statistics in Medicine*, 18:1833–1848.

Bauer, P. and Koenig, F. (2005). The reassessment of trial perspectives from interim data—A critical view. *Statistics in Medicine*, 25:23–36.

Bauer, P., Koenig, F., Brannatha, W., and Poscha M. (2010). Selection and bias—Two hostile brothers. *Statistics in Medicine*, 29:1–13.

Bauer, P. and Kohne K. (1994). Evaluation of experiments with adaptive interim analyses. *Biometrics*, 50:1029–1041.

Bauer, P. and Köhne, K. (1996). Evaluation of experiments with adaptive interim analyses. *Biometrics*, 52:380 (Correction).

Bauer, P. and König, F. (2006). The reassessment of trial perspectives from interim data—A critical view. *Statistics in Medicine*, 25, 23–36.

Bauer, P. and Rohmel, J. (1995). An adaptive method for establishing a dose-response relationship, *Statistics in Medicine*, 14:1595–1607.

Bebu, I., Dragalin, V., and Luta, G. (2008). Confidence intervals for con rmatory adaptive two-stage designs with tretament selection. *Biometrical Journal*, 55:294–309.

Bechhofer, R.E., Kiefer, J., and Sobel, M. (1968). *Sequential Identification and Ranking Problems*. University of Chicago Press, Chicago, Illinois.

Beck, R.W., Maguire, M.G., Bressler, N.M., Glassman, A.R., Lindblad, A.S., and Ferris, F.L. (2007). Visual acuity as an outcome measure in clinical trials of retinal diseases. *Ophthalmology*, 114(10):1804–9.

Benjamini, Y. and Hochberg, Y. (1995). Controlling the false discovery rate: A practical and powerful approach to multiple testing. *Journal of the Royal Statistical Society Series B*, 57:289–300.

Berger, R. (1982). Multiparameter hypothesis testing and acceptance sampling. *Technometrics*, 295–300.

Berry, D.A. (2005a). Introduction to Bayesian methods III: Use and interpretation of Bayesian tools in design and analysis. *Clinical Trials*, 2:295–300.

Berry, D.A. (2005b). Statistical innovations in cancer research. In Holland, J. et al., editors. *Cancer Medicine*. 7th ed. pp. 411–425. London: BC Decker.

Berry, D.A. and Eick, S.G. (1995). Adaptive assignment versus balanced randomization in clinical trials: a decision analysis. *Statistics in Medicine*, 14:231–246.

Berry, D.A. and Fristedt, B. (1985). *Bandit Problems: Sequential Allocation of Experiments*. Chapman & Hall, London, UK.

Berry, D.A. et al. (2001). Adaptive Bayesian designs for dose-ranging drug trials. In Gatsonis, C. et al., editors. *Case Studies in Bayesian Statistics V.* pp. 99–181. New York: Springer-Verlag.

Berry, D.A., Mueller. P., Grieve, A.P. et al. (2002). Adaptive Bayesian designs for dose-ranging drug trials. In *Case Studies in Bayesian Statistics V. Lecture Notes in Statistics*. pp. 162–181. New York: Springer.

Berry, D.A. and Stangl, D.K. (1996). *Bayesian Biostatistics*, Marcel Dekker, Inc., New York.

Birkett, N.J. (1985). Adaptive allocation in randomized controlled trials. *Controlled Clinical Trials*, 6:146–155.

Birnbaum, A. (1962). On the foundations of statistical inference. *Journal of American Statistical Association*, 57:269–306.

Bischoff, W. and Miller, F. (2005). Adaptive two-stage test procedures to find the best treatment in clinical trials. *Biometrika*, 92:197–212.

Blackwell, D. and Hodges, J.L., Jr. (1957). Design for the control of selection bias. *Annals of Mathematical Statistics*, 28:449–460.

Blume, J.D. (2002). Likelihood methods for measuring statistical evidence. *Statistics of Medicine*, 21:2563–2599.

Bowden, J. and Glimm, E. (2008). Unbiased estimation of selected treatment means in two-stage trials. *Biometrical Journal*, 50(4):515–527.

Brannath, W. and Bauer, P. (2004). Optimal conditional error functions for the control of conditional power. *Biometrics*, 60:715–723.

Brannath, W., Bauer, P., Maurer, W., and Posch, M. (2003). Sequential tests for non-inferiority and superiority. *Biometrics*, 59:106–114. DOI: 10.1111=1541-0420.00013

Brannath, W., Koenig, F., and Bauer, P. (2003). Improved repeated confidence bounds in trials with a maximal goal. *Biometrical Journal*, 45:311–324.

Brannath, W., Koenig, F., and Bauer, P. (2006). Estimation in flexible two-stage designs. *Statistics of Medicine*, 25:3366–3381.

Brannath, W., Posch, M., and Bauer, P. (2002). Recursive combination tests. *Journal of American Statistical Association*, 97(457):236–244.

Branson, M. and Whitehead, W. (2002). Estimating a treatment effect in survival studies in which patients switch treatment. *Statistics in Medicine*, 21:2449–2463.

Breslow, N.E. and Haug, C. (1977). Sequential comparison of exponential survival curves. *JASA*, 67:691–697.

Bretz, F. and Hothorn, L.A. (2002). Detecting dose-response using contrasts: Asymptotic power and sample-size determination for binary data. *Statistics in Medicine*, 21:3325–3335.

Bretz, F., Schmidli, H., König, F., Racine, A., and Maurer, W. (2006). Confirmatory seamless phase II/III clinical trials with hypotheses selection at interim: General concepts. *Biometrical Journal*, 48(4):623–634. DOI: 10.1002/bimj.200510232.

Brittain, E. and Hu, Z. (2009). Noninferiority trial design and analysis with an ordered three-level categorical endpoint. *Journal of Biopharmaceutical Statistics*, 19:685–699.

Bronshtein, I.N. et al., (2004). *Handbook of Mathematics*. Springer-Verlag, Berlin, Heidelberg.

Brophy, J.M. and Joseph, L. (1995). Placing trials in context using Bayesian analysis. GUSTO revisited by Reverend Bayes. *Journal of American Medical Association*, 273:871–875.

Burman, C.F. and Sonesson, C. (2006). Are flexible designs sound? (with discussion). *Biometrics*, 62:664–683.

Buyse, M. and Molenberghs, G. (1998). Criteria for the validation of surrogate endpoints in randomized experiments. *Biometrics*, 54:1014–1029.

Buyse, M. et al. Statistical validation of surrogate endpoint. *Drug Information Journal*, 34:49–67, 447–454.

Campbell, M.J., Julious, S.A., and Altman, D.G. (1995). Estimating sample sizes for binary, ordered categorical, and continuous outcomes in two group comparisons. *British Medical Journal*, 311:1145–1148.

Canner, P.L. (1997). Monitoring treatment differences in long-term clinical trials. *Biometrics*, 33:603–615.

Carreras, M. and Brannath, W. (2012). Shrinkage estimation in two-stage adaptive designs with midtrial treatment selection. *Statistics of Medicine*.

Casella, G. and Berger, R. (2001). *Statistical Inference*. Duxbury Press.

Chakravarty, A. (2005). Regulatory aspects in using surrogate markers in clinical trials. In The evaluation of surrogate endpoint, Burzykowski, Molenberghs, and Buyse, editors. Springer.

Chaloncr, K. and Larntz, K. (1989). Optimal Bayesian design applied to logistic regression experiments. *Journal of Planning and Inference*, 21:191–208.

Chan, I.S. (2002). Power and sample size determination for noninferiority trials using an exact method. *Journal of Biopharmaceutical Statistics*, 12(4): 457–469.

Chang, M. (2005a). Adaptive clinical trial design. In *Proceedings of the XIth International Symposium on Applied Stochastic Models and Data Analysis*. Janssen, J. and Lenca, P., editors. Brest, France, ENST Bretagne.

Chang, M. (2005b). Bayesian adaptive design with biomarkers. Presented at IBC's Second Annual Conference on Implementing Adaptive Designs for Drug Development, November 7-8, 2005, Princeton, New Jersey.

Chang, M. (2006a). Adaptive design based on sum of stagewise $p$-values. *Statistics in Medicine* (in press). DOI: 10.1002/sim.2755.

Chang, M. (2006b). Adaptive design with biomarkers. Conference on Innovating Clinical Drug Development, January 24-25, 2006, London, UK.

Chang, M. (2006c). Bayesian Adaptive Design Method with Biomarkers. Biopharmaceutical Report 14.

Chang, M. (2006d). Phase II/III seamless adaptive design. International Chinese Statistical Association Bulletin January, 42–47.

Chang, M. (2006e). Recursive two-stage adaptive design, submitted.

Chang, M. (2007a). Clinical trial simulations in early development phases. In *Encyclopedia of Biopharmaceutical Statistics*, Chow, S.C., editor. Taylor & Francis, New York.

Chang, M. (2007b). Multiple-arm superiority and noninferiority designs with various endpoints. *Pharmaceutical Statistics*, 6:43–52.

Chang, M. (2007c). Multiple-endpoint adaptive design, submitted.

Chang, M. et al. (2007). BIO White Paper: Innovative approaches in drug develpment. Submitted.

Chang, M. (2010). *Monte Carlo Simulation for the Pharmaceutical Industry.* Chapman & Hall/CRC: Boca Raton, FL.

Chang, M. and Chow, S.C. (2006b). Power and sample-size for dose response studies. In Dose Finding in Drug Development. Ting, N. editor. Springer, New York.

Chang, M. (2012). Adaptive Design and Simulation. Deming Conference 2012. December 2012, New Jersey.

Chang, M. and Chow, S.C. (2005). A hybrid Bayesian adaptive design for dose response trials. *Journal of Biopharmaceutical Statistics,* 15:667–691.

Chang, M. and Chow, S.C. (2006a). An innovative approach in clinical development—utilization of adaptive design methods in clinical trials. Submitted.

Chang, M. (2011). *Modern Issues and Methods in Biostatistics.* Springer, New York.

Chang, M., Chow, S.C., and Pong, A. (2006). Adaptive design in clinical research - issues, opportunities, and recommendations. *Journal of Biopharmaceutical Statistics,* 16(3):299–309.

Chang, M.N. (1989). Confidence intervals for a normal mean following group sequential test. *Biometrics,* 45:249–254.

Chang, M.N., Gould, A.L., and Snapinn, S.M. (1995). P-values for group sequential testing, *Biometrika,* 82:650–654.

Chang, M.N. and O'Brien, P.C. (1986). Confidence intervals following group sequential test. *Controlled Clinical Trials,* 7:18–26.

Chang, M.N., Wieand, H.S., and Chang, V.T. (1989). The bias of the sample proportion following a group sequential phase II trial. *Statistics in Medicine,* 8:563–570.

Chang and Wang (2014). The Add-Arm Design for Unimodal Response Curve with Unknown Mode. *Journal of Biopharmaceutical Statistics.* In press.

Chen, J., and Quan, H. (2013). Comment: The PLATO Trial Case Study. *Statistics in Biopharmaceutical Research,* 5:102–104.

Chen, J., Quan, H., Binkowitz, B., Ouyang, S.P., Tanaka, Y., Li, G., Menjoge, S., and Ibia, E. (2010). Assessing consistent treatment effect in a multiregional clinical trial: A systematic review. *Pharmaceutical Statistics,* 9: 242–253.

Chen, J., Quan, H., Gallo, P., Menjoge, S., Luo, X., Tanaka, Y., Li, G., Ouyang, S.P., Binkowitz, B., Ibia, E., Talerico, S., and Ikeda, K. (2011). Consistency of treatment effect across regions in multiregional clinical trials, Part 1: design considerations. *Drug Information Journal,* 45:595–602.

Chen, J., Quan, H., Gallo, P., Ouyang, S.P., and Binkowitz, B. (2012). An adaptive strategy for assessing regional consistency in multiregional clinical trials. *Clinical Trials,* 9:330–339.

Chen, J., Zheng, H., Quan, H., Li, G., Gallo, P., Ouyang, S.P., Binkowitz, B., Ting, N., Tanaka, Y., Luo, X., and Ibia, E. (2013). Graphical assessment of consistency in treatment effect among countries in multi-regional clinical trials. *Clinical Trials,* 10:842–851.

Chen, J.J., Tsong, Y., and Kang, S. (2000). Tests for equivalence or noninferiority between two proportions. *Drug Information Journal,* 34:569–578.

Chen, T.T. (1997). Optimal three-stage designs for phase II cancer clinical trials. *Statistics in Medicine*, 16:2701–2711.

Chen, T.T. and Ng, T.H. (1998). Optimal flexible designs in phase II cancer clinical trials. *Statistics in Medicine*, 17:2301–2312.

Chen, X.Y., Lu, N., Nair, R., Xu, Y.L., Kang, C.L., Huang, Q., Li, N., and Chen, H.Z. (2012). Decision Rules and Associated Sample Size Planning for Regional Approval Utilizing Multiregional Clinical Trials. *Journal of Biopharmaceutical Statistics*, 22(5):1001–1018.

Chen, Y.F., Wang, S.J., Khin, N.A., Hung, H.M.J., and Laughren, T.P. (2010). Trial design issues and treatment effect modelling in multi-regional schizophrenia trials. *Pharmaceutical Statistics*, 9(3):217–229.

Chen, Y.F, Yang, Y., Hung, H.J., and Wang, S.J. (2011). Evaluation of performance of some enrichment designs dealing with high placebo response in psychiatric clinical trials. *Contemporary Clinical Trials*, 32:592–604.

Chen, Y.H.J., DeMets, D.L., and Lan, K.K.G. (2004). Increasing the sample size when the unblinded interim result is promising. *Statistics in Medicine*, 23(7):1023–1038.

Cheng, Y. and Shen, Y. (2004). Estimation of a parameter and its exact confidence interval following sequential sample-size re-estimation trials. *Biometrics*, 60:910–918.

Cheng, Y.S. (2014). Some recent advances in multivariate statistics: Modality inference and statistical monitoring of clinical trials with multiple co-primary endpoints. Graduate School of Art and Sciences, Boston University, Boston, MA.

Cheng, Y.S., Menon, S., and Chang, M. (2014). Group sequential design and monitoring using multivariate B-value tool for clinical trials with multiple co-primary endpoints. *Statistics in Biopharmaceutical Research*.

Chevret, S. (1993). The continual reassessment method in cancer phase I clinical trials: A simulation study. *Statistics in Medicine*, 12:1093–1108.

Chevret, S. (2006). (Ed.). *Statistical Methods for Dose-Finding Experiments*. John Wiley & Sons Ltd. West Sussex, England.

CHMP. (2005). Guideline on the choice of the noninferiority margin, EMEA/EWP/2158/99. London.

CHMP. (2009). Guideline on missing data in confirmatory clinical trials/1776/99 Rev. 1.

Chow, S.C. (2013). Biosimilars: Design and Analysis of Follow-on Biologics. Chapman & Hall/CRC: Boca Raton, FL.

Chow, S.C. and Chang, M. (2005). Statistical consideration of adaptive methods in clinical development. *Journal of Biopharmaceutical Statistics*, 15:575–591.

Chow, S.C., and Chang, M. (2006). *Adaptive Design Methods in Clinical Trials*. Chapman & Hall/CRC.

Chow, S.C., Chang, M., and Pong, A. (2005). Statistical consideration of adaptive methods in clinical development. *Journal of Biopharmaceutical Statistics*, 15:575–91.

Chow, S.C. and Ju, C. (2013). Assessing biosimilarity and interchangeability of biosimilar products under the Biologics Price Competition and Innovation Act. *Generics and Biosimilars Initiative Journal*, 2(1):20–25.

Chow, S.C., Hsieh, E., Chi, E., and Yang, J. (2010). A comparison of moment-based and probability-based criteria for assessment of follow-on biologics. *Journal Biopharm Statistics*, 20(1):31–45.

Chow, S.C. and Liu, J.P. (1999). *Design and Analysis of Bioavailable and Bioeqivalence Studies*, 3rd ed. Chapman & Hall/CRC: Boca Raton, FL.

Chow, S.C. and Liu, J.P. (2003). *Design and Analysis of Clinical Trials*. 2nd edition, John Wiley & Sons, New York.

Chow, S.C., Lu, Y., and Yang, L.Y. (2013). Assessing similarity using the reproducibility and generalizability probabilities and the sensitivity index, in Design and Analysis of Bridging Studies, Liu, Chow, and Hsiao, editors. CRC Press, Boca Raton, FL.

Chow, S.C. and Shao, J. (2002). *Statistics in Drug Research*. Marcel Dekker, Inc., New York.

Chow, S.C. and Shao, J. (2005). Inference for clinical trials with some protocol amendments. *Journal of Biopharmaceutical Statistics*, 15:659–666.

Chow, S.C. and Shao, J. (2006). On margin and statistical test for noninferiority in active control trials. *Statistics in Medicine*, 25:1101–1113.

Chow, S.C., Shao, J., and Hu, Y.P. (2002). Assessing sensitivity and similarity in bridging studies. *Journal of Biopharmaceutical Statistics*, 12:385–400.

Chow, S.C., Shao, J., and Wang, H. (2003). *Sample Size Calculation in Clinical Research*. Marcel Dekker, Inc., New York.

Chow, S.C., Shao, J., and Wang, H. (2011). *Sample Size Calculations in Clinical Research*, 2nd ed. Chapman & Hall/CRC: Boca Raton, FL.

Chuang, S.C. and Agresti, A. (1997). A review of tests for detecting a monotone dose-response relationship with ordinal response data. *Statistics in Medicine*, 16:2599–2618.

Chuang, S.C. et al., (2006). Sample size re-estimation. Submitted.

Chuang-Stein, C., Stryszak, P., Dmitrienko, A., and Offen, W. (2007). Challenge of multiple co-primary endpoints: A new approach. *Statistics in Medicine*, 26(6):1181–1192.

Chuang-Stein, C. et al. (2013). Design and sample size consideration for global trials. In *Design and Analysis of Bridging Studies*, Liu, Chow, and Hsuao, edirors. CRC Press, Boca Raton, FL.

Clayton, D.G. (1978). A model for association in bivariate life tables and its application in epidemiological studies of familial tendency in chronic disease incidence. *Biometrika*, 65:141–151.

Coad, D.S. and Rosenberger, W.F. (1999). A comparison of the randomized play-the-winner and the triangular test for clinical trials with binary responses. *Statistics in Medicine*, 18:761–769.

Coburger, S. and Wassmer, G. (2001). Conditional point estimation in adaptive group sequential test designs. *Biometrical Journal*, 43:821–833.

Coburger, S. and Wassmer, G. (2003). Sample size reassessment in adaptive clinical trials using a bias corrected estimate. *Biometrical Journal*, 45:812–825.

Cochran, W.G. (1954). Some methods for strengthening the common $\chi^2$ tests. *Biometrics*, 10:417–451.

Code of Federal Regulations, Title21, Section 312.21 Phases of an Investigation.

Cohen, A. and Sackrowitz, H.B. (1989a). Exact tests that recover interblock information in balanced incomplete block design. *Journal of American Statistical Association*, 84, 556–559.

Cohen, A., and Sackrowitz, H. (1989b). Two stage conditionally unbiased estimators of the selected mean. *Statistics and Probability Letters*, 8: 273–278.

Collette, L. et al. (2005). Is Prostate-Specific Antigen a Valid Surrogate End Point for Survival in Hormonally Treated Patients with Metastatic Prostate Cancer? Joint Research of the European Organisation for Research and Treatment of Cancer, the Limburgs Universitair Centrum, and AstraZeneca Pharmaceuticals. *Journal Clinical Oncology*, 23:6139–6148.

Conawav, M.R. and Petroni, G. R. (1996). Designs for phase II trials allowing for a trade-off between response and toxicity. *Biometrics*, 52:1375–1386.

Conley, B.A. and Taube, S.E. (2004). Prognostic and predictive marker in cancer. *Disease Markers*, 20:35–43.

Cook, R.J., Lee, K.A., and Li, H. (2007). Noninferiority trial design for recurrent events. *Statistics in Medicine*, 26:4563–4577.

Cornfield, J. (1976). Recent methodological contributions to clinical trials. *American Journal of Epidemiology*, 104(4):408–421.

Cox, D.R. (1952). A note of the sequential estimation of means. *Proc. Camb. Phil. Soc.*, 48:447–450.

Cox, D.R. (2006). *Principles of Statistical Inference*. Cambridge University Press, Cambridge, UK.

Cox, D.R. (1972). Regression Models and Life-Tables. *Journal of the Royal Statistical Society B*, 34:187–220.

Cox, D.R. and Oakes, D. (1984). *Analysis of Survival Data*. Monographs on Statistics and Applied Probability. Chapman & Hall, London.

Crowley, J. (2001). *Handbook of Statistics in Clinical Oncology*, Marcel Dekker, Inc., New York.

Crowder, M.J. (2001). *Classical Competing Risks*, Chapman & Hall/CRC: Boca Raton, FL.

CTriSoft International (2002). *Clinical Trial Design with ExpDesign Studio*®. www.ctrisoft.net.

Cui, L., Hung, H.M.J., and Wang, S.J. (1999). Modification of sample-size in group sequential trials. *Biometrics*, 55:853–857.

D'Agostino, R.B. (2003). Editorial/noninferiority trials: Advances in concepts and methodology, *Statistics in Medicine*, 22:165–167.

Dargie, H.J. (2001). Effect of carvedilol on outcome after myocardial infarction in patients with left-ventricular dysfunction: the CAPRICORN randomised trial. *Lancet*, 357:1385–1390.

De Gruttola, V.G. et al. (2001). Considerations in the evaluation of surrogate endpoints in clinical trials: Summary of a National Institutes of Health Workshop. *Controlled Clinical Trials*, 22:485–502.

DeMets, D.L. and Lan, K.K.G. (1994). Interim analysis—the alpha-spending function-approach. *Statistics in Medicine*, 13:1341–1352.

DeMets, D.L. and Ware, J.H. (1980). Group sequential methods for clinical trials with a one-sided hypothesis. *Biometrika*, 67:651–660.

DeMets, D.L. and Ware, J.H. (1982). Asymmetric group sequential boundaries for monitoring clinical trials. *Biometrika*, 69:661–663.

Denne, J.D. (2001). Sample size recalculation using conditional power. *Statistics in Medicine*, 20:2645–2660.

Denne, J. S. and Jennison, C. (2000). A group sequential t-test with updating of sample-size. *Biometrika*, 87:125–134.

Dent, S.F. and Fisenhauer, F.A. (1996). Phase I trial design: Are new methodologies being put into practice? *Annals of Oncology*, 6:561–566.

Di, S.L. and Glimm, E. (2011). Time-to-event analysis with treatment arm selection at interim. *Statistics in Medicine*, 30(26):3067–3081.

Dittrich, R., Francis, B. Hatzinger, R., and Katzenbeisser, W. (2012). Missing observations in paired comparison data. *Statistical Modelling*, 12:117–143.

Dmitrienko, A. et al. (2005), *Analysis of Clinical Trials Using SAS*. SAS Institute Inc., Cary, North Carolina.

Dmitrienko, A. and Tamhane, A.C. (2007). Gatekeeping procedures with clinical trial applications. *Pharmaceutical Statistics*, 6:171–180.

Dmitrienko, A. and Wang, M.D. (2006). Bayesian predictive approach to interim monitoring in clinical trials. *Statistics in Medicine*, 25:2178–2195.

Dmitrienko, A., Tamhane, A.C., and Bretz, F. (2010). *Multiple Testing Problems in Pharmaceutical Statistics*. Chapman & Hall/CRC: Boca Raton, FL.

Dmitrienko, A., Wiens, B.L., Tamhane, A.C., and Wang, X. (2007). Tree-structured gatekeeping tests in clinical trials with hierarchically ordered multiple objectives. *Statistics in Medicine*, 26:2465–2478.

Doros, G., Pencina, M., Rybin, D., Meisnera, A., and Favad, M. (2013). A repeated measures model for analysis of continuous outcomes in sequential parallel comparison design studies. *Statistics in Medicine*, 32(16):2767–2789.

Dragalin, V. (2006). Adaptive designs: Terminology and classification. *Drug Information Journal*, 40:425–435.

Dragalin, V., and Fedorov, V. (2006). Adaptive designs for dose-finding based on efficacy–toxicity response. *Journal of Statistical Planning and Inference*, 136:1800–1823.

Dunnett, C.W. (1955). A multiple comparison procedure for comparing several treatments with a control. *Journal of the American Statistical Association*, 50:1096–1121.

Dragalin, V., Fedorov, V., and Wu, Y. (2008). Adaptive designs for selecting drug combinations based on efficacy-toxicity response. *Journal of Statistical Planning and Inference*, 138:352–373.

Dunnett C.W. (1964). New tables for multiple comparisons with a control, *Biometrics*, 20:482–491.

Efron, B. (1971). Forcing a sequential experiment to be balanced. *Biometrika*, 58:403–417.

620     *Adaptive Design Theory and Implementation*

Efron, B. (1980). Discussion of "minimum chi-square, not maximum likelihood." *Annal of Statistics*, 8:469–471.

Ellenberg, S.S., Fleming, T.R., and DeMets, D.L. (2002). *Data Monitoring Committees in Clinical Trials—A Practical Perspective*, John Wiley & Sons, New York.

Ellision, A.M. (1987). Effect of seed dimorphism on the density-dependent dynamics of experimental populations of Atriplex triangularis (Chenopodiaceae). *American Journal of Botany*, 74(8):1280–1288.

EMEA (2002). Point to Consider on Methodological Issues in Confirmatory Clinical Trials with Flexible Design and Analysis Plan. The European Agency for the Evaluation of Medicinal Products Evaluation of Medicines for Human Use. CPMP/EWP/2459/02, London, UK.

EMEA (2004). Point to Consider on the Choice of Non-inferiority Margin. The European Agency for the Evaluation of Medicinal Products Evaluation of Medicines for Human Use. London, UK.

EMEA (2006). Reflection Paper on Methodological Issues in Confirmatory Clinical Trials with Flexible Design and Analysis Plan. The European Agency for the Evaluation of Medicinal Products Evaluation of Medicines for Human Use. CPMP/EWP/2459/02, London, UK.

Emerson, S.S. and Fleming, T.R. (1990). Parameter estimation following group sequential hypothesis testing. *Biometrika*, 77:875–892.

Emerson, S.S. and Kittelson, J.M. (1997). A computationally simpler algorithm for the UMVUE of a normal mean following a group sequential test. *Biometrics*, 53:365–369.

Ensign, L.G. et al. (1994). An optimal three-stage design for phase II clinical trials. *Statistics in Medicine*, 13:1727–1736.

European Medicines Agency (EMEA). (2005, December). Committee for Medicinal Products for Human Use (CHMP). Guideline on the Evaluation of Anticancer Medicinal Products in Man. Available from http://www.emea.eu.int /pdfs/human/ewp/ 020595en.pdf. Date of access: 10 August 2006.

European Medicines Agency (EMA). (2007). Reflection Paper on Methodological Issues In Confirmatory Clinical Trials Planned with an Adaptive Design (October 2007).

Fairbanks, K. and Madsen, R. (1982). P values for tests using a repeated significance test design, *Biometrika*, 69:69–74.

Fan, X. and DeMets, D.L. (2006). Conditional and unconditional confidence intervals following a group sequential test. *Journal of Biopharmaceutical Statistics*, 16:107–122.

Fan, X., DeMets, D. L., and Lan, K.K.G. (2004). Conditional bias of point estimates following a group sequential test. *Journal of Biopharmaceutical Statistics*, 14:505–530.

Fan, S.K., Venook, A.P., and Lu, Y. (2009). Design issues in dose-finding phase I trials for combinations of two agents. *Journal of Biopharmaceutical Statistics*, 19(3):509–523.

Faries, D. (1994). Practical modifications of the continual reassessment method for phase I cancer clinical trials. *Journal of Biopharmaceutical Statistics*, 4:147–164.

Farrington, C.P. and Manning, G. (1990). Test statistics and sample size formulae for comparative binomial trials with null hypothesis of non-zero risk difference or non-unity relative risk. *Statistics in Medicine*, 9:1447–1454.

Fava, M., Evins, A.E., Dorer, D.J., and Schoenfeld, D.A. (2003). The problem of the placebo response in clinical trials for psychiatric disorders: Culprits, possible remedies, and a novel study design approach. *Psychotherapy and Psychosomatics* 2003; 72:115–127.

Fava M., Schoenfeld, D., (2010). System and method for reducing the placebo effect in controlled clinical trials. Available at http://www.patentlens.net/patentlens/patent/US_7840419/en/ [Accessed on 20 July 2012].

FDA. (1988). Guideline for Format and Content of the Clinical and Statistical Sections of New Drug Applications. The United States Food and Drug Administration, Rockville, Maryland.

FDA. (1998). Providing clinical evidence of effectiveness for human drug and biological products, guidance for industry [online]. Available from http://www.fda.gov/cder/guidance/index.htm [Accessed 2005 July 20]

FDA. (2000). Guidance for Clinical Trial Sponsors On the Establishment and Operation of Clinical Trial Data Monitoring Committees. The United States Food and Drug Administration, Rockville, Maryland.

FDA. (2001). Guidance for Industry, Statistical Approaches to Establishing Bioequivalence January.

FDA. (2005). Guidance for Clinical Trial Sponsors. Establishment and Operation of Clinical Trial Data Monitoring Committees (Draft). Rockville, Maryland. http://www.fda.gov/ cber/qdlns/ clintrialdmc.htm

FDA Guidance for Industry. (2005, April). Clinical Trial Endpoints for the Approval of Cancer Drug and Biologiecs. FDA. Available from http://www.fda.gov/cder/Guidance/6592dft.htm. Accessed: 11 August 2006.

FDA. (2006, March). Innovation Stagnation, Critical Path Opportunities List. www.fda.gov

FDA. (2006). Draft Guidance for the use of Bayesian statistics in Medical Device Clinical Trials. www.fda.gov/cdrh/osb/guidance/1601.pdf Accessed 22 May 2006.

FDA. (2010). Guidance for Industry Non-Inferiority Clinical Trials (draft). Food and Drug Administration, Department of Health and Human Services: Washingtom, DC.

Felson D.T., Anderson J.J., Boers, M. et al. (1993). The American College of Rheumatology preliminary core set of disease activity measures for rheumatoid arthritis clinical trials. *Arthritis Rheumatology*, 36:729–740.

Fisher, R.A. (1956). *Statistical Methods and Scientific Inference*. New York: Hafner.

Fisher, L. D. (1998). Self-designing clinical trials. *Statistics in Medicine*, 17:1551–1562.

Fisher, L.D. (1999). Carvedilol and the Food and Drug Administration (FDA) approval process: The FDA paradigm and reflections on hypothesis testing. *Controlled Clinical Trials*, 20:16–39.

Fisher, L.D. and Moyé, L.A. (1999). Carvedilol and the Food and Drug Administration (FDA) approval process: An introduction. *Controlled Clinical Trials*, 20: 1–15.

Fleming, T.R. and DeMets, D.L. (1996) Surrogate endpoint in clinical trials: are we being misled? *Annals of Internal Medicine*, 125, 605–613.

Fiore, L.D., Brophy, M., Ferguson, R.E. et al. (2011). A point-of-care clinical trial comparing insulin administered using a sliding scale versus a weight-based regimen. *Clinical Trials*, 8:183–195.

Follman, D.A., Proschan, M.A., and Geller, N.L. (1994). Monitoring pairwise comparisons in multi-armed clinical trials. *Biometrics*, 50:325–336.

Freedman, L.S., Graubard. B.I., and Schatzkin, A. (1992). Statistical validation of intermediate endpoints for chronic diseases. *Statistics in Medicine*, 11:167–178.

Freidlin, B. and Simon, R. (2005). Adaptive signature design: An adaptive clinical trial design for generating and prospectively testing a gene expression signature for sensitive patients. *Clinical Cancer Research*, 11(21).

Friede, T. et al. (2003). A comparison of procedures for adaptive choice of location tests in flexible two-stage designs. *Biometrical Journal*, 45:292–310.

Friede, T. and Kieser, M. (2003). Blinded sample size reassessment in non-inferiority and equivalence trials. *Statistics in Medicine*, 22:995–1007.

Friede, T. and Kieser, M. (2006). Sample size recalculation in internal pilot study designs: A review. *Biometrical Journal*, 48:537–555.

Friede, T., Parsons, N., Stallard, N., Todd, S., Valdes, M.E., Chataway, J., and Nicholas, R. (2011). Designing a seamless phase II/III clinical trial using early outcomes for treatment selection: An application in multiple sclerosis. *Statistics in Medicine*, 30(13):1528–1540.

Friedman, B. (1949). A simple urn model. *Comm. Pure Appl. Math*, 2:59–70.

Gallo, P. et al. (2006). Adaptive designs in clinical drug development—An executive summary of the PhRMA Working Group. *Journal of Biopharmaceutical Statistics*, 16:275–283.

Gallo, P. (2006a). Confidentiality and trial integrity issues for adaptive designs, *Drug Information Journal*, 40:445–450.

Gallo, P. (2006b). Operational challenges in adaptive design implementation. *Pharm. Statist*, 5:119–124.

Gallo, P., Chen, J., Quan, H., Menjoge, S., Luo, X., Tanaka, Y., Li, G., Ouyang, S.P., Binkowitz, B., Ibia, E., Talerico, S., and Ikeda, K. (2011). Consistency of treatment effect across regions in multiregional clinical trials, Part 2: Monitoring, reporting, and interpretation. *Drug Information Journal*, 45:603–608.

Gasprini, M. and Eisele, J. (2000). A curve-free method for phase I clinical trials. *Biometrics*, 56:609–615.

Gaydos, B. et al. (2006). Adaptive Dose Response Studies. *Drug Inf J.* 2006.

Gelman, A., Carlin, J.B., and Rubin, D.B. (2003). *Bayesian Data Analysis*. 2nd ed., Chapman & Hall/CRC. New York.

Genest, C. and Rivest, L.P. (1993). Statistical inference procedures for bivariate Archimedean copulas, *Journal of the American Statistical Association*, 88:1034–1043.

Gilbert, N. (1976). *Statistics*. WB Saunders, Philadelphia (PA).

Gillis, P.R. and Ratkowsky, D.A. (1978). The behaviour of estimators of the parameters of various yield-density relationships. *Biometrics*, 34: 191–198.

Goodman, S.N. (2005). Introduction to Bayesian methods I: Measuring the strength of evidence. *Clinical Trials*, 2:282–290.

Goodman, S.N. (1999). Towards evidence-based medical statistics, I: The $p$-value fallacy. *Annals of Internal Medicine*, 130:995–1004.

Goodman, S.N., Lahurak, M.L., and Piantadosi, S. (1995). Some practical improvements in the continual reassessment method for phase I studies. *Statistics in Medicine*, 5:1149–1161.

Gottlieb, S. (2006). Speech before 2006 Conference on Adaptive Trial Design, Washington, DC. http://www.fda.gov/ oc/speeches/ 2006/ trialdesign0710.html.

Gould, A.L. (1992). Interim analyses for monitoring clinical trials that do not maternally affect the type-I error rate. *Statistics in Medicine*, 11:55–66.

Gould, A.L. (1995). Planning and revising the sample-size for a trial. *Statistics in Medicine* 14:1039–1051.

Gould, A.L. (2001). Sample size re-estimation: recent developments and practical considerations. *Statistics in Medicine*, 20:2625–2643.

Gould, A.L. and Shih, W.J. (1992). Sample size re-estimation without unblinding for normally distributed outcomes with unknown variance. *Communications in Statistics—Theory and Methodology*, 21:2833–2853.

Gould, A.L. and Shih, W.J. (1998). Modifying the design of ongoing trials without unblinding, *Statistics in Medicine*, 17:89–100.

Govindarajulu, Z. (2003). Robustness of sample size re-estimation procedure in clinical trials (arbitrary populations). *Statistics in Medicine*, 22: 1819–1828.

Hallstron, A. and Davis, K. (1988). Imbalance in treatment assignments in stratified blocked randomization. *Controlled Clinical Trials*, 9:375–382.

Hardwick, J.P. and Stout, Q.F. (1991). Bandit strategies for ethical sequential allocation. *Computing Science and Statistics*, 23:421–424.

Hardwick, J.P. and Stout, Q.F. (1993). Optimal allocation for estimating the product of two means. *Computing Science and Statistics*, 24:592–596.

Hardwick, J.P. and Stout, Q.F. (2002). Optimal few-stage designs. *Journal of Statistical Planning and Inference*, 104:121–145.

Hartung, J. (2001). A self-designing rule for clinical trials with arbitrary response variables. *Controlled Clinical Trials*, 22:111–116.

Hartung, J. (2006). Flexible designs by adaptive plans of generalized Pocock- and O'Brien–Fleming-type and by self-designing clinical trials. *Biometrical Journal*, 48:521–536.

Hartung, J. and Knapp G. (2003). A new class of completely self-designing clinical trials. *Biometrical Journal*, 45:3–19.

Hauben, M. and Reich, L. (2004). Safety related drug-labelling changes findings from two data mining algorithms. *Drug Safety*, 27(10):735–744.

Hauben, M. et al. (2005). Data mining in pharmacovigilance—The need for a balanced perspective. *Drug Safety*, 28(10): 835–842.

624    *Adaptive Design Theory and Implementation*

Hawkins, M. J. (1993). Early cancer clinical trials: Safety, numbers, and consent. *Journal of the National Cancer Institute*, 85:1618–1619.

Hedges, L.V. and Olkin, I. (1985). *Statistical Methods for Meta-Analysis*. Academic Press, New York.

Heinemann, L. and Hompesch, M. (2011). Biosimilar insulins: How similar is similar? *Journal of Diabetes Science and Technology*, 5(3):

Hellmich, M. (2001). Monitoring clinical trials with multiple arms. *Biometrics*, 57:892–898.

Heritier, S., Lô, S. N., and Morgan, C.C. (2011). An adaptive confirmatory trial with interim treatment selection: Practical experiences and unbalanced randomization. *Statistics in Medicine*, 30:1541–1554.

Hochberg, Y. (1988). A sharper Bonferroni procedure for multiple tests of significance. *Biometrika*, 75:800–802.

Hochberg, Y. and Benjamini, Y. (1990), More powerful procedures for multiple significance testing. *Statistics in Medicine*, 9:811–818.

Hochberg, Y. and Tamhane, A.C. (1987). *Multiple Comparison Procedure*. John Wiley & Son, Inc. New York.

Holm, S. (1979). A simple sequentially rejective multiple test procedure. *Scand. J. Statist.* 6:65–70.

Holmgren, E.B. (1999). Establishing equivalence by showing that a specified percentage of the effect of the active control over placebo is maintained. *Journal of Biopharmaceutical Statistics* 9:651–659.

Holzmann, H. and Vollmer, S. (2008). A likelihood ratio test for bimodality in two-component mixtures—with application to regional income distribution in the EU. *AStA* 2(1):57–69.

Hommel, G. (1988). A stagewise rejective multiple test procedure based on a modified Bonferroni test. *Biometrika*, 75:383–386.

Hommel G. (2001). Adaptive modifications of hypotheses after an interim analysis. *Biometrical Journal*, 43:581–589.

Hommel, G. and Bretz, F. (2008). Aesthetics and power considerations in multiple testing—a contradiction? *Biometrical Journal*, 50:657–666.

Hommel, G. and Kropf, S. (2001). Clinical trials with an adaptive choice of hypotheses. *Drug Information Journal*, 33:1205–1218.

Hommel, G., Lindig, V., and Faldum, A. (2005). Two-stage adaptive designs with correlated test statistics. *Journal of Biopharmaceutical Statistics*, 15:613–623.

Horwitz, R.I. and Horwitz, S.M. (1993). Adherence to treatment and health outcomes. *Annals of Internal Medicine*, 153:1863–1868.

Hothorn, L.A. (2000). Evaluation of animal carcinogenicity studies: Cochran-Armitage trend test vs. Multiple contrast tests. *Biometrical Journal*, 42:553–567.

Houede, N., Thall, P.F., Nguyen, H. (2010). Paoletti X, Kramar A. Utility-based optimization of combination therapy using ordinal toxicity and efficacy in Phase I/II trials. *Biometrics*, 66(2):532–540.

Hsu, J.C. (1996). *Multiple Comparisons: Theory and Methods*. Chapman & Hall: London.

Hsu, J. and Berger, R.L. (1999). Stepwise confidence intervals without multiplicity adjustment for dose-response and toxicity studies. *Journal of the American Statistical Association*, 94:468–482.

Huang, W.S., Liu, J.P., and Hsiao, C.F. (2011). An alternative phase II/III design for continuous endpoints. *Pharmaceut. Statist.*, 10:105–114.

Huang, X., Biswas, S., Oki, Y., Issa, J.-P., and Berry, D. (2007). A parallel phase I/II dose-finding trial design for combination therapies, *Biometrics*, 63:429–436.

Hu, F. and Rosenberger, W.F.(2006). *The Theory of Response-Adaptive Randomization in Clinical Trials*. John-Wiley, Hoboken, NJ.

Hughes, M.D. (1993). Stopping guidelines for clinical trials with multiple treatments. *Statistics in Medicine*, 12:901–913.

Hughes, M.D. and Pocock, S.J. (1988). Stopping rules and estimation problems in clinical trials. *Statistics in Medicine*, 7:1231–1242.

Hung, H.M.J., O'Neill, R.T., Wang, S.J., and Lawrence, J. (2006). A regulatory view on adaptive/flexible clinical trial design. *Biometrical Journal*, 48:565–573.

Hung, H.M.J. et al. (2003). Some fundemental issues with non-inferiority testing in active controlled trials. *Statistics in Medicine*, 22:213–225.

Hung, H.M.J. et al. (2005). Adaptive statistical analysis following sample-size modification based on interim review of effect size. *Journal of Biopharmaceutical Statistics*, 15:693–706.

Hung, H.M.J. and Wang, S.J. (2004). Multiple testing of noninferiority hypotheses in active controlled trials. *Journal of Biopharmaceutical Statistics*, 14:327–335.

Hung, H.M.J. and Wang, S.J. (2012). Sample size adaptation in fixed-dose combination drug trial. *Journal of Biopharmaceutical Statistics*, 22(4):679–86.

Hung, H.M.J., Wang, S.J., and O'Neill, R. (2006). Methodological issues with adaptation of clinical trial design. *Pharmaceutical Statistics*, 4(1):1–16.

Hung, H.M.J., Wang, S.J., and O'Neill, R.T. (2010). Consideration of regional difference in design and analysis of multi-regional trials. *Pharmaceutical Statistics*, 9(3):173–178.

Hung, H.M.J., Wang, S.J., and O'Neill, R. (2013). Issues of sample size in bridging trials and global clinical trials. In *Design and Analysis of Bridging Studies*, Liu, J.P., Chow, S.C., and Hsiao, C.F., editors, CRC Press, Boca Raton, FL.

Huque M. and Röhmel, J. (2010), Multiplicity problems in clinical trials: A regulatory perspective, In *Multiple Testing Problems in Pharmaceutical Statistics*, Dmitrienko, A., Tamhane, A.C., and Bretz, F., editors. Chapman & Hall/CRC Press: Boca Raton, FL.

ICH. (1996). International Conference on Harmonization Tripartite Guideline for Good Clinical Practice.

ICH. E9 Expert Working Group. (1999). Statistical principles for clinical trials (ICH Harmonized Tripartite Guideline E9). Statistics in Medicine 18:1905–1942.

ICH. (1998). ICH Harmonised Tripartite Guideline Statistical Principles for Clinical Trials E9 Current Step 4 version.

Iglesias, C.P. and Claxton, K. (2006). Comprehensive decision-analytic model and Bayesian value-of-information analysis. *Pharmacoeconomics*, 24(5):465–78.

Ikeda, K. and Bretz, F. (2010). Sample size and proportion of Japanese patients in multi-regional trials. *Pharmaceutical Statistics*, 9(3):207–216.

Inoue, L.Y.T., Thall, P.F., and Berry, D.A. (2002). Seamlessly expanding a randomized phase II trial to phase III. *Biometrics*, 58:823–831.

Ivanova, A. and Flournoy, N. (2001). A birth and death urn for ternary outcomes: stochastic processes applied to urn models. In *Probability and Statistical Models with Applications*. Charalambides, C.A., Koutras, M.V., and Balakrishnan, N., editors. pp. 583–600. Chapman & Hall/CRC Press, Boca Raton, FL.

Ivanova, A., Liu, K., Snyder, E., and Snavely, D. (2009). An adaptive design for identifying the dose with the best efficacy/tolerability profile with application to a crossover dose finding study. *Statistics in Medicine*, 28:2941–2951.

Ivanova, A., Xiao, C., and Tymofyeyev, Y. (2012). Two-stage designs for Phase 2 dose-finding trials. *Statistics in Medicine*, 31:2872–2881.

Ivanova, A., and Wang, K. (2004). A non-parametric approach to the design and analysis of two-dimensional dose-finding trials. *Statistics in Medicine*, 23(12):1861–1870.

Ivanova, A., Xiao, C., and Tymofyeyev, Y. (2011). Two-stage designs for phase 2 dose-finding trials. *Statistics in Medicine*, 31:2872–2881.

Jackson, P.R., Tucker, G.T., and Woods, H.F. (1989). Testing for bimodality in frequency distributions of data suggesting polymorphisms of drug metabolism–hypothesis testing. *Br. J. Clin. Pharmacol.*, 28(6):655–662.

Jeffery, H. (1961). *Theory of Probability*. 3rd ed. Oxford: Oxford University Press.

Jenkins, M., Stone, A., and Jennison, C. (2011). An adaptive seamless phase II/III design for oncology trials with subpopulation selection using correlated survival endpoints. *Pharmaceut. Statist.* 10:347–356.

Jennison, C. and Turnbull, B.W. (1984). Repeated confidence intervals for group sequential clinical trials. *Controlled Clinical Trials*, 5:33–45.

Jennison, C. and Turnbull, B.W. (1989). Interim analyses: the repeated confidence interval approach (with discussion). *Journal of the Royal Statistical Society*, Series B 51:305–361.

Jennison, C. and Turnbull, B.W. (1990). Statistical approaches to interim monitoring of medical trials: a review and commentary. *Statistics in Medicine*, 5:299–317.

Jennison, C. and Turnbull, B.W. (2000a). Efficient group sequential designs when there are several effect sizes under consideration. *Statistics in Medicine*, 00:1–6.

Jennison, C. and Turnbull, B.W. (2000b). Group Sequential Tests with Applications to Clinical Trials. Chapman & Hall: London/Boca Raton, Florida.

Jennison, C. and Turnbull, B.W. (2003). Mid-course sample-size modification in clinical trials. *Statistics in Medicine*, 22:971–993.

Jennison, C. and Turnbull, B.W. (2005). Meta-analysis and adaptive group sequential design in the clinical development process. *Journal of Biopharmaceutical Statistics*, 15:537–558.

Jennison, C. and Turnbull, B.W. (2006a). Adaptive and non-adaptive group sequential tests. *Biometrika*, 93: 1–21.

Jones, B. and Kenward, M. (2003). Design and Analysis of Cross-Over Trials, 2nd Edition. Chapman & Hall/CRC, Boca Raton, FL.

Johnson, N.L., Kotz, S. and Balakrishnan, N. (1994). *Continuous Univariate Distributions*, vol. 1, John Wiley & Sons, New York.

Joseph Moon Wai Wu. (2014). Adaptive Methodologies in Multi-Arm Dose Response and Biosimilarity Clinical Trials. Ph.D. Dissertation. Boston University.

Julious, S.A. (2004). Tutorial in biostatistics: Sample sizes for clinical trials with normal data. *Statistics in Medicine*, 23:1921–86.

Kaitin, K.I. (2010). Deconstructing the drug development process: The new face of innovation. *Clinical Pharmacology & Therapeutics*, 87:356–361.

Kalbfleisch, J.D. and Prentice, R.L. (1980). *The Statistical Analysis of Failure Time Data*. Wiley, New York.

Kalbfleisch, J.D. and Prentice, R.L. (2002). *The Statistical Analysis of Failure Time Data*, 2nd ed., John Wiley & Sons, New York.

Kanji, G.K. (2006). *100 Statistical Tests*, 3rd ed., Sage Publications: London, UK.

Kathman, S.J. and Hale, M.D. (2007). Combining estimates from multiple early studies to obtain estimates of response: Using shrinkage estimates to obtain estimates of response. *Pharmaceut. Statist.*, 6:297–306.

Kawai, N., Stein, C., Komiyama, O., Li, Y. (2008). An approach to rationalize partitioning sample size into individual regions in a multi-regional trial. *Drug Information Journal*, 42:139–147.

Kelly, P.J., et al. (2005). A practical comparison of group-sequential and adaptive designs. *Journal of Biopharmaceutical Statistics*, 15:719–738.

Kelly, P., Stallard, N., and Todd, S. (2003). An adaptive group sequential design for clinical trials that involve treatment selection. Technical Report 03=1, School of Applied Statistics, The University of Reading.

Kelly, P.J., Stallard, N., and Todd, S. (2005). An adaptive group sequential design for phase II/III clinical trials that select a single treatment from several. *Journal of Biopharmaceutical Statistics*, 15:641–658.

Kieser, M. (2006). Inference on multiple endpoints in clinical trials with adaptive interim analyses. *Biometrical Journal*, 41(3):261–277.

Kieser, M., Bauer, P., and Lehmacher, W. (1999). Inference on multiple endpoints in clinical trials with adaptive interim analyses. *Biometrical Journal*, 41:261–277.

Kieser, M. and Friede, T. (2000). Re-calculating the sample-size in internal pilot study designs with control of the type-I error rate. *Statistics in Medicine*, 19:901–911.

Kieser, M. and Friede, T. (2003). Simple procedures for blinded sample-size adjustment that do not affect the type-I error rate. *Statistics in Medicine*, 22:3571–3581.

Kieser, M., Schneider, B., and Friede, T. (2002). A bootstrap procedure for adaptive selection of the test statistic in flexible two-stage designs. *Biometrical Journal*, 44:641– 652.

Kim, K. and DeMets, D.L. (1992). Sample size determination for group sequential clinical trial with immediate responses. *Statistics in Medicine*, 11: 1391–1399.

Kim, K. (1989). Point estimation following group sequential tests. *Biometrics*, 45:613–617.

Kim, K. and DeMets, D. L. (1987a). Confidence intervals following group sequential tests in clinical trials. *Biometrics*, 43:857–864.

Kim, K. and DeMets, D. L. (1987b). Design and analysis of group sequential tests based on the type-I error spending rate function. *Biometrika*, 74:149–154.

Kimko, H.C. and Duffull, S.B. (2003). *Simulation for Designing Clinical Trials*, Marcel Dekker, Inc., New York.

Ko, F.S., Tsou, H.H., Liu, J.P., and Hsiao, C.F. (2010). Sample size determination for a specific region in a multi-regional trial. *Journal of Biopharmaceutical Statistics*, 20(4):870–885.

Koch, A. (2006). Confirmatory clinical trials with an adaptive design. *Biometrical Journal*, 48:574–585.

Koenig, F., Brannath, W., Bretz, F., and Posch, M. (2008). Adaptive Dunnett tests for treatment selection. *Statistics in Medicine*, 27(10):1612–1625.

Kokoska, S. and Zwillinger, D. (2000). *Standard Probability and Statistics Table and Formulae, Student Edition*. Chapman & Hall/CRC, Boca Raton, Florida.

Kong, L., Kohberger, R.C., and Koch, G.G. (2004). Type I error and power in noninferiority/equivalence trials with correlated multiple endpoints: An example from vaccine development trials. *Journal of Biopharmaceutical Statistics*, 14:893–907.

Kramar, A., Lehecq, A., and Candalli, E. (1999). Continual reassessment methods in phase I trials of the combination of two drugs in oncology. *Statistics in Medicine*, 18:1849–1864.

Lachin, J.M. (1988). Statistical properties of randomization in clinical trials. *Controlled Clinical Trials*, 9:289–311.

Lachin, J.M. (2005). A review of methods for futility stopping based on conditional power. *Statistics in Medicine*, 24(18):2747–2764.

Lachin, J.M. and Foukes, M.A. (1986). Evaluation of sample-size and power for analysis of survival with allowance for nonuniform patient entry, losses to follow-up, noncompliance, and stratification. *Biometrics*, 42:507–19.

Lan, K.K.G (2002). Problems and issues in adaptive clinical trial design. Presented at New Jersey Chapter of the American Statistical Association, Piscataway, NJ, June 4.

Lan, K.K.G. and DeMets, D.L. (1983). Discrete sequential boundaries for clinical trials. *Biometrika*, 70:659–663.

Lan, K.K.G. and DeMets, D.L. (1987). Group sequential procedures: Calendar versus information time. *Statistics in Medicine*, 8:1191–1198.

Lan, K.K.G. and DeMets, D.L. (1989). Changing frequency of interim analysis in sequential monitoring. *Biometrics*, 45:1017–1020.

Lan, K.K.G., Reboussin, D., and DeMets, D. (1994). Information and information fractions for design and sequential monitoring of clinical trials. *Communications in Statistics—Theory and Methods*, 23(2):403–420.

Lan, K.K.G. and Wittes, J. (1988). The B-value: A tool for monitoring data, *Biometrics*, 44:579–585.

Lan, K.K.G. and Zucker, D. (1993). Sequential monitoring of clinical trials: The role of information in Brownian motion. *Stat. Med.* 12:753–765.

Lang, T., Auterith, A., and Bauer, P. (2000). Trend tests with adaptive scoring. *Biometrical Journal*, 42:1007–1020.

Lawrence, J. (2002). Strategies for changing the test statistics during a clinical trial. *Journal of Biopharmaceutical Statistics*, 12:193–205.

Lawrence, J. and Hung, H.M.J. (2003). Estimation and confidence intervals after adjusting the maximum information. *Biometrical Journal*, 45:143–152.

Lee, B.L and Fan, S.K. (2012). A two-dimensional search algorithm for dose-finding trials of two agents. *J. Biopharm. Stat.* 22(4):802–818.

Lee, M.L.T., Chang, M., and Whitmore, G.A. (2008). A Threshold regression mixture model for assessing treatment efficacy in multiple myeloma clinical trial. *Journal of Biopharmaceutical Statistics*, 18:1136–1149.

Lee, M.-L.T., DeGruttola, V., and Schoenfeld, D. (2000). A model for markers and latent health status, *J. Royal. Statist. Soc., Series B*, 62:747–762.

Lee, M.-L.T. and Whitmore G.A. (2004). First hitting time models for lifetime data. In Handbook of Statistics: Volume 23, Advances in Survival Analysis, C. R. Rao, N. Balakrishnan, editors, pp. 537–543.

Lee, M.L.T. and Whitmore, G.A. (2006). Threshold Regression for Survival Analysis: Modeling Event Times by a Stochastic Process Reaching a Boundary. *Statistical Science*, 21(4):501–513.

Lehmacher, W., Kieser, M. and Hothorn, L. (2000). Sequential and multiple testing for dose-response analysis. *Drug Information Journal*, 34:591–597.

Lehmacher, W. and Wassmer G. (1999). Adaptive sample-size calculations in group sequential trials. *Biometrics*, 55:1286–1290.

Lehmann, E.L. (1975). *Nonparametric: Statistical Methods Based on Ranks*. Holden-Day, San Francisco, California.

Lehmann, E.L. (1983). *The Theory of Point Estimation*. Wiley, New York.

Li, G., Chen, J., Quan, H., and Shentu, Y. (2013). Consistency assessment with global and bridging development strategies in emerging markets. *Contemporary Clinical Trials*, 36:687–696.

Li, G., Wang, Y., and Ouyang, S.P. (2009). Interim treatment selection in drug development. *Statist. Biosci.* 1(2):268–88.

Li, G., Zhu, J., Ouyang, S.P., Xie, J., Deng, L., and Law, G. (2009). Adaptive designs for interim dose selection. *Statist. Biopharm. Res.* 1(4):366–376.

Li, H.I. and Lai, P.Y. (2003). Clinical trial simulation. In *Encyclopedia of Biopharmaceutical Statistics*, Chow, S.C., editors. pp. 200–201. Marcel Dekker, Inc., New York.

Li, M., Quan, H., Chen, J., Tanaka, Y., Ouyang, P., Luo, X., Li, G.R. (2012). Functions for sample size and probability calculations for assessing consistency of treatment effects in multi-regional clinical trials. *Journal of Statistical Software* 47, online journal.

Li, N. (2006). Adaptive trial design—FDA statistical reviewer's view. Presented at the CRT 2006 Workshop with the FDA, Arlington, Virginia, April 4, 2006.

Li, W.J., Shih, W.J., and Wang, Y. (2005), Two-stage adaptive design for clinical trials with survival data. *Journal of Biopharmaceutical Statistics*, 15:707–718.

Lilford, R.J. and Braunholtz, D. (1996). For debate; The statistical basis of public policy: a paradigm shift is overdue. *British Medical Journal*, 313:603–607.

Lin, Y. and Shih, W.J. (2001). Statistical properties of the traditional algorithm-based designs for phase I cancer clinical trials. *Biostatistics* 2:203–215.

Lindley, D.V. (1957). A statistical paradox. *Biometrika*, 44:187–192.

Lindley, D.V. (1962). Discussion of Professor Stein's paper "Confidence sets for the mean of a multivariate normal distribution." *Journal of the Royal Statistical Society, Series B*, 24:265–296.

Little, R.J. (2010). *Panel on Handling Missing Data in Clinical Trial: The Prevention and Treatment of Missing Data in Clinical Trials*. The National Academies Press, Washington, D.C.

Little, R.J. and Rubin, D.B. (2002). *Statistical Analysis with Missing Data*, 2nd edition. Wiley: New York.

Liu, A. (2000). Maximum likelihood estimate following sequential probability ratio tests. *Sequential Analysis*, 19:63–75.

Liu, A. and Hall, W.J. (1998). Minimum variance unbiased estimation of the drift of Brownian motion with linear stopping boundaries. *Sequential Analysis*, 17: 91–107.

Liu, A. and Hall, W.J. (1999). Unbiased estimation following a group sequential test. *Biometrika*, 86:71–78.

Liu, A. and Hall, W.J. (2001). Unbiased estimation of secondary parameters following a sequential test. *Biometrika*, 88:895–900.

Liu, A., Troendle, J.F., Yu, K.F., and Yuan, V. (2004). Conditional maximum likelihood estimation following a group sequential test. *Biometrical Journal*, 46: 760–768.

Liu, J.P., Chow, S.C., and Hsiao, C.F. (2013). *Design and Analysis of Bridging Studies*, Chapman & Hall/CRC, Boca Raton, FL.

Liu, J.P., Hsueh, H.M., Hsieh, E., and Chen, J.J. (2002). Tests for equivalence or noninferiority for paired binary data. *Statistics in Medicine*, 21:231–245.

Liu, Q. (1998). An order-directed score test for trend in ordered 2xK tables. *Biometrics*, 54:1147–1154.

Liu, Q. and Chang, M. (2010). Note on Special Technical Issue on Adaptive Designs for Clinical Trials. In Special Issue: Adaptive Designs for Clinical Trials: Considerations about and beyond the FDA Adaptive Designs Guidance, *Journal of Biopharmaceutical Statistics*.

Liu, Q. and Chi, G.Y.H (2001). On sample-size and inference for two-stage adaptive designs. *Biometrics*, 57:172–177.

Liu, Q. and Pledger, G.W. (2005). Phase 2 and 3 combination designs to accelerate drug development. *Journal of American Statistical Association*, 100:493–502.

Liu, Q., Proschan, M.A., and Pledger, G.W. (2002). A unified theory of two-stage adaptive designs. *Journal of American Statistical Association*, 97:1034–1041.

Liu, S. and Ning, J. (2013). A Bayesian dose-finding design for drug combination trials with delayed toxicities. *Bayesian Analysis*, 8(3):703–722.

Lokhnygina, Y. (2004). Topics in design and analysis of clinical trials. Ph.D. Thesis, Department of Statistics, North Carolina State Univeristy. Raleigh, NC.

Looker, A.C. et al. (1997). Prevalence of iron deficiency in the United States. *JAMA*, 277:973–976.

Louis, T.A. (2005). Introduction to Bayesian methods II: Fundamental concepts. *Clinical Trials*, 2:291–294.

Lu, Y., and Bean, J.A. (1995). On the sample size for one-sided equivalence of sensitivities based upon McNemar's Test. *Statistics in Medicine*, 14:1831–1839.

Lu, Y., Jin, H. and Genant, H.K. (2003). On the noninferiority of a diagnostic test based on paired observations, *Statistics in Medicine*, 22:3029–3044.

Luo, X., Shih, W.J., Ouyang, S.P., and Delap, R.J. (2010). An optimal adaptive design to address local regulations in global clinical trials. *Pharmaceutical Statistics*, 9:179–189.

Luo, X., Wu, S.S., and Xiong, J. (2010). Parameter estimation following an adaptive treatment selection trial design. *Biometrical Journal*, 52, 823–835.

Lynch, T.J. et al. (2004). Activating mutations in the epidermal growth factor receptor underlying responsiveness of non-small-cell lung cancer to gefitinib. *New England Journal of Medicine*, 350:2129–2139.

Maca, J. et al. (2006). Adaptive seamless phase II/III designs—background, operational aspects, and examples.

Machin, D. et al. (1997). *Statistical Tables for the Design of Clinical Studies*. 2nd ed. Blackwell Scientific Publications: Oxford.

Maitournam, A. and Simon, R. (2005). On the efficiency of targeted clinical trials. *Statistics in Medicine*, 24:329–339.

Marcus, R., Peritz, E., and Gabriel, K.R. (1976). On closed testing procedures with special reference to ordered analysis of variance. *Biometrika*, 63:655–660.

Marubini, E. and Valsecchi, M.G. (1995). *Analysis Survival Data from Clinical Trials and Observational Studies*, John Wiley & Sons, New York.

Maxwell, C., Domenet, J.G., and Joyce, C.R.R. (1971). Instant experience in clinical trials: A novel aid to teaching by simulation. *J. Clin. Pharmacol*, 11:323–331.

Mehta, C.R. and Patel, N.R. (2006). Adaptive, group sequential and decision theoretic approaches to sample-size determination. *Stat. Med.* 25(19):3250–3269.

Mehta, C.R., and Pocock, S.J. (2011). Adaptive increase in sample size when interim results are promising: a practical guide with examples. *Stat. Med.* 30(28):3267–3284.

Mehta, C.R. and Tsiatis, A.A. (2001). Flexible sample-size considerations using information-based interim monitor. *Drug Information Journal*, 35:1095–1112.

Melfi, V. and Page, C. (1998). Variability in adaptive designs for estimation of success probabilities. In *New Developments and Applications in Experimental Design, IMS Lecture Notes Monograph Series*, 34:106–114.

Mendelhall, W. and Hader, R.J. (1985). Estimation of parameters of mixed exponentially distributed failure time distributions from censored life test data. *Biometrika*, 45:504–520.

Menon, S. and Chang, M. (2012). Optimization of adaptive designs: efficiency evaluation. *J. Biopharm. Stat.* 22(4):641–61.

Meyerson, L., Muirhead, R., Stryszak, P., Boddy, A., Chen, K., Copley-Merriman, K. et al. (2007). Multiple co-primary endpoints: Medical and statistical solutions a report from the multiple endpoints expert team of the pharmaceutical research and manufacturers of america. *Drug Information Journal*, 41:31–46.

Miller, F., Guilbaud, O., and Dette, H. (2007). Optimal designs for estimating the interesting part of a dose-effect curve. *Journal of Biopharmaceutical Statistics*, 17:1097–1115.

Ministry of Health, Labor, and Welfare (2007). *Basic Concepts for Joint International Clinical Trials.* September 28, 2007.

Molenberghs, G., Geys, H., and Buyse, M. (2001). Evaluation of surrogate endpoints in randomized experiments with mixed discrete and continuous outcomes. *Statistics in Medicine*, 20:3023–3038.

Molenberghs, G., Buyse, M. and Burzykowski, T. (2005). The history of surrogate endpoint validation, In *The Evaluation of Surrogate Endpoint*, Burzykowski, Molenberghs, and Buyse, editors. Springer, New York.

Montori, V.M. et al. (2005). Randomized trials stopped early for benefit—a systematic review. *Journal of American Medical Association*, 294: 2203–2209.

Moyé, L.A. (2003). *Multiple Analysis in Clinical Trials.* Springer-Verlag, New York, Inc.

Müller, H.H. and Shäfer, H. (2001). Adaptive group sequential designs for clinical trials: Combining the advantages of adaptive and classical group sequential approaches. *Biometrics*, 57:886–891.

Müller, H.H. and Shäfer, H. (2004). A general ststistical principle of changing a design any time during the course of a trial. *Statist. Med.* 23: 2497–2508.

Nam, J. (1987). A simple approximation for calculating sample sizes for detecting linear tend in proportions. *Biometrics*, 43:701–705.

Nam, J. (1997). Establishing equivalence of two treatments and sample size requirements in matched-pairs design. *Biometrics*, 53:1422–1430.

Neuhauser, M. (2001). An adaptive location-scale test. *Biometrical Journal*, 43:809–819.

Neuhauser, M. and Hothorn, L. (1999). An exact Cochran—Armitage test for trend when dose-response shapes are a priori unknown. *Computational Statistics & Data Analysis*, 30:403–412.

Newey, W.K. and McFadden, D. (1994). Large sample estimation and hypothesis testing. In *Handbook of Econometrics, Volume IV*, Elsevier Science, pp. 2111–2245.

O'Brien, P.C. and Fleming, T.R. (1979). A multiple testing procedure for clinical trials. *Biometrika*, 35:549–556.

Offen, W. et al. (2006). Multiple co-primary endpoints: Medical and statistical solutions. *Drug Information Journal.*

Offen, W., Chuang-Stein C., Dmitriendko, A. et al. (2007). Multiple co-primary endpoints: medical and statistical solutions. A report from the multiple endpoints expert team of the pharmaceutical research and manufacturers of America. *Drug Information Journal*, 41:31–46.

Offen, W.W. (2003). Data Monitoring Committees (DMC). In *Encyclopedia of Biopharmaceutical Statistics*. Chow, S.C., editor. Marcel Dekker, Inc., New York.

Ohman, J., Strickland, P. A., and Casella, G. (2003). Conditional inference following group sequential testing. *Biometr. J.* 45:515–526.

O'Neill, R.T. (1997). The primary endpoint does not demonstrate clear statistical significance. *Controlled Clinical Trials*, 18:550–556.

O'Neill, R.T. (2004). A perspective on contributions of biostatistics to the critical path initiative. Presentation given at Workshop on "Model-based drug development—A cornerstone of the FDA's Critical Path Initiative,"Basel Biometric Society, December 2004, available at http://www.psycho.unibas.ch/BBS/slides/ONeill2.ppt.zip

O'Quigley, J., Pepe, M. and Fisher, L. (1990). Continual reassessment method: A practical design for phase I clinical trial in cancer. *Biometrics*, 46:33–48.

O'Quigley, J. and Shen, L. (1996). Continual reassessment method: A likelihood approach. *Biometrics*, 52:673–684.

Packer, M. et al. Effect of carvedilol on survival in severe chronic heart failure. *New England Journal of Medicine*, 344:1651–1658.

Paez, J.G. et al. (2004). EGFR mutations in lung cancer: correlation with clinical response to gefitinib therapy. *Science*, 304:1497–1500.

Pahl, R., Ziegler, A., and Koenig, I.K. (2006). Designing clinical trials using group sequential designs. *Rnews*, 6:21–26.

PAREXEL. (2003). *PAREXEL's Pharmaceutical R & D Statistical Sourcebook 2002/2003*. Waltham, MA.

Park, S.K. and Miller, K.W. (1988). *Communications of the ACM*, 31:1192–1201.

Parmigiani, G. (2002). *Modeling in Medical Decision Making*. John Wiley & Sons, West Sussex, England.

Paulson, E. (1964). A selection procedure for selecting the population with the largest mean from k normal populations. *Annal of Mathematical Statistics*, 35:174–180.

Pearson, K. (1916). Mathematical contributions to the theory of evolution, XIX: Second supplement to a memoir on skew variation. *Phil. Trans. Roy. Soc. London, Series A*, 216(538–548):429–457.

Pickard, M. and Chang, M (2014). A flexible method using a parametric bootstrap for reducing bias in adaptive designs with treatment selection. *Statistics in Biopharmaceutical Research*, 6(2):

Pocock, S.J. (1977). Group sequential methods in the design and analysis of clinical trials. *Biometrika*, 64:191–199.

Pocock, S.J. (1982). Interim analyses for randomized clinical trials: The group sequential approach. *Biometrics*, 38:153–162.

Pocock, S.J. (2005). When (not) to stop a clinical trial for benefit. *Journal of American Medical Association*, 294:2228–2230.

Pocock, S.J. and Simon, R. (1975). Sequential treatment assignment with balancing for prognostic factors in the controlled clinical trials. *Biometrics*, 31:103–115.

Pong, A. and Luo, Z. (2005). Adaptive design in clinical research. A special issue of the *Journal of Biopharmaceutical Statistics*, 15(4):

Posch, M. and Bauer, P. (1999). Adaptive two-stage designs and the conditional error function. *Biometrical Journal*, 41:689–696.

Posch, M. and Bauer, P. (2000). Interim analysis and sample-size reassessment. *Biometrics*, 56:1170–1176.

Posch, M., and Bauer, P. (2003). Dealing with the unexpected: Modification of ongoing trials. *Proceedings ROES Seminar*, St. Gallen, Switzerland.

Posch, M., Bauer, P., and Brannath, W. (2003). Issues in designing flexible trials. *Statistics in Medicine*, 22:953–969.

Posch, M., Maurer, W., and Bretz, F. (2011). Type I error rate control in adaptive designs for confirmatory clinical trials with treatment selection at interim. *Pharmaceut. Statist.* 10:96–104.

Posch, M. et al. (2005). Testing and estimation in flexible group sequential designs with adaptive treatment selection. *Statistics in Medicine*, 24:3697–3714.

Prentice, R.L. (1989). Surrogate endpoints in clinical trials: definitions and operational criteria. *Statistics in Medicine*, 8:431–440.

Proschan, M.A. (2003). The geometry of two-stage tests. *Statistica Sinica* 13:163–177.

Proschan, M.A. (2005). Two-stage sample-size re-estimation based on a nuisance parameter: a review. *Journal of Biopharmaceutical Statistics*, 15:559–574.

Proschan, M.A., Follmann, D.A., and Geller, N.L. (1994). Monitoring multiarmed trials. *Statistics in Medicine*, 13:1441–1452.

Proschan, M.A., Follmann, D.A., and Waclawiw, M.A. (1992). Effects of assumption violations on type-I error rate in group sequential monitoring. *Biometrics*, 48:1131–1143.

Proschan, M.A. and Hunsberger, S.A. (1995). Designed extension of studies based on conditional power. *Biometrics*, 51:1315–1324.

Proschan, M.A., Lan, K.K.G., and Wittes, J.T. (2006). *Statistical Monitoring of Clinical Trials—A Uniform Approach*. Springer, New York.

Proschan, M.A., Leifer, E., and Liu, Q. (2005). Adaptive regression. *Journal of Biopharmaceutical Statistics*, 15:593–603.

Proschan, M.A., Liu, Q.L. and Hunsberger, S. (2003). Practical midcourse sample-size modification in clinical trials. *Controlled Clinical Trials*, 24:4–15.

Proschan, M.A. and Wittes, J. (2000). An improved double sampling procedure based on the variance. *Biometrics*, 56:1183–1187.

Qu, Y. and Case, M. (2006). Quantifying the indirect treatment effect via surrogate markers. *Statist. Med.* 2006:25:223–23. Published online 5 September 2005 in Wiley InterScience. DOI: 10.1002/sim.2176. www.interscience.wiley.com

Quan, H., Li, M.Y., Chen, J., Gallo, P., Binkowitz, B., Ibia, E., Tanaka, Y., Ouyang, S.P., Luo, X.l., Li, G., Menjoge, S., Talerico, S., and Ikeda, K. (2010). Assessment of Consistency of Treatment Effects in Multiregional Clinical Trials. *Drug Information Journal*, 44(5):617–632.

Quan, H., Li, M., Shih, W.J., Ouyang, S.P., Chen, J., Zhang, J., and Zhao, P.L. (2012). Empirical shrinkage estimator for consistency assessment of treatment effects in multi-regional clinical trials. *Statistics in Medicine*, 32(10):1691–1706.

Quan, H., Mao, X., Chen, J., Shih, W.J., Ouyang, S.P., Zhang, J., Zhao, P.L., and Binkowitz, B. (2014). Multi-regional clinical trial design and consistency assessment of treatment effects. *Statistics in Medicine*—Early Online February 11, 2014.

Quan, H., Li, M., Shih, W.J., Ouyang, S.P., Chen, J., Zhang, J., and Zhao, P.L. (2013). Empirical shrinkage estimator for consistency assessment of treatment effects in multi-regional clinical trials. *Statistics in Medicine*, 32:1691–1706.

Quan, H., Zhao, P.L., Zhang, J., Roessner, M., and Aizawa, K. (2010). Sample size considerations for Japanese patients in a multi-regional trial based on MHLW guidance. *Pharmaceutical Statistics*, 9(1):100–112.

Quinlan, J.A., Gallo, P., and Krams, M. (2006). Implementing adaptive designs: logistical and operational consideration.

R Development Core Team. (2005). R: A language and environment for statistical computing. R Foundation for Statistical Computing, Vienna, Austria. www.R-project.org

Raiffa, H. and Schlaifer, R. (2000). *Applied Statistical Decision Theory*. Wiley-Interscience. NJ.

Raiffa, H. and Schlaifer, R. (1961). *Applied Statistical Decision Theory*. Harvard Business School, 356, xxviii.

Ravaris, C.L. et al. (1976). Multiple dose controlled study of phenelzine in depression anxiety states. *Areh Gen Psychiatry*, 33:347–350.

Ricciardi. M. and Sato, S. (1988). First-passage-time density and moments of the Ornstein–Uhlenbeck process. *Journal of Applied Probability*, 25:43–57.

Robert, C.P. (1997). *The Bayesian Choice*. Springer-Verlag, New York.

Robins, J.M. and Tsiatis, A.A. (1991). Correcting for non-compliance in randomized trials using rank preserving structural failure time models. *Communications in Statistics—Theory and Methods*, 20:2609–2631.

Roderick, J.A., Little, Donald, and B. Rubin. (2002). *Statistical Analysis with Missing Data*, 2nd ed. Wiley-Interscience, New Jersey.

Rom, D.M. (1990). A sequentially rejective test procedure based on a modified Bonferroni inequality. *Biometrika*, 77:663–665.

Rosenberger, W.F. et al. (2001). Optimal adaptive designs for binary response trials. *Biometrics*, 57:909–913.

Rosenberger, W.F. and Lachin, J. (2002). *Randomization in Clinical Trials*, John Wiley & Sons, New York.

Rosenberger, W.F. and Seshaiyer, P. (1997). Adaptive survival trials. *Journal of Biopharmaceutical Statistics*, 7:617–624.

Rosner, G.L. and Tsiatis, A.A. (1988). Exact confidence intervals following a group sequential trial: A comparison of methods. *Biometrika*, 75:723–729.

Rothmann, M., Li, N., Chen, G., Chi1, G.Y.H., Temple, R., and Tsou, H.H. (2003). Design and analysis of noninferiority mortality trials in oncology. *Statistics in Medicine*, 22:239–264.

Rothmann, M.D., Wiens, B.L., and Chan, I.S.F. (2011). *Design and Analysis of Non-Inferiority Trials*. Chapman & Hall/CRC, Boca Raton, FL.

Royall, R. (1997). *Statistical Evidence: A Likelihood Paradigm*. London, Chapman & Hall.

Ruberg, S.J. (1995). Dose response studies: I. Some design considerations. *Journal of Biopharmaceutical Statistics*, 5:1–14.

Ruberg, S.J. (1998). Contrasts for identifying the minimum effective dose. *Journal of the American Statistical Association*, 84:816–822.

Rubin, D.B. (1976). Inference and missing data. *Biometrika* 63:581–592.

Sampson, A. and Sill, M.W. (2005). Drop-the-losers design: Normal case. *Biometrical Journal*, 47:257–268.

Sargent, D.J. and Goldberg, R.M. (2001). A flexible design for multiple armed screening trials. *Statistics in Medicine*, 20:1051–1060.

Satagopan, J.M. and Elston, R.C. (2003). Optimal two-stage genotyping in population-based association studies. *Genetic Epidemiology*, 25:149–157.

Schafer, H. and Muller, H.H. (2001). Modification of the sample-size and the schedule of interim analyses in survival trials based on data inspections. *Statistics in Medicine*, 20:3741–3751.

Schafer, H., Timmesfeld, N., and Muller, H.H. (2006). An overview of statistical approaches for adaptive designs and design modifications. *Biometrical Journal* 48:507–520. DOI: 10.1002/bimj.200510234

Schaid, D.J., Wieand, S., and Therneau, T.M. (1990). Optimal two-stage screening designs for survival comparisons. *Biometrika*, 77:507– 513.

Scherag, A., et al. (2003). Data adaptive interim modification of sample sizes for candidate-gene association studies. *Human Heredity*, 56:56–62.

Schmitz, N. (1993). *Optimal Sequentially Planned Decision Procedures*, vol. 79 of Lecture Notes in Statistics, Springer, New York.

Schneider, S., Schmidli, H., and Friede, T. (2013). Robustness of methods for blinded sample size re-estimation with overdispersed count data. Published online 18 April 2013 in Wiley Online Library.

Sellke, T. and Siegmund, D. (1983). Sequential analysis of proportional hazards model. *Biometrika*, 70:315–326.

Shaffer, J.P. (1986). Modified sequentially rejective multiple test procedures. *Journal of the American Statistical Association*, 81:826–831.

Shaffer, J.P. (1995). Multiple hypothesis testing. *Ann. Rev. Psychol.* 46:561–84.

Shao, J., Chang, M., and Chow, S.C. (2005). Statistical inference for cancer trials with treatment switching. *Statistics in Medicine*, 24:1783–1790.

Shein-Chung Chow. (2013). *Biosimilars: Design and Analysis of Follow-on Biologics*. Chapman & Hall/CRC, Boca Raton, FL.

Shen, L. (2001). An improved method of evaluating drug effect in a multiple dose clinical trial. *Statistics in Medicine* 20:1913–1929. DOI: 10.1002=sim.842.

Shen, Y. and Fisher, L. (1999). Statistical inference for self-designing clinical trials with a one-sided hypothesis. *Biometrics*, 55:190–197.

Sherman, R.E. (2012). Biosimilar Biological Products. Biosimilar Guidance Webinar. February 15, 2012.

Shih, W.J. (2001). Sample size re-estimation—A journey for a decade. *Statistics in Medicine*, 20:515–518.

Shih, W.J. and Lin, Y. (2006). Traditional and modified algorithm-based designs for phase I cancer clinical trials. In Cheveret S., editor. *Statistical Methods for Dose-Finding Experiments*. John Wiley & Sons. New York.

Shih, W.J. and Quan, H. (2013). Consistency of treatment efects in bridging studies and global multiregional trials. In *Design and Analysis of Bridging Studies*, Liu, Chow, and Hsiao, editors. CRC Press, Boca Raton, FL.

Shih, W.J. and Zhao, P.L. (1997). Design for sample size re-estimation with interim data for double-blind clinical trials with binary outcomes, *Statistics in Medicine*, 16:1913–1923.

Shirley, E. (1977). A non-parametric equivalent of William's test for contrasting increasing dose levels of treatment. *Biometrics*, 33:386–389.

Shun, Z., Lan, G., and Soo, Y. (2008). Interim treatment selection using the normal approximation approach in clinical trials. *Statist. Med.* 27: 597–618.

Šidák, Z. K. (1967). Rectangular Confidence Regions for the Means of Multivariate Normal Distributions. *Journal of the American Statistical Association*, 62(318):626–633.

Sidik, K. (2003). Exact unconditional tests for testing noninferiority in matched-pairs design. *Statistics in Medicine*, 22:265–278.

Siegmund, D. (1978). Estimation following sequential tests. *Biometrika*, 65:341–349.

Siegmund, D. (1985). *Sequential Analysis: Tests and Confidence Intervals*. Springer. New York.

Simes, R.J. (1986). An improved Bonferroni procedure for multiple test procedures. *Journal of American Statistical Association*, 81:826–831.

Simon, R. (1979). Restricted randomization designs in clinical trials. *Biometrics*, 35:503–512.

Simon, R. (1989). Optimal two-stage designs for phase II clinical trials. *Controlled Clinical Trials*, 10:1–10.

Simon, R. and Maitournam, A. (2004). Evaluating the efficiency of targeted designs for randomized clinical trials. *Clinical Cancer Research*, 10:6759–6763.

Singpurwalla, N.D. (1995). Survival in dynamic environments. *Statistical Science*, 10:86–103.

Sommer, A. and Zeger, S.L. (1991). On estimating efficacy from clinical trials. *Statistics in Medicine*, 10:45–52.

Sozu, T., Kanou, T., Hamada, C., and Yoshimura, I. (2006). Power and sample size calculations in clinical trials with multiple primary variables. *Japanese Journal of Biometrics*, 27:83–96.

Sozu, T., Sugimoto, T., and Hamasaki, T. (2010). Sample size determination in clinical trials with multiple co-primary binary endpoints. *Statistics in Medicine*, 29(21):2169–2179.

Sozu, T., Sugimoto, T., and Hamasaki, T. (2011). Sample size determination in superiority clinical trials with multiple co-primary correlated endpoints. *Journal of Biopharmaceutical Statistics*, 21(4):650–668.

Spiegelhalter, D.J., Abrams, K.R. and Myles, J.P. (2004). *Bayesian Approach to Clinical Trials and Health-Care Evaluation*. Chichester: John Wiley & Sons, Ltd.

Spiegelhalter, D.J., Freedman, L., and Blackburn, P. (1986). Monitoring clinical trials: conditional or predictive power? *Controlled Clinical Trials*, 7(1):8–17.

Stallard, N. (2010). A confirmatory seamless phase II/III clinical trial design incorporating short-term endpoint information. *Statist. Med.* 29(9): 959–71.

Stallard, N. and Friede, T. (2008). A group-sequential design for clinical trials with treatment selection. *Statist. Med.* 27(29):6209–6227.

Stallard, N. and Rosenberger, W.F. (2002). Exact group-sequential designs for clinical trials with randomized play-the-winner allocation. *Statist. Med.* 21:467–480.

Stallard, N. and Todd, S. (2003). Sequential designs for phase III clinical trials incorporating treatment selection. *Statistics in Medicine*, 22:689–703.

Stallard, N. and Todd, S. (2005). Point estimates and confidence regions for sequential trials involving selection. *Journal of Statistical Planning and Inference*, 135:402–419.

Stallard, N., Todd, S., and Whitehead, J. (2008). Estimation following selection of the largest of two normal means. *Journal of Statistical Planning and Inference*, 138:1629–1638.

Stewart, W. and Ruberg, S.J. (2000). Detecting dose response with contrasts. *Statist. Med.* 19:913-921.

Strickland, P.A. and Casella, G. (2003). Conditional inference following group sequential testing. *Biometr. J.* 45:515–526.

Stuart, A. and Ord, K. (1998). *Kendall's Advanced Theory of Statistics.* 6th edition. Wiley.

Susarla, V. and Pathala, K.S. (1965). A probability distribution for time of first birth. *Journal of Scientific Research*, Banaras Hindu University, 16:59–62.

Tanaka, Y., Li, G., Wang, Y., and Chen, J. (2012). Qualitative consistency of treatment effects in multiregional clinical trials. *Journal of Biopharmaceutical Statistics*, 2012:22:988–1000.

Tang, D. and Geller, N.L. (1999). Closed testing procedures for group sequential clinical trials with multiple endpoints. *Biometrics*, 55:1188–1192.

Tang, D., Gnecco, C., and Geller, N.L. (1989). An approximate likelihood ratio test for a normal mean vector with nonnegative components with application to clinical trials. *Biometrika*, 76:577–583.

Tang, M.L. and Tang, N.S. (2004). Tests of noninferiority via rate difference for three-arm clinical trials with placebo. *Journal of Biopharmaceutical Statistics*, 14:337–347.

Tango, T. (1998). Equivalence test and confidence interval for the difference in proportions for the paired-sample design. *Statistics in Medicine*, 17:891–908.

Tappin, L. (1992). Unbiased estimation of the parameter of a selected binomial population. *Communications in Statistics: Theory and Methods*, 21:1067–1083.

Taves, D.R. (1974). Minimization—A new method of assessing patients and control groups. *Clinical Pharmacol. Ther.* 15:443–453.

Taylor, H.M. and Karlin, S. (1998). *An Introduction to Stochastic Modeling.* Academic Press Limited, London, UK.

Temple, R. (2005). How FDA currently make decisions on clinical studies. *Clinical Trials*, 2:276–281.

Temple, R. (2006). FDA perspective on trials with interim efficacy evaluations. *Statist. Med.* 25:3245–3249.

Thach, C.T. and Fisher, L.D. (2002). Self-designing two-stage trials to minimize expected costs. *Biometrics*, 58:432–438.

Thall, P.F. and Cook, J.D. (2004) Dose-finding based on efficacy–toxicity trade-offs. *Biometrics*, 60:684–693.

Thall, P., Millikan, R., and Sung, H.G. (2000). Evaluating multiple treatment courses in clinical trials. *Statisti. Med.* 19:1011–1028.

Thall, P., Simon, R., and Ellenberg, S.S. (1989). A two-stage design for choosing among several experimental treatments and a control in clinical trials. *Biometrics*, 45:537–547.

Thall, P.F., Millikan, RE., Mueller, P., and Lee, S.J.J. (2003). Dose-finding with two agents in phase I oncology trials. *Biometrics*, 59(3):487–496.

Thall, P.F. and Nguyen, H.Q. (2012). Adaptive randomization to improve utility-based dose-finding with bivariate ordinal outcomes. *J. Biopharm. Stat.* 22(4):785–801.

Thall, P.F. and Russell, K.E. (1998). A strategy for dose finding and safety monitoring based on efficacy and adverse outcomes in phase I/II clinical trials. *Biometrics*, 54:251–264.

Thall, P.F., Simon R., and Ellenberg S.S. (1988). Two-stage selection and testing designs for comparative clinical trials. *Biometrika*, 75:303–310.

The International Conference on Harmonisation of Technical Requirements for Registration of Pharmaceuticals for Human Use (ICH). (10 March 1994) Harmonised Tripartite Guideline E4: Dose-Response Information to Support Drug Registration. http://www.ich.org/LOB/media/MEDIA480.pdf. Accessed: 10 August 2006.

Thomas, D., Xie, R.R., and Gebregziabher, M. (2004). Two-stage sampling designs for gene association studies. *Genetic Epidemiology*, 27:401–414.

Thomas, D.C., Haile, R.W., and Duggan, D. (2005). Recent developments in genomewide association scans: A workshop summary and review. *American Journal of Human Genetics*, 77:337–345.

Tibeiro, J.J.S. and Murdoch, D.J. (2010). Correspondence analysis with incomplete paired data using Bayesian imputation. *Bayesian Analysis*, 5(3):519–532.

Tiemannn, R., Machnig, T., and Neuhaus, K.L. (2001). The Na+=H+ exchange inhibitor eniporide as an adjunct to early reperfusion therapy for acute myocardial infarction. *Journal of the American College of Cardiology*, 38:1644-1651.

Timmesfeld, N., Schafer, H., and Muller, H. H. (2007). Increasing the sample-size during clinical trials with t-distributed test statistics without inflating the type-I error rate. *Statistics in Medicine*, 26:244–246.

Ting, N. (2006) (Ed.). *Dose Finding in Drug Development.* Springer Science+Business Media Inc., New York.

Todd, S. (2003). An adaptive approach to implementing bivariate group sequential clinical trial designs. *Journal of Biopharmaceutical Statistics*, 13(4):605–619.

Todd, S. and Stallard, N. (2005). A new clinical trial design combining Phases 2 and 3: sequential designs with treatment selection and a change of endpoint. *Drug Information Journal*, 39:109–118.

Tonkens, R. (2005). An overview of the drug development process. *The Physician Executive*, May/June, p. 51.

Torres, M. and Moayedi, S. (2007). Evaluation of the acutely dyspneic elderly patient. *Clin. Geriatr. Med.* 23(2):307–325, vi.

Tsiatis, A.A. and Mehta, C. (2003). On the inefficiency of the adaptive design for monitoring clinical trials. *Biometrika*, 90:367–378.

Tsiatis, A.A., Rosner G.L, and Metha, C.R. (1984). Exact confidence intervals following a group sequential test. *Biometrics*, 40:797– 803.

Tsou, H.H., Hung, H.M.J., Chen, Y.M., Huang, W.S., Chang, W.J., and Hsiao, C.F. (2012). Establishing consistency across all regions in a multi-regional clinical trial. *Pharmaceutical Statistics*, 11(4):295–299.

Tsong, Y., Chang, W.J., Dong, X.Y., and Tsou, H.H. (2012). Assessment of regional treatment effect in a multiregional clinical trial. *Journal of Biopharmaceutical Statistic*, 22(5):1019–1036.

Tukey, J.W. and Heyse, J.F. (1985). Testing the statistical certainty of a response to increasing doses of a drug, *Biometrics*, 41:295–301.

Uchida, T. (2006). Adaptive trial design—FDA view. Presented at the CRT 2006 Workshop with the FDA, Arlington, Virginia, April 4.

Uesaka, H. (2009). Sample Size Allocation to Regions in a Multiregional Clinical Trials. *Journal of Biopharmaceutical Statistics*, 19(4):580–594.

United States Department of Health and Human Services. Food and Drug Administration. (2005 April) Guidance for Industry: Clinical Trial Endpoints for the Approval of Cancer Drugs and Biologics. Available from http://www.fda.gov /cder/Guidance/6592dft.pdf. Date of access: 10 August 2006.

US Food and Drug Administration (FDA) (2010). Draft Guidance – Guidance for Industry Adaptive Design Clinical Trials for Drugs and Biologics (February).

US Food and Drug Administration (FDA) (2010). – Guidance for the Use of Bayesian Statistics in Medical Device Clinical Trials (February).

US Food and Drug Administration (FDA) (2012). – Draft Guidance- Guidance for Industry on Enrichment Strategies for Clinical Trials to Support Approval of Human Drugs and Biological Products (December).

Vaupel, J.W., Manton, K.G., and Stallard, E. (1979). The impact of heterogeneity in individual frailty on the dynamics of mortality. *Demography* 16:439–454.

Wald, A. (1947). *Sequential Analysis*. Dover Publications, New York.

Walsh, T.B., Seidman, S.N., Sysko, R., and Gould, M. (2002). Placebo response in studies of major depression. *JAMA*, 287(14):1840–1847.

Walton, M.K. (2006). PhRMA-FDA Adaptive Design Workshop.

Wang and Chang (2014). Biomarker-informed adaptive design. Submitted.

Wang, J. (2001). Modeling and generating daily changes in market variables using a multivariate mixture of normal distributions. Proceedings of the 2001 Winter Simulation Conference.

Wang, J. (2006). Generating multivariate mixture of normal distributions using a modified cholesky decomposition. Proceedings of the 2006 Winter Simulation Conference.

Wang, J. (2013). Biomarker informed adaptive seamless phase II/III design. PhD thesis, Boston University, Boston, MA.

Wang, J., Chang, M., Menon, S., and Wang L. (2013). Biomarker informed adaptive seamless phase II/III design. *SIM.*

Wang, J., Menon, S., and Chang, M. (2013). Finding critical values to control type I error for a biomarker informed two-stage winner design. *JBS.*

Wang, K., and Ivanova, A. (2005). Two-dimensional dose finding in discrete dose space. *Biometrics*, 61(1):217–222.

Wang, S.J. (2006). Regulatory experience of adaptive designs in well-controlled clinical trials. Presented at Adaptive Designs: Opportunities, Challenges and Scope in Drug Development, Washington, DC, November.

Wang, S.J. and Hung, H.M.J. (2005). Adaptive covariate adjustment in clinical trials. *Journal of Biopharmaceutical Statistics*, 15:605–611.

Wang, S.J., Hung, H.M.J., and O'Neill, R.T. (2006). Adapting the sample-size planning of a phase III trial based on phase II data. *Pharmaceut. Statist.* 5:85–97, Published online in Wiley InterScience, DOI: 10.1002/pst.217. www.interscience.wiley.com.

Wang, S.J., Hung, H.M., Tsong, Y., and Cui, L. (2001). Group sequential test strategies for superiority and noninferiority hypotheses in active controlled clinical trials. *Statistics in Medicine*, 20:1903–1912.

Wang, S.K. and Tsiatis, A.A. (1987). Approximately optimal one-parameter boundaries for a sequential trials. *Biometrics*, 43:193–200.

Wang, Y. and McDermott, M.P. (1998). Conditional likelihood ratio test for a nonnegative normal mean vector. *Journal of the American Statistical Association*, 93:380–386.

Wang, Y.C., Chen, G., and Chi, G.Y.H. (2006). A ratio test in active control noninferiority trials with time-to-event endpoint. *Journal of Biopharmaceutical Statistics*, 16:151–164.

Wassmer, G. (1998)0, A Comparison of two methods for adaptive interim analyses in clinical trials. *Biometrics*, 54:696–705.

Wassmer, G. (1999). Multistage adaptive test procedures based on Fisher's product criterion. *Biometrical Journal*, 41:279–293.

Wassmer, G., Eisebitt, R., and Coburger, S. (2001). Flexible interim analyses in clinical trials using multistage adaptive test designs. *Drug Information Journal*, 35:1131–1146.

Wassmer, G. and Vandemeulebroecke, M. (2006). A brief review on software developments for group sequential and adaptive designs. *Biometrical Journal*, 48:732–737.

Wei, L.J. (1977). A class of designs for sequential clinical trials. *Journal of American Statistical Association*, 72:382–386.

Wei, L.J. (1978). The adaptive biased-coin design for sequential experiments. *Annals of Statistics*, 9:92–100.

Wei, L.J. et al. (1990). Statistical inference with data-dependent treatment allocation rules. *JASA*, 85:156–162.

Wei, L.J. and Durham, S. (1978). The randomized play-the-winner rule in medical trials. *Journal of American Statistical Association*, 73:840–843.

Wei, L.J., Smythe, R.T., Lin, D.Y. and Park, T.S. (1990). Statistical inference with data-dependent treatment allocation rules. *J. Amer. Statist. Assoc.* 85:156–162.

Wei, L.J., Smythe, R.T., and Smith, R.L. (1986). K-treatment comparisons with restricted randomization rules in clinical trials. *Annals of Statistics*, 14:265–274.

Wiens, B.L. (2003). A fixed-sequence Bonferroni procedure for testing multiple endpoints. *Pharmaceutical Statistics*, 2:211–215.

Wiens, B.L. and Dmitrienko, A. (2005). The fallback procedure for evaluating a single family of hypotheses. *Journal of Biopharmaceutical Statistics*, 15:929–942, 26.

Weinthrau, M. et al. (1977). Piroxicam (CP 16171) in rheumatoid arthritis: A controlled clinical trial with novel assessment features. *J. Rheum.* 4:393–404.

Weir, C.J. and Walley, R.J. (2006). Statistical evaluation of biomarkers as surrogate endpoints: A literature review. *Statist. Med.* 25:183–203. Published online 26 October 2005 in Wiley InterScience (www.interscience.wiley.com). DOI: 10.1002/sim.2319.

Westfall, P.H. and Young, S.S. (1993). *Resampling-Based Multiple Testing: Examples and Methods for p-value Adjustment*. Wiley, New York, 1993.

Westfall, P.H. et al. (1999). *Multiple Comparisons and Multiple Tests*, SAS Institute Inc., Cary, North Carolina.

White, I.R. et al. (1999). Randomisation-based methods for correcting for treatment changes: examples from the Concorde trial. *Statistics in Medicine* 18:2617–2634.

White, I.R., Walker, S., and Babiker, A.G. (2002). Randomisation-based efficacy estimator. *Stata Journal*, 2:140–150.

Whitehead, J. (1986). On the bias of maximum likelihood estimation following a sequential test. *Biometrika*, 73:573–581.

Whitehead, J. (1993). Sample size calculation for ordered categorical data. *Statistics in Medicine*, 12:2257–71.

Whitehead, J. (1994). Sequential methods based on the boundaries approach for the clinical comparison of survival times (with discussions). *Statistics in Medicine*, 13:1357–1368.

Whitehead, J. (1997a). Bayesian decision procedures with application to dose-finding studies. *International Journal of Pharmaceutical Medicine*, 11:201–208.

Whitehead, J. (1997b). *The Design and Analysis of Sequential Clinical Trials*. rev. edition. Chichester, UK, John Wiley.

Whitehead, J. and Stratton, I. (1983). Group sequential clinical trials with triangular continuation regions. *Biometrics*, 39:227–236.

Whitmore, G.A. (1983). A regression method for censored inverse-Gaussian data, *Canadian. J. Statist.* 11:305–315.

Whitmore, G.A., Crowder, M. J., and Lawless J. F. (1998). Failure inference from a marker process based on a bivariate Wiener model. *Lifetime Data Analysis*, 4:229–251.

Wiens, B.L. and Heyes, J.F. (2003). Testing for interactions in studies of noninferiority. *Journal of Biopharmaceutical Statistics*, 13:103–115.

Williams, D.A. (1971). A test for difference between treatment means when several dose levels are compared with a zero dose control. *Biometrics*, 27:103–17.

Williams, D.A. (1972). Comparison of several dose levels with a zero dose control. *Biometrics*, 28:519–31.

Williams, G., Pazdur, R., and Temple, R. (2004). Assessing tumor-related signs and symptoms to support cancer drug approval. *Journal of Biopharmaceutical Statistics*, 14:5–21.

Wittes, J. and Brittain, E. (1990). The role of internal pilot studies in increasing the effciency of clinical trials, *Statistics in Medicine*, 9:65–72.

Wittes, J., Schabenberger, O., Zucker, D., Brittain, E., and Proschan, M. (1999). Internal pilot studies I: Type I error rate of the naive t-test. *Statistics in Medicine*, 18:3481–3491.

Woodcock, J. (2005). FDA introductory comments: clinical studies design and evaluation issues. *Clinical Trials*, 2:273–75.

Woodcock, J. (2004). *FDA's Critical Path Initiative*. www.fda.gov/oc/ initiatives/criticalpath/woodcock0602/woodcock0602.html

Wu, Y. and Zhao, P.L. (2012). Interim treatment selection with a flexible selection margin in clinical trials. *Statistics in Medicine*. 32(15):2529–2543.

Xiong, C., Yu, K., Gao, F. et al. (2005). Power and sample size for clinical trials when efficacy is required in multiple endpoints: Application to an alzheimer's treatment trial. *Clinical Trials*, 2(5):387–393.

Yasuda, N. (2012). Consideration on mutual recognition of clinical trials: Study on ethnic factors in China, Japan and Korea. ICDRA: Workshop H, 25 October.

Yin, G., Li, Y., and Ji, Y. (2006). Bayesian dose-finding in phase I/II dose-finding trials using toxicity and efficacy odds ratios, *Biometrics*, 62:777–787.

Yin, G. and Yuan, Y. (2011). Bayesian approach for adaptive design. In *Handbook of Adaptive Designs in Pharmaceutical and Clinical Development*. Pong and Chow, editors. CRC Press, Boca Raton, FL.

Yin, G. and Yuan, Y. (2009). Bayesian dose finding in oncology for drug combinations by copula regression. *Journal of the Royal Statistical Society: Series C (Applied Statistics)*, 58(2):211–224.

Zehetmayer, S., Bauer, P., and Posch, M. (2005). Two-stage designs for experiments with a large number of hypotheses. *Bioinformatics*, 21:3771–3777.

Zelen, M. (1969). Play the winner rule and the controlled clinical trial. *JASA*, 80:974–984.

Zelen, M. (1974). The randomization and stratification of patients to clinical trials. *Journal of Chronic Diseases*, 28:365–375.

Zhang, W., Sargent, D.J., and Mandrekar, S. (2006). An adaptive dose-finding design incorporating both toxicity and efficacy. *Statistics in Medicine*, 25:2365–2383.

Zucker, D.M. et al. (1999). Internal pilot studies II: Comparison of various procedures. *Statistics in Medicine*, 19:901–911.

Zwillinger, D. and Kokoska, S. (2000). *Standard Probability and Statistics Tables and Formulae*. Chapman & Hall/CRC, Boca Raton, FL.

# Index

Printed in the United States
by Baker & Taylor Publisher Services